Principles of Pulmonary Medicine

Principles of Pulmonary Medicine

Edited by **Michael Glass**

hayle
medical

New York

Published by Hayle Medical,
30 West, 37th Street, Suite 612,
New York, NY 10018, USA
www.haylemedical.com

Principles of Pulmonary Medicine
Edited by Michael Glass

International Standard Book Number: 978-1-63241-403-8 (Hardback)

The publisher's policy is to use permanent paper from mills that operate a sustainable forestry policy. Furthermore, the publisher ensures that the text paper and cover boards used have met acceptable environmental accreditation standards.

Trademark Notice: Registered trademark of products or corporate names are used only for explanation and identification without intent to infringe.

Printed in the United States of America.

Contents

Preface

This book discusses the fundamentals as well as modern approaches of pulmonary medicine. It strives to provide a fair idea about this discipline and to help develop a better understanding of the latest advances within this field. It is a specialized branch of medicine that deals with the diagnosis and treatment of diseases related to respiratory system and respiratory tract. Pulmonology also addresses the chronic breathing problems with the help of ventilator support. In this book, using case studies and examples, constant effort has been made to make the understanding of the difficult concepts as easy and informative as possible, for the readers. Pulmonologists, researches and students will benefit alike from this book.

This book unites the global concepts and researches in an organized manner for a comprehensive understanding of the subject. It is a ripe text for all researchers, students, scientists or anyone else who is interested in acquiring a better knowledge of this dynamic field.

I extend my sincere thanks to the contributors for such eloquent research chapters. Finally, I thank my family for being a source of support and help.

Editor

Effect and Safety of Mycophenolate Mofetil or Sodium in Systemic Sclerosis-Associated Interstitial Lung Disease: A Meta-Analysis

Argyris Tzouvelekis,[1] Nikolaos Galanopoulos,[2] Evangelos Bouros,[3] George Kolios,[3] George Zacharis,[1] Paschalis Ntolios,[1] Andreas Koulelidis,[1] Anastasia Oikonomou,[4] and Demosthenes Bouros[1]

[1] *Department of Pneumonology, University Hospital of Alexandroupolis, Democritus University of Thrace, 68100 Alexandroupolis, Greece*
[2] *Department of Rheumatology, University Hospital of Alexandroupolis, Democritus University of Thrace, 68100 Alexandroupolis, Greece*
[3] *Laboratory of Pharmacology, Democritus University of Thrace, 68100 Alexandroupolis, Greece*
[4] *Department of Radiology, University Hospital of Alexandroupolis, Democritus University of Thrace, 68100 Alexandroupolis, Greece*

Correspondence should be addressed to Argyris Tzouvelekis, atzouvelekis@yahoo.gr

Academic Editor: Athol Wells

Background. Interstitial lung disease (ILD) is the most common complication of systemic sclerosis (SSc) with treatment ineffective. Objective: The aim of this meta-analysis was to provide an estimate of the safety and efficacy profile of Mycophenolate Mofetil (MMF) or sodium (MMS) in SSc-ILD patients. *Materials and Methods.* All studies were reviewed systematically. The main end-points were safety and efficacy profile as estimated by forced vital capacity (FVC)% and diffusion capacity of the lung for carbon monoxide (DL_{CO})% of the predicted normal value (%pred.) before and after treatment in patients with SSc-ILD. Quality assessment and data extraction were performed independently by two reviewers. *Results.* Seventeen studies were reviewed systematically. Six studies, one prospective, were eligible for analysis encompassing 69 patients, including 10 subjects from our, yet unpublished, retrospective study. There was no statistically significant difference in both efficacy outcomes of interest, including FVC% pred. (weighted mean difference 1.48, 95% confidence interval (CI): -2.77 to 5.72, $P = 0.49$) and DL_{CO}% pred. (weighted mean difference -0.83, 95% CI: -4.75 to 3.09, $P = 0.93$). No cases of clinically significant side effects were documented. *Conclusions.* Meta-analysis data suggest that MMF is a safe therapeutic modality which was associated with functional stabilization in patients with SSc-ILD.

1. Introduction

Interstitial lung disease (ILD) is one the most common complications of systemic sclerosis (SSc) with a prevalence of 40%–84% and represents the major source of morbidity and mortality [1–5]. Thus, lung involvement has been the target of several clinical studies estimating safety and efficacy of a significant number of therapeutic agents, including corticosteroids and cyclophosphamide [6–11]. So far, only the latter has been proven of some benefit in patients with SSc-ILD [12], as has been demonstrated in a large

multicenter-randomized controlled clinical trial. Nevertheless, follow-up studies reported a rather temporary beneficial functional effect that began to partially fade 6 months after drug discontinuation [13]. In addition, assessment of HRCT findings in the same cohort of patients recorded amelioration of the extent of fibrosis in the cyclophosphamide arm [14–16]. Despite relative enthusiasm arising from the above data, the modest and temporary functional and radiological improvement in patients under cyclophosphamide treatment coupled with the potential toxicity associated with drug usage, raises crucial dilemmas of whether and for how long all patients with SSc-ILD should be treated with aggressive cytotoxic drugs and whether we should reserve these regimens for patients at greatest risk for progression and search for safer alternatives in mild-to-moderate disease patterns.

Mycophenolate mofetil (MMF) and mycophenolate sodium (MS) are commercialised drugs containing the active moiety of mycophenolate acid, an inhibitor of lymphocytes proliferation acting through blockage of inosine monophosphate dehydrogenase and interference with purine biosynthesis, that is commonly used to prevent rejection following solid-organ transplantation as well as for the treatment of several autoimmune and renal disorders [17–21]. In addition to its anti-inflammatory activity, MA acts also as anti-proliferating agent by downregulating the expression of several fibrotic growth factors such as transforming growth factor (TGF)-β, evidence that makes it an attractive candidate drug for the treatment of fibrotic lung diseases of different causes [22, 23]. Currently, its utility has been investigated in the context of one prospective [24] and four retrospective studies [25–28] encompassing, in total, 59 patients with SSc-ILD of mild-to-moderate disease severity, and a modest beneficial effect in functional and radiological status has been demonstrated.

While awaiting for the results of the, only so far, large multicentric-randomized clinical trial (Scleroderma Lung Study II) to compare the functional effect of MMF with oral cyclophosphamide in patients with SSc-ILD, we performed a meta-analysis of the current knowledge coupled with results from our, yet unpublished, retrospective cohort, to provide a more rigid estimate of the safety and efficacy profile of MMF and MS in SSC-ILD patients.

2. Materials and Methods

2.1. Study Selection. A MEDLINE, Embase, Ovid, and Cochrane database search was performed on all studies between 2006 and 2011 comparing the safety and efficacy of the administration of mycophenolate mofetil or sodium in patients with systemic sclerosis-associated interstitial lung disease. The following Mesh search headings were used: mycophenolate mofetil, mycophenolate sodium, scleroderma, systemic-sclerosis, interstitial lung disease, effect, safety, and lung function. The related article function from PubMed was used to broaden the search, and all abstracts, studies, and citations scanned were reviewed. No language restrictions were made. The latest date for this search was September 1, 2011. We have also enrolled in the pooled published data results from our, yet unpublished, retrospective study of the safety and efficacy profile of a 12-month MMF treatment in SSc-ILD patients.

2.2. Data Extraction. Two reviewers (AT and DB) independently extracted the following from each study: first author, year of publication, study population characteristics, study design, inclusion and exclusion criteria, and male-to-female ratio.

2.3. Inclusion Criteria. To be included in the analysis, studies had to (1) compare functional data including FVC% and DL$_{CO}$% of the predicted normal value prior and at least 6 months after MMF or MS treatment, (2) report at least one of the outcome measures mentioned below; (3) clearly document MMF or MS administration in patients with SSc-ILD. When two studies were reported by the same institution and/or authors, they were included only if there was no overlap between the results of the studies. Otherwise, the larger higher-quality studies were included in the analysis.

2.3.1. Exclusion criteria. Studies were excluded from the analysis if: (1) it was impossible to extrapolate or calculate the necessary data from the published results that is absent from spirometry raw data; (2) there was considerable overlap between authors, centers, or patient cohorts evaluated in the published literature.

2.4. Outcomes of Interest. The following outcomes were used to compare the effect of mycophenolate mofetil or sodium in the same group of patients with systemic sclerosis-associated interstitial lung disease who were firstly off treatment and then administered the drug:

(1) safety profile as assessed by cases of clinically significant infection, leucopenia, or elevated liver enzymes;

(2) efficacy profile as assessed by functional data including FVC% and DL$_{CO}$% of the predicted normal value.

2.5. Statistical Analysis. The meta-analysis was performed in line with recommendations from the Cochrane Collaboration and the Quality of Reporting of Meta-analyses guidelines. Weighted mean difference (WMD) was used to analyze continuous variables. It was reported with 95% confidence intervals (CIs). WMDs summarize the differences between the two groups with respect to continuous variables, accounting for sample size. Statistical algorithms were used to calculate the standard deviations (SDs) for studies that presented continuous data as means and range values, thus standardizing all continuous data for analysis. Analysis was conducted by use of Review Manager version 5.0.14 (The Cochrane\Collaboration, Software Update, Oxford, UK). Results were analyzed by paired Student's *t*-test.

3. Results

3.1. Eligible Studies. By using the search key words listed above, we identified 50 publications. Thirty-four studies were excluded after title and abstract review. These included 14 review articles, one study in experimental model of scleroderma, and 19 letters or case reports. The remaining 16 articles were carefully evaluated and eleven were referring to studies estimating the safety and efficacy profile of MMF either in diffuse cutaneous systemic sclerosis or in other connective tissue disorders including systemic sclerosis, rheumatoid arthritis, lupus erythematosus, and polymyositis and, therefore, were excluded from further analysis since it was impossible to extrapolate or calculate the necessary data from the published results. A total of five studies encompassing one prospective [24] and four retrospective studies [25–28] evaluating safety and efficacy of MS and MMF, retrospectively, in an overall of 59 patients with SSc-ILD were included in this meta-analysis. We have also included 10 patients with SSc-ILD from our retrospective, yet unpublished, study to estimate the safety and effect of a 12-month oral administration of MMF. All patients included in the meta-analysis met American College of Rheumatology Criteria for SSc and had evidence of SSc-ILD based on HRCT findings with no other apparent cause for ILD.

As depicted in Table 1, the majority of patients enrolled in the studies included in meta-analysis were middle-aged, women of mean age 53 years old, with a mean time of SSc diagnosis and study enrolment, meaning drug initiation, ranging from 2–7.7 years. In addition, 26/42 patients (62%) were under cytotoxic treatment with either cyclophosphamide and/or azathioprine prior MMF administration. There was no data available regarding this issue for the remaining 27 patients included in the studies of Zamora et al. [28] and Koutroumpas et al. [26].

All of the studies included presented with major limitations due to the limited number of patients enrolled and their retrospective single-center nature (apart one prospective) and, therefore, their power to identify important differences in efficacy outcomes such as functional parameters could be questioned. As it is easily understandable, none of the studies was randomized, controlled evidence that further diminished the scientific rigidity of the data extracted. Five studies, all retrospectives, estimated safety and efficacy profile of MMF, while the remaining one prospective study evaluated similar outcomes of interest in SSc-ILD patients after a 12-month oral administration of MS.

3.2. Safety Outcomes. In the five retrospective studies no cases of liver toxicity, clinically significant infection and leucopenia were recorded during MMF treatment. In addition, MMF was well tolerated by the vast majority patients with development of nausea that led to drug discontinuation in only one patient and abdominal pain and nausea that were transient and required no further interventions in another patient. There was only one case of a patient presented *Aspergillus terreus* pulmonary infection that required treatment with voriconazole and MS suppression. She did not require admission and recovered completely. No other adverse effects were noted. The above data suggest that MMF or MS present with a readily acceptable safety and tolerability profile (Table 1).

3.3. Efficacy Outcomes. Four studies, all retrospective, (Tzouvelekis et al. mean difference of 4.73%, and 64.71% versus 69.44% of the predicted normal value from baseline, or 215 mL, CI: −7 to 1.4%, P = 0.001) and (Liossis et al. [27], Gerbino et al. [25] and Koutroumpas et al. [26]) reported statistically significant differences in FVC% predicted at baseline and 12 months after treatment with MMF. In the remaining two trials, a disease stabilization as assessed by nonstatistically significant differences in FVC%

predicted at baseline and 12 months of treatment with MMF (and Zamora et al. [28]) or MS (Simeon-Aznar et al. [24]) (Figure 1, Table 2). With regards to DL_{CO}, all studies, except of Liossis et al. [27] who reported a statistically significant improvement 6 months after MMF administration (75.4% pred. versus 64.2% pred., P = 0.033), clearly demonstrated nonstatistically significant alterations either increase (Gerbino et al. [25] 52.5% pred. versus 51% pred., Koutroumpas et al. [26] 86.67% pred. versus 80.67% pred., Zamora et al. [28] 51.4% pred. versus 50% pred.) or decrease (Tzouvelekis et al. 51.41% pred. versus 49.38% pred. and Simeon-Aznar et al. [24] 40% pred. versus 37% pred.) of DL_{CO} following MMF or MS oral administration compared to baseline (Figure 2, Table 2). As depicted in Table 2, all included studies enrolled patients with mild-to-moderate disease severity as assessed by functional parameters prior MMF or MS administration (FVC ranging from 64–79.5% pred. and DL_{CO} ranging from 40–64.2% pred.).

Despite the above findings, meta-analysis of the data showed no statistically significant difference favoring MMF or MS administration in both FVC% pred. (weighted mean difference 1.48, 95% confidence interval (CI): −2.77 to 5.72, P = 0.49) and DL_{CO}% pred. (weighted mean difference −0.83, 95% CI: −4.75 to 3.09, P = 0.93).

4. Discussion

This is the first meta-analysis in the literature reporting the safety and efficacy profile of MMF and MS administration in patients with SSc-ILD. Pooled extracted data by detailed review of 6 eligible studies, encompassing 69 patients, clearly demonstrated that MMF and MS are safe therapeutic modalities, and their administration was linked with disease stabilization regarding functional parameters in patients with SSc-ILD.

Interstitial lung disease commonly complicates with various radiological, functional and histopathological patterns of disease severity, the lung of scleroderma patients and currently represents the leading cause of morbidity and mortality [1, 2, 4, 5, 29]. Its natural history is greatly downhill with therapeutic options limited and yet ineffective. So far, there is only one randomized controlled trial showing a modest beneficial effect of 2.53% in the mean absolute difference in adjusted 12-month FVC% predicted following oral cyclophosphamide therapy [12]. The above evidence of modest and temporary effectiveness of cyclophosphamide coupled with substantial drug toxicities over time highlight the need to search for safer alternatives especially for younger patients with mild disease that would benefit from longitudinal administration of therapeutic modalities with minimal side effects and reserve more aggressive and potentially more beneficial cytotoxic regimens for later stages of the disease course.

MMF and a newly commercialised delayed-release tablet containing mycophenolate acid, called MS, may represent such options. Based on the versatile anti-inflammatory, antifibrotic [22, 23] and immunomodulatory properties of its active metabolite, mycophenolic acid, MMF and MS

TABLE 1: Baseline characteristics of the patients included per study.

Study/year	Number of patients	Age (years)	Female	Prior cytotoxic treatment received	Diffuse SSc	Disease duration (years)
Liossis et al., 2006 [27]	6	46	4/6	1/6	4/6	3.4
Gerbino et al., 2008 [25]	13	52	5/13	9/13	9/13	5
Koutroumpas et al., 2010 [26]	10	59	8/10	NA	10/10	7.7
Zamora et al., 2008 [28]	17	51	10/17	NA	15/17	2
Simeon-Aznar, 2011 [24]	14	54	13/14	10/14	8/14	6.5
Tzouvelekis et al., 2012	10	56	4/10	6/10	10/10	1.5
Total	69	53	44/69	26/42	56/69	4.7

Data are presented as mean unless otherwise stated.
Abbreviations: SSc: systemic sclerosis and NA: nonapplicable.

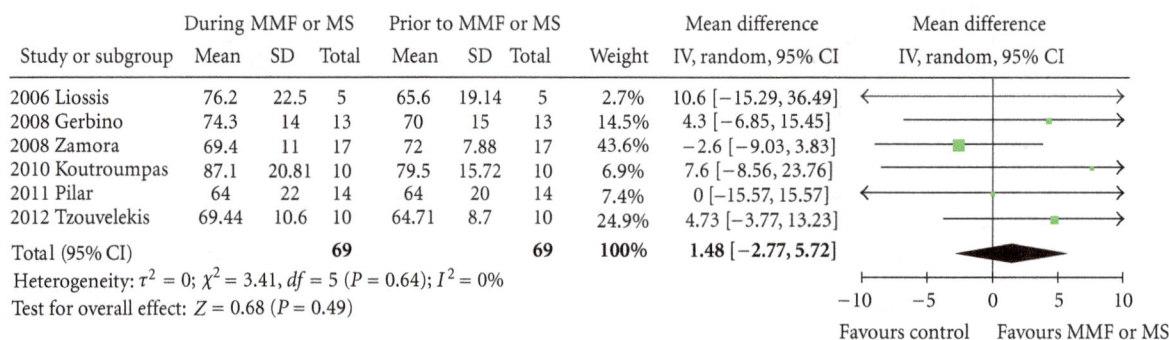

	During MMF or MS			Prior to MMF or MS				Mean difference	Mean difference
Study or subgroup	Mean	SD	Total	Mean	SD	Total	Weight	IV, random, 95% CI	IV, random, 95% CI
2006 Liossis	76.2	22.5	5	65.6	19.14	5	2.7%	10.6 [−15.29, 36.49]	
2008 Gerbino	74.3	14	13	70	15	13	14.5%	4.3 [−6.85, 15.45]	
2008 Zamora	69.4	11	17	72	7.88	17	43.6%	−2.6 [−9.03, 3.83]	
2010 Koutroumpas	87.1	20.81	10	79.5	15.72	10	6.9%	7.6 [−8.56, 23.76]	
2011 Pilar	64	22	14	64	20	14	7.4%	0 [−15.57, 15.57]	
2012 Tzouvelekis	69.44	10.6	10	64.71	8.7	10	24.9%	4.73 [−3.77, 13.23]	
Total (95% CI)			69			69	100%	1.48 [−2.77, 5.72]	

Heterogeneity: $\tau^2 = 0$; $\chi^2 = 3.41$, $df = 5$ ($P = 0.64$); $I^2 = 0\%$
Test for overall effect: $Z = 0.68$ ($P = 0.49$)

−10 −5 0 5 10
Favours control   Favours MMF or MS

FIGURE 1: Forest plot of pooled data on FVC prior (favours control arm) and during treatment with MMF or MS (favours MMF or MS arm). Abbreviations: CI: confidence interval, DL_{CO}: diffusing capacity for carbon monoxide, MMF: mycophenolate mofetil, MS: mycophenolate sodium, and SD: standard deviation.

TABLE 2: Extracted data on outcomes of interest from all studies.

Study/year	Number of patients	Design	Side effects	FVC		DL_{CO}	
				Prior MMF/MS	During MMF/MS	Prior MMF/MS	During MMF/MS
Liossis et al., 2006 [27]	6	RT	0/6	65.6 (19.14)	76.2 (22.5)	64.2 (22.55)	75.4 (26.73)
Gerbino et al., 2008 [25]	13	RT	2/13	70 (15)	74.3 (14)	51 (13)	52.5 (12)
Zamora et al., 2008 [28]	17	RT	0/17	72 (7.8)	69.4 (11)	50 (7)	48.6 (9)
Koutroumpas et al., 2010 [26]	10	RT	0/10	79.5 (15.72)	87.1 (20.81)	80.67 (33.52)	86.67 (25.58)
Simeon-Aznar et al., 2011 [24]	14	PT	1/14	64 (20)	64 (22)	40 (13)	37 (13)
Tzouvelekis et al., 2012	10	RT	0/10	64.71 (8.7)	69.44 (10.6)	51.41 (13.2)	49.38 (9.2)
Total	69		3/69				

Data are presented as mean (SD) unless otherwise stated.
Abbreviations: DL_{CO}: diffusing capacity for carbon monoxide, FVC: forced vital capacity, RT: retrospective, PT: prospective, MMF: mycophenolate mofetil, and MS: mycophenolate sodium.

Study or subgroup	During MMF or MS			Prior to MMF or MS			Weight	Mean difference IV, random, 95% CI	Mean difference IV, random, 95% CI
	Mean	SD	Total	Mean	SD	Total			
2006 Liossis	75.4	26.73	5	64.2	22.55	5	1.6%	11.2 [−19.45, 41.85]	
2008 Gerbino	52.5	12	13	51	13	13	16.6%	1.5 [−8.12, 11.12]	
2008 Zamora	48.6	9	17	50	7	17	52.3%	−1.4 [−6.82, 4.02]	
2010 Koutroumpas	86.67	25.58	10	80.67	33.52	10	2.2%	6 [−20.13, 32.13]	
2011 Pilar	37	13	10	40	13	10	11.8%	−3 [−14.39, 8.39]	
2012 Tzouvelekis	49.38	9.2	10	51.41	13.2	10	15.4%	−2.03 [−12, 7.94]	
Total (95% CI)			65			65	100%	−0.83 [−4.75, 3.09]	

Heterogeneity: $\tau^2 = 0$; $\chi^2 = 1.32$, $df = 5$ ($P = 0.93$); $I^2 = 0\%$
Test for overall effect: $Z = 0.42$ ($P = 0.68$)

−50 −25 0 25 50

Favours control   Favours MMF or MS

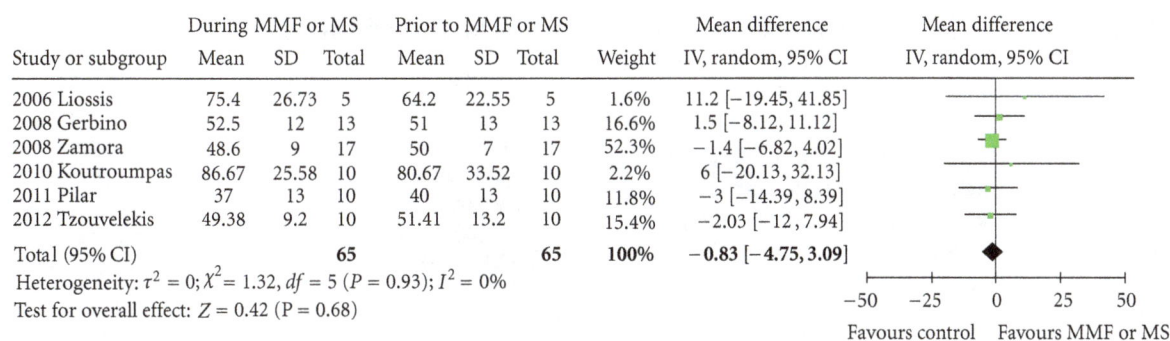

FIGURE 2: Forest plot of pooled data on DL_{CO} prior (favours control arm) and during treatment with MMF or MS (favours MMF or MS arm). Abbreviations: CI: Confidence Interval, DL_{CO}: Diffusing Capacity for carbon monoxide, MMF: Mycophenolate mofetil, MS: Mycophenolate Sodium, SD: Standard deviation.

treatments have been recently applied with promising results in patients with SSc and interstitial lung involvement [24–28, 30–32]. Although most of these studies reported a beneficial effect of MMF or MS in patients with SSc-ILD; however, all of them were unicentric, underpowered with limited number of patients enrolled, retrospective and nonrandomized controlled. Therefore, rigid conclusions regarding MMF or MS safety and efficacy profile cannot be drawn based on these studies.

While anticipating the results of the, only so far, large multicentric-randomized clinical trial (Scleroderma Lung Study II) to compare the beneficial effect in lung function parameters of a 2-year course of MMF with those of a 1-year course of oral cyclophosphamide, in patients with symptomatic scleroderma-related ILD, we performed a meta-analysis of the current knowledge coupled with results from our, yet unpublished, retrospective cohort, to provide a more rigid estimate of the safety and efficacy profile of MMF and MS in SSC-ILD patients.

After scrutinized review of the literature and using outcomes of interest safety and functional efficacy profile of mycophenolate acid in patients with scleroderma-associated ILD, a total of 6 studies fulfilling our inclusion criteria, encompassing a total number of 69 patients were enrolled in the final meta-analysis.

With regards to safety outcomes, all studies demonstrated an excellent safety profile for MMF or MS, and this finding was further supported by pooled analysis since there were only 3 patients presenting with side effects resulting in only case to drug discontinuation and in another to treatment suppression.

Regarding drug efficacy, despite the fact that 4 out of 6 studies reported on the primary analysis statistically significant functional improvement following a 12-month oral administration of MMF or MS, and the remaining two stated disease stabilization; nevertheless, pooled analysis failed to corroborate this finding. In particular, in the overall analysis of 69 patients, MMF or MS treatment failed to be associated with a statistically significant beneficial functional effect as assessed by both FVC and DL_{CO}.

On the other hand, the latter observation merits further investigation since by analyzing data one can easily report

that MMF or MS usage resulted in disease stabilization or reduced rate of annual functional decline compared to prior treatment with cytotoxic agents including cyclophosphamide and/or azathioprine. Meta-analysis demonstrated a mean difference of 1.48% and −0.83% of the predicted normal value in FVC and DL_{CO}, respectively, while at the same time in three studies by Gerbino et al., Tzouvelekis et al., and Simeon-Aznar et al. a decline of 5.4%, 6.45%, and 6% in FVC at baseline and 12 months after administration of cytotoxic agents was reported, indicating a rather beneficial effect of MMF usage. Although a direct comparison of these percentages was impossible to be performed in this meta-analysis due to the fact that they reflect mean differences, and they do not represent raw data; nevertheless, these results may potentially indicate a favorable outcome associated with MMF administration. In line with this, given the fact that the reported annual rate of lung function deterioration over time for patients with SSc-ILD is 32% loss for VC during the first two years of the disease, 12% for 2–4 years and 3% for 4–6 years [33], it is conceivable to state that a marginal increase in FVC or even a stabilization of functional status through disease course is of vital importance for this category of patients especially when the therapeutic agent used presents with an excellent safety profile tested on a longitudinal basis.

One final issue to be clarified in our meta-analysis was the absence of a beneficial effect of MMF or MS treatment in DL_{CO} values while at the same time, as reported previously, a clear trend towards FVC improvement following mycophenolate acid administration was highly notable. At this point it is of critical importance to highlight the major problems arising when interpreting treatment effects and using DL_{CO} as an end-point for interstitial lung disease in SSc, since this variable is so often influenced by other confounding factors closely related to vascular issues including pulmonary hypertension. In particular the two largest studies [8, 11], so far, estimating efficacy of a therapeutic agent, namely cyclophosphamide, in patients with SSc-ILD, demonstrated an almost marginal statistically significant difference in FVC levels favoring drug usage, while no beneficial effect in gas-transfer indicators was reported in both studies. Our personal view is that gas-transfer capacity should not be used as primary outcome of interest in clinical trials estimating drug efficacy in patients with SSc-ILD, since major data misinterpretations may easily arise given the high incidence of pulmonary hypertension (almost 50%) that so often complicates disease natural course and influences functional parameters such as DL_{CO}. Alternatively, if used, results should be cautiously concluded and extrapolated according to the presence and the severity of right-heart dysfunction.

Despite relative enthusiasm arising from the above observations, our review presents with some limitations that should be addressed cautiously. The quality of the evidence was limited; no study met all standard quality criteria since all of the studies were nonrandomized controlled, unicentric and underpowered with limited number of patients enrolled, and therefore their power to identify important differences in efficacy outcomes such as functional parameters could be questioned. Furthermore, it is important to underline that all the included studies enrolled middle-aged female patients with mild-to-moderate disease severity as assessed by functional parameters (FVC ranging from 64–79.5% pred. and DL_{CO} ranging from 40–64.2% pred.) prior MMF or MS administration. Thus, based on our data it is rather unknown whether stabilization of functional parameters could be attributed to therapeutic intervention or the former simply represents a bystander of disease clinical course. Alternatively, the majority of the patients included in the meta-analysis could be considered as slow progressors regarding their lung involvement indicating a potentially more favorable prognosis irrespective of therapeutic approach.

In conclusion, based on cumulative data from this meta-analysis our statement is that MMF or MS could wonderfully couple cyclophosphamide in the treatment of patients with SSc-ILD, since administration of the latter has been starkly demonstrated to be associated with statistically significant functional improvement in patients with SSc-ILD. On the other hand, mycophenolate acid could be administered as maintenance treatment, since it seems to represent a safe therapeutic agent that has been linked with disease stabilization regarding functional parameters overcoming the fear for potential side effects arising from longitudinal administration of aggressive cytotoxic agents or limited for patients with mild disease pattern. Slowing down disease progression and modulating disease natural history with less cost seems to be of paramount significance for this dismal disease. Larger randomized controlled studies are sorely needed to support this premise.

List of Abbreviations

DL_{CO}: Diffusion capacity of the lung for carbon monoxide
FVC: Forced vital capacity
HRCT: High-resolution computed tomography
ILD: Interstitial lung disease
MMF: Mycophenolate mofetil
MS: Mycophenolate sodium
NA: Nonapplicable
SSc: Systemic sclerosis
WMD: Weighted mean difference.

Authors' Contribution

Argyris Tzouvelekis, George Kolios, and Demosthenes Bouros were involved in the study conception. Argyris Tzouvelekis wrote the paper and performed the meta-analysis. Argyris Tzouvelekis and Evangelos Bouros performed laboratory and functional data acquisition. Argyris Tzouvelekis, Nikolaos Galanopoulos, George Zacharis, Andreas Koulelidis, Paschalis Ntolios and Demosthenes Bouros were involved in patients' recruitment and followup. Anastasia Oikonomou performed HRCT data acquisition and interpretation. Demosthenes Bouros and George Kolios were involved in revising the paper for its important intellectual content. All authors read and approved the final paper.

Conflict of Interests

Argyris Tzouvelekis is a recipient of an unrestricted grant provided by Hellenic Thoracic Society for the years 2009–2011.

Acknowledgments

The authors are thankful to Nikolaos Gouvas, Resident in General Surgery Department, "Agia Olga" hospital, Athens and Vassileios Vasdekis, Assistant Professor, Department of Statistics, Athens University of Economic and Business, for their valuable comments in the statistical analysis of the study.

References

[1] V. D. Steen, C. Conte, G. R. Owens, and T. A. Medsger, "Severe restrictive lung disease in systemic sclerosis," *Arthritis and Rheumatism*, vol. 37, no. 9, pp. 1283–1289, 1994.

[2] V. D. Steen, "The Many Faces of Scleroderma," *Rheumatic Disease Clinics of North America*, vol. 34, no. 1, pp. 1–15, 2008.

[3] U. A. Walker, A. Tyndall, L. Czirják et al., "Clinical risk assessment of organ manifestations in systemic sclerosis: a report from the EULAR Scleroderma Trials and Research group database," *Annals of the Rheumatic Diseases*, vol. 66, no. 6, pp. 754–763, 2007.

[4] D. Bouros, A. U. Wells, A. G. Nicholson et al., "Histopathologic subsets of fibrosing alveolitis in patients with systemic sclerosis and their relationship to outcome," *American Journal of Respiratory and Critical Care Medicine*, vol. 165, no. 12, pp. 1581–1586, 2002.

[5] A. U. Wells and N. Hirani, "Interstitial lung disease guideline: the British thoracic society in collaboration with the thoracic society of Australia and New Zealand and the Irish thoracic society," *Thorax*, vol. 63, supplement 5, pp. v1–v58, 2008.

[6] P. J. Clements, D. E. Furst, W. K. Wong et al., "High-dose versus low-dose D-penicillamine in early diffuse systemic sclerosis: analysis of a two-year, double-blind, randomized, controlled clinical trial," *Arthritis and Rheumatism*, vol. 42, no. 6, pp. 1194–1203, 1999.

[7] P. J. Clements, J. R. Seibold, D. E. Furst et al., "High-dose versus low-dose D-penicillamine in early diffuse systemic sclerosis trial: lessons learned," *Seminars in Arthritis and Rheumatism*, vol. 33, no. 4, pp. 249–263, 2004.

[8] R. K. Hoyles, R. W. Ellis, J. Wellsbury et al., "A multicenter, prospective, randomized, double-blind, placebo-controlled trial of corticosteroids and intravenous cyclophosphamide followed by oral azathioprine for the treatment of pulmonary fibrosis in scleroderma," *Arthritis and Rheumatism*, vol. 54, no. 12, pp. 3962–3970, 2006.

[9] M. Matucci-Cerinic, V. D. Steen, D. E. Furst, and J. R. Seibold, "Clinical trials in systemic sclerosis: lessons learned and outcomes," *Arthritis Research and Therapy*, vol. 9, no. 2, p. S7, 2007.

[10] L. Mouthon, A. Berezne, L. Guillevin, and D. Valeyre, "Therapeutic options for systemic sclerosis related interstitial lung diseases," *Respiratory Medicine*, vol. 104, supplement 1, pp. S59–S69, 2010.

[11] D. P. Tashkin, R. Elashoff, P. J. Clements et al., "Cyclophosphamide versus placebo in scleroderma lung disease," *New England Journal of Medicine*, vol. 354, no. 25, pp. 2655–2666, 2006.

[12] D. P. Tashkin, R. Elashoff, P. J. Clements et al., "Cyclophosphamide versus placebo in scleroderma lung disease," *New England Journal of Medicine*, vol. 354, no. 25, pp. 2655–2666, 2006.

[13] D. P. Tashkin, R. Elashoff, P. J. Clements et al., "Effects of 1-year treatment with cyclophosphamide on outcomes at 2 years in scleroderma lung disease," *American Journal of Respiratory and Critical Care Medicine*, vol. 176, no. 10, pp. 1026–1034, 2007.

[14] J. Goldin, R. Elashoff, H. J. Kim et al., "Treatment of scleroderma-interstitial lung disease with cyclophosphamide is associated with less progressive fibrosis on serial thoracic high-resolution CT scan than placebo: findings from the scleroderma lung study," *Chest*, vol. 136, no. 5, pp. 1333–1340, 2009.

[15] J. G. Goldin, D. A. Lynch, D. C. Strollo et al., "High-resolution CT scan findings in patients with symptomatic scleroderma-related interstitial lung disease," *Chest*, vol. 134, no. 2, pp. 358–367, 2008.

[16] M. D. Roth, C.-H. Tseng, P. J. Clements et al., "Predicting treatment outcomes and responder subsets in scleroderma-related interstitial lung disease," *Arthritis and Rheumatism*, vol. 63, no. 9, pp. 2797–2808, 2011.

[17] A. C. Allison and E. M. Eugui, "Mycophenolate mofetil and its mechanisms of action," *Immunopharmacology*, vol. 47, no. 2-3, pp. 85–118, 2000.

[18] A. C. Allison and E. M. Eugui, "Mechanisms of action of mycophenolate mofetil in preventing acute and chronic allograft rejection," *Transplantation*, vol. 80, no. 2, pp. S181–S190, 2005.

[19] A. C. Allison, "Mechanisms of action of mycophenolate mofetil," *Lupus*, vol. 14, no. 1, pp. s2–s8, 2005.

[20] G. Ciancio, G. W. Burke, J. J. Gaynor et al., "A randomized long-term trial of tacrolimus and sirolimus versus tacrolimus and mycophenolate mofetil versus cyclosporine (neoral) and sirolimus in renal transplantation. I. Drug interactions and rejection at one year," *Transplantation*, vol. 77, no. 2, pp. 244–251, 2004.

[21] G. Ciancio, J. Miller, and T. A. Gonwa, "Review of major clinical trial with mycophenolate mofetil in renal transplantation," *Transplantation*, vol. 80, no. 2, pp. S191–S200, 2005.

[22] E. L. Altschuler, "Consideration of mycophenolate mofetil for idiopathic pulmonary fibrosis," *Medical Hypotheses*, vol. 57, no. 6, pp. 701–702, 2001.

[23] J. R. Waller, N. R. Brook, G. R. Bicknell, G. J. Murphy, and M. L. Nicholson, "Mycophenolate mofetil inhibits intimal hyperplasia and attenuates the expression of genes favouring smooth muscle cell proliferation and migration," *Transplantation Proceedings*, vol. 37, no. 1, pp. 164–166, 2005.

[24] C. P. Simeon-Aznar, V. Fonollosa-Pla, C. Tolosa-Vilella, A. Selva-O'Callaghan, R. Solans-Laqué, and M. Vilardell-Tarres, "Effect of mycophenolate sodium in scleroderma-related interstitial lung disease," *Clinical Rheumatology*, vol. 30, no. 11, pp. 1393–1398, 2011.

[25] A. J. Gerbino, C. H. Goss, and J. A. Molitor, "Effect of mycophenolate mofetil on pulmonary function in scleroderma-associated interstitial lung disease," *Chest*, vol. 133, no. 2, pp. 455–460, 2008.

[26] A. Koutroumpas, A. Ziogas, I. Alexiou, G. Barouta, and L. I. Sakkas, "Mycophenolate mofetil in systemic sclerosis-associated interstitial lung disease," *Clinical Rheumatology*, pp. 1–2, 2010.

[27] S. N. C. Liossis, A. Bounas, and A. P. Andonopoulos, "Mycophenolate mofetil as first-line treatment improves clinically evident early scleroderma lung disease," *Rheumatology*, vol. 45, no. 8, pp. 1005–1008, 2006.

[28] A. C. Zamora, P. J. Wolters, H. R. Collard et al., "Use of mycophenolate mofetil to treat scleroderma-associated interstitial lung disease," *Respiratory Medicine*, vol. 102, no. 1, pp. 150–155, 2008.

[29] V. D. Steen, G. Graham, C. Conte, G. Owens, and T. A. Medsger, "Isolated diffusing capacity reduction in systemic sclerosis," *Arthritis and Rheumatism*, vol. 35, no. 7, pp. 765–770, 1992.

[30] S. I. Nihtyanova, G. M. Brough, C. M. Black, and C. P. Denton, "Mycophenolate mofetil in diffuse cutaneous systemic sclerosis - A retrospective analysis," *Rheumatology*, vol. 46, no. 3, pp. 442–445, 2007.

[31] S. C. Plastiras, P. G. Vlachoyiannopoulos, and G. E. Tzelepis, "Mycophenolate mofetil for interstitial lung disease in scleroderma [1]," *Rheumatology*, vol. 45, no. 12, p. 1572, 2006.

[32] J. J. Swigris, A. L. Olson, A. Fischer et al., "Mycophenolate mofetil is safe, well tolerated, and preserves lung function in patients with connective tissue disease-related interstitial lung disease," *Chest*, vol. 130, no. 1, pp. 30–36, 2006.

[33] V. Steen, "Predictors of end stage lung disease in systemic sclerosis," *Annals of the Rheumatic Diseases*, vol. 62, no. 2, pp. 97–99, 2003.

Significant Differences in Markers of Oxidant Injury between Idiopathic and Bronchopulmonary-Dysplasia-Associated Pulmonary Hypertension in Children

Kimberly B. Vera,[1] Donald Moore,[1] English Flack,[1] Michael Liske,[1] and Marshall Summar[2]

[1] Division of Cardiology, Department of Pediatrics, Vanderbilt University School of Medicine, Nashville, TN 37232, USA
[2] Center for Genetic Medicine Research, Children's National Medical Center, Washington, DC 20010, USA

Correspondence should be addressed to Kimberly B. Vera, kimberly.vera@vanderbilt.edu

Academic Editor: Serpil Erzurum

While oxidant stress is elevated in adult forms of pulmonary hypertension (PH), levels of oxidant stress in pediatric PH are unknown. The objective of this study is to measure F_2-isoprostanes, a marker of oxidant stress, in children with idiopathic pulmonary hypertension (IPH) and PH due to bronchopulmonary dysplasia (BPD). We hypothesized that F_2-isoprostanes in pediatric IPH and PH associated with BPD will be higher than in controls. Plasma F_2-isoprostanes were measured in pediatric PH patients during clinically indicated cardiac catheterization and compared with controls. F_2-Isoprostane levels were compared between IPH, PH due to BD, and controls. Five patients with IPH, 12 with PH due to BPD, and 20 control subjects were studied. Patients with IPH had statistically higher isoprostanes than controls 62 pg/mL (37–210) versus 20 pg/mL (16–27), $P < 0.01$. The patients with PH and BPD had significantly lower isoprostanes than controls 15 pg/ml (8–17) versus 20 pg/mL (16–27), $P < 0.02$. F_2-isoprostanes are elevated in children with IPH compared to both controls and patients with PH secondary to BPD. Furthermore, F_2-isoprostanes in PH secondary to BPD are lower than control levels. These findings suggest that IPH and PH secondary to BPD have distinct mechanisms of disease pathogenesis.

1. Introduction

It has long been recognized that patients with pediatric idiopathic pulmonary hypertension (IPH) have poor long-term survival. More recently pulmonary hypertension (PH) associated with bronchopulmonary dysplasia (BPD) has been identified as a significant cause of mortality among BPD patients [1, 2]. Few studies have evaluated the mechanisms and optimal treatment of PH due to BPD, resulting in management strategies for these patients which mirror the better studied pharmacologic treatments of IPH. The use of similar therapeutic strategies in these two populations relies on the unproven assumption that the diseases share similar molecular pathophysiologies.

Oxidant stress appears to play a role in the molecular mechanism of adult IPH. Multiple studies measuring F_2-isoprostanes, a stable marker of oxidant stress resulting from the oxidation of cell-membrane arachidonic acid, have shown adult IPH patients, have higher F_2-isoprostane levels than do control patients [3, 4]. Elevated F_2-isoprostane levels suggest enhanced oxidant stress in IPH patients and may also directly contribute to pulmonary vasoconstriction [5]. There are no published data on oxidant stress or F_2-isoprostane levels in pediatric patients with PH secondary to BPD or IPH. The objective of this study is to measure F_2-isoprostanes in children with IPH and PH due to BPD and to compare them to normal controls to assess the role of oxidant stress in pediatric populations with PH. We hypothesize that children with IPH and PH due to BPD will have F_2-isoprostane levels higher than those measured in healthy control subjects. Evidence supporting similar biochemical mechanisms between these pediatric populations with PH would support the practice of utilizing similar therapeutic strategies in these children.

2. Materials and Methods

2.1. Study Population. All patients who presented to the pediatric catheterization laboratory at Vanderbilt Children's Hospital for evaluation of pulmonary hypertension between December 2007 and December 2008 were approached for participation in the study. Patients were excluded if they had ventricular septal defects; patients with an atrial septal defect or hemodynamically insignificant patent ductus arteriosus were allowed. Other exclusion criteria were pulmonary vein stenosis, valvar stenosis of any kind, aortic arch obstruction, left ventricular dysfunction, active infection of any kind, and autoimmune disease. All catheterizations were performed for clinical reasons in accordance with the standard of care at the Vanderbilt Pulmonary Hypertension Center.

Two groups of control patients were enrolled. The primary control group was recruited from the general pediatric clinic at Vanderbilt Children's Hospital. Patients without acute or chronic illness who required a routine blood draw for health maintenance were approached for enrollment in the study. In addition, in order to assess the effect of general anesthesia and the general impact of the catheterization on F_2-isoprostane levels, patients presenting to the pediatric catheterization laboratory for atrial septal defect (ASD) device closure were also approached to participate as controls. Patients undergoing device ASD closure were chosen because they typically do not have elevation of their pulmonary artery pressure and are in good general health. Exclusion criteria for both control groups were a history of prematurity, ventricular septal defect, pulmonary vein stenosis, valvar stenosis of any kind, aortic arch obstruction, left ventricular dysfunction, active infection of any kind, and autoimmune disease.

2.2. Echocardiography. All consenting control subjects recruited from the general pediatric clinic underwent echocardiography to screen for undiagnosed pulmonary hypertension. Right ventricular pressure was assessed by interrogation of the tricuspid regurgitation jet and utilization of the Bernoulli equation. The right atrial pressure was assumed to be 5 mmHg. Any right ventricular pressure measurement of greater than 30 mmHg was deemed elevated. In the absence of tricuspid regurgitation, flattening of the ventricular septum during systole in the parasternal short axis was defined as evidence of elevated right ventricular pressure. The echocardiograms were independently reviewed by two pediatric cardiologists. Evidence of elevated right ventricular pressure found by one or more reviewer excluded a patient from participation as a control subject.

2.3. Cardiac Catheterization. At the Vanderbilt Pediatric Pulmonary Hypertension Center, the timing of cardiac catheterization is specific to each type of PH. IPH patients undergo cardiac catheterization with vasodilatory testing at diagnosis and every 3–12 months thereafter depending on their clinical status and changes in therapy. Patients with PH and BPD are not routinely catheterized at diagnosis

unless structural abnormalities are suspected such as pulmonary vein stenosis. Our center uses echocardiography to identify and follow elevated pulmonary artery pressure in neonates with BPD in the neonatal ICU and in follow up after discharge from the ICU. Tricuspid regurgitation velocity and systolic flattening of the ventricular septum are the primary echocardiographic features used to assess pulmonary artery pressure. BPD patients with persistent echocardiographic evidence of elevated pulmonary artery pressure are followed in the PH clinic as outpatients and undergo catheterization within 3–6 months if on vasodilator therapy. BPD-PH patients may also undergo catheterization prior to discontinuation of vasodilator therapy.

Consenting participants with PH and the ASD control patients underwent their clinically indicated cardiac catheterization under general anesthesia. All patients underwent a right heart catheterization with directly measured saturations and pressures at the lowest FiO₂ were required to maintain oxygen saturations of above 95% by pulse oximetry. In patients with an ASD, a catheter was placed across the ASD from the right heart to obtain a pressure in the left atrium and a saturation measurement from a pulmonary vein. A femoral artery sheath was placed in all patients to directly measure the systemic blood pressure and the descending aortic saturation. Pulmonary flows were calculated using the Fick equation with assumed oxygen consumption in all BPD patients, in the IPH patients with an atrial septal defect, and in all the ASD control patients. Thermodilution was used to measure pulmonary flow in IPH patients without an atrial septal defect. All pulmonary flows were indexed to body surface area. Pulmonary vascular resistance (PVR) was calculated in Woods units (WU) and indexed to body surface area.

2.4. Blood Sampling. In control patients recruited from the general pediatric clinic, 5 mLs of study blood was drawn by routine phlebotomy. ASD control patients and PH patients had 5 mls of study blood drawn during the baseline hemodynamic measurements. If patients undergoing catheterization had a pulmonary venous sample obtained, the study blood was taken from a pulmonary vein. Catheterized patients without an ASD had study blood obtained in the descending aorta through the femoral arterial sheath or arterial catheter. All blood samples were obtained before any pulmonary vasodilator testing was performed. All study blood was collected on ice in an EDTA tube and immediately transported to the laboratory for isoprostane analysis.

2.5. F_2-Isoprostane Analysis. F_2-isoprostanes were measured using a method pioneered by Drs. Morrow and Roberts [6]. Briefly this involves passing the sample through two Waters Corporation Sep-Pak cartridges to remove much of the unwanted impurities. First one uses a C-18 packing material and the second uses a silica packing material. The final elution is then esterified with pentafluorobenzyl bromide and silated with bis(trimethylsilyl)trifluoroacetamide before being subjected to GC/MS analysis on an Agilent 5973 inert

TABLE 1: Subjects' demographics.

	Control	IPH	PH due to BPD	P value
N	18	4	12	
Age§ (years)	7.5 (3.8–15.3)	11 (3–16.8)	2 (1–2.8)	<.01*
Gender (# male)	10	2	10	.63**, .12†, .25¶
BMI§ (kg/m²)	17.9 (16.6–25.2)	23.1 (15.4–27.1)	16.1 (15.7–16.7)	.02*
Race (# Caucasian)	10	4	8	.14**, .41†, .27¶

*P value based on the Kruskal-Wallis test.
**P value based on the Fisher's exact test of control versus IPH.
†P value based on the Fisher's exact test of control versus PH due to BPD.
¶P value based on the Fisher's exact test of IPH versus PH due to BPD.
§Data expressed as median (IQR).

MSD coupled with and Agilent 6890N Network GC from Agilent Technologies in Wilmington, Delaware.

2.6. Statistical Analysis. Study data were collected and managed using the REDCap electronic data capture tools hosted at Vanderbilt University [7]. Data are presented as medians with interquartile ranges (IQR) due to lack of normal distribution. The Mann-Whitney U test was performed to determine the statistical significance of the difference between any two groups. The Kruskal-Wallis test was used to analyze differences between all three groups. Categorical variables between groups were assessed with the Fisher's exact test. Spearman's test was used to analyze correlations. A two-tailed α of <0.05 was considered statistically significant. Bonferroni correction was not used due to its conservative nature and the small number of comparisons done in this study. SPSS was used to perform the statistical analysis (IBM SPSS statistics, version 20).

This study was approved by the Institutional Review Board of the Vanderbilt University Medical Center.

3. Results

We enrolled 5 patients with IPH and 12 patients with PH secondary to BPD. All PH patients approached consented to participate in the study. Twenty controls, including 5 ASD patients and 15 healthy controls from the primary care clinic, consented to participate in the study. Three eligible control patients approached in the primary care clinic refused to participate because they did not have time to undergo echocardiography. All ASD patients approached to participate consented. None of the healthy control subjects had abnormal echocardiograms. One of the 5 IPH patients underwent diagnostic catheterization while the remainder underwent routine follow-up catheterizations. All of the BPD patients were catheterized for purposes of treatment follow-up. The F_2-isoprostane data could not be obtained in one IPH patient and two controls due to sample problems.

Table 1 describes the baseline characteristics of the study groups. The median age of control patients did not statistically differ from IPH patients ($P = 0.99$), but those with PH due to BPD were significantly younger than controls ($P < 0.01$). There was no statistical difference in gender distribution between the controls and the two PH groups.

TABLE 2: Medical therapy of pulmonary hypertension patients.

	IPH	PH due to BPD	P value
N	4	12	
Home Oxygen (No. of patients)	1	8	.13*
Epoprostenol (No. of patients)	3	2	.06*
Bosentan (No. of patients)	1	1	.52*
Sildenafil (No. of patients)	3	11	.45*
Months on Therapy†	17.5 (4–27.5)	20 (12–29)	.99**

*P value based on Fisher's exact test.
**P values based on Mann-Whitney U test.
†Data expressed as median (IQR).

While the body mass index (BMI) of the IPH patients did not significantly differ from the controls, the BMI of those with PH due to BPD was significantly less than controls ($P = 0.01$).

The medical treatments of patients with PH are described in Table 2. There were significantly more IPH patients treated with epoprostenol than patients with PH due to BPD, although this did not reach statistical significance ($P = 0.06$). There was no difference in the number of subjects on bosentan, sildenafil, and home oxygen in the two PH groups.

The hemodynamic data from the cardiac catheterizations are presented in Table 3. The control patients undergoing ASD device closure had normal right ventricular pressure and pulmonary vascular resistance which were significantly lower than in both the IPH group ($P < 0.01$) and the BPD-PH group ($P < 0.01$). The right and left ventricular end diastolic pressures, cardiac index, and baseline FiO_2 in ASD controls were not different from either PH group. As expected, those undergoing ASD device closure had a larger pulmonary to systemic blood flow ratio than those with IPH ($P < 0.01$) and PH due to BPD ($P < 0.01$). The median right ventricular pressure as a percentage of left ventricular pressure (RVP/LVP ratio) and the median PVR were distinctly lower in those with PH due to BPD

TABLE 3: Hemodynamics of subjects in catheterization laboratory[¶].

	IPH	PH due to BPD	ASD controls	P value IPH versus BPD
N	4	12	5	
RVP/LVP (%)	83 (80–1.1)	46 (38–59)	.24 (.22–.25)	.08*
Pulmonary vascular resistance (WUs)[†]	17.2 (16.2–19.6)	4 (3.5–5.4)	1.4 (1.1–1.6)	.08*
Mean PAP[††] (mmHg)	61 (53–63)	25 (22–36)	17 (14–19)	.08*
RVEDP[‡] (mmHg)	10 (8–10)	7.5 (6.3–9)	8 (7.5–8.5)	.26*
LVEDP[6] (mmHg)	8 (8–9)	8 (7–9)	10 (8–10)	.99*
Cardiac index (L/min/m²)	3.6 (3.1–3.6)	3.6 (3.5–3.8)	3.0 (2.7–3.5)	.99*
Qp : Qs[§]	.87 (0.8-.94)	1.0 (1.0-1.0)	2.1 (1.6–4.1)	.53*
Baseline FiO_2 (%)	21 (21–26)	21 (21-22)	21 (21–21)	.52*
ASD (# patients)	2	7	5	.62**

[*] Value based on Mann-Whitney U test.
[**] Value based on Fisher's exact test.
[†] Indexed to body surface area.
[††] Pulmonary artery pressure.
[‡] Right ventricular end diastolic pressure.
[‡‡] Left ventricular end diastolic pressure.
[§] Ratio of pulmonary to systemic blood flow.
[¶] Interval data expressed as median (IQR).

compared to those with IPH, but the differences did not quite reach statistical significance. The median right ventricular end diastolic pressure (RVEDP), left ventricular end diastolic pressure (LVEDP), and baseline FiO_2 were not significantly different among the two groups with PH. A patent foramen ovale was found in 5 patients with PH secondary to BPD, and a moderate atrial septal defect was found in one patient with PH secondary to BPD. One patient with PH secondary to BPD had a patent foramen ovale in addition to a small patent ductus arteriosus. In those with IPH, two patients had small atrial septal defects.

Patients with IPH had significantly higher F_2-isoprostanes than controls (62 pg/mL (37–210) versus 20 pg/mL (16–27), $P \leq 0.01$) (Figure 1) . The patients with PH due to BPD had significantly lower F_2- isoprostanes than controls (15 pg/mL (8–17) versus 20 pg/mL (16–27), $P = 0.02$). F_2-Isoprostane levels in IPH patients were significantly higher than those with PH secondary to BPD ($P = 0.002$). No correlation was found between F_2-isoprostane levels and age ($R_S^2 = 0.02$) or between F_2-isoprostane levels and BMI ($R_S^2 = 0.09$) in the study cohort. Among all PH patients, no correlation was found between F_2-isoprostanes and RVP/LVP ratio ($R_S^2 = 0.02$) or any other hemodynamic measure. When analyzing only BPD patients with RVP/LVP >50%, those with PH due to BPD still had lower F_2-isoprostanes ((8.7 pg/mL (6.3–12.7)) than controls ($P \leq 0.01$) and those with IPH ($P = 0.02$). No significant difference was found between the F_2-isoprostane levels of the control subjects undergoing ASD device closure and those undergoing routine phlebotomy ($P = 0.95$). Similarly, the F_2-isoprostanes drawn from the pulmonary veins were not significantly different from those drawn from the descending aorta among those with PH due to BPD ($P = 0.09$) or among those with IPH ($P = 0.44$).

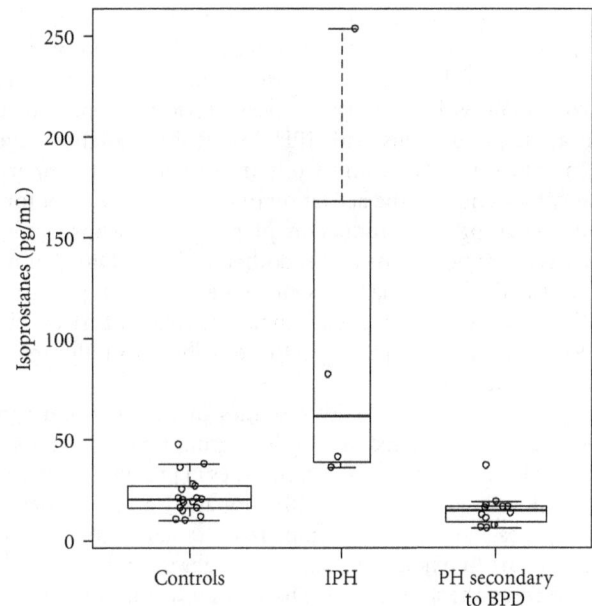

FIGURE 1: Box plot of plasma F_2-isoprostanes in IPH, PH due to BPD, and controls. F_2-Isoprostanes are significantly higher in children with IPH compared to pediatric controls and children with PH secondary to BPD. Plasma F_2-isoprostanes are statistically lower in children with PH secondary to BPD compared to those with IPH and pediatric controls.

Both the IPH and BPD-PH groups had one outlier with a high F_2-isoprostane level. The BPD patient with the high isoprostane value had only mildly elevated pulmonary artery pressures with a RVP/LVP ratio of .38 and a PVR of 3.6 WU and was only being treated with sildenafil and home oxygen. The IPH patient with the high isoprostane value had similar hemodynamics to the other IPH patients with a RVP/LVP ratio of .83, a PVR of 17.1 WU, a RVEDP of 10 mmHg, and a LVEDP of 10 mmHg. This IPH patient was on epoprostenol and sildenafil similar to the remaining IPH patients but was the only one on bosentan. When repeating the analysis without the two outlier, the F_2-isoprostanes of the IPH group are still significantly higher than the BPD-PH group ($P = 0.01$), and the control F_2-isoprostanes are still significantly lower than the IPH group ($P = 0.02$) and higher than the BPD-PH group ($P < 0.01$).

4. Discussion

F_2-isoprostanes are elevated in pediatric patients with IPH but not in those with PH secondary to BPD. In fact, F_2-isoprostanes in the BPD-PH group seem to be lower than controls. Anesthesia and the general effect of the catheterization did not appear to influence F_2-isoprostane levels as there was no difference between the ASD controls and the clinic controls. To our knowledge, this is the first time F_2-isoprostane levels have been studied in pediatric patients with IPH and PH secondary to BPD. Different F_2-isoprostane levels suggest that IPH and PH secondary to BPD have distinct molecular pathophysiologies with different degrees of chronic oxidant injury. This suggests that these entities may be amenable to different pharmacologic approaches. The finding of elevated F_2-isoprostanes in children with IPH is consistent with the elevated levels previously reported in the adult populations with IPH [3]. F_2-isoprostanes have been shown to have a direct role in producing pulmonary vasoconstriction by the activation of thromboxane receptors and increasing the production of potent vasoconstrictors such as thromboxane A_2 and endothelin 1 [3, 8]. Our finding of elevated circulating F_2-isoprostane levels in pediatric patients with IPH suggests enhanced oxidant stress in these patients which may directly contribute to pulmonary vasoconstriction.

The low levels of F_2-isoprostanes in PH secondary to BPD was an unexpected finding. Two groups have previously shown elevated levels of F_2-isoprostanes in premature infants in the first weeks of life [9, 10]. Impaired and disordered angiogenesis and resultant impaired alveolarization due at least in part to oxidant damage is thought to underlie much of the BPD phenotype [11]. The natural history of oxidant stress in premature infants with or without PH due to BPD is unknown. In this study, there was no difference in months on treatment between the IPH group and the BPD-PH group suggesting the two cohorts are at reasonably similar points in disease time course. Even if the F_2-isoprostane levels are elevated early in the course of PH secondary to BPD, the low levels we found in these established BPD-PH patients is in marked contrast to the elevated levels we found in IPH patients at a similar point in disease course.

The etiology of low levels of F_2-isoprostanes in children with PH secondary to BPD is unknown. F_2-isoprostanes are formed by the free-radical-induced peroxidation of arachidonic acid in cell membranes [4, 12]. This would suggest that PH secondary to BPD does not generate

the oxidant stress seen in IPH at the molecular level and/or that BPD enhances compensatory mechanisms to scavenge free radicals. An alternative possibility would be the preferential production of other isoprostane molecules from arachidonic acid, such as E_2 and D_2 isoprostanes, in children with BPD-associated PH. Polyunsaturated fatty acids such as linoleic acid, DHA, and EPA may be oxidized to form isoprostane like molecules more efficiently than arachidonic acid [12]. Children with PH due to BPD may have an unknown mechanism to encourage oxidation of these polyunsaturated fats over arachidonic acid. This is another potential explanation of the low F_2-isoprostane levels in children with BPD-associataed PH, although there is no data on this possibility. Another alternative is inhibition of F_2-isoprostane formation by very high oxygen tension with diversion to isofuran production; however, those with BPD-associated PH in this study were not on significantly higher FiO_2 than the other groups [13]. In fact, all of the groups were breathing a FiO_2 of near 21% making hyperoxic suppression of F_2-isoprostanes very unlikely. The inevitable pO_2 difference between the pulmonary venous samples and systemic venous samples did not appear to influence F_2-isoprostane levels as there was no difference in the F_2-isoprostane levels between the ASD controls, who all had pulmonary venous samples, and the clinic controls, who all had systemic venous samples. Regardless of any potential mechanism to lower F_2-isoprostane levels below normal controls, this study strongly supports the absence of a high level of uncompensated oxidant stress in this population of children with PH secondary to BPD.

The limitations of this study include the fact that the patients with PH due to BPD are younger and have a lower BMI than both the controls and those with IPH. The age difference is difficult to remedy as IPH typically presents later in childhood while PH due to BPD is a disease of infants and toddlers. If the patient survives infancy, PH secondary to BPD tends to improve or even resolve with age leaving few older children with active disease to study [2]. The lower BMI in the PH due to BPD is likely a function of both the younger age in this group and the commonly seen feature of failure to thrive early in life in patients with BPD. The absence of correlation of age or BMI with F_2-isoprostane level suggests the age and BMI differences do not explain the difference in F_2-isoprostanes seen in this study.

Another limitation of the study is the different PH severity among the IPH group and those with PH due to BPD. If infants survive the initial malignant phase of PH secondary to BPD, pulmonary artery pressures tend to decrease over time [2]. This natural history of improvement in PH due to BPD explains the lower pulmonary vascular resistance and RVP/LVP in those with PH secondary to BPD compared to those with IPH. The fact that no correlation exists between hemodynamic measures of elevated pulmonary pressures and F_2-isoprostanes suggests the F_2-isoprostane difference between IPH and PH due to BPD is not caused by the difference in PH severity. Similarly, analysis of only the BPD PH patients with RVP/LVP >50% continues to show significantly lower F_2-isoprostanes than IPH patients and controls. While clinical function data, such as New York

Heart Association class, was not collected due to the difficulty in applying these measures to infants and toddlers, normal ventricular filling pressures, and normal cardiac outputs in both groups demonstrate similar stable hemodynamic states despite the difference in PH severity. A greater percentage of those with IPH were on treatment with epoprostenol when compared to those with PH due to BPD. Evidence exists that this drug lowers F_2-isoprostane levels in patients; thus, this bias would act to lessen the difference between IPH patients and the other 2 study groups [3]. Finally, it would be optimal to increase the number of patients in the IPH group, but the rarity of this disease in children makes obtaining larger numbers difficult.

5. Conclusion

We found that pediatric patients with IPH have elevated F_2-isoprostane levels while children being followed for PH secondary to BPD have low F_2-isoprostane levels. This marked difference in oxidant stress suggests each disease has a unique pathophysiology. Future studies are needed to better elucidate these differences thereby leading to better targeted therapies for pediatric patients with a broad spectrum of pulmonary hypertensive diseases.

Abbreviations

PH:	Pulmonary hypertension
IPH:	Idiopathic pulmonary hypertension
BPD:	Bronchopulmonary dysplasia
ASD:	Atrial septal defect
PVR:	Pulmonary vascular resistance
WU:	Woods units
IQR:	Interquartile range
RVP/LVP:	Right ventricular pressure as a percentage of left ventricular pressure
RVEDP:	Right ventricular end diastolic pressure
LVEDP:	Left ventricular end diastolic pressure.

References

[1] D. Yung, A. C. Widlitz, E. B. Rosenzweig, D. Kerstein, G. Maislin, and R. J. Barst, "Outcomes in children with idiopathic pulmonary arterial hypertension," *Circulation*, vol. 110, no. 6, pp. 660–665, 2004.

[2] E. Khemani, D. B. McElhinney, L. Rhein et al., "Pulmonary artery hypertension in formerly premature infants with bronchopulmonary dysplasia: clinical features and outcomes in the surfactant era," *Pediatrics*, vol. 120, no. 6, pp. 1260–1269, 2007.

[3] I. M. Robbins, J. D. Morrow, and B. W. Christman, "Oxidant stress but not thromboxane decreases with epoprostenol therapy," *Free Radical Biology and Medicine*, vol. 38, no. 5, pp. 568–574, 2005.

[4] L. J. M. Roberts and J. D. Morrow, "Measurement of F_2-isoprostanes as an index of oxidative stress in vivo," *Free Radical Biology and Medicine*, vol. 28, no. 4, pp. 505–513, 2000.

[5] L. J. Janssen, "Isoprostanes and lung vascular pathology," *American Journal of Respiratory Cell and Molecular Biology*, vol. 39, no. 4, pp. 383–389, 2008.

[6] J. D. Morrow and L. J. Roberts, "Mass spectrometric quantification of F_2-isoprostanes in biological fluids and tissues as measure of oxidant stress," *Methods in Enzymology*, vol. 300, pp. 3–12, 1998.

[7] P. A. Harris, R. Taylor, R. Thielke, J. Payne, N. Gonzalez, and J. G. Conde, "Research electronic data capture (REDCap)-A metadata-driven methodology and workflow process for providing translational research informatics support," *Journal of Biomedical Informatics*, vol. 42, no. 2, pp. 377–381, 2009.

[8] K. M. Kang, J. D. Morrow, L. J. Roberts, J. H. Newman, and M. Banerjee, "Airway and vascular effects of 8-epi-prostaglandin F(2α) in isolated perfused rat lung," *Journal of Applied Physiology*, vol. 74, no. 1, pp. 460–465, 1993.

[9] T. Ahola, V. Fellman, I. Kjellmer, K. O. Raivio, and R. Lapatto, "Plasma 8-isoprostane is increased in preterm infants who develop bronchopulmonary dysplasia or periventricular leukomalacia," *Pediatric Research*, vol. 56, no. 1, pp. 88–93, 2004.

[10] M. Comporti, C. Signorini, S. Leoncini, G. Buonocore, V. Rossi, and L. Ciccoli, "Plasma F_2-isoprostanes are elevated in newborns and inversely correlated to gestational age," *Free Radical Biology and Medicine*, vol. 37, no. 5, pp. 724–732, 2004.

[11] K. R. Stenmark and S. H. Abman, "Lung vascular development: implications for the pathogenesis of bronchopulmonary dysplasia," *Annual Review of Physiology*, vol. 67, pp. 623–661, 2005.

[12] G. L. Milne, H. Yin, and J. D. Morrow, "Human biochemistry of the isoprostane pathway," *Journal of Biological Chemistry*, vol. 283, no. 23, pp. 15533–15537, 2008.

[13] J. P. Fessel, N. A. Porter, K. P. Moore, J. R. Sheller, and L. J. Roberts, "Discovery of lipid peroxidation products formed in vivo with a substituted tetrahydrofuran ring (isofurans) that are favored by increased oxygen tension," *Proceedings of the National Academy of Sciences of the United States of America*, vol. 99, no. 26, pp. 16713–16718, 2002.

Prevalence of Occupational Asthma and Respiratory Symptoms in Foundry Workers

Servet Kayhan,[1] **Umit Tutar,**[2] **Halit Cinarka,**[1] **Aziz Gumus,**[1] **and Nurhan Koksal**[3]

[1] *Department of Chest Disease, Faculty of Medicine, Recep Tayyip Erdogan University, 53100 Rize, Turkey*
[2] *Department of Chest Disease, Hospital of Chest Disease and Thoracic Surgery, 55090 Samsun, Turkey*
[3] *Department of Chest Disease, Faculty of Medicine, Ondokuz Mayis University, 55139 Samsun, Turkey*

Correspondence should be addressed to Servet Kayhan; kayhanservet@gmail.com

Academic Editor: Stefano Centanni

This cross-sectional study was conducted in a foundry factory to assess the prevalence of respiratory symptoms and occupational asthma in foundry workers. Physical examination, spirometric evaluation, chest radiograph, and a questionnaire related to respiratory symptoms were performed. Monitoring of peak expiratory flow rates, spirometric reversibility test, and high-resolution computed tomographies were performed for the participants having respiratory symptoms and/or impaired respiratory function test. A total of 347 participants including 286 workers from production department and 61 subjects who worked in nonproduction departments were enrolled in this study. It is found that phlegm (n: 71, 20.46%) and cough (n: 52, 14.98%) were the most frequent symptoms. The other symptoms were breathlessness (n: 28, 8.06%), chest tightness (n: 14, 4.03%), and wheezing (n: 7, 2.01%). The prevalence of occupational asthma was found to be more frequent among the subjects who worked in the production department (n: 48, 16.78%) than the other persons who worked in the nonproduction department (n: 3, 4.91%) by chi-square test (P: 0.001). To prevent hazardous respiratory effects of the foundry production, an early diagnosis of occupational asthma is very important. Cessation of cigarette smoking and using of protective masks during the working time should be encouraged.

1. Introduction

The prevalence of occupational diseases shows the quality of working conditions and health of working environment. Respiratory diseases are common entities in occupational industries, because the lungs are the route of entry for noxious particles and gases. These agents can be inhaled in the form of fibers or dusts. The development of occupational respiratory disease is dependent on several factors including the chemical nature and physical state of the inhaled substance, the size and concentration of the dust particles, the duration of exposure, and individual susceptibility [1]. Respiratory irritants represent a major cause of occupational obstructive airway diseases related to irritative agents causing occupational asthma.

Work-related or occupational asthma is defined as a chronic inflammatory disorder of the airways with recurrent episodes of respiratory symptoms such as coughing, wheezing, chest tightness, dyspnea, shortness of breath at rest, and reversible airflow limitations caused by a particular occupational environment. The foundry workers are potentially exposed to a number of noxious particles and gases including asbestos, silica, diphenylmethane diisocyanate, polycyclic aromatic hydrocarbons, benzene, and sulfuric acid mist and toxic metals including zinc, chromium, nickel, and cadmium [2]. They have a risk of having respiratory symptoms and life-long chronic obstructive airway diseases including asthma, COPD, pneumoconiosis, and cancers [3–7].

This study was designed to evaluate the effects of the foundry production on respiratory health of workers.

2. Materials and Methods

2.1. Study Design, Study Population, and Definitions. This is a cross-sectional study, and it was conducted at one of the foundry factories localized in the industrial region of Samsun, Turkey. A total of 347 workers including 286 workers from production department who were exposed to dust and noxious gases and 61 subjects from the other departments were enrolled in the study. The study was approved by the Local Ethics Committee. The participants were informed about the aim of the study. All participants were assessed with a modified questionnaire adopted from the European Community Respiratory Health Survey (ECRHS) by face-to-face interviews [8]. The relationships between work department and using of protective masks and respiratory symptoms including cough, phlegm, wheezing, chest tightness, breathlessness, and smoking history (pack/year) were evaluated.

A physician of pulmonary disease examined all participants, and an experienced technical staff for measuring the respiratory function test performed the test in the factory. Standard posteroanterior chest X-rays were taken for all subjects. High-resolution computed tomographies (HRCT) were also obtained in cases presenting with respiratory symptoms and obstructive and restrictive disorders in respiratory function tests and for the subjects with abnormal chest X-ray findings.

In the diagnosis of occupational asthma, the internationally recommended criteria are used. Subjects with one of the asthma symptoms that lessen or disappear when the subject leaves the work environment, with variability in PEF > 20%, and did not have a previous history of asthma before their employment were considered as occupational asthma [9, 10].

2.2. Working Environment. The foundry based factory is located in Samsun Industrial Zone and has an annual casting capacity of 30.000 tons. The production program of the factory covers the design and manufacture of the pumping and piping equipment such as the centrifugal, mixed, and axial flow pumps for water; gate, butterfly, check and air valves, ductile iron pipe fittings, tapping valves, and fire hydrants.

2.3. Exposure Assessment. Foundry workers are classified into 5 categories for exposure assessments: (1) core making, (2) moulding, (3) melting and pouring, (4) fettling (cleaning castings), and (5) after processing groups. Some workers in this study population had worked in more than one department at their shifts, and they have not worked in the separate locations according to the job categories. Job area was classified as the longest-held job during their foundry work. Thus, the workers in production department have been exposed to similar hazards regardless of job categories. And individual exposure assessment could not be done in this study. Core makers are exposed to isocyanate, but the concentrations of isocyanate could not be measured in this study. The working environment with a dust concentration was measured in 16 different parts of the factory, and dust concentration was reported as below maximum allowable concentration (MAC $<10 \, mg/m^3$) in 14 departments and higher than MAC level in two departments; those were core making department ($10.122 \, mg/m^3$) and fettling (cleaning casting) department ($10.448 \, mg/m^3$). Workers in furnace and fettling were classified into the high-exposure group. Average respirable dust concentration was $0.216 \, mg/m^3$ for the moulding group, $0.322 \, mg/m^3$ for the melting and pouring group, and

$0.216 \, mg/m^3$ for after processing group. The workers in moulding, melting and pouring, and after processing departments were classified into low-exposure group. Job categories were mainly classified into two groups as production and non-production according to working area.

2.4. Pulmonary Function Tests. Pulmonary function tests of all subjects were performed using an MIR Spirolab-II vitalograph (Italy) device in a sitting position and in accordance with the test procedures recommended by the American Thoracic Society [11]. Spirometric tests were performed at least three times for each worker and the best values were accepted. Forced vital capacity (FVC), forced expiratory volume at one second (FEV_1), FEV_1/FVC, peak expiratory flow (PEF), and forced expiratory flow 25–75% (FEF_{25-75}) were measured. All measurements were expressed as the percentage of predicted values. The workers were evaluated in terms of respiratory diseases according to consensus reports of GINA for asthma and GOLD for COPD. It was considered to be abnormal if the tested FVC and PEF values were found to be below 80% of predicted value or FEV_1/FVC was found to be below 70%. Reversibility test and peak expiratory flow (PEF) meter (SpiroFlow, PEF meter, USA) followup were used to diagnose occupational asthma in subjects with respiratory symptoms and restrictive or obstructive spirometric disorder. In reversibility test, pulmonary function tests were repeated 15 minutes later from the first test inhalation of $400 \, \mu g$ salbutamol. A 12% increase in FEV_1 percent of predicted or an absolute volume of 200 mL increase in FEV_1 was considered as positive. The subjects were trained to use PEF meter, PEF measurements were performed 4 times daily, PEF variability was calculated, and the values >20% were considered to be positive [10].

2.5. Statistical Analysis. All statistical analyses were performed by using SPSS 16 programme. Descriptive analysis of data expressed as mean ± standard deviation (SD), range and percentage, and a P-value of <0.05 was used as the level of statistical significance. Between-group comparisons of parametric variables were made by a Student's t-test, and chi-square test was used for nonparametric variables.

3. Results

A total of 347 participants including 286 workers from the department of foundry production with the mean age 33.57 ± 7.0 and 61 subjects with the mean age 37.55 ± 9.3 who worked in non-production departments were enrolled in the study. It is found that phlegm (n: 71, 20.46%) and cough (n: 52, 14.98%) were the most frequent symptoms among the workers. The other symptoms were breathlessness (n: 28, 8.06%), chest tightness (n: 14, 4.03%), and wheezing in (n: 7, 2.01%) persons. Cough and phlegm were found to be related to smoking habit (P: 0.029). The symptoms of cough, phlegm, breathlessness, and chest tightness were found to be more frequent in the workers of foundry production department as is shown in Table 1 (P: 0.023, P: 0.001, P: 0.048, and P: 0.054, resp.). The prevalence of occupational asthma was found to be more

TABLE 1: The distribution of respiratory symptoms among the foundry workers.

Respiratory symptoms	Workers in production departments ($n = 286$)	Workers in other departments ($n = 61$)	Total ($n = 347$)	P
Cough	48	4	52 (14.98%)	0.008*
Phlegm	66	5	71 (20.46%)	0.001*
Breathlessness	26	2	28 (8.06%)	0.041*
Chest tightness	13	1	14 (4.03%)	0.154
Wheezing	6	1	7 (2.01%)	0.803

*Statistically significant.

TABLE 2: The number of workers with occupational asthma and airway obstruction (based on FEV_1).

Working department	OA (%)	Decrease in FEV_1 (% of predicted)		
		Mild	Moderate	Severe
Production department ($n = 286$)	48 (16.78%)*	5	38	5
Nonproduction department ($n = 61$)	3 (4.91%)	—	3	—
Total ($n = 347$)	51 (14.69%)	5	41	5

OA: occupational asthma; the airway obstruction was classified according to forced expiratory volume in one second (FEV_1, % of predicted) results and divided into 3 groups as mild (>79%), moderate (60–79%), and severe (40–59%).
*$P = 0.001$ compared to non-production department.

frequent among the subjects who worked in foundry production department (n: 48, 16.78%) than the other persons who worked in non-production department (n: 3, 4.91%) (P: 0.003) as shown in Table 2. The workers who used protective masks all the time had a lower prevalence rate of respiratory symptoms and occupational asthma than those not using them (P: 0.039 and P: 0.001 respectively) as it is shown in Table 3.

The reversibility test with the variability in mean PEF records (>20%) was found during working days in these 51 individuals. Diurnal PEF variability (>20%) was also found in most of these groups (n: 32, 62.7%).

We found that smoking also increased the risk of occupational asthma in foundry workers. It is found that smokers were more frequent among asthmatics (P: 0.021), and degree of smoking (pack/year) was higher than that of nonasthmatics (P: 0.037). We did not diagnose any cancer and pneumoconiosis at study time by chest X-ray and HRCT. The prevalence of occupational asthma was found to be increased in the workers who were exposed to high concentrations of respirable dust, and the results of pulmonary function tests (FEV_1% of predicted) with occupational asthma prevalence according to dust exposure are shown in Table 4.

TABLE 3: The prevalance of respiratory symptoms among the foundry workers according to the use of protective mask.

Parameter	Presence of protective mask ($n = 178$)	Absence of protective mask ($n = 104$)	Total ($n = 286$)	P
Respiratory symptoms (any one or more)	44 (24.7%)	38 (36.5%)	82	0.039
Occupational asthma	19 (10.6%)	29 (27.8%)	48	0.001

4. Discussion

Occupational asthma became the second prevalent occupational lung disease following pneumoconiosis. Occupational asthma has been reported to be associated with several occupation groups in the literature including automobile and furniture painters, textile workers, plastics manufacturers, hairdressers, food processors, paper factory workers, farm workers, welders, and chemical processors [8]. The foundry workers also have a risk of occupational asthma. Furthermore, it was previously reported that there are an increased number of lung cancer cases among foundry workers [12]. The prevalence of pneumoconiosis was reported as 3.7% in 950 foundry workers, and they were classified as stage 1/0 or more advanced according to the International Labor Organization (ILO) classification [13]. In the present study, we observed that there is an increase in occupational asthma in foundry workers, and we did not find any pneumoconiosis and lung cancer cases. But long-term followup is needed to analyze the risk of neoplastic disease and pneumoconiosis in foundry workers. Cigarette smoking adversely affects the lung function of the workers, and exposure to air contaminants in the foundry may also impair the lung function additively, and we found similar results in this study.

We used questionnaire and PEF monitoring as an alternative method to nonspecific bronchial provocation test to demonstrate airway hyperreactivity [11]. Nonspecific bronchial provocation test requires experienced staff and can be performed in specific centers [14, 15]. According to the fact that the most of our study population did not give their consent to bronchial provocation test, we could not use the nonspecific bronchial provocation test to diagnose occupational asthma in this study.

A reduction in FEV_1/FVC and FEV_1 is an indicator of obstructive abnormalities, and a reduction in FEF_{25-75} is an indicator of small airway obstruction [16]. In a controlled study involving 166 workers exposed to chemicals in a paper factory, spirometric results (FEV_1%, FVC%, FEF_{25-75}%, and FEV_1/FVC) were found to be lower in the workers compared to controls [17]. In another study involving the workers exposed to chemicals in a paper production factory, PFT was monitored for 3 years in certain intervals and the reductions in FEV_1 and FVC were associated with the duration of employment [18].

TABLE 4: The distribution of occupational asthma and mean FEV_1 (%) in foundry workers according to dust exposure.

Exposure	Department	Mean respirable dust concentration	OA ($n = 51$)	Mean FEV_1 (% of predicted)[a]
High-exposure groups	Fettling, cleaning castings ($n = 64$)	10.448 mg/m^3	15 (23.4%)[b,*]	87.8
	Core making, furnace ($n = 53$)	10.122 mg/m^3	14 (26.4%)[c,*]	89.5
Low-exposure groups	Moulding, melting, and pouring ($n = 83$)	0.322 mg/m^3	11 (13.2%)[d]	94.2
	After processing ($n = 86$)	0.216 mg/m^3	8 (9.3%)[e]	91.8
Unexposed group	Nonproduction ($n = 61$)	Non	3 (4.9%)	93.1

OA: occupational asthma, FEV_1: forced expiratory volume in one second; [a]the mean FEV_1 (% of predicted) results of the workers were not found to be different compared to unexposed group ($P > 0.05$). [b]P: 0.002, [c]P: 0.001, [d]P: 0.294, [e]P: 0.072 compared to unexposed group; *statistically significant.

Limitation of the present study is the fact that it is a cross-sectional study, and long-term followup results of the foundry workers are not studied. We used only the respirable dust concentrations for exposure analysis. Foundry workers are exposed to some other chemicals and gases such as isocyanates. But individual dust and gas exposure assessment could not be done in this study.

As a conclusion, we found a high prevalence of occupational asthma in foundry workers and smoking had an additive effect on respiratory symptoms. Encouragement of smoking cessation, occupational health education to reduce the dust exposure, using protective masks during work period, and periodical medical examination are needed to control occupational asthma.

Acknowledgments

The authors thank the managers of the foundry factory and the directors of Samsun Public Health Management for their support to the study.

References

[1] D. A. Schwartz and M. W. Peterson, "Occupational lung disease," *Disease*, vol. 44, no. 2, pp. 44–84, 1998.

[2] Y.-S. Ahn, J.-U. Won, and R. M. Park, "Cancer morbidity of foundry workers in Korea," *Journal of Korean Medical Science*, vol. 25, no. 12, pp. 1733–1741, 2010.

[3] R. Hahn and B. Beck, "Prevalence of chronic bronchitis among foundries' workers," *Zeitschrift fur Erkrankungen der Atmungsorgane*, vol. 166, no. 3, pp. 267–280, 1986.

[4] G. M. Liss, D. I. Bernstein, D. R. Moller, J. S. Gallagher, R. L. Stephenson, and I. L. Bernstein, "Pulmonary and immunologic evaluation of foundry workers exposed to methylene diphenyldiisocyanate (MDI)," *Journal of Allergy and Clinical Immunology*, vol. 82, no. 1, pp. 55–61, 1988.

[5] H. Löfstedt, H. Westberg, A. I. Seldén, I.-L. Bryngelsson, and M. Svartengren, "Respiratory symptoms and lung function in foundry workers using the Hot Box method: a 4-year followup," *Journal of Occupational and Environmental Medicine*, vol. 53, no. 12, pp. 1425–1429, 2011.

[6] A. Johnson, C. Y. Moira, L. MacLean et al., "Respiratory abnormalities among workers in an iron and steel foundry," *British Journal of Industrial Medicine*, vol. 42, pp. 94–100, 1985.

[7] X. Baur, P. Bakehe, and H. Vellguth, "Bronchial asthma and COPD due to irritants in the workplace an evidence based approach," *Journal of Occupational Medicine and Toxicology*, vol. 7, p. 19, 2012.

[8] Global Strategy for Asthma Management and Prevention, "Global Initiative for Asthma (GINA)," 2012, http://www.gin-asthma.org/local/uploads/files/GINA_Report_March13.pdf.

[9] M. Chan-Yeung, "Assessment of asthma in the workplace," *Chest*, vol. 108, no. 4, pp. 1084–1117, 1995.

[10] O. Brandli, C. Schindler, P. H. Leuenberger et al., "Re-estimated equations for 5th percentiles of lung function variables," *Thorax*, vol. 55, no. 2, pp. 173–174, 2000.

[11] P. S. Burge, I. M. O'Brien, and M. G. Harries, "Peak flow rate records in the diagnosis of occupational asthma due to isocyanates," *Thorax*, vol. 34, no. 3, pp. 317–323, 1979.

[12] Y. S. Ahn, J. S. Song, S. K. Kang, and H. K. Chung, "Understanding the occurrence of lung cancer in foundry workers through health insurance data," *Korean Journal of Preventive Medicine*, vol. 33, pp. 299–305, 2000.

[13] Y. S. Ahn, "Respiratory diseases in foundry workers," in *Training Materials for Occupational Respiratory Diseases*, Korea Occupational Safety Health Agency, Ed., pp. 171–190, Korea Occupational Safety Health AgencyIncheon, 2005, (Korean).

[14] A. Cartier, "Definition and diagnosis of occupational asthma," *European Respiratory Journal*, vol. 7, no. 1, pp. 153–160, 1994.

[15] D. E. Banks, S. M. Tarlo, F. Masri, R. J. Rando, and D. N. Weissman, "Bronchoprovocation tests in the diagnosis of isocyanate-induced asthma," *Chest*, vol. 109, no. 5, pp. 1370–1379, 1996.

[16] R. Pellegrino, G. Viegi, V. Brusasco et al., "Interpretative strategies for lung function tests," *European Respiratory Journal*, vol. 26, no. 5, pp. 948–968, 2005.

[17] A. Orman, H. Ellidokuz, H. Esme, M. Unlu, and A. Ay, "Evaluation of pulmonary system symptoms with pulmonary functional tests in workers in pulp and paper industry," *Respiratory Diseases*, vol. 15, pp. 165–169, 2004 (Turkish).

[18] A. J. Mehta, P. K. Henneberger, K. Torén, and A.-C. Olin, "Airflow limitation and changes in pulmonary function among bleachery workes," *European Respiratory Journal*, vol. 26, no. 1, pp. 133–139, 2005.

4

Delineating a Retesting Zone Using Receiver Operating Characteristic Analysis on Serial QuantiFERON Tuberculosis Test Results in US Healthcare Workers

Wendy Thanassi,[1, 2, 3, 4] Art Noda,[4, 5] Beatriz Hernandez,[4, 5] Jeffery Newell,[4] Paul Terpeluk,[6] David Marder,[7] and Jerome A. Yesavage[4, 5]

[1] Department of Medicine, Veterans Affairs Palo Alto Health Care System, 3801 Miranda Avenue MC-, Palo Alto, CA 94304-1207, USA
[2] Occupational Health Strategic Health Care Group, Office of Public Health, Veterans Health Administration, Washington, DC 20006, USA
[3] Division of Emergency Medicine, Stanford University School of Medicine, Stanford, CA 94304, USA
[4] War Related Illness and Injury Study Center (WRIISC) and Mental Illness Research Education and Clinical Center (MIRECC), Department of Veterans Affairs, Palo Alto, CA 94304, USA
[5] Department of Psychiatry and Behavioral Sciences, Stanford University School of Medicine, Stanford, CA 94304, USA
[6] Department of Occupational Health, The Cleveland Clinic, Cleveland, OH 44195, USA
[7] University Health Services, University of Illinois Chicago, Chicago, IL 60612, USA

Correspondence should be addressed to Wendy Thanassi, wendy.thanassi@gmail.com

Academic Editor: Anete Trajman

Objective. To find a statistically significant separation point for the QuantiFERON Gold In-Tube (QFT) interferon gamma release assay that could define an optimal "retesting zone" for use in serially tested low-risk populations who have test "reversions" from initially positive to subsequently negative results. *Method*. Using receiver operating characteristic analysis (ROC) to analyze retrospective data collected from 3 major hospitals, we searched for predictors of reversion until statistically significant separation points were revealed. A confirmatory regression analysis was performed on an additional sample. *Results*. In 575 initially positive US healthcare workers (HCWs), 300 (52.2%) had reversions, while 275 (47.8%) had two sequential positive tests. The most statistically significant (Kappa = 0.48, chi-square = 131.0, $P < 0.001$) separation point identified by the ROC for predicting reversion was the tuberculosis antigen minus-nil (TBag-nil) value at 1.11 International Units per milliliter (IU/mL). The second separation point was found at TBag-nil at 0.72 IU/mL (Kappa = 0.16, chi-square = 8.2, $P < 0.01$). The model was validated by the regression analysis of 287 HCWs. *Conclusion*. Reversion likelihood increases as the TBag-nil approaches the manufacturer's cut-point of 0.35 IU/mL. The most statistically significant separation point between those who test repeatedly positive and those who revert is 1.11 IU/mL. Clinicians should retest low-risk individuals with initial QFT results < 1.11 IU/mL.

1. Introduction

We report the findings of a multisite study of United States healthcare workers (HCWs) that began as a quality control initiative in the Veterans Administration Palo Alto Health Care System (VAPAHCS) when QuantiFERON Gold In-Tube (QFT) serial screening tests were observed to be initially positive and were subsequently negative in those low-risk individuals. This seemingly spontaneous "reversion" has been reported around the world in the literature, and the variability that occurs mostly around the baseline is recognized [1–6].

This study design was driven by the clinical experience: when an HCW presents with a positive QFT result, what can the clinician do to discern whether the next test is likely to remain positive or become negative?

The foundation of the problem lies in the dichotomous nature of the results reported. Currently, a QuantiFERON tuberculosis antigen minus-nil (TBag-nil) ≥ 0.35 International Units per milliliter (IU/mL) is reported as "positive." At that point the provider has a decision to make, one that is generally to investigate further with a chest radiograph, seek specialty consultation, and/or recommend medical treatment. Whereas positive tuberculin skin tests (TSTs) were often felt to be erroneous due to prior BCG vaccination, and compliance and treatment rates were low; studies are showing that positive interferon-gamma release assay (IGRA) results are more likely to lead to both the recommendation and the acceptance of chemotherapy [7–10]. Chemotherapy puts the patient at risk for side effects including hepatotoxicity [11], as well as social stigma or workplace discrimination [12]. The presumptive diagnosis of tuberculosis infection in HCWs, particularly when interpreted as an occupational conversion, can trigger Occupational Safety and Health Administration, National Institute for Occupational Safety, and Health or hospital infection control contact investigations that are both time consuming and costly. Thus the presence of spontaneous "reversions" implies that clinicians and patients are experiencing unnecessary concern, action, or expense and potentially placing patients in harm's way for transiently positive results which are forced by the binary nature of the current reporting structure. There is a need for increased accuracy and efficiency in the screening process to reduce the burdens to the patient and the system, and utilization of this predictive tool may lend some assistance.

In response to the persistent concerns regarding reversions near the cut-point of 0.35 IU/mL, a 2010 Morbidity and Mortality Weekly Report published by the Centers for Disease Control and Prevention (CDC) recommended that quantitative QFT results should be reported. The CDC did not, however, provide guidance for either the interpretation or the use of these values [13]. We investigated reversions in US HCWs in order to develop a validated model, using receiver operating characteristic analysis, to define the range of results that best predicts a transiently positive result. With the ability to predict the likelihood of reversion, clinicians and patients could choose to retest rather than to pursue costly and time-consuming consultations and therapies.

2. Materials and Methods

2.1. Participants and Variables. Data were obtained from a retrospective review of available clinical laboratory records from three different sites: (1) Veterans Administration Palo Alto Health Care System (VAPAHCS), California, (2) University of Illinois Chicago (UIC) Il, and the (3) Cleveland Clinic (CC), Ohio, where each HCW undergoes preemployment and annual QFT testing irrespective of previous results. All subjects are US HCWs who were serially tested by QFT Gold-in-Tube in their hospital's laboratory. All HCWs at least 18 years of age with available records were included. The study's date range was January 2009 through June 2011 at VAPAHCS, from August 2008 through June 2011 at UIC, and

Table 1: Test results for analyzed HCWs from VA Palo Alto Health Care System (VAPAHCS), University of Illinois Chicago (UIC) and the Cleveland Clinic (CC).

Test results	VAPAHCS	UIC	CC	Total (n)
Repeat positive result	113	338	25	476
Reversion	73	275	38	386
Total (n)	186	613	63	862

Note: HCWs were excluded if their only positive test result was their last test taken or if data for only one test result was available.

from October 2009 through December 2011 at the Cleveland Clinic.

HCWs who tested consistently negative and those with only a single test result were excluded. Results reported without the QFT TBag-nil numerical value, as well as HCWs with negative-to-positive discordance/conversion at the conclusion of their testing series were removed from the dataset (22/195 from VAPAHCS, 124/742 from UIC, and 61/127 from CC). To be included in the analysis, at least two QFT tests were required, one of which was a positive result that was followed by either a positive or a negative result. This reproduces the clinician's actionable decision point; that is, when a patient presents with a positive result, the action to test further, to refer, or to treat is initiated. Patients were only included once (see Table 1).

2.2. Participant Sites. The VAPAHCS is a suburban teaching hospital located in Palo Alto, California. The county in which it resides, Santa Clara, has the 3rd highest tuberculosis (TB) rate in California [14] at 11.4% from 2006–2011 [15], and California is ranked 3rd in USA for TB cases behind Alaska and Hawaii [16]. All VAPAHCS HCWs are United States citizens. The HCW population is approximately 3,500. The lab performed over 16,000 QFT-GIT tests (including patient testing) during this period. Of the 4,019 HCWs who were tested between January 1, 2009 and June 30, 2011, 2,706 (67%) tested negative one time and 293 (7%) tested positive one time, without repeat testing. (Note that VAPA also tests researchers, students, volunteers, and Peace Corps personnel, most of whom are on campus for only one testing cycle). Of the 4,019 unique HCWs, 781 (19%) tested negative more than once and never tested positive. Thus the overall negative rate at VAPA is (67% + 19%) = 86%, while 14% of personnel tested positive at least once in their series. The indeterminate rate in this lab is 0.4%.

The University of Illinois, Chicago (UIC) is a public, urban academic teaching hospital. The HCW population is approximately 5,000. Their laboratory performed over 50,000 QFT-GIT tests by June 2011; 20,543 of these were on HCWs. Annual HCW TB screening is mandated and compliance is 99%, with most HCWs tested annually, but some who are on surveillance are tested every six months. UIC reports a HCW QFT negative rate of 89.5%, with 1.1% indeterminate and 9.4% positive at some point in their series. Illinois ranks 21st for tuberculosis cases in the nation [16], and Chicago itself had a TB incidence rate recorded at 7.4% during 2006–2010 [17].

The Cleveland Clinic Foundation (Cleveland, OH, USA) is an urban teaching hospital. The laboratory had performed over 10,000 QFT-GIT tests by June 2011. This includes patient and HCW testing. Cleveland Clinic hires approximately 2,500 HCWs annually. The HCW population is 98.5% negative with 0.5% indeterminate and 1% positive at some point in their series. Ohio ranks 35th in the nation for tuberculosis cases [16] with Cleveland itself having a 6.4% case rate from 2006–2010 [18].

2.3. QuantiFERON Gold In-Tube Blood Assay (Qiagen, Inc). The interferon gamma released was measured by enzyme-linked immunosorbent assay (ELISA) according to the manufacturer's protocol though with an 8-point standard curve for each microplate. The results were read at 450 nm by the Diamedix DS2 Automated ELISA System (Diamedix Corporation, Miami, FL) at VAPAHCS, by the Diamedix DSX Automated ELISA System (Diamedix Corporation, Miami, FL) at UIC, and by a BioTek ELx800 Absorbance Microplate Reader (BioTek Instruments, Winooski, VT) at CC. All tests in this series met the nil, mitogen, and the equation criteria for test validity delineated in the manufacturer's package insert [19].

2.4. Measures. In the absence of a gold standard against which to evaluate latent tuberculosis infection, the expected probability of two consecutive positive tests was employed as a proxy for corroboration of the test result in question, which is the implied presence of latent tuberculosis disease. In seeking what would best predict whether an individual was likely to be a "reverter", the initial TBag-nil value in the series of two sequential tests was evaluated as a possible predictor variable. Note that the QFT result was considered positive if the TBag-nil was ≥0.35 IU/mL, so all TBag-nil values were at least 0.35 IU/mL in this analysis.

2.5. Data Analytic Approach. We used a two-step data analytic approach. First, we employed a receiver operating characteristic analysis (ROC) [20, 21] on two-thirds (the Exploratory Group) of the 862 HCW sample to identify characteristics that might significantly differentiate reversions from those with two consecutively positive results. An ROC analysis is an exploratory process that searches every value of every predictor variable entered to identify the variable and value that results in the highest sensitivity and specificity (using the weighted kappa statistic) for identifying the targeted criterion. The targeted criterion in this case is reversion. Second, because ROC is an exploratory technique, we conducted a confirmatory logistic regression analysis and chi-square tests using the remaining one-third of the HCWs (the Confirmatory Group) to examine whether the predictor that had been identified in the first step did in fact predict reversion in an independent sample.

Regarding the details of the ROC analysis, once the optimal variable and associated separation point are identified, the association with the success criterion is tested against a stopping rule. Stopping rules include a subgroup sample size too small for further analysis ($n < 20$) and/or when no further variables are selected because the P value associated with the Chi-square statistic is ≥0.01. If the association does not meet the criteria for the stopping rule, the sample is divided into two groups based on the optimal variable and identified separation point. The ROC analysis is then restarted, separately, for each of these two subgroups. The result is a decision tree identifying the HCW characteristics and associated separation points that best predict reversions, with P values, chi-square, and Kappa values calculated and reported. The ROC software developed by Drs. Yesavage and Kraemer is publicly available [21], and the logistic regression and Chi-square tests were performed using SAS software (Version 9.3, Cary, NC, USA).

3. Results and Discussion

3.1. Results. HCWs from each site had undergone between 2 and 9 tests in series. The most recent positive test that was followed by either a positive (no reversion) or negative (reversion) result defined the two test results in the series that were analyzed (see Table 1). The mean number of days between tests was 434 for VAPAHCS, 261 for UIC, and 235 for CC.

The 862 HCWs who met inclusion criteria were randomly assigned to one of two groups: the Exploratory Group ($n = 575$) or the Confirmatory Group ($n = 287$). The Exploratory Group of tested HCWs had a 52.2% (300/575) reversion rate. The results of the ROC analysis performed on the Exploratory Group are presented as a decision tree shown in Figure 1. TBag-nil in IU/mL was most statistically significant for predicting reversion at the separation point 1.11 IU/mL (Kappa = 0.48, chi-Square = 131.0, $P < 0.001$). Two groups of HCWs were identified:

> group 1: 75% reversions: 225/300 HCWs with TBag-nil <1.11 IU/mL;
>
> group 2: 27% reversions: 75/275 HCWs with Tbag-nil ≥1.11 IU/mL.

The ROC analysis further identified two subgroups of HCWs derived from group 1 above with a TBag-nil at 0.72 IU/mL (Kappa = 0.16, chi-square = 8.2, $P < 0.01$):

> group a: 80% reversions: 163/204 HCWs with TBag-nil <0.72 IU/mL;
>
> group b: 65% reversions: 62/96 HCWs with TBag-nil ≥0.72 and <1.11 IU/mL.

Two subgroups of HCWs were also identified from group 2 above with TBag-nil at 2.17 IU/mL (Kappa = 0.27, chi-Square = 20.4, $P < 0.001$):

> group c: 43% reversions: 43/99 HCWs with TBag-nil ≥ 1.11 and <2.17 IU/mL;
>
> group d: 18% reversions: 32/176 HCWs with TBag-nil ≥ 2.17 IU/mL.

Figure 2 contains a decision tree classifying the 575 HCWs in the Exploratory Group as Reversions or No Reversions and by TBag-nil values using the ROC selected

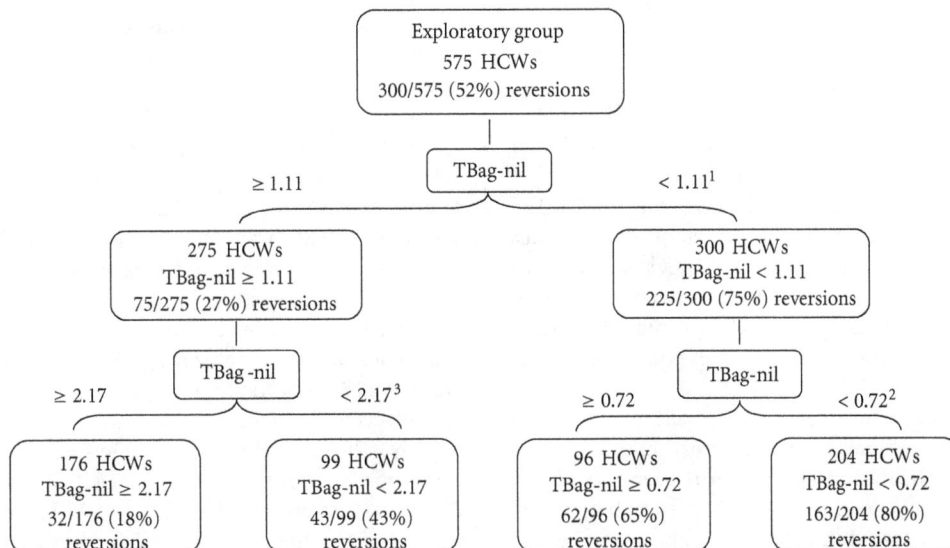

FIGURE 1: Receiver operating characteristic (ROC) decision tree identifying statistically significant TBag-nil (in IU/mL) separation points which predict those HCWs with a positive TB test result at time one who retest negative at time two. Logistic regression analysis on a separate Confirmatory sample of 287 HCWs validated all 3 separation points at 0.72, 1.11, and 2.17 IU/mL and remained statistically significant for all subgroups by chi-square ($P < 0.001$). 1 Kappa = 0.48, chi-square = 131.0, $P < 0.001$, 2 Kappa = 0.16, chi-square = 8.2, $P < 0.01$, 3 Kappa = 0.27, chi-square = 20.4, $P < 0.001$.

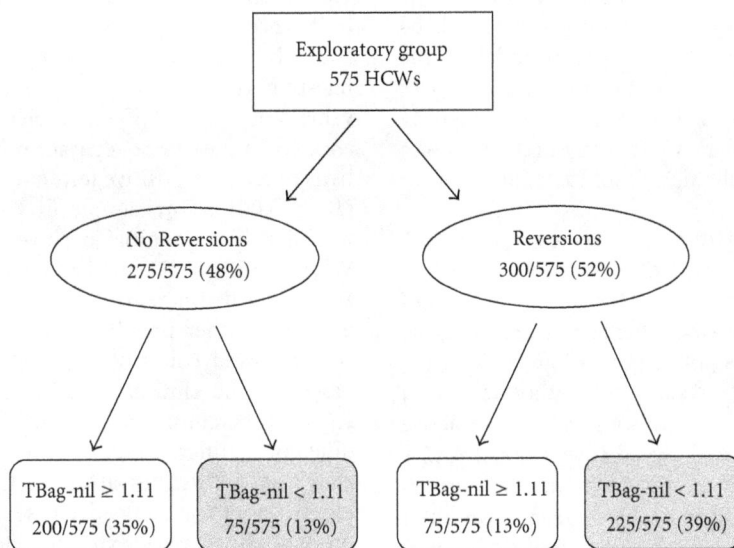

FIGURE 2: Exploratory group with 575 HCWs classified as No Reversions (those with two positive tests) or Reversions (with a positive TB test result at time one and who retest negative at time two). The two groups are further classified by TBag-nil values using the ROC selected separation point of 1.11 IU/mL (Kappa = 0.48, chi-square = 131.0, $P < 0.001$). Highlighted boxes emphasize the difference in number of No Reversions versus Reversions when TBag-nil < 1.11 IU/mL, the identified retesting zone.

separation point of 1.11 IU/mL. Note that 225 of the 300 "reverters" are identified at this separation point.

A logistic regression analysis was conducted in the Confirmatory Group ($n = 287$) using the same dependent measure (reversion) and predictor variable (TBag-nil) identified in the primary ROC analysis. The relationship remained statistically significant ($P < 0.001$). All three separation points at 0.72, 1.11, and 2.17 IU/mL (4 subgroups) identified

in the ROC analysis also remained statistically significant for all subgroups by chi-square ($P < 0.001$).

4. Discussion

Multiple papers have reported within-subject variability in serial QFT results [1, 3, 6, 22, 23], and much work has been done to unmask a retesting zone by suggesting alternative separation points of 0.5, 0.7 [6], or 1.0 IU/mL [23]. In Europe, employing a borderline zone between 0.2–0.7 IU/mL decreased conversions and reversions from 1.9 to 0.6% and from 6.1 to 2.6%, respectively, with no active tuberculosis cases occurring in the "positive" population in a 2-year follow-up period [24].

Further, it is both observed and understood that QFT reversions are much more common than conversions. Among the many studies published and reviewed on this topic [25], Schablon et al. [22] reports a conversion to reversion ratio of 6.1 versus 32.6% in 287 German healthcare workers, which is the same range as studies conducted in the United States (6.3 versus 33%) [26].

The predominance of reversions is likely explained in part by the statistical phenomenon of regression to the mean [24]. Regression to the mean (RTM) is the tendency of observations to move closer to the mean when repeated. When measurements are repeated in individuals, and measures are selected based on exceeding an absolute threshold in an inherently continuous range of values, influence by RTM should be considered. Examples of RTM are common in clinical medicine. In this case, since the observed mean result in these US HCWs is <0.35 IU/mL, retesting a population subset that is initially above that mean will likely yield values that are closer to the population mean (in this case, in the negative range). The population "conversion" rate will be a mix of both true incident disease (proportional to the epidemiology of TB in the US HCWs) and false positives that will likely have reversions. The challenge is to identify a retesting zone with an upper value that minimizes noise while still identifying clinically significant cases for followup in a cost-effective manner.

As for the reliability of that negative result, the QFT Gold In-Tube has a specificity of 99% [19], reflecting the measurement of persons correctly identified as not having the condition (in this case tuberculosis). Further, the prevalence of disease in this population is low, making the pretest probability of positive results low. Additionally, Diel et al. conducted a study of 954 persons exposed to active tuberculosis and report a negative predictive value of 99.7% after 5 years [27]. With all of this in mind, the authors conclude that while the decision on how to act upon a test result lays with the clinician and never purely with numerical data, a negative QFT result is significantly more reliable than a low positive result in its ability to predict disease or the lack thereof.

To help clarify a practice algorithm, there is a call in the literature for a statistically based, data-driven retesting zone. Zwerling et al. in a 2011 review article in *Thorax* concluded that "the use of IGRAs for serial testing is complicated by lack of data on optimum cut-offs for serial testing …" [28], and a 2012 editorial in *Chest* stated that "it is quite arbitrary to limit true conversion to those with a QFT-GIT of >1.0 IU/mL, since that value, though a nice round figure, has not been validated" [29]. Here we offer that a statistically driven optimal separation point between consistently positive serially tested US healthcare workers and healthcare workers who are likely to revert is 1.11 IU/mL.

We focus on 1.11 IU/mL as the border of a retesting zone because it was determined by the Kappa statistic in the ROC software as the optimally sensitive and specific separation point between the "reversions" from those who did not "revert" in this multisite cohort. At a separation point of 1.11 IU/mL, sensitivity is 0.75 and specificity is 0.73, whereas at a separation point of 0.72 IU/mL sensitivity is 0.54 and specificity is 0.85. The respective Kappas are 0.48 versus 0.39. As is the case by lowering the retesting separation point to 0.72 IU/mL, further lowering it to 0.50 IU/mL would increase the specificity of the measure to 0.93 and capture 84/103 (82%) of reversions in this range, but this would include only 103/575 (18%) of the total population and 84/300 (28%) of the "reverters." The sensitivity of this separation point would be only 0.28 and its Kappa 0.21. Thus with the ROC there are trade-offs in sensitivity versus specificity, depending upon the separation points selected. The 1.11 IU/mL measurement was chosen by the ROC analysis for this population because that value maximizes the percentage of "reverters" while optimizing sensitivity and specificity.

5. Conclusion

We present a validated model on a sample of 862 US healthcare workers from three major US hospitals that could be used to define a QuantiFERON Gold In-Tube retesting zone between 0.35 and 1.11 IU/mL. The upper value was selected by a receiver operating characteristic analysis to maximize separation between HCWs who have two consecutive positive tests and those who have reversions ($P < 0.001$). Our sample of HCWs had a 75% risk for reversion if their initial positive test fell within this range. While 0.35–1.11 IU/mL is therefore the optimal retesting zone identified here, 0.35–0.72 IU/mL (80% reversion; $P < 0.01$) is another possible separation point also selected by the ROC and could be reasonably employed by providers based on the clinical situation much like the 5, 10, and 15 mm tuberculin skin test cut-off points that are used in different settings. Acceptance of TBag-nil values reported above as the delineators of a QFT retesting zone could lessen patient anxiety, decrease unnecessary radiographs, prevent unnecessary exposure investigations, and possibly spare patients from inappropriate medical treatment due to transiently "positive" QFT test results.

6. Limitations and Future Directions

Limitations of the study include that while the current analyses incorporated over 850 positive HCW records, these data are from only three facilities. Furthermore, results in this study are weighted towards UIC, since their data comprise the majority of the sample group. While there could be selection bias among those HCWs who present for serial testing, it is not clear how that could influence these results. Finally, it should also be noted that prospective long-term followup would be required to provide thorough validation of the results.

Future analyses using the same statistical methods could include additional data from other institutions in USA, Europe, or from countries with higher risk for HCWs. There is a possibility that there could be local variation based on biologic or regional laboratory differences that would be exposed when more data are analyzed.

Conflict of Interests

The authors declare that they have no Conflict of interests.

Acknowledgments

The authors thank Leah Friedman, Senior Research Associate, Stanford University School of Medicine, for editorial assistance and Professor Helena Kraemer, Stanford University (Emerita) and University of Pittsburgh, for her writing of the data analysis software and advice regarding methodology. Additional thanks are to Dr. Drew Levy for methodological review and Dr. George Todaro for his original data review and insights. This work was supported in part by the Department of Veterans Affairs, Veterans Health Administration, Office of Research and Development and by the Department of Veterans Affairs Sierra-Pacific Mental Illness Research, Education, and the War Related Illness and Injury Study Center (MIRECC).

References

[1] R. Belknap, J. Kelaher, K. Wall et al., "Diagnosis of latent tuberculosis infection in U.S. health care workers: reproducibility, repeatability and 6 month follow-up with interferon-γ release assays (IGRAs)," *American Journal of Respiratory and Critical Care Medicine*, vol. 179, Article ID A4101, 2009.

[2] A. K. Detjen, L. Loebenberg, H. M. S. Grewal et al., "Short-term reproducibility of a commercial interferon γ release assay," *Clinical and Vaccine Immunology*, vol. 16, no. 8, pp. 1170–1175, 2009.

[3] M. Pai, R. Joshi, S. Dogra et al., "Serial testing of health care workers for tuberculosis using interferon-γ assay," *American Journal of Respiratory and Critical Care Medicine*, vol. 174, no. 3, pp. 349–355, 2006.

[4] S. Rafiza and K. G. Rampal, "Serial testing of Malaysian health care workers with QuantiFERON(R)-TB gold in-tube," *The International Journal of Tuberculosis and Lung Disease*, vol. 16, no. 2, pp. 163–168, 2012.

[5] F. C. Ringshausen, A. Nienhaus, J. T. Costa et al., "Within-subject variability of *Mycobacterium tuberculosis*-specific γ interferon responses in German health care workers," *Clinical and Vaccine Immunology*, vol. 18, no. 7, pp. 1176–1182, 2011.

[6] J. T. Costa, R. Silva, R. Sá, M. J. Cardoso, and A. Nienhaus, "Serial testing with the interferon-γ release assay in Portuguese healthcare workers," *International Archives of Occupational and Environmental Health*, vol. 84, no. 4, pp. 461–469, 2011.

[7] R. Sahni, C. Miranda, B. Yen-Lieberman et al., "Does the implementation of an interferon-γ release assay in lieu of a tuberculin skin test increase acceptance of preventive therapy for latent tuberculosis among healthcare workers?" *Infection Control and Hospital Epidemiology*, vol. 30, no. 2, pp. 197–199, 2009.

[8] R. Diel, R. Loaddenkemper, and A. Nienhaus, "Evidence-based comparison of commercial Interferon-γ release assays for detecting active TB: a metaanalysis," *Chest*, vol. 137, no. 4, pp. 952–968, 2010.

[9] Y. Hirsch-Moverman, A. Daftary, J. Franks, and P. W. Colson, "Adherence to treatment for latent tuberculosis infection: systematic review of studies in the US and Canada," *International Journal of Tuberculosis and Lung Disease*, vol. 12, no. 11, pp. 1235–1254, 2008.

[10] C. R. Horsburgh Jr., "Priorities for the treatment of latent tuberculosis infection in the United States," *The New England Journal of Medicine*, vol. 350, no. 20, pp. 2060–2067, 2004.

[11] F. F. Fountain, E. Tolley, C. R. Chrisman, and T. H. Self, "Isoniazid hepatotoxicity associated with treatment of latent tuberculosis infection: a 7-year evaluation from a public health tuberculosis clinic," *Chest*, vol. 128, no. 1, pp. 116–123, 2005.

[12] U.S. Equal Employment Opportunity Commission, *Health Partners, Inc. To Pay $25, 000 to Resolve EEOC Disability Discrimination Case*, 2012, http://www.eeoc.gov/eeoc/newsroom/release/5-30-12.cfm.

[13] G. H. Mazurek, J. Jereb, A. Vernon, P. LoBue, S. Goldberg, and K. Castros, "Updated guidelines for using interferon γ release assays to detect *Mycobacterium tuberculosis* infection—United States, 2010," *Morbidity and Mortality Weekly Report*, vol. 59, no. 5, pp. 1–25, 2010.

[14] Tuberculosis Control Branch, California Department of Public Health, *California Tuberculosis Data, 2011*, 2011, http://www.cdph.ca.gov/programs/tb/Documents/TBCB-CA-TB-2011-Data-Tables.pdf.

[15] Tuberculosis Control Branch, California Department of Public Health, *Tuberculosis Cases and Case Rates Per 100, 000 Population: California, 1985–2011*, 2011, http://www.cdph.ca.gov/programs/tb/Documents/TBCB-CA-TB-2011-Data-Tables.pdf.

[16] CDC, *Reported Tuberculosis in the United States, 2011*, 2011, http://www.cdc.gov/tb/statistics/reports/2011/table19.htm.

[17] Health and Human Services Unit, Chicago Department of Innovation and Technology, *Tuberculosis Cases and Average Annual Incidence Rate, Chicago, 2007–2011*, 2011, https://data.cityofchicago.org/Health-Human-Services/Public-Health-Statistics-Tuberculosis-cases-and-av/ndk3-zftj.

[18] Center for Public Statisitics and Informatics, Ohio Department of Health, *Ohio TB Morbidity by County and Seven Major Cities, 2006–2011*, 2012, http://www.odh.ohio.gov/~/media/ODH/ASSETS/Files/hst/tuberculosis surveillance/countyratetable2011.ashx.

[19] Cellestis Inc, QuantiFERON-TB Gold (In-Tube Method) [package insert], Note: the above is the official onlinxe package insert from the manufacturer, not a patient product/counseling notice, The date (July 2011) is the last modification date, normally found at the end of the package insert file, Doc. No. US05990301K, http://www.cellestis.com.

[20] H. C. Kraemer, *Evaluating Medical Tests: Objective and Quantitative Guidelines*, Sage, Newbury Park, Calif, USA, 1992.

[21] J. A. Yesavage and H. C. Kraemer, "Signal detection software for receiver operator characteristics," Version 4. 22 [Computer software], 2007, http://www.stanford.edu/~yesavage/ROC.html.

[22] A. Schablon, M. Harling, R. Diel et al., "Serial testing with an interferon-γ release assay in German healthcare workers," *GMS Krankenhhygiene Interdisziplinär*, vol. 5, no. 2, Article ID Doc05, 2010.

[23] K. S. Fong, J. W. Tomford, L. Teixeira et al., "Challenges of interferon-γ release assay conversions in serial testing of health

care workers in a tuberculosis control program," *Chest*, vol. 142, no. 1, pp. 55–62, 2012.

[24] F. C. Ringshausen, A. Nienhaus, A. Schablon, S. Schlösser, G. Schultze-Werninghaus, and G. Rohde, "Predictors of persistently positive Mycobacterium-tuberculosis-specific interferon-γ responses in the serial testing of health care workers," *BMC Infectious Diseases*, vol. 10, article 220, 2010.

[25] F. C. Ringshausen, A. Schablon, and A. Nienhaus, "Interferon-γ release assays for the tuberculosis serial testing of health care workers: a systematic review," *Journal of Occupational Medicine and Toxicology*, vol. 7, no. 1, article 6, 2012.

[26] S. Perry, L. Sanchez, S. Yang, Z. Agarwal, P. Hurst, and J. Parsonnet, "Reproducibility of QuantiFERON-TB gold in-tube assay," *Clinical and Vaccine Immunology*, vol. 15, no. 3, pp. 425–432, 2008.

[27] R. Diel, R. Loddenkemper, S. Niemann, K. Meywald-Walter, and A. Nienhaus, "Negative and positive predictive value of a whole-blood interferon-γ release assay for developing active tuberculosis: an update," *American Journal of Respiratory and Critical Care Medicine*, vol. 183, no. 1, pp. 88–95, 2011.

[28] A. Zwerling, S. van den Hof, J. Scholten et al., "Interferon-γ release assays for tuberculosis screening of healthcare workers: a systematic review," *Thorax*, vol. 67, no. 1, pp. 62–70, 2012.

[29] R. Loddenkemper, R. Diel, and A. Nienhaus, "To repeat or not to repeat-that is the question!: serial testing of health-care workers for TB infection," *Chest*, vol. 142, no. 1, pp. 10–11, 2012.

5

Test-Retest Reliability and Physiological Responses Associated with the Steep Ramp Anaerobic Test in Patients with COPD

Robyn L. Chura,[1] Darcy D. Marciniuk,[2] Ron Clemens,[2] and Scotty J. Butcher[1]

[1] *School of Physical Therapy, University of Saskatchewan, 1121 College Dr, Saskatoon, SK, Canada S7N 0W3*
[2] *Respirology, Critical Care and Sleep Medicine, University of Saskatchewan, Canada*

Correspondence should be addressed to Scotty J. Butcher, scotty.butcher@usask.ca

Academic Editor: Roland Wensel

The Steep Ramp Anaerobic Test (SRAT) was developed as a clinical test of anaerobic leg muscle function for use in determining anaerobic power and in prescribing high-intensity interval exercise in patients with chronic heart failure and Chronic Obstructive Pulmonary Disease (COPD); however, neither the test-retest reliability nor the physiological qualities of this test have been reported. We therefore, assessed test-retest reliability of the SRAT and the physiological characteristics associated with the test in patients with COPD. 11 COPD patients (mean FEV$_1$ 43% predicted) performed a cardiopulmonary exercise test (CPET) on Day 1, and an SRAT and a 30-second Wingate anaerobic test (WAT) on each of Days 2 and 3. The SRAT showed a high degree of test-retest reliability (ICC = 0.99; CV = 3.8%, and bias 4.5 W, error −15.3–24.4 W). Power output on the SRAT was 157 W compared to 66 W on the CPET and 231 W on the WAT. Despite the differences in workload, patients exhibited similar metabolic and ventilatory responses between the three tests. Measures of ventilatory constraint correlated more strongly with the CPET than the WAT; however, physiological variables correlated more strongly with the WAT. The SRAT is a highly reliable test that better reflects physiological performance on a WAT power test despite a similar level of ventilatory constraint compared to CPET.

1. Introduction

Individuals with Chronic Obstructive Pulmonary Disease (COPD) are often prescribed aerobic exercise to enhance function and reduce shortness of breath during activities of daily living. General guidelines for this exercise prescription suggest patients should exercise continuously at moderate intensities [1–3]. There is evidence, however, to suggest that exercise at higher intensities may be more beneficial for this population [4].

Traditionally, results from cardiopulmonary exercise testing (CPET) involving an incremental, graded exercise test (GXT) of 8–12 minutes in duration, have been used to prescribe exercise for individuals with COPD and are widely considered to be the gold standard for measurement of cardiopulmonary function and aerobic performance [5]. CPET, however, may underestimate the workload required for optimal physiological benefit from exercise training due

to ventilatory limitations causing early test cessation and a blunted peak work rate [6, 7]. High-intensity interval exercise intensity may be prescribed for healthy individuals based on tests of anaerobic power and capacity, such as a 30-second Wingate Anaerobic Test (WAT), which is considered to be the gold standard measure of anaerobic capacity [8]; however, these types of tests have not been widely used, nor would be appropriate in typical clinical use for individuals with COPD. However, the steep ramp anaerobic test (SRAT) has been proposed as a clinical test that may more accurately reflect leg muscle capabilities and better set interval training intensities for individuals with chronic heart failure [7, 9, 10] and COPD [11].

The SRAT was developed by Meyer et al. [7] for use by patients with heart failure to specifically challenge the muscles maximally before patients reached a cardiovascular limit. Unlike the WAT, in which subjects must pedal as fast as possible against a fixed resistance for 30 seconds, the SRAT is an incremental GXT where the workload increases by 25 watts every 10 seconds until patient exhaustion [7, 10]. Much higher work rates are typically achieved with the SRAT compared to the incremental CPET, and a percentage of the peak work rate (PWR) from the SRAT can be used to prescribe intervals for training in this population [10]. The SRAT has also been used in COPD patients to prescribe intensity for high intensity interval exercise [11]. The SRAT may be better tolerated for use in populations that become short of breath quickly during exercise because, and rather than being a timed test like the WAT, it is patient-limited. The test-retest reliability and the physiological responses of the SRAT in this population remain unknown.

The purposes of this study were to determine (a) the test-retest reliability of the SRAT in patients with COPD and (b) the physiologic, ventilatory, and perceptual parameters obtained on the SRAT compared with performance on a traditional CPET or WAT in COPD patients.

2. Materials and Methods

2.1. Subjects. 11 patients (7 males and 4 females) with moderate and severe COPD (11) were recruited through the Saskatoon Pulmonary Rehabilitation Program and through the Division of Respirology, Critical Care and Sleep Medicine, University of Saskatchewan. Subjects had a respirologist confirmed diagnosis of COPD [12], did not require the use of supplemental oxygen at rest or during exercise, and had not been in hospital with an acute exacerbation within the previous 6 weeks. Subjects were excluded if they had cardiovascular or musculoskeletal disease that would prevent them from completing heavy exercise.

This research was approved by the University of Saskatchewan Biomedical Ethics Committee. All subjects signed a consent form and were advised that they could freely withdraw from the study at any time.

2.2. Research Design. A randomized cross-over design was used to assess subjects' physiological, ventilatory, and perceptual responses to the SRAT as compared to the CPET and WAT. The subjects attended 3 sessions for testing, within a 3 week period, with at least 48 hours separating sessions. An initial baseline assessment session included screening, assessment of criteria for study admission, pulmonary function tests, and an incremental CPET. The following 2 visits each included a 30-second WAT and a SR test separated by one hour. The second of these 2 visits was included in order to establish the test-retest reliability of these measures. The order of the tests was constant between visits but randomized between subjects.

2.3. Pulmonary Function Testing and CPET. Resting pulmonary function testing (FEV$_1$, FVC, RV, TLC, D$_L$CO) was performed according to established standards [13] (V6200C Autobox and V_{max} 229D gas analyzer, SensorMedics Corp., Yorba Linda, California, USA). CPET was performed using established protocols [5] with a workrate increment of 5–15 W/min on a mechanically braked cycle ergometer

(800 S, SensorMedics). The test was terminated when the subject indicated voluntary exhaustion, or the revolutions per minute fell below 60 and could not be increased with encouragement. Peak work rate (CPET$_{peak}$), and all physiologic, ventilatory, and perceptual measures were collected and used in the analysis.

2.4. 30-Second Wingate Anaerobic Test (WAT). The WAT was performed as per established protocol [8]. Subjects completed a self-paced 5 minute warm-up on the cycle ergometer (Monark 894 E, Ergomedic). Subjects were given two practice trials where they were asked to pedal as fast as possible, and one half the brake weight used for the actual WAT was applied to the flywheel for two seconds. This protocol was repeated for a second practice trial. After a two minute rest, the WAT was performed. Patients were instructed to maintain the maximal velocity for 30 seconds against the full break weight (females: 35 g/kg [14] and males: 45 g/kg [15]). Continual standardized encouragement was given to the patient throughout the entire test. The average power output (WAT$_{avg}$) over the 30 seconds (which reflects anaerobic capacity), and all physiologic, ventilatory, and perceptual measures were collected and used in the analysis.

2.5. The Steep Ramp Anaerobic Test (SRAT). The SRAT was performed as described by Meyer et al. [7]. Testing was performed using the same equipment, with monitoring of the same parameters as for the CPET and WAT. After a 2 minute unloaded warm-up, the intensity increased by 25 watts every 10 seconds. The test was terminated when the subject indicated they could no longer continue or if the revolutions per minute fell below 60 rpm. Continual standardized encouragement was given to the patient throughout the entire test. The peak work rate (SRAT$_{peak}$), and all physiologic, ventilatory, and perceptual measures were collected and used in the analysis.

2.6. Physiologic, Ventilatory, and Perceptual Measures. For all three exercise tests, physiologic measurements (blood pressure, heart rate (HR) and rhythm (3-lead ECG), oxygen saturation (SpO$_2$) (N-395, Nellcor)), and perceptual measures (ratings of perceived exertion (RPE) for dyspnea and fatigue (0–10 modified Borg scale)), were obtained at baseline, during exercise, and end-exercise. Measurements including oxygen consumption (V_{O_2}), carbon dioxide production (V_{CO_2}), tidal volume (V_T), minute ventilation (V_E), and respiratory rate (RR) were recorded on a breath-by-breath basis and were averaged in 10 second increments. Inspiratory capacity (IC) maneuvers [16] were performed at baseline, during exercise, and end-exercise. From these maneuvers, operational lung volumes (end-expiratory lung volume (EELV) and end-inspiratory lung volume (EILV)) were calculated at each time point. EELV was estimated as the difference between TLC and IC, whereas EILV was estimated as the EELV plus V_T. The degree of ventilatory constraint at peak exercise was evaluated by the inspiratory reserve volume (IRV; equals TLC−EILV) and by the V_T/IC ratio.

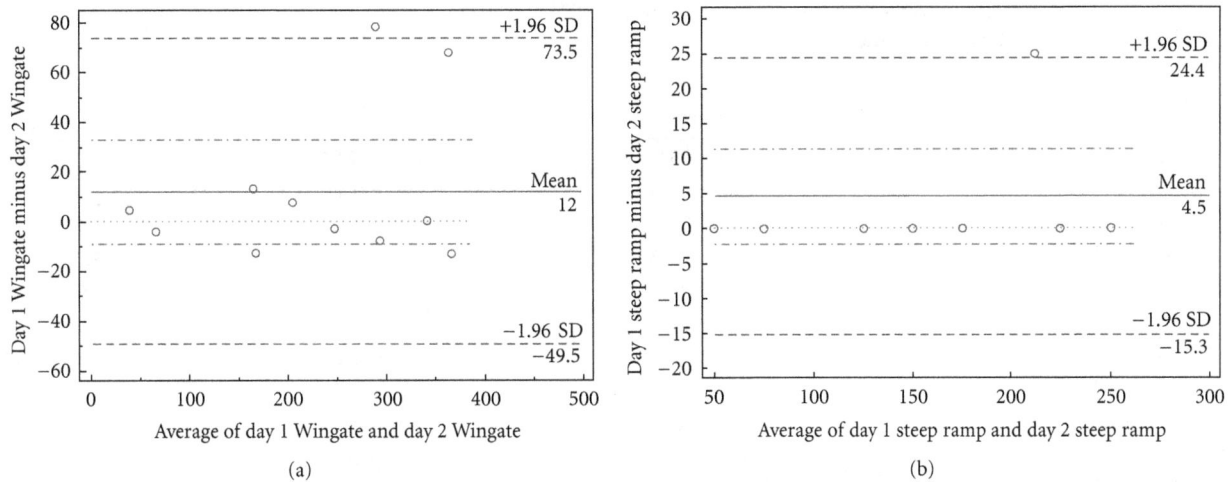

(a)

(b)

FIGURE 1: (a) Bland-Altman plot of reliability of Wingate average power measurements (W_{avg}) between both sessions. Y-axis: The difference between W_{avg} from one day to the next. X-axis: The average of W_{avg} between both days. (b) Bland-Altman plot of reliability of the steep ramp peak power measurements (SR_{peak}) between both sessions. Y-axis: The difference between SR_{peak} from one day to the next. X-axis: The average of SR_{peak} between both days.

TABLE 1: Subject characteristics.

Subject characteristics ($n = 11$)	
Male : Female, (n)	7 : 4
Age, years	71 ± 3
Weight, kg	84.6 ± 21.0
BMI, kg/m^2	29.3 ± 5.9
TLC, L (% predicted)	6.56 ± 1.21 (108 ± 10)
RV, L (% predicted)	3.42 ± 0.91 (151 ± 32)
FEV$_1$, (L) (% predicted)	1.08 ± 0.26 (43 ± 15)
FVC (L), (% predicted)	2.73 ± 0.68 (83 ± 15)
FEV$_1$/FVC, %	41 ± 10

Mean ± standard deviation. Abbreviations: TLC: total lung capacity, RV: residual volume, FEV$_1$: forced expiratory volume in 1 second, FVC: forced vital capacity, pred = predicted.

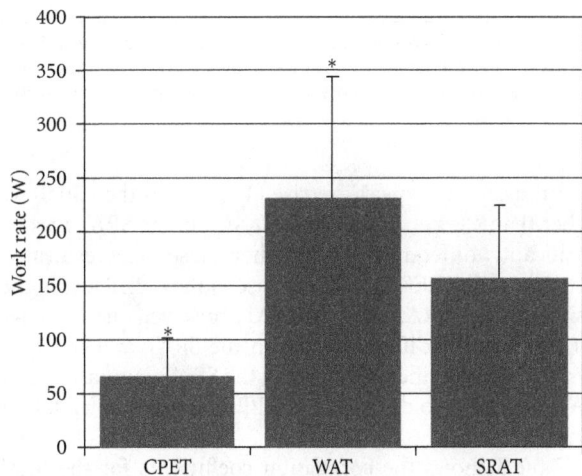

FIGURE 2: Comparison of the cardiopulmonary exercise test peak power (CPET), the steep ramp test (SRAT) peak power, and the average power in the 30-second Wingate anaerobic test (WAT) in watts. Results are presented as mean ±0.95 confidence interval. * = $P < 0.05$ versus SRAT.

2.7. Statistical Analysis. Test-retest reliability of the SRAT and the WAT was analyzed using Intraclass correlations (ICC), coefficient of variation (CV), and Bland-Altman plots. The analysis of the data comparing the CPET$_{peak}$, SRAT$_{peak}$, and the W_{avg}, as well as the ventilatory, physiological, and perceptual measures for each of the three tests included repeated measures analysis of variance (ANOVA). Tukey's post hoc analysis was performed where significant differences were found. Pearson r correlations for the work rate, ventilatory, physiological, and perceptual measures of each of the three tests were also performed to determine significant relationships between measures. All statistical analyses were performed using a significance level of $P < 0.05$.

3. Results

Subject characteristics are presented in Table 1. Both the WAT and the SRAT demonstrated a high degree of test-retest reliability. ICC was 0.99 and 0.98, and the CV was 3.8% and 8.6% for the SRAT and WAT, respectively. Bland-Altman plots demonstrated a small degree of bias and error between the 2 sessions for the SRAT (4.5 W; −15.3–24.4 W, resp.) and the WAT (12.0 W; −49.5–73.5 W, resp.) (See Figures 1(a) and 1(b)).

Between-test physiological, ventilatory, and perceptual data are presented in Table 2. In addition, Figure 2 shows the mean work rates for the 3 tests. There were significant differences between CPET$_{peak}$, SRAT$_{peak}$, and W_{avg} (65.9 ± 35.6, 156.8 ± 67.9, and 231.2 ± 113.4 W, resp.). There were no differences between V_{O_2}, RR, SpO$_2$, HR, V_E, IC, IRV, EELV, and V_T/IC measurements at peak exercise in each of

TABLE 2: End-exercise measures for cardiopulmonary exercise test (CPET), steep ramp test (SR), and Wingate anaerobic test (WAT) presented with means and standard deviations.

End-exercise measures	Tests		
	CPET	SRAT	WAT
PWR (CPET & SR) Wavg (WAT)	65.9 ± 35.9	$156.8 \pm 67.9^{*\dagger}$	$231.2 \pm 113.4^*$
V_{O_2} (L/min)	1.11 ± 0.46	1.07 ± 0.41	0.99 ± 0.45
V_{CO_2} (L/min)	1.13 ± 0.52	0.97 ± 0.40	$0.90 \pm 0.42^*$
V_E (L/min)	40.436 ± 13.33	38.94 ± 13.01	39.73 ± 14.73
RER	1.00 ± 0.13	$0.90 \pm 0.07^*$	$0.89 \pm 0.08^*$
V_T (L)	1.19 ± 0.31	1.12 ± 0.24	1.09 ± 0.33
V_T/IC (%)	76.5 ± 13.0	$70.1 \pm 12.0^*$	70.4 ± 13.8
IC/TLC (%)	24.1 ± 4.7	25.1 ± 5.5	23.5 ± 4.0
EELV/TLC (%)	75.9 ± 4.7	74.9 ± 5.5	76.5 ± 4.0
EILV/TLC (%)	94.0 ± 4.7	92.0 ± 5.1	92.9 ± 4.2
IRV/TLC (%)	6.0 ± 4.7	8.0 ± 5.1	7.1 ± 4.2
RR (breaths per minute)	34 ± 6	35 ± 8	37 ± 8
SpO_2 (%)	91.5 ± 3.0	92.3 ± 1.5	93.3 ± 3.9
HR (beats per minute)	111.9 ± 20.9	109.8 ± 19.7	116.9 ± 22.0
HR (%pred)	75.3 ± 14.7	73.7 ± 13.0	78.5 ± 14.5
Dyspnea	5.6 ± 1.8	$5.5 \pm 2.1^{\dagger}$	6.8 ± 2.3
Leg Fatigue	5.7 ± 1.7	5.6 ± 1.8	6.2 ± 1.9

Mean $\pm$ standard deviation. *: $P < 0.05$. †indicates significance from WAT. PWR: peak work rate, V_{O_2}: oxygen consumption, V_{CO_2}: carbon dioxide elimination, V_E: minute ventilation, RER: respiratory exchange ratio, V_T: tidal volume, IC: inspiratory capacity, TLC: total lung capacity, EELV: end expiratory lung volume, EILV: end inspiratory lung volume, IRV: inspiratory reserve volume, RR: respiratory rate, SpO_2: oxygen saturation, HR: heart rate.

the 3 tests. V_{CO_2} at peak exercise ($V_{CO_{2peak}}$) in the CPET was higher than $V_{CO_{2peak}}$ in the WAT. $V_{CO_{2peak}}$ in the SRAT was not significantly different from the other 2 tests. The respiratory exchange ratio (RER) at end exercise in the CPET was higher than both the SRAT and the WAT; however, the RER was not significantly different between the SRAT and the WAT. Dyspnea was significantly lower in the SRAT compared to the WAT; however, no difference in RPE in regards to leg fatigue between the tests.

Table 3 shows the correlation coefficients for the SRAT test data with respect to the corresponding data on each of the CPET and WAT tests. SRAT$_{peak}$ correlated strongly with both the CPET$_{peak}$ and the W$_{avg}$. Most ventilatory and physiological parameters for the SRAT were found to correlate significantly with those on the CPET and WAT. Physiologic exercise performance variables tended to correlate better with the WAT, whereas ventilatory parameters tended to correlate better with the CPET.

4. Discussion

The primary purpose of this study was to determine the test-retest reliability of the SRAT. Our data demonstrate excellent retest consistency. All subjects but one obtained the same peak score on the SRAT between both test sessions. The reliability of the WAT was similarly assessed to determine the appropriateness of this test to be used as a criterion measure of anaerobic capacity in patients with COPD. Although reliability analysis of this test was not part of the purposes of this study, we demonstrated that the WAT was

TABLE 3: Pearson's r correlation coefficients between end-exercise measures during the SRAT and the cardiopulmonary exercise test (CPET) and Wingate anaerobic test (WAT).

End-exercise measures	Tests	
	CPET	WAT
PWR (CPET & SR) W$_{avg}$ (WAT)	0.887^*	0.887^*
V_{O_2} (L/min)	0.891^*	0.939^*
V_{CO_2} (L/min)	0.837^*	0.926^*
V_E (L/min)	0.800^*	0.930^*
RER	0.549	0.615^*
V_T (L)	0.907^*	0.954^*
V_T/IC (%)	0.838^*	0.806^*
IC/TLC (%)	0.905^*	0.873^*
EELV/TLC (%)	0.905^*	0.873^*
EILV/TLC (%)	0.916^*	0.880^*
IRV/TLC (%)	0.916^*	0.880^*
RR (breaths per minute)	0.559	0.877^*
SpO_2 (%)	0.499	-0.017
HR (bpm)	0.684^*	0.955^*

* indicates significant correlation ($P < 0.05$).

also a reliable measure. Reliability of the WAT has been previously established in health individuals [17] and patients with COPD using an abbreviated WAT [8]. Although the reliability of the SRAT has not yet been reported, incremental exercise tests of a smaller increment have demonstrated excellent reliability [18]; therefore, it is not surprising that the SRAT would also do so. The SRAT has been used in previous studies examining the effects of exercise training [9–11]; therefore, the results of the present study lend credibility to the use of the SRAT as an outcome measure in these previous, and future studies.

The secondary purpose of the present study was to compare the exercise responses and performance variables on the SRAT with those on the CPET and WAT. We demonstrated that the SRAT results in higher peak power output than the aerobic-based CPET, but lower than the anaerobic-based WAT. Despite these work load disparities, there were no differences in end-test oxygen consumption, heart rate, ventilation, and levels of ventilatory constraint between the tests. These findings complement those of Miyahara et al. [19] who demonstrated that, during CPET, higher ramp increments resulted in higher power outputs than lower ramp increments, despite similar cardiorespiratory responses; however, the ramp increment used in the SRAT was much higher than that used previously. As has been observed in patients with COPD during a CPET, limitations on the ability of patients to increase ventilation during exercise constrain performance, and consequently, oxygen consumption and heart rate [20]. Our study supports this assertion because we also found that mean values for peak heart rate were not maximal at end-exercise. The similar levels of metabolic demand and ventilatory limitation found in the present study suggest subjects performing any of the three tests are primarily limited by the inability to increase ventilation, rather than by a physiologically maximal oxygen consumption. Due to the short amount of time to complete the SRAT (67 ± 27 seconds) [21] and the high power output compared to the CPET, however, the SRAT elicits a greater degree of leg muscle anaerobic power than the CPET. In addition, the SRAT peak power was also strongly correlated with WAT average power output. These factors combined suggest that the SRAT may be a practical test of anaerobic power, even in the setting of ventilatory limitation.

Ventilatory constraint at end-exercise is suggested by an inability to further increase tidal volume due in part to dynamic hyperinflation [20] and by nearing predicted maximal ventilation. With dynamic hyperinflation, EELV increases, IRV decreases, and therefore V_T during exercise occupies a large percentage of IC [20]. In the present study, it was assumed that the patients would be limited by ventilatory factors during the CPET, in part due to reliance upon aerobic metabolism and the requirement to ventilate in proportion to aerobic demands. Therefore, it was also assumed that patients would hyperinflate less, demonstrate less ventilatory constraint (i.e., increased ventilatory reserve), and be limited more by peripheral muscle performance during tests lasting only 30–90 seconds (i.e., the SRAT). Despite the varying exercise durations, however, the similar level of ventilatory restriction observed at the end of the 3 tests suggests this may be a shared limiting factor in all of the tests. This common limitation may help to explain the high degree of correlation between the three tests.

The WAT_{avg} was significantly larger than the $SRAT_{peak}$, and this may be partially related to the protocol design of the tests. The anaerobic metabolism present at the beginning of the WAT encourages high work rates without immediately driving ventilation. The patients gave maximal effort across the 30 seconds without realizing the degree of dyspnea they would incur due to the requirement for acid buffering, which was often near the end, or after cessation, of the WAT. Although not objectively measured in our study protocol, posttesting dyspnea scores were often reported to increase beyond the end-test values during immediate recovery from the WAT. In contrast, the SRAT, although also at a very high power output, builds incrementally to a patient-limited maximum. Patients were better able to control the amount of work performed prior to the development of disabling dyspnea, and the posttest increase observed in the WAT did not occur in the SRAT. For this reason, the SRAT seems to be an appropriate compromise between the low peak work rate of the CPET and the high work rate, but demanding recovery, of the WAT. The power output on the SRAT, albeit statistically lower than the WAT_{avg}, combined with the short duration of the SRAT suggest that the SRAT reflects performance on an anaerobic power test (WAT), while allowing the patients to appropriately and safely manage their symptoms.

Since ventilation may have been a common limiting factor between the 3 tests, stratifying the population into categories of disease severity may have elicited different results in this study. Similarly, stratifying according to gender may have shown some differences. These options may be available in a study with a larger sample size.

This study demonstrates that the SRAT is a highly reliable measure of high-intensity muscle performance. In addition, it supports the assertion that leg power is often markedly underestimated in the traditional incremental design of the CPET, and that exercise is frequently terminated before a maximal muscular response has been achieved because of ventilatory limitations [6, 7, 22, 23]. Performance on the SRAT resulted in peak work rates 238% higher than that of the CPET. This is comparable to the findings of both Meyer et al. [10] and Puhan et al. [11], where $SRAT_{peak}$ was approximately double the $CPET_{peak}$ in chronic heart failure and COPD patients, respectively. Although further research is required, it is likely the SRAT would be more useful than the CPET in assessing and establishing intensities for exercise training that are sufficiently high to elicit clinical gains in leg muscle power and high-intensity performance.

5. Conclusions

The SRAT is a highly reliable, feasible, high-power test in patients with COPD and may be useful in estimating leg muscle power. CPET underestimates the capabilities of the leg muscles to perform high levels of work, due to the attainment of ventilatory limitations in COPD patients. Despite similar degrees of ventilatory constraint, the SRAT demonstrates markedly greater work rates and better reflects anaerobic performance in this population. The SRAT may thus be more suitable for prescribing high-intensity interval exercise in order to increase the potential for training benefit in COPD patients.

References

[1] J. L. Durstine and G. E. Moore, *ACSM's Exercise Management for Persons with Chronic Diseases and Disabilities*, American College of Sports Medicine, Indianapolis, Ind, USA, 2nd edition, 2003.

[2] A. L. Ries, G. S. Bauldoff, B. W. Carlin et al., "Pulmonary rehabilitation: joint ACCP/AACVPR evidence-based clinical practice guidelines," *Chest*, vol. 131, no. 5, supplement, pp. 4S–42S, 2007.

[3] L. Nici, C. Donner, E. Wouters et al., "American thoracic society/European respiratory society statement on pulmonary rehabilitation," *American Journal of Respiratory and Critical Care Medicine*, vol. 173, no. 12, pp. 1390–1413, 2006.

[4] R. Casaburi, J. Porszasz, M. R. Burns, E. R. Carithers, R. S. Y. Chang, and C. B. Cooper, "Physiologic benefits of exercise training in rehabilitation of patients with severe chronic obstructive pulmonary disease," *American Journal of Respiratory and Critical Care Medicine*, vol. 155, no. 5, pp. 1541–1551, 1997.

[5] I. M. Weisman, K. Beck, R. Casaburi et al., "ATS/ACCP statement on cardiopulmonary exercise testing," *American Journal of Respiratory and Critical Care Medicine*, vol. 167, no. 2, pp. 211–277, 2003.

[6] S. J. Butcher and R. L. Jones, "The impact of exercise training intensity on change in physiological function in patients with chronic obstructive pulmonary disease," *Sports Medicine*, vol. 36, no. 4, pp. 307–325, 2006.

[7] K. Meyer, L. Samek, W. Schwaibold et al., "Physical responses to different modes of interval exercise in patients with chronic heart failure—application to exercise training," *European Heart Journal*, vol. 17, no. 7, pp. 1040–1047, 1996.

[8] O. Bar-Or, "The Wingate anaerobic test: an update on methodology, reliability and validity," *Sports Medicine*, vol. 4, no. 6, pp. 381–394, 1987.

[9] K. Meyer, M. Schwaibold, S. Westbrook et al., "Effects of short-term exercise training and activity restriction on functional capacity in patients with severe chronic congestive heart failure," *American Journal of Cardiology*, vol. 78, no. 9, pp. 1017–1022, 1996.

[10] K. Meyer, L. Samek, M. Schwaibold et al., "Interval training in patients with severe chronic heart failure: analysis and recommendations for exercise procedures," *Medicine and Science in Sports and Exercise*, vol. 29, no. 3, pp. 306–312, 1997.

[11] M. A. Puhan, G. Büsching, H. J. Schünemann, E. VanOort, C. Zaugg, and M. Frey, "Interval versus continuous high-intensity exercise in chronic obstructive pulmonary disease: a randomized trial," *Annals of Internal Medicine*, vol. 145, no. 11, pp. 816–825, 2006.

[12] K. F. Rabe, S. Hurd, A. Anzueto et al., "Global strategy for the diagnosis, management, and prevention of chronic obstructive pulmonary disease: GOLD executive summary," *American Journal of Respiratory and Critical Care Medicine*, vol. 176, no. 6, pp. 532–555, 2007.

[13] "Standardization of Spirometry, 1994 Update. American Thoracic Society," *American Journal of Respiratory and Critical Care Medicine*, vol. 152, no. 3, pp. 1107–1136, 1995.

[14] T. Kostka, M. Bonnefoy, L. M. Arsac, S. E. Berthouze, A. Belli, and J. R. Lacour, "Habitual physical activity and peak anaerobic power in elderly women," *European Journal of Applied Physiology and Occupational Physiology*, vol. 76, no. 1, pp. 81–87, 1997.

[15] M. Bonnefoy, T. Kostka, L. M. Arsac, S. E. Berthouze, and J. R. Lacour, "Peak anaerobic power in elderly men," *European Journal of Applied Physiology and Occupational Physiology*, vol. 77, no. 1-2, pp. 182–188, 1998.

[16] D. E. O'Donnell and K. A. Webb, "Exertional breathlessness in patients with chronic airflow limitation: the role of lung hyperinflation," *American Review of Respiratory Disease*, vol. 148, no. 5, pp. 1351–1357, 1993.

[17] J. A. Evans and H. A. Quinney, "Determination of resistance settings for anaerobic power testing," *Canadian Journal of Applied Sport Sciences*, vol. 6, no. 2, pp. 53–56, 1981.

[18] N. J. M. Cox, J. C. M. Hendriks, R. A. Binkhorst, T. H. M. Folgering, and C. L. A. Van Herwaarden, "Reproducibility of incremental maximal cycle ergometer tests in patients with mild to moderate obstructive lung diseases," *Lung*, vol. 167, no. 2, pp. 129–133, 1989.

[19] N. Miyahara, R. Eda, H. Takeyama et al., "Cardiorespiratory responses during cycle ergometer exercise with different ramp slope increments in patients with chronic obstructive pulmonary disease," *Internal Medicine*, vol. 39, no. 1, pp. 15–19, 2000.

[20] D. E. O'Donnell, S. M. Revill, and K. A. Webb, "Dynamic hyperinflation and exercise intolerance in chronic obstructive pulmonar-y disease," *American Journal of Respiratory and Critical Care Medicine*, vol. 164, no. 5, pp. 770–777, 2001.

[21] American College of Sports Medicine, *ACSM's Resource Manual for Guidelines for Exercise Testing and Prescription*, Lippincott Williams & Wilkins, Baltimore, Md, USA, 4th edition, 2001.

[22] I. Vogiatzis, S. Nanas, E. Kastanakis, O. Georgiadou, O. Papazahou, and C. Roussos, "Dynamic hyperinflation and tolerance to interval exercise in patients with advanced COPD," *European Respiratory Journal*, vol. 24, no. 3, pp. 385–390, 2004.

[23] I. Vogiatzis, O. Georgiadou, S. Golemati et al., "Patterns of dynamic hyperinflation during exercise and recovery in patients with severe chronic obstructive pulmonary disease," *Thorax*, vol. 60, no. 9, pp. 723–729, 2005.

6

Abnormalities of the Ventilatory Equivalent for Carbon Dioxide in Patients with Chronic Heart Failure

Lee Ingle,[1] Rebecca Sloan,[1] Sean Carroll,[1] Kevin Goode,[2] John G. Cleland,[2] and Andrew L. Clark[2]

[1] *Department of Sport, Health & Exercise Science, University of Hull, Cottingham Road, Kingston-upon-Hull HU6 7RX, UK*
[2] *Department of Cardiology, Hull York Medical School, Daisy Building, University of Hull, Castle Hill Hospital, Cottingham, Kingston-upon-Hull HU16 5JQ, UK*

Correspondence should be addressed to Lee Ingle, l.ingle@hull.ac.uk

Academic Editor: Roland Wensel

Introduction. The relation between minute ventilation (VE) and carbon dioxide production (VCO_2) can be characterised by the instantaneous ratio of ventilation to carbon dioxide production, the ventilatory equivalent for CO_2 ($VEqCO_2$). We hypothesised that the time taken to achieve the lowest $VEqCO_2$ (time to VEqCO2 nadir) may be a prognostic marker in patients with chronic heart failure (CHF). *Methods.* Patients and healthy controls underwent a symptom-limited, cardiopulmonary exercise test (CPET) on a treadmill to volitional exhaustion. *Results.* 423 patients with CHF (mean age 63 ± 12 years; 80% males) and 78 healthy controls (62% males; age 61 ± 11 years) were recruited. Time to VEqCO2 nadir was shorter in patients than controls (327 ± 204 s versus 514 ± 187 s; $P = 0.0001$). Univariable predictors of all-cause mortality included peak oxygen uptake ($X^2 = 53.0$), $VEqCO_2$ nadir ($X^2 = 47.9$), and time to $VEqCO_2$ nadir ($X^2 = 24.0$). In an adjusted Cox multivariable proportional hazards model, peak oxygen uptake ($X^2 = 16.7$) and $VEqCO_2$ nadir ($X^2 = 17.9$) were the most significant independent predictors of all-cause mortality. *Conclusion.* The time to $VEqCO_2$ nadir was shorter in patients with CHF than in normal subjects and was a predictor of subsequent mortality.

1. Introduction

Cardiopulmonary exercise testing (CPET) is used to stratify risk in patients with cardiorespiratory disease [1]. In patients with chronic heart failure (CHF), the normal linear relation between ventilation (VE) and carbon dioxide production (VCO_2) is maintained, but the slope of the relation is greater than normal, so that, for a given volume of carbon dioxide production, the ventilatory response is greater [2–6]. Another way of characterising the relation between minute ventilation and carbon dioxide production is the instantaneous ratio of ventilation to carbon dioxide production, the ventilatory equivalent for CO_2 ($VEqCO_2$). Recently, we have shown that the lowest $VEqCO_2$ ($VEqCO_2$ nadir) provides greater prognostic value than other CPET-derived variables in patients with suspected CHF [7]. Other studies have reported that the lowest $VEqCO_2$ has similar prognostic power to the VE/VCO_2 slope derived from the whole of exercise [8].

During an incremental CPET, as exercise intensity increases, both VCO_2 and VE increase linearly. However, $VEqCO_2$ falls at the onset of exercise, possibly due to a reduction in dead space ventilation. Beyond the ventilatory compensation point (VCP), lactic acid production causes an increase in ventilation relative to carbon dioxide production, and thus the $VEqCO_2$ rises. Although patients with CHF have the same pattern of $VEqCO_2$ during exercise as normal subjects, with more severe heart failure, the increase in $VEqCO_2$ towards the end of exercise becomes more marked [9]. In the most severely affected patients, $VEqCO_2$ increases from the start of exercise [9]. We hypothesised that the time taken to reach $VEqCO_2$ nadir would be shorter in patients with CHF compared to healthy controls and thus may be an important prognostic indicator.

2. Methods

The Hull and East Riding Ethics Committee approved the study, and all patients provided informed consent. We recruited consecutive patients referred to a community heart failure clinic with symptoms of breathlessness (NYHA functional class II-III) who were found to have left ventricular systolic dysfunction on investigation. Clinical information obtained included past medical history and drug and smoking history. Clinical examination included assessment of body mass index (BMI), heart rate, rhythm, and blood pressure. Patients were excluded if they were unable to exercise because of noncardiac limitations (such as osteoarthritis) or had significant respiratory disease (defined as a predicted $FEV_1 < 70\%$).

Heart failure was defined as the presence of current symptoms of HF, or a history of symptoms controlled by ongoing therapy, and impaired left ventricular systolic function. Left ventricular function was determined from 2D echocardiography which was carried out by one of three trained operators. Left ventricular function was assessed by estimation on a scale of normal, mild, mild-to-moderate, moderate, moderate-to-severe, and severe impairment and was assessed by a second operator blind to the assessment of the first; where there was disagreement on the severity of left ventricular (LV) dysfunction, the echocardiogram was reviewed jointly with the third operator and a consensus reached. Where possible, left ventricular ejection fraction (LVEF) was calculated using the Simpson's formula from measurements of end-diastolic and end-systolic volumes on apical 2D views, following the guidelines of Schiller and colleagues [10], and LVSD was diagnosed if LVEF was ≤45%. When LVEF could not be calculated, LVSD was diagnosed if LVEF ≤45 or there was at least "mild-to-moderate" impairment.

Patients underwent a symptom-limited, maximal CPET on a treadmill using the Bruce protocol modified by the addition of a Stage 0 (2.74 km·h^{-1} and 0% gradient) at the onset of exercise. Metabolic gas exchange was measured with an Oxycon Delta metabolic cart (VIASYS Healthcare Inc., Philadelphia, PA, USA). Peak oxygen uptake (pVO$_2$) was calculated as the average VO$_2$ for the final 30 s of exercise. The ventilatory anaerobic threshold (AT) was calculated by the V-slope method [11]. The gradient of the relationship between VE and VCO$_2$ (VE/VCO$_2$ slope) was calculated by linear regression analysis using data acquired from the whole test. The VEqCO$_2$ relation was plotted from start to the finish of exercise. Each consecutive 30-second reading was averaged, and the lowest point was defined as the VEqCO$_2$ nadir [7]. The time taken to reach the VEqCO$_2$ nadir was reported in seconds (s). The peak respiratory exchange ratio (pRER) was calculated as the mean VCO$_2$/VO$_2$ ratio for the final 30 s of exercise. For comparative purposes, we also included a healthy control group who had no evidence of cardiac, respiratory, or musculoskeletal limitation. Healthy controls were randomly invited to participate from two local GP practices.

2.1. Statistical Analysis. We used SPSS (version 17.0) for statistical analysis. Continuous variables are presented as mean ± SD, and categorical data are presented as percentages. Continuous variables were assessed for normality by the Kolmogorov-Smirnov test. An arbitrary level of 5% statistical significance was used throughout (two tailed). An independent *t*-test was used to measure differences between CHF patients and healthy controls. All survivors were followed for a minimum of 12 months, and we therefore give the probability of 12-month survival. Receiver operator characteristic (ROC) curves were used to identify the value of the strongest predictor variables of survival to 12 months. We reported the area under the curve (AUC) with 95% confidence intervals (CI), sensitivity, specificity, and optimal cut-points in our ROC analysis. To define the optimal cut-point, we used the point closest to the upper left corner of the ROC curve, often known as the (0, 1) criterion.

All baseline variables (Table 1) were entered as potential univariable predictors of mortality using Cox analysis, and we adjusted for age, sex, BMI, aetiology of heart failure, and severity of LV dysfunction (none, trivial, mild, mild-to-moderate, moderate, moderate-to-severe, severe). Model building was based on backward elimination (*P* value for entry was <0.05; *P* value for removal >0.1). A multivariable Cox proportional hazards model using the backward likelihood ratio method was used to identify independent predictors of all-cause mortality from all significant candidate predictor variables. The outcome measure was all-cause mortality. Kaplan-Meier survival curves were plotted for the strongest candidate predictors; data were dichotomised by optimal cut-points.

3. Results

423 patients with CHF (mean age 63 ± 12 years; 80% males; LVEF 36 ± 6%; peak VO$_2$ 22.3 ± 8.1 mL·kg^{-1}·min^{-1}; VE/VCO$_2$ slope 34 ± 8) were included in the study. Of these, 75% were taking ACE inhibitors, 77% beta blockers, and 67% loop diuretics. Seventy eight healthy subjects (62% males; age 61 ± 11 years) were recruited as a control group. The healthy controls had a higher peak oxygen uptake, lower VE/VCO$_2$ slope, and lower VEqCO$_2$ nadir (Table 1). Time to VEqCO$_2$ nadir was shorter in patients than controls (327 ± 204 s versus 514 ± 187 s; *P* = 0.0001) but was similar as a percentage of the total exercise duration in both groups (55 ± 23% versus 60 ± 17%; *P* = 0.077). We performed a subgroup analysis in 62 NYHA class III patients and found that the time to VEqCO$_2$ nadir was significantly lower (199 ± 59 s) compared to other less symptomatic patients (344 ± 202 s; *P* < 0.0001). We also performed a subgroup analysis by sex and found that the time to VEqCO$_2$ nadir was very similar between males (327 ± 209 s) and females (328 ± 94 s; *P* > 0.05; *n* = 85).

In patients, time to VEqCO$_2$ nadir correlated with age (*r* = −0.17; *P* = 0.0001) and LVEF (*r* = 0.24; *P* = 0.0001) but was not associated with BMI (*r* = 0.001; *P* = 0.98). Time to VEqCO$_2$ nadir correlated with peak oxygen uptake (*r* = 0.59; *P* = 0.001) and showed an inverse association with both VE/VCO$_2$ slope (*r* = −0.55; *P* = 0.001) and VEqCO$_2$ nadir (*r* = −0.56; *P* = 0.001). Scatter plots showing the association between time to VEqCO$_2$ nadir, peak oxygen uptake, and

TABLE 1: Baseline clinical characteristics between CHF patients and healthy controls.

Variable (mean ± SD)	CHF patients	Healthy controls	P value*
N	423	78	—
Males (%)	80	62	0.0001*
Age (years)	63 (12)	61 (11)	0.529
BMI (kg·m^{-2})	28 (5)	26 (3)	0.001*
LVEF (%)	36 (6)	60 (6)	0.0001*
pVO$_2$ (mL·kg^{-1}·min^{-1})	22.3 (8.1)	36.2 (8.8)	0.0001*
VE/VCO$_2$ slope (full)	33.8 (7.7)	27.7 (3.0)	0.0001*
VEqCO$_2$ nadir	32.4 (6.2)	26.5 (3.0)	0.0001*
Time to VEqCO$_2$ nadir(s)	327 (514)	514 (187)	0.0001*
AT (mL·kg^{-1}·min^{-1})	15.2 (5.7)	23.4 (6.6)	0.0001*
Peak RER	1.07 (0.10)	1.08 (0.06)	0.223
Exercise duration (s)	564 (250)	881 (256)	0.0001*
Heart rate (rest) (beats·min^{-1})	76 (15)	72 (12)	0.079
Heart rate (peak) (beats·min^{-1})	136 (30)	165 (20)	0.0001*
Systolic BP (rest) (mmHg)	137 (25)	148 (20)	0.0001*
Systolic BP (peak) (mmHg)	172 (36)	199 (22)	0.0001*
Diastolic BP (rest) (mmHg)	84 (15)	90 (9)	0.0001*
Diastolic BP (peak) (mmHg)	93 (22)	101 (21)	0.003*
Loop diuretic (%)	67	—	—
ACE-I (%)	75	—	—
Beta-blocker (%)	77	—	—

BMI: body mass index; LVEF: left ventricular ejection fraction; pVO$_2$: peak oxygen uptake; ACE-I: ACE inhibitor; peak RER: peak respiratory exchange ratio; AT: anaerobic threshold; BP: blood pressure; *differences between CHF and healthy controls, $P < 0.05$.

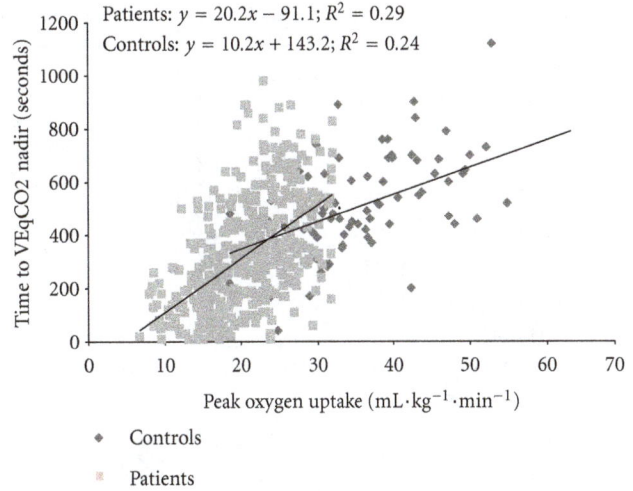

FIGURE 1: Relation between time to VEqCO2 nadir and peak oxygen uptake in patients with CHF and controls.

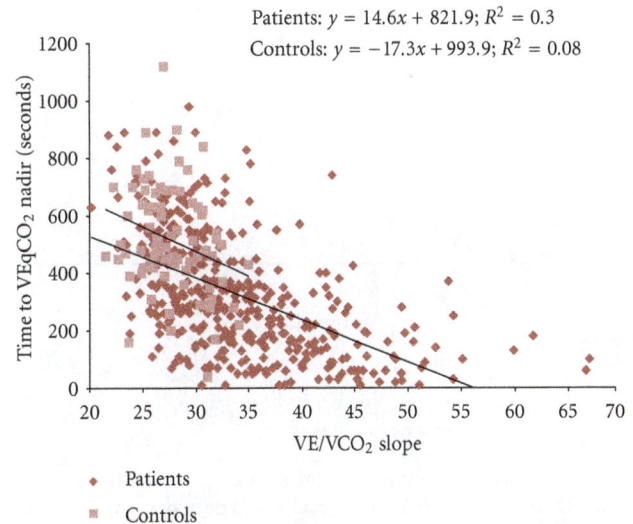

FIGURE 2: Relation between time to VEqCO$_2$ nadir and VE/VCO$_2$ slope in patients with CHF and controls.

VE/VCO$_2$ slope in patients and controls are shown in Figures 1 and 2.

One hundred and eighteen patients (28%) died during followup. The median followup in survivors was 8.6 ± 2.1 years. Univariable predictors of outcome derived from CPET are shown in Table 2. With the exception of resting heart rate, all candidate variables were significant univariable predictors. The strongest univariable predictors of all-cause mortality were peak oxygen uptake ($\chi^2 = 53.0$), VEqCO$_2$ nadir ($\chi^2 = 47.9$), VE/VCO$_2$ slope ($\chi^2 = 31.7$), and time to VEqCO$_2$ nadir ($\chi^2 = 24.0$). In a Cox multivariable proportional hazards model adjusted for age, sex, BMI, and severity of LV dysfunction, peak oxygen uptake ($\chi^2 = 16.7$; HR = 0.91; 95% CI 0.88–0.95; $P = 0.0001$) and VEqCO$_2$ nadir ($\chi^2 = 17.9$; HR = 1.12; 95% CI 1.04–1.20; $P = 0.0001$) were the most significant independent predictors of mortality.

ROC curve analysis of the relation between time to VEqCO$_2$ nadir (and both VEqCO$_2$ nadir and peak VO$_2$) and all-cause mortality at 12 months is shown in Figure 3. Time to VEqCO$_2$ nadir (AUC = 0.75; $P < 0.0001$; 95% CI = 0.67–0.84; sensitivity = 81; specificity = 62; optimal cut-point = 250 s); VEqCO$_2$ nadir (AUC = 0.81; $P < 0.0001$; 95% CI = 0.74–0.89; sensitivity = 86; specificity = 62; optimal cut-point = 33); peak VO$_2$ (AUC = 0.76; $P < 0.0001$; 95% CI = 0.67–0.85; sensitivity = 86; specificity = 57; optimal cut-point = 20 mL·kg^{-1}·min^{-1}) were similar in their relation to all-cause mortality at 12 months. Optimal cut-points determined from ROC analysis were used to construct Kaplan-Meier survival curves for time to VEqCO$_2$ nadir (Figure 4), VEqCO$_2$ nadir (Figure 5), and peak VO$_2$ (Figure 6).

TABLE 2: Unadjusted univariable predictors of outcome (in order of Chi-square value).

Variables	P value	HR		95% CI	Chi-square
Peak oxygen uptake	0.0001	0.891	0.862	0.920	53.0
VEqCO$_2$ nadir	0.0001	1.095	1.068	1.122	47.9
VE/VCO$_2$ slope	0.0001	1.060	1.041	1.079	31.7
Time to VEqCO$_2$ nadir*	0.0001	0.705	0.523	0.905	24.0
Heart rate at peak exercise	0.0001	0.995	0.978	0.992	18.5
Systolic blood pressure (rest)	0.001	0.986	0.978	0.994	12.0
Diastolic blood pressure (rest)	0.02	0.977	0.963	0.991	9.3
Heart rate (rest)	0.744	1.002	0.990	1.014	0.1

HR: hazard ratio; 95% CI: 95% confidence intervals; *adjusted HR associated with 10 s increase in time to VEqCO$_2$ nadir.

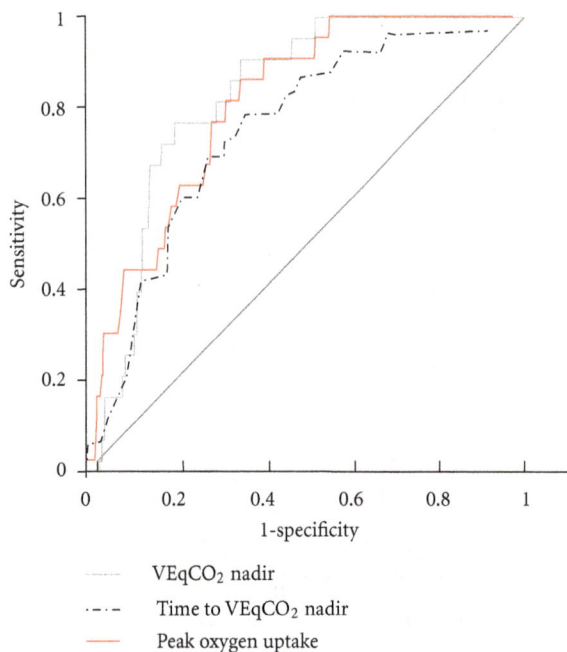

FIGURE 3: Receiver operating characteristic curve showing value of VEqCO$_2$ nadir, time to VEqCO$_2$ nadir, and peak oxygen uptake for predicting all-cause mortality at 12 months. VEqCO$_2$ nadir: AUC = 0.81; $P < 0.0001$; 95% CI = 0.74–0.89; sensitivity = 86; specificity = 62; optimal cut-point = 33; time to VEqCO$_2$ nadir: AUC = 0.75; $P < 0.0001$; 95% CI = 0.67–0.84; sensitivity = 81; specificity = 62; optimal cut-point = 250 s; peak VO$_2$: AUC = 0.76; $P < 0.0001$; 95% CI = 0.67–0.85; sensitivity = 86; specificity = 57; optimal cut-point = 20 mL·kg^{-1}·min^{-1}.

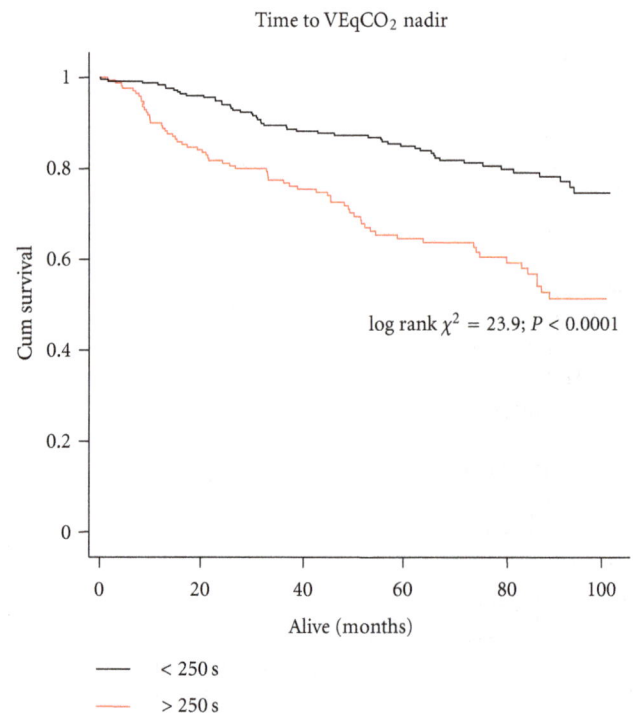

FIGURE 4: Kaplan-Meier survival curve showing time to VEqCO$_2$ nadir-data dichotomised by optimal cut-points (<250 s; $n = 170$, event free survival 61%; ≥ 250 s $n = 254$ patients, event free survival 80%).

4. Discussion

We have shown that the time to VEqCO$_2$ nadir is significantly lower in patients with CHF compared to controls. To our knowledge, no previous study has evaluated the prognostic value of time to VEqCO$_2$ nadir. Sun and colleagues [12] showed that the lowest VEqCO$_2$ (VEqCO$_2$ nadir) was the most stable marker of ventilatory inefficiency in healthy controls. During maximal exercise testing, the VEqCO$_2$ nadir was achieved at around the ventilatory anaerobic threshold and occurred during "moderate" exercise intensity. Both VE and VCO$_2$ are linearly related up to the ventilatory

compensation point (VCP). Beyond this point (during heavy to maximal exertion), an increase in VE relative to VCO$_2$ is dependent upon the fall in pH and PaCO$_2$ [12].

The exaggerated ventilatory response of patients with CHF is seen at the outset of exercise; that is, the VE/VCO$_2$ slope is abnormal from the moment exercise starts. A wide variety of factors has been proposed as the reason for the increase in VE/VCO$_2$ slope including an increased dead space and resultant "wasted" ventilation [13–15], early metabolic acidosis [16], and overactivation of chemoreceptors and ergoreceptors [17, 18]. The fall in the VEqCO$_2$ at the onset of exercise is at least in part due to the reduction in fixed anatomical dead space ventilation as a proportion of total ventilation at the onset of exercise, but the increase after

VEqCO$_2$ nadir

Log rank $\chi^2 = 61.9$; $P < 0.0001$

Alive (months)

— < 33
— ≥ 33

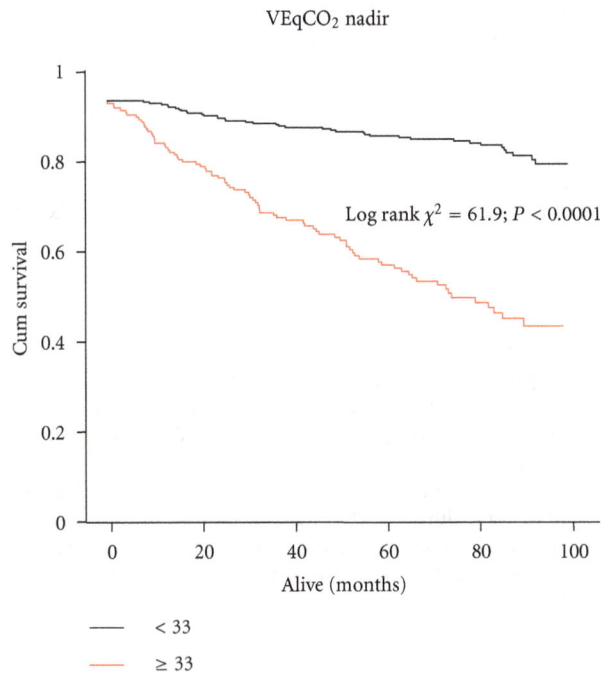

FIGURE 5: Kaplan-Meier survival curve showing VEqCO$_2$ nadir-data dichotomised by optimal cut-points (<33 $n = 252$ patients, event free survival 85%; ≥ 33 $n = 171$ patients, event free survival 54%).

Peak VO$_2$

log rank $\chi^2 = 44.8$; $P < 0.0001$

Alive (months)

— $\geq 20\,\text{mL} \cdot \text{kg}^{-1} \cdot \text{min}^{-1}$
— $< 20\,\text{mL} \cdot \text{kg}^{-1} \cdot \text{min}^{-1}$

FIGURE 6: Kaplan-Meier survival curve showing peak VO$_2$-data dichotomised by optimal cut-points ($<20\,\text{mL} \cdot \text{kg}^{-1} \cdot \text{min}^{-1}$ $n = 184$ patients, event free survival 60%; $\geq 20\,\text{mL} \cdot \text{kg}^{-1} \cdot \text{min}^{-1}$ $n = 239$ patients, event free survival 82%).

the plateau phase is due to a non-CO$_2$ stimulus to ventilation, wheather lactate production or an alternative stimulus to ventilation, such as the ergoreflex [9, 19]. The shorter time to VEqCO$_2$ nadir reflects the earlier onset (and more important influence of) the non-CO$_2$ stimulus to ventilation in patients with CHF.

We found a strong relation between the time to VEqCO$_2$ nadir and mortality. The time to VEqCO$_2$ nadir was an important univariable predictor of all-cause mortality although it was outperformed by peak oxygen uptake and VEqCO$_2$ nadir in a multivariable survival model. We have previously shown that peak oxygen uptake [20] and VEqCO$_2$ nadir [7] are independent predictors of all-cause mortality in patients with CHF. Other investigators have also reported similar findings [8, 21].

A limitation of our study is that we do not have test-retest CPET data for individual patients/controls; therefore, we cannot determine the reproducibility of the time to VEqCO$_2$ nadir in either healthy or diseased populations.

Cardiopulmonary exercise testing provides two broad types of prognostic variable: a measure of exercise capacity, such as peak VO$_2$, reflecting the complex relation between pump, ventilator, and muscle extraction; and a measure of the ventilatory response to exercise, such as the VE/VCO$_2$ slope or time to VEqCO$_2$ nadir, reflecting the abnormal stimulus to ventilation in CHF. The time to VEqCO$_2$ nadir following maximal CPET was shorter in patients with CHF than in normal subjects and is a predictor of subsequent mortality.

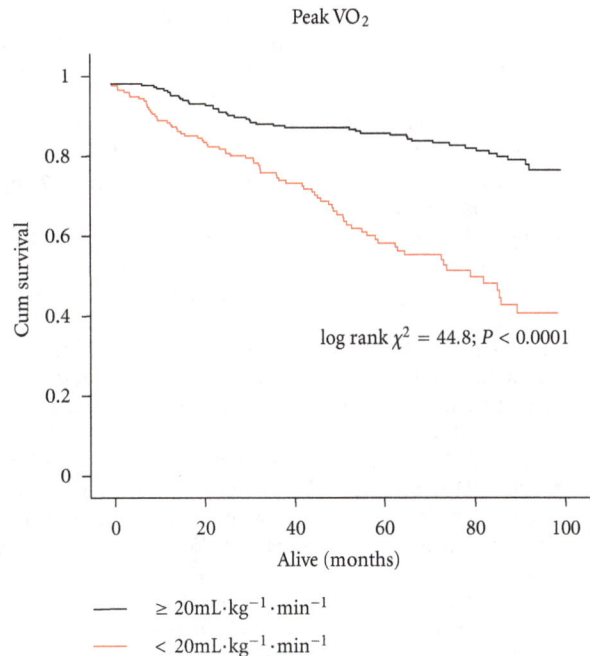

5. Clinical Messages

(i) Cardiopulmonary exercise testing is becoming increasingly important for prescribing appropriate exercise training volumes in patients with cardiovascular disease including CHF.

(ii) The ventilatory response to exercise is abnormal in patients with CHF compared to age-matched controls.

(iii) Metabolic responses to exercise are important predictors of risk and should be monitored prior to and following a program of rehabilitation in patients with CHF.

Conflict of interests

The authors declare that there is no conflict of interests.

Acknowledgment

This research received no specific grant from any funding agency in the public, commercial, or not-for-profit sectors.

References

[1] G. J. Balady, R. Arena, K. Sietsema et al., "Clinician's guide to cardiopulmonary exercise testing in adults: a scientific statement from the american heart association," *Circulation*, vol. 122, no. 2, pp. 191–225, 2010.

[2] T. P. Chua, P. Ponikowski, D. Harrington et al., "Clinical correlates and prognostic significance of the ventilatory response to exercise in chronic heart failure," *Journal of the American College of Cardiology*, vol. 29, no. 7, pp. 1585–1590, 1997.

[3] A. Clark and A. Coats, "The mechanisms underlying the increased ventilatory response to exercise in chronic stable heart failure," *European Heart Journal*, vol. 13, no. 12, pp. 1698–1708, 1992.

[4] L. Ingle, K. Goode, S. Carroll et al., "Prognostic value of the VE/VCO_2 slope calculated from different time intervals in patients with suspected heart failure," *International Journal of Cardiology*, vol. 118, no. 3, pp. 350–355, 2007.

[5] A. L. Clark, M. Volterrani, J. W. Swan, and A. J. S. Coats, "The increased ventilatory response to exercise in chronic heart failure: relation to pulmonary pathology," *Heart*, vol. 77, no. 2, pp. 138–146, 1997.

[6] R. L. Bard, B. W. Gillespie, N. S. Clarke, T. G. Egan, and J. M. Nicklas, "Determining the best ventilatory efficiency measure to predict mortality in patients with heart failure," *Journal of Heart and Lung Transplantation*, vol. 25, no. 5, pp. 589–595, 2006.

[7] L. Ingle, R. Sloan, S. Carroll, K. Goode, J. G. Cleland, and A. L. Clark, "Prognostic significance of different measures of the ventilation-carbon dioxide relation in patients with suspected heart failure," *European Journal of Heart Failure*, vol. 13, no. 5, pp. 537–542, 2011.

[8] J. Myers, R. Arena, R. B. Oliveira et al., "The lowest VE/VCO_2 ratio during exercise as a predictor of outcomes in patients with heart failure," *Journal of Cardiac Failure*, vol. 15, no. 9, pp. 756–762, 2009.

[9] A. L. Clark, A. Poole-Wilson AP. A., and A. J. S. Coats, "Relation between ventilation and carbon dioxide product in patients with chronic heart failure," *Journal of the American College of Cardiology*, vol. 20, no. 6, pp. 1326–1332, 1992.

[10] N. B. Schiller, P. M. Shah, M. Crawford et al., "Recommendations for quantitation of the left ventricle by two-dimensional echocardiography. American society of echocardiography committee on standards, subcommittee on quantitation of two-dimensional echocardiograms," *Journal of the American Society of Echocardiography*, vol. 2, no. 5, pp. 358–367, 1989.

[11] W. L. Beaver, K. Wasserman, and B. J. Whipp, "A new method for detecting anaerobic threshold by gas exchange," *Journal of Applied Physiology*, vol. 60, no. 6, pp. 2020–2027, 1986.

[12] X. G. Sun, J. E. Hansen, N. Garatachea, T. W. Storer, and K. Wasserman, "Ventilatory efficiency during exercise in healthy subjects," *American Journal of Respiratory and Critical Care Medicine*, vol. 166, no. 11, pp. 1443–1448, 2002.

[13] K. Wasserman, Y. Y. Zhang, A. Gilt et al., "Lung function and exercise gas exchange in chronic heart failure," *Circulation*, vol. 96, no. 7, pp. 2221–2227, 1997.

[14] M. Guazzi, G. Reina, G. Tumminello, and M. D. Guazzi, "Exercise ventilation inefficiency and cardiovascular mortality in heart failure: the critical independent prognostic value of the arterial CO_2 partial pressure," *European Heart Journal*, vol. 26, no. 5, pp. 472–480, 2005.

[15] J. R. Wilson and N. Ferraro, "Exercise intolerance in patients with chronic left heart failure: relation to oxygen transport and ventilatory abnormalities," *American Journal of Cardiology*, vol. 51, no. 8, pp. 1358–1363, 1983.

[16] J. Myers, A. Salleh, N. Buchanan et al., "Ventilatory mechanisms of exercise intolerance in chronic heart failure," *American Heart Journal*, vol. 124, no. 3, pp. 710–719, 1992.

[17] T. Tomita, H. Takaki, Y. Hara et al., "Attenuation of hypercapnic carbon dioxide chemosensitivity after postinfarction exercise training: possible contribution to the improvement in exercise hyperventilation," *Heart*, vol. 89, no. 4, pp. 404–410, 2003.

[18] A. Ciarka, N. Cuylits, J. L. Vachiery et al., "Increased peripheral chemoreceptors sensitivity and exercise ventilation in heart transplant recipients," *Circulation*, vol. 113, no. 2, pp. 252–257, 2006.

[19] A. L. Clark, P. A. Poole-Wilson, and A. J. S. Coats, "Exercise limitation in chronic heart failure: central role of the periphery," *Journal of the American College of Cardiology*, vol. 28, no. 5, pp. 1092–1102, 1996.

[20] L. Ingle, K. K. Witte, J. G. F. Cleland, and A. L. Clark, "Combining the ventilatory response to exercise and peak oxygen consumption is no better than peak oxygen consumption alone in predicting mortality in chronic heart failure," *European Journal of Heart Failure*, vol. 10, no. 1, pp. 85–88, 2008.

[21] E. A. Jankowska, T. Witkowski, B. Ponikowska et al., "Excessive ventilation during early phase of exercise: a new predictor of poor long-term outcome in patients with chronic heart failure," *European Journal of Heart Failure*, vol. 9, no. 10, pp. 1024–1031, 2007.

7

Stereotactic Body Radiotherapy for Metastatic Lung Cancer as Oligo-Recurrence: An Analysis of 42 Cases

Wataru Takahashi,[1] Hideomi Yamashita,[1] Yuzuru Niibe,[2] Kenshiro Shiraishi,[1] Kazushige Hayakawa,[2] and Keiichi Nakagawa[1]

[1] Department of Radiology, University of Tokyo Hospital, 7-3-1, Hongo, Bunkyo-ku, Tokyo 113-8655, Japan
[2] Department of Radiology and Radiation Oncology, Kitasato Universtiy, Kanagawa 252-0374, Japan

Correspondence should be addressed to Hideomi Yamashita, yamachan07291973@yahoo.co.jp

Academic Editor: Takao Hiraki

Purpose. To investigate the outcome and toxicity of stereotactic body radiotherapy (SBRT) in patients with oligo-recurrence cancer in the lung (ORCL). *Methods and Materials.* A retrospective review of 42 patients with ORCL who underwent SBRT in our two hospitals was conducted. We evaluated the outcome and adverse effects after SBRT for ORCL. *Results.* All patients finished their SBRT course without interruptions of toxicity reasons. The median follow-up period was 20 months (range, 1–90 months). The 2-year local control rate and overall survival were 87% (95% CI, 75–99%) and 65% (95% CI, 48–82%). As for prognostic factor, the OS of patients with a short disease-free interval (DFI) < 31.9 months, between the initial therapy and SBRT for ORCL, was significantly worse than the OS of long DFI ≥ 31.9 months ($P < 0.05$). The most commonly observed late effect was radiation pneumonitis. One patient had grade 4 gastrointestinal toxicity (perforation of gastric tube). No other ≥ grade 3 acute and late adverse events occurred. There were no treatment-related deaths during this study. *Conclusions.* In patients with ORCL, radical treatment with SBRT is safe and provides a chance for long-term survival by offering favorable local control.

1. Introduction

Lung is one of the common sites of metastasis after definitive therapy for a primary cancer. So far, recurrent or metastatic lung cancers have been considered to uniformly carry a poor prognosis because multiple metastases tend to be difficult to treat intensively. Chemotherapy has been broadly applied as a standard management at these conditions. On the other hand, the innovation of methods of early detection of recurrence, such as positron-emission tomography (PET), allows the detection of limited site recurrent, called oligo-recurrence. Oligo-recurrence, proposed by Niibe et al. in 2006 [1–4], was the condition of one or a few metastatic or recurrent lesions occurred with controlled primary lesion. For case with oligo-recurrence cancer in the lung (ORCL), the controversy exists regarding the optimal approach of these metastatic sites. Despite surgical approach is considered as an alternative for a single metastasis, there are many patients with ORCL who were not amenable for metasta-sectomy. For them, less invasive techniques such as SBRT

have been used to treat ORCL. In cases considered to have a favorable prognosis, radical treatment with SBRT seems to be beneficial for prolonging the survival time. However, the role of radiotherapy and the prognostic factors for oligo-recurrence have not yet been clearly elucidated [5]. In this study, we evaluated the efficacy and toxicity of SBRT for patients with oligo-recurrence cancer treated from 2001 through 2011 in two hospitals.

2. Materials and Methods

2.1. Patient Eligibility and Pretreatment Evaluation. A retrospective review of all patients with ORCL treated with SBRT after prior therapy at University of Tokyo Hospital and Kitasato University Hospital from April 2001 to July 2011 was conducted. Patients with ORCL who were not suitable for surgery due to medical or functional reasons were included in this analysis. Pretreatment evaluation included a complete medical history, physical examination, computed tomography (CT), pulmonary function tests, and laboratory tests. In addition, 36 of 42 patients (86%) were evaluated with ^{18}F fluorodeoxyglucose (FDG)-PET before treatment. Inclusion criteria of this study were as follows: (a) primary cancer was completely treated; (b) the number of lung metastases were up to three; (c) there was no other distant metastasis or other distant metastasis was scheduled to be treated with curative intent after SBRT. As long as these evaluations fulfilled the inclusion criteria, there was no restriction regarding tumor size, location, or general pulmonary function. Radiotherapy was the exclusive treatment modality in all patients.

2.2. Radiotherapy. SBRT was given with 6 MV X-ray of a linear accelerator. In curative intention, hypofractionated SBRT was delivered to a median dose of 48 Gy (range, 20–56 Gy) with a median daily dose of 12 Gy (range, 8–30 Gy). Dose and fractionation schedules were chosen depending on location and institution. In University of Tokyo Hospital, SBRT was performed using the Synergy linear accelerator (ELEKTA), which fully integrates IGRT by means of kV-CT scanning. In Kitasato University Hospital, real-time tumor-tracking radiotherapy was used for SBRT. The gross tumor volume (GTV) or internal target volume (ITV) included the visible gross tumor mass on CT were delineated on a three-dimensional radiation treatment planning system (3D RTPS) using the lung window. The planning target volume (PTV) was created by adding five mm margin to the ITVs in all directions.

2.3. Follow-Up. After completion of therapy, patients were scheduled for regular follow-up visits 3 monthly during the first year, 6 monthly thereafter. Those who did not appear for a routine follow-up were contacted by phone. Follow-up evaluations included a history and physical examination and CT scans of the thorax. Additional imaging investigations such as FDG-PET were only required if there was clinical suspicion of recurrence. In this study, we define local recurrence as an increase in opacity size on CT imaging, along with either increased maximum standardized uptake values (SUVmax) $\geq$ 5 on FDG-PET, or biopsy proof of disease [6]. Toxicity was evaluated and scored according to the National Cancer Institute Common Terminology Criteria for Adverse Events (NCI CTCAE) version 4.0, with toxicity occurring within 3 months after the initiation of RT classified as acute toxicity. Late toxicity was graded using the RTOG/EORTC criteria.

2.4. Statistical Analysis. The baseline follow-up date was the first day of radiotherapy, and the last follow-up date was the last Hospital visit or phone day. Overall survival (OS) was calculated from the start of the SBRT to the date of death, censoring the last follow-up date. Local control rate (LCR) was calculated from the start of the SBRT to the first local recurrence date, censoring death or last follow-up date.

To discuss risk factors for OS and LCR, the patients of ORCL were classified into two groups: early recurrence group and late recurrence group. The former group consisted of 21 patients whose disease-free interval (DFI), meaning interval between the start date of initial therapy and the start date of SBRT for ORCL, was shorter than 31.9 months (median

DFI time). In addition, we compared OS and LCR following SBRT for ORCL from colorectal cancer (CRC) and other origins. OS and LCR curves were plotted using the Kaplan-Meier method. Log-rank testing was used to compare OS and LCR between the subsets of patients analyzed. All analyses were performed using SPSS software version 12.0 (SPSS Inc., Chicago, IL).

3. Results

From April 2001 to July 2011, we identified 42 patients with ORCL who were treated with SBRT. The median age was 69 years (range, 25–84 years). There were 30 men and 12 women. The median maximum diameter of metastatic tumor was 19 mm (range, 9–40 mm). Patient characteristics are shown in Table 1. One patient underwent chemotherapy for ORCL before SBRT and the other 41 patients did not undergo neoadjuvant, concurrent, or adjuvant chemotherapy for ORCL. Sites of primary disease included lung ($n = 16$), colon and rectum ($n = 7$), head and neck (6), esophagus ($n = 4$), uterus ($n = 4$), kidney ($n = 2$), and others (renal pelvis, breast, sarcoma; $n = 3$). Of these, 32 patients had lung metastasis alone, 8 patients had another lung metastasis treated with SBRT after initial SBRT, and 2 patients had a distant metastasis in addition to lung lesion (retroperitoneal node and adrenal gland). These distant metastases in both patients were also treated with SBRT after completing SBRT for lung lesion. At the time to analysis, they were alive without evidence of any recurrence.

All patients finished their SBRT course without interruptions of toxicity reasons. Acute toxicities were mild and tolerable except for one case. Grade 4 acute adverse event were observed in only 1 patient (2%), which displayed the perforation of the pulled-up gastric tube. This patient was a 59-year-old man, with esophageal cancer after total esophagectomy with esohageal replacement by means of a gastric tube, had undergone SBRT, consisting of 50 Gy in four fractions in 4 days. The D2 cc, the minimum dose in the most irradiated 2 cc of the gastric tube, was 48.66 Gy. He was a heavy smoker and had an alcohol problem. Two months later, he developed perforation of the gastric tube.

No other grade $\geq$ 3 acute side effects occurred. Twenty-one patients (50%) and 5 patients (12%) experienced grade 1 and 2 adverse event after irradiation of metastases, respectively. Of the 42 patients, 21 patients (50%) and 3 patients (7%) displayed grade 1 pneumonitis (asymptomatic, radiographic findings only) and grade 2 pneumonitis (symptomatic, not interfering with activities of daily living), respectively. No grade $\geq$ 3 late adverse events occurred until now. The median duration of follow-up was 20 months (range, 1–90 months) for all patients and 24 months (range, 6–90 months) for those alive. The 1- and 2-year local control rates were 91% (95% CI, 82–100%) and 87% (95% CI, 75–99%), respectively (Figure 1). At the time of last follow-up, 16 patients had died. The causes of death were recurrence ($n = 9$), other diseases ($n = 7$). The overall 1- and 2-year survival rates were 81% (95% CI, 69–94%) and 65% (95% CI, 48–82%), respectively (Figure 1), with a median survival time

TABLE 1: Patients characteristics ($n = 42$).

Variable	Distribution	No. of patients	%
Sex	Male	30	71
	Female	12	29
Age	Median	69 years	
	Range	25–84 years	
Karnofsky Performance status	Median	90	
	Range	50–90	
Number of metastases	1	32	76
	2	10	24
	$\geqq 3$	0	0
Maximum diameter (mm)	Median	19 mm	
	Range	9–40 mm	
Primary site	Lung	16	38
	Colon and rectum	7	17
	Head and neck	6	14
	Esophagus	4	10
	Uterus	4	10
	Kidney	2	5
	Other	3	5
Follow-up (months)	Median	20 months	
	Range	1–90 months	

of 40 months. Seventeen of 42 patients showed a long-term survival of longer than 2 years.

In present study, seven patients with ORCL originated from CRC and 35 patients originated from other origins were treated by SBRT. The 1- and 2-year LCR in ORCL from CRC and in ORCL from other origins were 83% and 67%, 89% and 89%, respectively (Figure 2). The overall 1- and 2-year survival rates in ORCL from CRC and in ORCL from other origins were 85% and 85%, 82% and 63%, respectively (Figure 3). These results showed no significant difference in LCR ($P = 0.31$) and OS ($P = 0.26$).

We also analyzed the LCR and OS differences stratified by DFI divided into < 31.9 or $\geq$ 31.9 months. As shown in Figure 4, the result indicated a negative correlation between DFI and LCR ($P = 0.29$). On the other hand, early recurrence group (short DFI) had significantly bad prognosis ($P < 0.05$; Figure 5).

4. Discussion

Although this is a retrospective study with a limited sample size, our results are also comparable to other studies in ORCL [7–9]. Norihisa et al. [10] also previously showed the results of SBRT for 43 metastatic lung cancers. In their series, the survival rates and local control rate at 2 years were reported to be 84.3% and 90%, respectively. Ricardi et al. [11] also reported a study of SBRT for oligometastatic lung tumors. Sixty-one patients treated with SBRT achieved 89% in local control and 66.5% in survival at 2 years.

Several studies have now shown that the local control after SBRT for lung metastases from CRC is worse than that from other origins. Takeda et al. [12] reported the difficulty of local control for ORCL from CRC. Norihisaet al. [10] proposed dose escalation in SBRT for CRC patients in order to achieve better local control. In the current study, there was no significant difference between CRC and other origins in LCR ($P = 0.31$) and OS ($P = 0.26$), respectively.

Furthermore, we also analyzed the OS and LCR differences stratified by DFI divided into < 31.9 or $\geq$ 31.9 months. As shown in Figure 5, short DFI was the prognostic factor ($P < 0.05$). Thus, even as oligo-recurrence, early metastasis may be bad prognostic factor.

It seems from these results that SBRT is an effective and safe treatment for patients with lung metastases as oligo-recurrence. In SBRT for lung metastases, limited toxicity rates are reported by several authors [12]. In our series, there was no patient with serious late toxicities except for one patient with perforation of gastric tube. Although it is likely that the perforation may be caused mainly by radiation to gastric tube, smoking and bad nutrition might have been partly related to this perforation. Several reports advocated that deterioration in smoking and bad nutritional status during radiotherapy could be associated with poorer short-term treatment outcomes and severe side effect [13, 14].

Several limitations of this study warrant mention. First, it was a retrospective review with a limited number of patients and limited follow-up. Second, we treated ORCL from various primary cancers by using different treatment

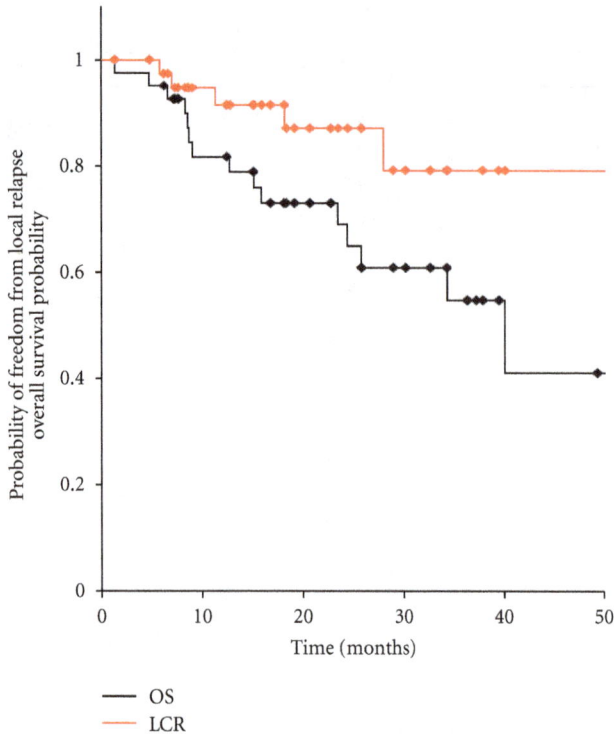

FIGURE 1: Overall survival and local control of 42 patients with oligo-recurrence cancer in the lung.

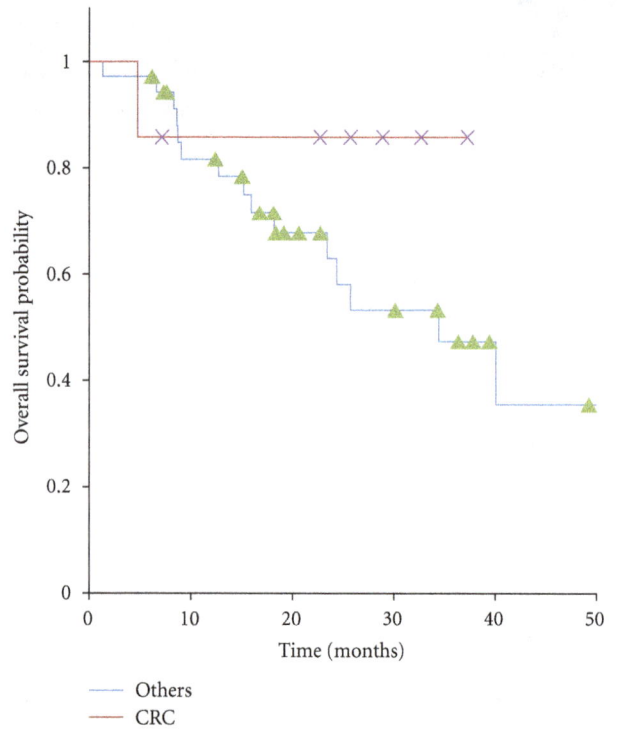

FIGURE 3: Kaplan-Meier curves for overall survival in 42 patients with oligo-recurrence cancer in the lung, cancers from colorectal cancer and ones from other origins.

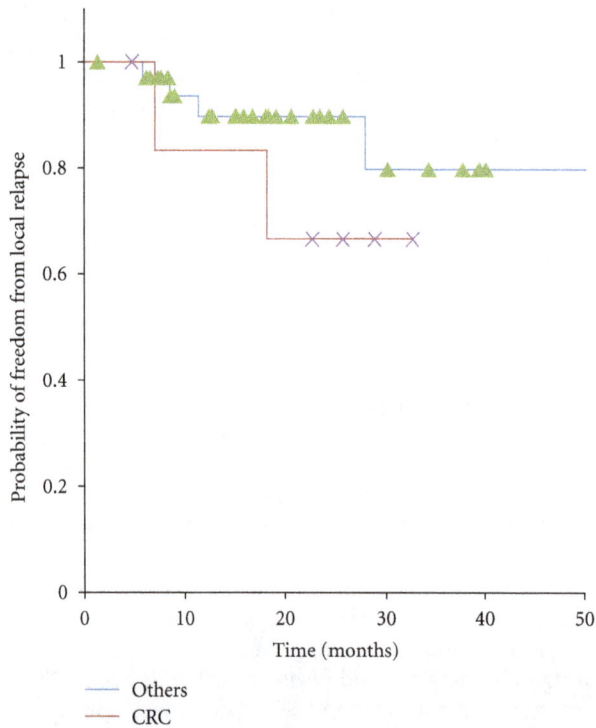

FIGURE 2: Kaplan-Meier curves for local control in 42 patients with oligo-recurrence cancer in the lung, cancers from colorectal cancer and ones from other origins.

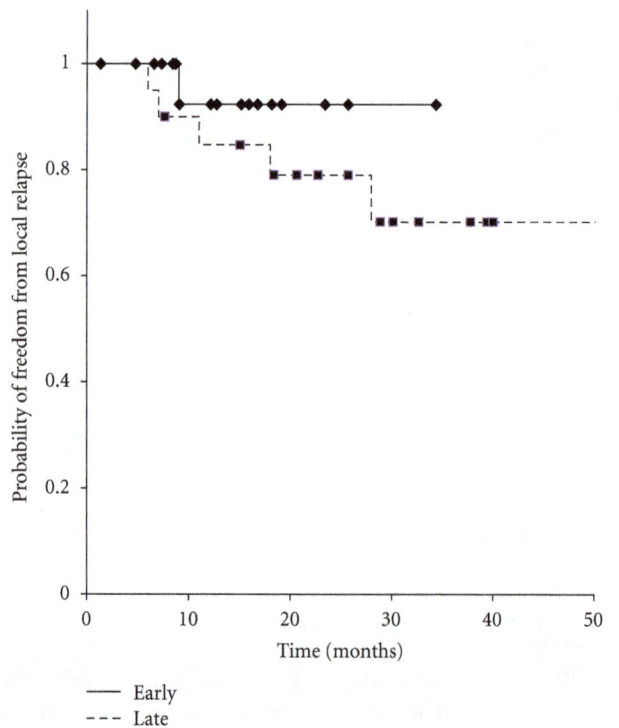

FIGURE 4: Kaplan-Meier curves for local control in 42 patients with oligo-recurrence cancer in the lung, early recurrence group versus late recurrence group.

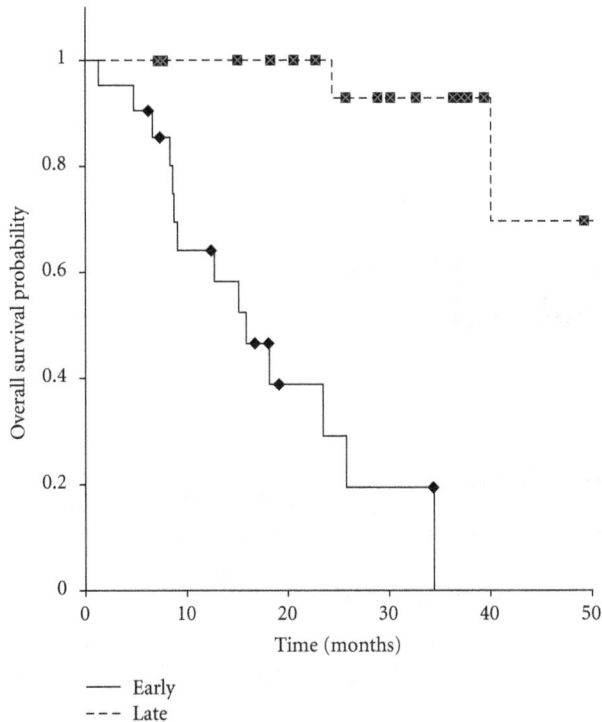

FIGURE 5: Kaplan-Meier curves for overall survival in 42 patients with oligo-recurrence cancer in the lung, early recurrence group versus late recurrence group.

protocol. There was a wide range of doses prescribed, and a variety of fractionation schema.

5. Conclusions

In patients with ORCL, radical treatment with SBRT offers good local control and provides a real chance for long-term survival. In addition, even in ORCL, SBRT is a safe and efficacious modality and appears to be well tolerated.

Conflict of Interests

The authors declare that they have no conflict of intrersts.

References

[1] Y. Niibe, T. Kazumoto, T. Toita et al., "Frequency and characteristics of isolated para-aortic lymph node recurrence in patients with uterine cervical carcinoma in Japan: a multi-institutional study," *Gynecologic Oncology*, vol. 103, no. 2, pp. 435–438, 2006.

[2] Y. Niibe, M. Kenjo, T. Kazumoto et al., "Multi-institutional study of radiation therapy for isolated para-aortic lymph node recurrence in uterine cervical carcinoma: 84 subjects of a population of more than 5,000," *International Journal of Radiation Oncology Biology Physics*, vol. 66, no. 5, pp. 1366–1369, 2006.

[3] Y. Niibe, M. Kuranami, K. Matsunaga et al., "Value of high-dose radiation therapy for isolated osseous metastasis in breast cancer in terms of oligo-recurrence," *Anticancer Research*, vol. 28, no. 6, pp. 3929–3931, 2008.

[4] Y. Niibe and K. Hayakawa, "Oligometastases and oligo-recurrence: the new era of cancer therapy," *Japanese Journal of Clinical Oncology*, vol. 40, no. 2, pp. 107–111, 2010.

[5] S. K. Jabbour, P. Daroui, D. Moore, E. Licitra, M. Gabel, and J. Aisner, "A novel paradigm in the treatment of oligometastatic non-small cell lung cancer," *Journal of Thoracic Disease*, vol. 3, no. 1, pp. 4–9, 2011.

[6] K. Huang, M. Dahele, S. Senan et al., "Radiographic changes after lung stereotactic ablative radiotherapy (SABR)—can we distinguish recurrence from fibrosis? A systematic review of the literature," *Radiotherapy & Oncology*, vol. 102, no. 3, pp. 335–342, 2012.

[7] P. Okunieff, A. L. Petersen, A. Philip et al., "Stereotactic body radiation therapy (SBRT) for lung metastases," *Acta Oncologica*, vol. 45, no. 7, pp. 808–817, 2006.

[8] K. E. Rusthoven, B. D. Kavanagh, S. H. Burri et al., "Multi-institutional phase I/II trial of stereotactic body radiation therapy for lung metastases," *Journal of Clinical Oncology*, vol. 27, no. 10, pp. 1579–1584, 2009.

[9] D. Oh, Y. C. Ahn, J. M. Seo et al., "Potentially curative stereotactic body radiation therapy (SBRT) for single or oligometastasis to the lung," *Acta Oncologica*, vol. 51, no. 5, pp. 596–602, 2012.

[10] Y. Norihisa, Y. Nagata, K. Takayama et al., "Stereotactic body radiotherapy for oligometastatic lung tumors," *International Journal of Radiation Oncology Biology Physics*, vol. 72, no. 2, pp. 398–403, 2008.

[11] U. Ricardi, A. R. Filippi, A. Guarneri et al., "Stereotactic body radiation therapy for lung metastases," *Lung Cancer*, vol. 75, no. 1, pp. 77–81, 2012.

[12] A. Takeda, E. Kunieda, T. Ohashi, Y. Aoki, N. Koike, and T. Takeda, "Stereotactic body radiotherapy (SBRT) for oligometastatic lung tumors from colorectal cancer and other primary cancers in comparison with primary lung cancer," *Radiotherapy & Oncology*, vol. 101, no. 2, pp. 255–259, 2011.

[13] A. Hill, N. Kiss, B. Hodgson, T. C. Crowe, and A. D. Walsh, "Associations between nutritional status, weight loss, radiotherapy treatment toxicity and treatment outcomes in gastrointestinal cancer patients," *Clinical Nutrition*, vol. 30, no. 1, pp. 92–98, 2011.

[14] C. M. Hoff, C. Grau, and J. Overgaard, "Effect of smoking on oxygen delivery and outcome in patients treated with radiotherapy for head and neck squamous cell carcinoma—a prospective study," *Radiotherapy & Oncology*, vol. 103, no. 1, pp. 38–44, 2012.

8

The Effects of Gas Humidification with High-Flow Nasal Cannula on Cultured Human Airway Epithelial Cells

Aaron Chidekel,[1,2,3] **Yan Zhu,**[1] **Jordan Wang,**[1]
John J. Mosko,[1] **Elena Rodriguez,**[1] **and Thomas H. Shaffer**[1,2,4]

[1] *Nemours Biomedical Research, Nemours Research Lung Center, Nemours/Alfred I. duPont Hospital for Children, 1600 Rockland Road, Wilmington, DE 19803, USA*
[2] *Department of Pediatrics, Jefferson Medical College, Thomas Jefferson University, 1025 Walnut Street, Suite 700, Philadelphia, PA 19107, USA*
[3] *Department of Pediatrics, Nemours/Alfred I. duPont Hospital for Children, 1600 Rockland Road, Wilmington, DE 19803, USA*
[4] *Departments of Physiology and Pediatrics, Temple University School of Medicine, 3420 North Broad Street, Philadelphia, PA 19140, USA*

Correspondence should be addressed to Aaron Chidekel, achidek@nemours.org

Academic Editor: S. L. Johnston

Humidification of inspired gas is important for patients receiving respiratory support. High-flow nasal cannula (HFNC) effectively provides temperature and humidity-controlled gas to the airway. We hypothesized that various levels of gas humidification would have differential effects on airway epithelial monolayers. Calu-3 monolayers were placed in environmental chambers at 37°C with relative humidity (RH) < 20% (dry), 69% (noninterventional comparator), and >90% (HFNC) for 4 and 8 hours with 10 L/min of room air. At 4 and 8 hours, cell viability and transepithelial resistance measurements were performed, apical surface fluid was collected and assayed for indices of cell inflammation and function, and cells were harvested for histology (n = 6/condition). Transepithelial resistance and cell viability decreased over time ($P < 0.001$) between HFNC and dry groups ($P < 0.001$). Total protein secretion increased at 8 hours in the dry group ($P < 0.001$). Secretion of interleukin (IL)-6 and IL-8 in the dry group was greater than the other groups at 8 hours ($P < 0.001$). Histological analysis showed increasing injury over time for the dry group. These data demonstrate that exposure to low humidity results in reduced epithelial cell function and increased inflammation.

1. Introduction

Humidification of inspired gas is important for patients receiving respiratory support with nasal cannulae or mechanical ventilation. During normal breathing, the inspired gas is heated and humidified by the nasal mucosa [1]. The ACCP-NHLBI National Conference on Oxygen Therapy concluded that it was not necessary to provide routine humidification at oxygen flow rates of 1–4 L/min when environmental humidity is adequate [2].

Medical gases contain only approximately six parts per million of water vapor [3]. Administering inadequately conditioned medical gases may shift the isothermic saturation boundary (ISB) farther down the bronchial tree [4]. The ISB is the point in the airway where the inspired air in the lung reaches 37°C and 100% relative humidity (RH), and the ISB is normally located just below the carina. If the ISB shifts downward, the lower respiratory tract becomes involved in heat and moisture change [5, 6] so that the airway mucosa is at risk for mucus membrane dehydration, impaired cilia function, and retention of secretions [7], which may lead to partial or complete airway obstruction and increased incidence of infection. Previous studies demonstrated that just five minutes of respiration using ambient gas with no heating or humidification in ventilated infants resulted in a significant decrease in both pulmonary compliance and conductance [8]; cool, dry air induces a bronchoconstriction response, which is associated with muscarinic receptors in the nasal mucosa [9]. Airway cooling and drying is also a potential mechanism of exercise-induced bronchospasm. A clinical study that compared the effect of heat and moisture exchangers and heated humidifiers showed that heat and moisture exchangers generated inadequate airway humidification resulting in high incidence of endotracheal tube occlusion [10].

Heated humidification is most often used during mechanical ventilation via an artificial airway. It is believed that 30 mg H_2O/L is the theoretical minimum humidity during invasive ventilation [11]. High-flow nasal cannula (HFNC) effectively provides temperature and humidity-controlled gas to the nasopharynx and airway. Humidification therapy plays an important role in the maintenance of the respiratory tract. However, while humidification therapy has been widely used in clinical practice, information regarding its effect on epithelial cell structure, function, and inflammatory indices is limited.

The Calu-3 cell line (American Type Culture Collection, ATCC HTB-55; ATCC, Manassas, VA) is a well-differentiated and characterized cell line derived from human bronchial submucosal glands [12]. Calu-3 cells form high-resistance monolayers when grown on air-interfaced culture (AIC) [13–15] and have demonstrated many of the characteristics of the bronchiolar epithelium [16], which, in vivo, serves as the barrier layer between inspired gas and other visceral tissues. This attribute is particularly advantageous for the evaluation of airway injury and response to medical treatments and respiratory therapeutic interventions [17]. Calu-3 cells have been used for drug delivery [18], pulmonary drug disposition [19], and bacterial invasiveness studies [20]. Devor et al. [21] used the Calu-3 cell line as a model system to study the mechanisms of HCO_3^- and Cl^- secretion, which reflects the transport properties of native submucosal gland serous cells. Other potential in vitro cell models have been employed for pulmonary research. Alveolar epithelial cells, such as A549 cells, lack many of the important secretory characteristics, do not form functional tight junction structure, and therefore generate very low epithelial resistance [22]. In a recent study, Stewart et al. [23] evaluated primary (human bronchial epithelial cells, HBEC) and nonprimary (Calu-3, BEAS-2B, BEAS-2B R1) bronchial epithelial cell lines as air-liquid interface-differentiated models for the in vitro study of asthma. These authors demonstrated that primary cells develop an inconsistent experimental phenotype and highly variable levels of transepithelial resistance (TER), thus highlighting the difficulties in utilizing primary cells for in vitro epithelial cell research. By contrast, Calu-3 cells formed high-resistance monolayers and expressed similar markers as compared to primary cells, suggesting that these cells may be the most suitable model cell line for air-liquid interface experiments.

In this study, Calu-3 cells served as an in vitro model to evaluate the effects of inspired gas humidification and high flow on the human airway epithelium. We hypothesized that levels of gas humidification would have differential effects on airway epithelial cell structure, function, and inflammatory indices from each other as well as compared with a noninterventional condition.

2. Materials and Methods

Calu-3 human airway epithelial cell monolayers were cultured on transwell plates with the apical surface exposed to gas and the basolateral surface exposed to culture medium. Following establishment of confluent monolayers, plates were exposed to environmental conditions as outlined below. At 4 and 8 hours, monolayer integrity and cell viability were determined by assessment of TER and CellTiter Blue Cell Viability Assay monolayer (Promega, Madison, WI). Apical surface wash fluid (ASF) samples were retrieved from additional wells for analysis of secreted inflammatory mediators. Enough wells were exposed to provide 6 observations ($n = 6$/condition) for each measured parameter. The total protein, interleukin (IL)-6, and IL-8 data were corrected by cell viability.

2.1. Calu-3 Cell Culture. Reagents were purchased from Invitrogen (Carlsbad, CA) and Transwell Permeable Supports from Corning Incorporated Life Sciences (Acton, MA). Calu-3 cells were cultured at 37°C and 5% CO_2 in a 50/50% mixture of Dulbecco's Modified Eagle's Medium/Ham's F-12 (DMEM/F12) supplemented with 15% fetal calf serum, 500 u/mL penicillin, and 50 μg/mL streptomycin. Cells were grown in 75 cm² tissue culture flasks and split when 90–95% confluent.

Calu-3 cell air-liquid interface culture was performed as previously described [24]. Calu-3 cells were plated at 2×10^6 cells/cm² onto Costar Transwell inserts (0.4 μm pore size, 12-mm diameter, clear polycarbonate membrane; Costar plate; Corning) treated with human type I collagen (Southern Biotech, Birmingham, AL). Apical culture medium was removed two days after plating, and monolayers were grown at an air-liquid interface and fed basolaterally with DMEM/F12 with 15% fetal calf serum. The basolateral medium was changed on alternate days.

After 11 days of transwell culture, full confluence was verified by measurement of TER with STX2 electrodes and an epithelial volt ohm meter (World Precision Instruments, Sarasota, FL). Calu-3 monolayers that exhibited TER values of at least 800 to 1,000 ohm·cm² were used for the experiments. For all conditions, one additional plate was placed in an incubator at RH 69% and 37°C as a noninterventional comparator group. Two plates of Calu-3 monolayers were placed in modular incubator chambers (MIC-101; Billups-Rothenberg, Del Mar, CA) and exposed to one of two levels of RH: less than 20% and more than 90% for 4 or 8 hours with 10 L/min of continuous room air flow at 37°C. To achieve the RH of less than 20%, the gas from 21% FiO_2 tank was flushed through the chamber using a Servo O_2-air 960 mixer (Siemens-Elema, Solna, Sweden) for 4 or 8 hours at a flow rate of 10 L/min in an incubator at 37°C. The HFNC (Vapotherm, Stevensville, MD) provided the gas at a flow

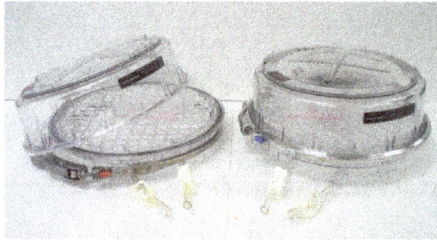

FIGURE 1: Cell-culture environmental chambers. Transwell plates were exposed to one of three levels of relative humidity: <20% (dry), 69% (noninterventional comparator), and >90% (HFNC) for 4 and 8 hours with 10 L/pm of room air at 37°C.

rate of 10 L/min and maintained the temperature at 37°C and the RH at 90%. Chamber oxygen level was monitored with an oxygen analyzer (MAXO$_2$; OM-25AE; Maxtec, Salt Lake City, UT). The modular incubator chamber was sealed, but the O ring was not compressed by a stainless steel ring clamp. This would allow the chambers to open in case the pressure inside exceeded atmospheric pressure. Pressure was confirmed by a Rüsch pressure monometer (Teleflex Medical, Duluth, GA), and the humidity was monitored by a humidity thermometer (Fisher Scientific, Cat no. S66279) inside the modular incubator chamber (Figure 1).

At each experimental time-point, monolayers were used for measurement of TER (n = 6/condition) or ASF collection (n = 6/condition). Six monolayers were then used for assessment of cell viability and cytomorphometry (n = 3/ condition).

The ASF samples were collected as previously described [15]. Monolayers were washed twice with 140 μL of normal saline. Washes from each insert were combined for a total volume of 280 μL and centrifuged for 15 min at 13,000 rcf and 4°C to remove debris. Supernatants were stored in aliquots at −70°C for subsequent assays.

2.2. Measurement of Cell Viability.
CellTiter Blue Cell Viability Assay (Promega, Madison, WI) was performed to estimate the number of viable cells and determine cell viability by the intensity of fluorescence. This assay is based on the reduction of resazurin to resorufin by living cells. Triplicate wells were set up without cells to serve as the negative control to determine background fluorescence. The monolayers exposed to RH 69% and 37°C served as a noninterventional comparator group. 200 μL of medium and 40 μL of CellTiter Blue reagent were added to the apical side of the transwell insert and 720 μL of medium to the basolateral side. The fluorescence was recorded using a plate-reading fluorometer at 550/590 nm.

2.3. Measurement of TER.
The TER measurements were made using STX2 electrodes and an epithelial volt ohm meter (World Precision Instruments). At baseline and after treatment, 0.5 mL of medium was added apically and 1 mL of medium was added basolaterally, and electrodes were inserted into each pool of medium to measure TER.

2.4. Measurement of Total Protein.
Total protein concentration was measured in duplicate using DC protein assay kit (Bio-Rad, Hercules, CA). Bovine serum albumin (standard II) was selected as a reference standard. Absorbance was measured at 655 nm.

2.5. Measurement of IL-6 and IL-8 Levels in Calu-3 ASF.
The ASF levels of IL-6 and IL-8 were measured in duplicate by quantitative enzyme-linked immunosorbent assay (ELISA) using human IL-6 and IL-8 Quantikine ELISA kits (R & D Systems, Minneapolis, MN). The test sensitivity for respective immunoassays was 0.039 pg/mL for IL-6 and 10 pg/mL for IL-8. Interassay and intraassay coefficients of variance were less than 10%. IL-6 and IL-8 data were corrected for cell viability.

2.6. Histology and Cytomorphology of Calu-3 Cells.
Cytospin slides were prepared using 100 μL of single-cell suspensions and stained for cell differentiation using Kwik-Diff solutions (Thermo Electron, Pittsburgh, PA). Cytomorphology was evaluated in a semiquantitative manner as the ratio of abnormal cells to total cells. Abnormal cells were defined by the following characteristics: (1) abnormal cellular appearance, (2) swollen nuclei, (3) intracellular and nuclear vacuoles, and/or (4) diffuse cytoplasm and cellular debris [25]. Two-hundred cells were evaluated for each experimental condition in the following fashion. Microscope slides were evaluated by the scorer in a blinded fashion to the experimental condition by randomly selecting four fields for visual observation. Fifty individual cells from each of four high-power fields were scored and only after each slide was scored was the experimental condition unblinded.

2.7. Statistical Analysis.
Statistical analysis was performed using Statistical Package for the Social Sciences (SPSS, Version 17, IBM, Armonk, NY) software. All data were expressed as mean ± SEM. Differences between conditions for each parameter were analyzed using two-way analyses of variance (ANOVA). Where applicable, one-way ANOVA was run across different treatments at each time interval (i.e., 24 and 72 hours), and post-hoc analyses were done using Bonferroni comparisons. Significance was accepted at $P < 0.05$. At least six samples were used for each group.

3. Results

After 11 days culture, Calu-3 cells developed a baseline TER of 1105.86 ± 43.8 ohm·cm^2 for all monolayers before the experiments. Calu-3 monolayers exposed to the gases with RH of less than 20% (dry group) and more than 90% (HFNC group) showed decreased TER ($P < 0.001$) over time. The TER in the noninterventional comparator group remained constant at the same level at 4 and 8 hours (Figure 2). Two-way ANOVA demonstrated an interaction for humidification and time of exposure ($P < 0.001$) whereby the TER did not change over time in the noninterventional comparator group but decreased in both the HFNC and dry groups. Post-hoc analysis revealed that the HFNC and

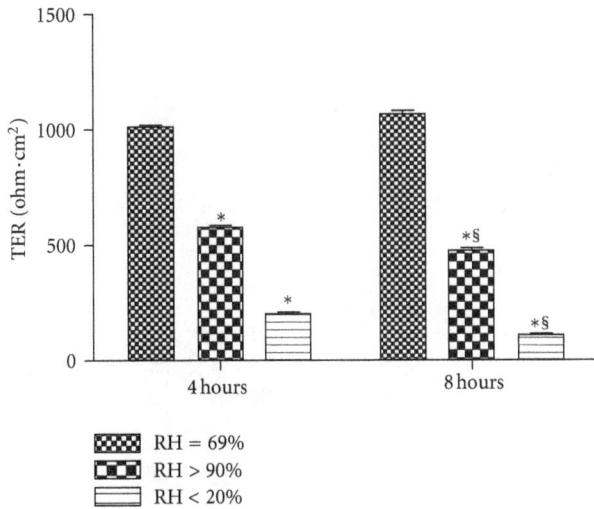

FIGURE 2: Transepithelial resistance (TER) for Calu-3 monolayers exposed to one of three levels of relative humidity: <20% (dry), 69% (noninterventional comparator), and >90% (HFNC). TER was less than the noninterventional comparator group in the HFNC and dry groups ($P < 0.001$). Data are mean ± SEM. *Group effect ($P < 0.001$). §Time effect ($P < 0.001$).

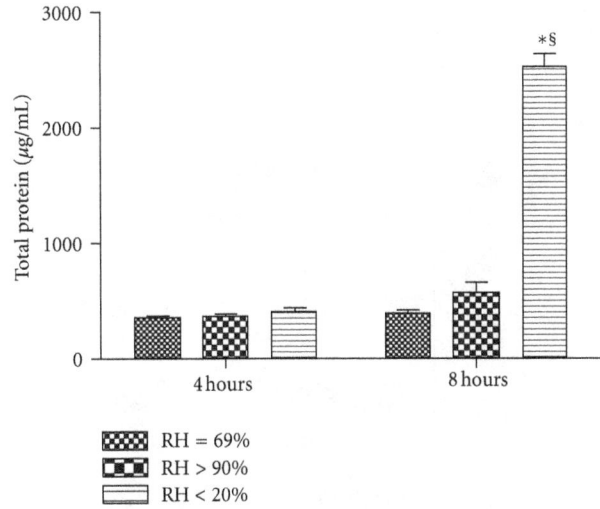

FIGURE 4: Total protein concentration in apical surface wash fluid from Calu-3 monolayers exposed to one of three levels of relative humidity: <20% (dry), 69% (noninterventional comparator), and >90% (HFNC). Secretion of total protein increased at 8 hours in the dry group ($P < 0.001$), but there was no difference between the noninterventional comparator group and the HFNC groups ($P > 0.05$) and no difference between groups at 4 hours ($P > 0.05$). Data are mean ± SEM. *Group effect ($P < 0.05$). §Time effect ($P < 0.05$). $n = 6$/condition.

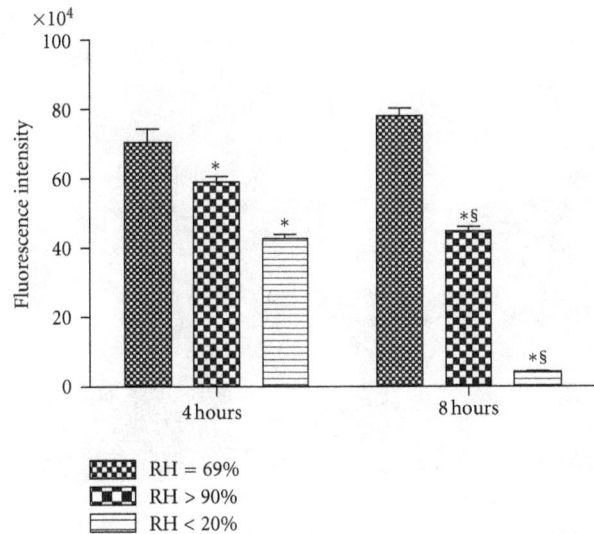

FIGURE 3: Cell viability for Calu-3 monolayers exposed to one of three levels of relative humidity: <20% (dry), 69% (noninterventional comparator), and >90% (HFNC). CellTiter Blue cell viability assay was performed to estimate the number of viable cells and determine cell viability by the intensity of fluorescence. Cell viability decreased over time ($P < 0.001$) for HFNC and dry groups. Data are mean ± SEM. *Group effect ($P < 0.05$). §Time effect ($P < 0.05$). $n = 6$/condition.

Cell viability also decreased over time ($P < 0.001$) for both of the intervention groups with a similar pattern noted as for the TER. Cell viability remained unchanged in the noninterventional comparator group, decreased 42.54% in the HFNC group, and decreased substantially (94.60%) in the dry group (Figure 3).

Secretion of total protein in the dry group ASF samples increased at 8 hours ($P < 0.001$), but there was no significant difference between the noninterventional comparator group and the HFNC groups ($P > 0.05$) and no significant difference between any of the groups at 4 hours ($P > 0.05$) (Figure 4).

Secretion of the inflammatory mediators IL-6 (Figure 5(a)) and IL-8 (Figure 5(b)) in the dry group was greater than in both the noninterventional comparator group and the HFNC groups at 8 hours ($P < 0.001$), with no significant difference noted between control and HFNC groups ($P > 0.05$) and no significant difference between any of the groups at 4 hours ($P > 0.05$).

At 4 hours and 8 hours, the monolayers of the dry group demonstrated a dry, rough, and granular appearance upon visual (naked eye) inspection. Representative histological photomicrographs at 4 and 8 hours are presented in Figure 6. The dry group showed abnormal cellular appearances, swollen nuclei, intracellular and nuclear vacuoles, diffused cytoplasm, and cellular debris. Semi-quantitative assessment of cell morphology (Figure 7) did not show injury for the noninterventional comparator group or HFNC groups at 4 and 8 hours, whereas the dry group demonstrated increasing histological evidence of injury over time.

dry groups were less than the noninterventional comparator group independent of time ($P < 0.01$). In addition, the TER of monolayers exposed to high humidity decreased less than those exposed to low humidity at both time points ($P < 0.001$).

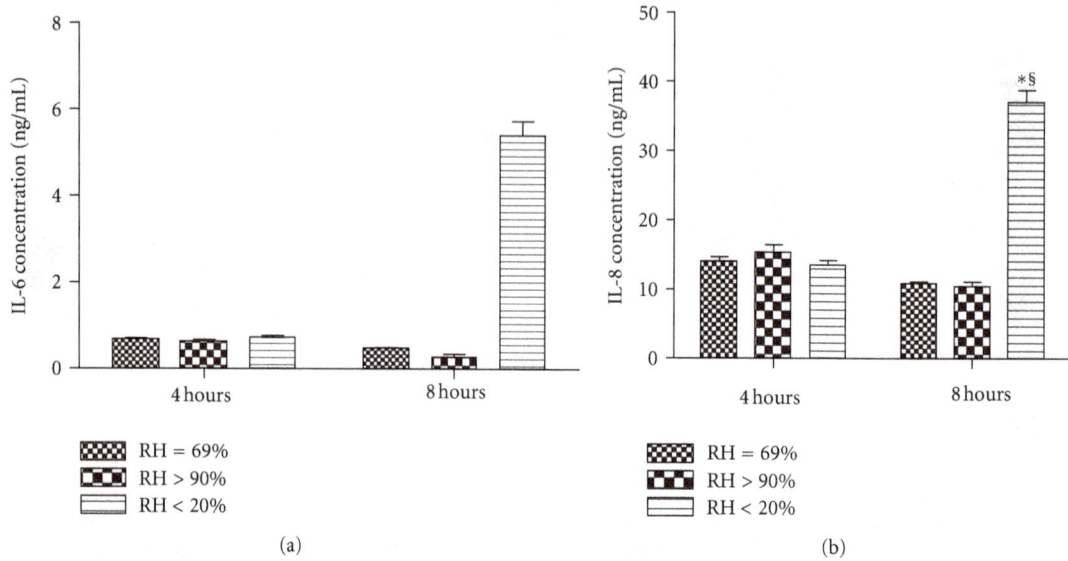

(a)

(b)

FIGURE 5: Proinflammatory mediator concentration in apical surface wash fluid from Calu-3 monolayers exposed to one of three levels of relative humidity: <20% (dry), 69% (noninterventional comparator), and >90% (HFNC). Secretion of interleukin (IL)-6 (5A) and IL-8 (5B) in the dry group was greater than the noninterventional comparator group and the HFNC groups at 8 hours ($P < 0.001$), with no difference between the noninterventional comparator group and the HFNC groups ($P > 0.05$) and no difference between any groups at 4 hours ($P > 0.05$). Data are mean ± SEM. *Group effect ($P < 0.05$). §Time effect ($P < 0.05$).

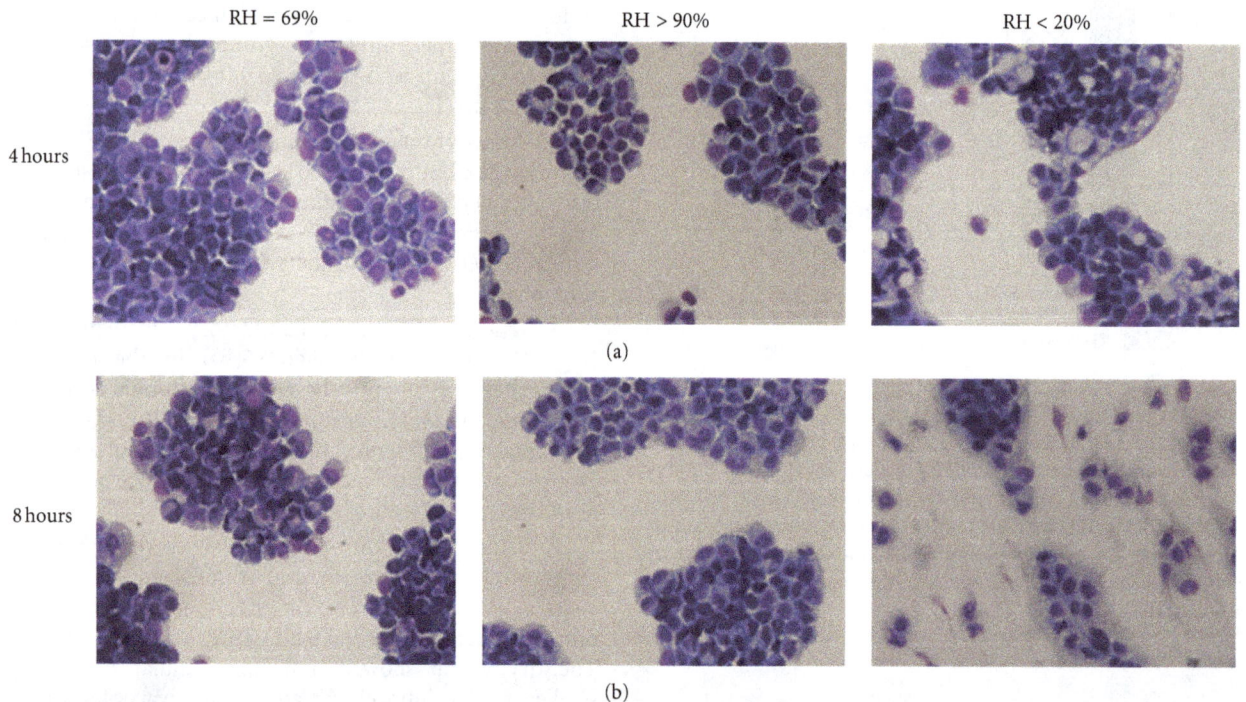

FIGURE 6: Cytomorphological examination of Calu-3 cell monolayers exposed to one of three levels of relative humidity: <20% (dry), 69% (noninterventional comparator), and >90% (HFNC). Representative cytomorphological examination of Calu-3 cells for both the noninterventional comparator group and the HFNC group demonstrated normal morphology. At 4 and 8 hours, the dry group showed abnormal cellular appearances, swollen nuclei, intracellular and nuclear vacuoles, diffused cytoplasm, and cellular debris. All cytospins were examined by light microscopy at 40x magnification.

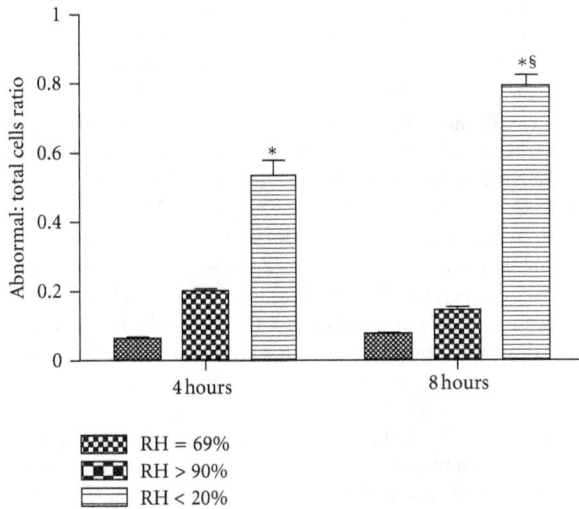

FIGURE 7: Semi-quantitative assessment of cell morphology as the ratio of abnormal cells to total cells. Histological analysis did not show injury for the noninterventional comparator or the high flow nasal cannula groups at 4 and 8 hours, whereas the dry group demonstrated increasing injury over time. Data are mean ± SEM. *Group effect ($P < 0.05$). §Time effect ($P < 0.05$). $n = 6$/condition.

4. Discussion

In this study, we used Calu-3 cells in an *in vitro* model to evaluate the effects of inspired gas humidification on the structure and function of cultured human airway epithelial cells. This study shows the effectiveness of maintaining a specific homeostatic temperature and level of humidity to optimize cell function in Calu-3 airway monolayers. These experiments demonstrate that humidification therapy is beneficial to the maintenance of cellular structure and function in that it enhances Calu-3 monolayer integrity, betters cell viability and morphology, and reduces airway epithelial inflammation compared to cells exposed to a dry condition over an 8-hour exposure time.

In this study, TER was measured for examination of the integrity of the monolayers [26] and the formation of functional intercellular tight junctions [27]. During the experiment, low humidity (less than 20%) decreased TER and cell viability over time compared with both HFNC-treated and noninterventional comparator groups. There was a partial deterioration in TER even in the HFNC-treated monolayers. This may be due to shear forces to which these monolayers are exposed, independently of gas humidification. A study showed that gas delivered by HFNC was more humid than nasal cannula and continuous positive airway pressure; however, the higher pressure and resistance delivered by the HFNC system may cause excessive expiratory pressure loading [28] and may also result in airway injury by this mechanism. We attempted to correct for pressure loading of the monolayers in our experiments by leaving the modular incubator chamber closed but unsealed by the pressure gasket.

These findings were also consistent with the findings in the histological analyses. Calu-3 cells in the dry group demonstrated disrupted morphology at 4 and 8 hours. Both the noninterventional comparator group and HFNC groups maintained normal cell morphology over 8 hours. Histological analysis did not show injury for the noninterventional comparator group or HFNC groups at 4 and 8 hours, whereas the dry group demonstrated increasing injury over time. In the current experiments, the decreased TER and cell viability indicated a loss of intracellular adhesion integrity, cellular membrane damage, and impaired cell metabolism after being exposed to low humidity for 8 hours.

In the dry group, the oxygen tank delivered the gas directly without adequate humidification at a flow rate of 10 L/min. This exacerbated the water evaporation from the surface of the monolayers in the modular incubator chamber. We speculate that the low humidity resulted in dehydration of Calu-3 cells, which was evident by the dry, rough, and granular appearance of the monolayers at 4 and 8 hours. The desiccation of the monolayers may have contributed to the disruption of intracellular adhesions and acute (necrotic) cell death with low humidity exposure.

Previous studies have shown that ASF and protein secretions in Calu-3 cultures are similar to those from primary airway cultures [29–31]. Total protein is a marker of cell membrane dysfunction and injury and is observed in noncardiogenic pulmonary edema states of acute lung injury in the clinical arena. In the current study, the secretion of total protein for Calu-3 monolayers increased over time in the dry group at 8 hours. There was no group effect between groups at 4 hours. These results demonstrate that low humidity induced higher protein secretion in the Calu-3 cells. We did not evaluate the mechanisms for this finding but speculate that it is also related to a nonspecific response to cell injury.

The pro-inflammatory mediators IL-6 and IL-8 are chemoattractant factors, which, *in vivo*, result in neutrophil infiltration and an exaggerated systemic inflammatory response [32]. IL-6 is a pleiotropic cytokine that is produced at sites of affected tissue. IL-8 plays an important role in the initiation and propagation of the inflammatory cascade and lung injury, primarily by neutrophil recruitment [30, 31, 33, 34]. The exposure of Calu-3 cell monolayers to low humidity (less than 20%) triggered Calu-3 cells to secrete increased levels of IL-6 and IL-8 compared with the noninterventional comparator group and HFNC group by 8 hours. In previous studies, we found that Calu-3 cells respond to pro-inflammatory stimuli, such as hyperoxia and pressure, in a graded fashion [25]. The results of the current experiments also suggest that airway drying causes an inflammatory response in a similar fashion. In addition, the inflammatory response observed in Calu-3 cell preparation was consistent with our previous animal study findings, which showed that physical and biological stimuli in the airway causes both systemic and local inflammation *in vivo*. In this regard, repeated intubation without mechanical ventilation and hyperoxia resulted in elevated levels of IL-6 in the tracheal tissue, aspirates, and plasma in a neonatal porcine model [35]. In another study, it was shown that after 4 hours of positive mechanical ventilation, secretion of heat shock protein (HSP70), a marker of tissue injury and inflammation modulation, increased in the tracheal wash fluid from a neonatal lamb airway [36].

In conclusion, after 4 hours, there was a significant detrimental effect of low humidification as a function of time on Calu-3 monolayers, TER, and cell viability for the dry group. After 8 hours, low humidity triggered Calu-3 cells to secrete increased levels of total protein, IL-6, and IL-8. These effects were ameliorated or eliminated with the use of HFNC. The study demonstrates findings that may have potential clinical relevance of inspired gas humidification for even short periods of time since exposure to low humidity results in worsened epithelial cell function and in inflammatory indices.

Acknowledgments

The authors thank Barbara E. Gray, BA, CPM, Administrative Manager, Nemours Research Lung Center, for her contribution to the research effort. This study was funded by NIH COBRE Grant no. 8 P20 GM103464 (the Center for Pediatric Research). This work was performed at the Nemours Research Lung Center, Nemours/Alfred I. duPont Hospital for Children, Wilmington, DE.

References

[1] M. P. Shelly, G. M. Lloyd, and G. R. Park, "A review of the mechanisms and methods of humidification of inspired gases," *Intensive Care Medicine*, vol. 14, no. 1, pp. 1–9, 1988.

[2] J. D. Fulmer, G. L. Snider, and R. K. Albert, "ACCP-NHLBI national conference on oxygen therapy," *Chest*, vol. 86, no. 2, pp. 234–247, 1984.

[3] E. J. Campbell, M. D. Baker, and P. Crites-Silver, "Subjective effects of humidification of oxygen for delivery by nasal cannula: a prospective study," *Chest*, vol. 93, no. 2, pp. 289–293, 1988.

[4] M. P. Shelly, "The humidification and filtration functions of the airways," *Respiratory Care Clinics of North America*, vol. 12, no. 2, pp. 139–148, 2006.

[5] E. R. McFadden Jr., "Heat and water exchange in human airways," *American Review of Respiratory Disease*, vol. 146, pp. S8–S10, 1992.

[6] E. R. McFadden Jr., B. M. Pichurko, and H. F. Bowman, "Thermal mapping of the airways in humans," *Journal of Applied Physiology*, vol. 58, no. 2, pp. 564–570, 1985.

[7] Z. J. Kubicka, J. Limauro, and R. A. Darnall, "Heated, humidified high-flow nasal cannula therapy: yet another way to deliver continuous positive airway pressure?" *Pediatrics*, vol. 121, no. 1, pp. 82–88, 2008.

[8] J. S. Greenspan, M. R. Wolfson, and T. H. Shaffer, "Airway responsiveness to low inspired gas temperature in preterm neonates," *Journal of Pediatrics*, vol. 118, no. 3, pp. 443–445, 1991.

[9] L. S. On, P. Boonyongsunchai, S. Webb, L. Davies, P. M. A. Calverley, and R. W. Costello, "Function of pulmonary neuronal M_2 muscarinic receptors in stable chronic obstructive pulmonary disease," *American Journal of Respiratory and Critical Care Medicine*, vol. 163, no. 6, pp. 1320–1325, 2001.

[10] A. Doyle, M. Joshi, P. Frank, T. Craven, P. Moondi, and P. Young, "A change in humidification system can eliminate endotracheal tube occlusion," *Journal of Critical Care*, vol. 26, pp. 673.e1–673.e4, 2011.

[11] R. D. Branson and M. A. Gentile, "Is humidification always necessary during noninvasive ventilation in the hospital?" *Respiratory Care*, vol. 55, no. 2, pp. 209–216, 2010.

[12] B. Q. Shen, W. E. Finkbeiner, J. J. Wine, R. J. Mrsny, and J. H. Widdicombe, "Calu-3: a human airway epithelial cell line that shows cAMP-dependent Cl- secretion," *American Journal of Physiology*, vol. 266, no. 5, pp. L493–L501, 1994.

[13] A. C. Da Paula, A. S. Ramalho, C. M. Farinha et al., "Characterization of novel airway submucosal gland cell models for cystic fibrosis studies," *Cellular Physiology and Biochemistry*, vol. 15, no. 6, pp. 251–262, 2005.

[14] N. S. Joo, D. J. Lee, K. M. Winges, A. Rustagi, and J. J. Wine, "Regulation of antiprotease and antimicrobial protein secretion by airway submucosal gland serous cells," *Journal of Biological Chemistry*, vol. 279, no. 37, pp. 38854–38860, 2004.

[15] Y. Zhang, W. W. Reenstra, and A. Chidekel, "Antibacterial activity of apical surface fluid from the human airway cell line Calu-3: pharmacologic alteration by corticosteroids and $\beta2$-agonists," *American Journal of Respiratory Cell and Molecular Biology*, vol. 25, no. 2, pp. 196–202, 2001.

[16] C. I. Grainger, L. L. Greenwell, D. J. Lockley, G. P. Martin, and B. Forbes, "Culture of Calu-3 cells at the air interface provides a representative model of the airway epithelial barrier," *Pharmaceutical Research*, vol. 23, no. 7, pp. 1482–1490, 2006.

[17] Y. Zhu, A. Chidekel, and T. H. Shaffer, "Cultured human airway epithelial cells (Calu-3): a model of human respiratory function, structure, and inflammatory responses," *Critical Care Research and Practice*, vol. 2010, Article ID 394578, 8 pages, 2010.

[18] B. Forbes and C. Ehrhardt, "Human respiratory epithelial cell culture for drug delivery applications," *European Journal of Pharmaceutics and Biopharmaceutics*, vol. 60, no. 2, pp. 193–205, 2005.

[19] J. L. Sporty, L. Horálková, and C. Ehrhardt, "In vitro cell culture models for the assessment of pulmonary drug disposition," *Expert Opinion on Drug Metabolism and Toxicology*, vol. 4, no. 4, pp. 333–345, 2008.

[20] Y. Hirakata, H. Yano, K. Arai et al., "Monolayer culture systems with respiratory epithelial cells for evaluation of bacterial invasiveness," *Tohoku Journal of Experimental Medicine*, vol. 220, no. 1, pp. 15–19, 2010.

[21] D. C. Devor, A. K. Singh, L. C. Lambert, A. DeLuca, R. A. Frizzell, and R. J. Bridges, "Bicarbonate and chloride secretion in Calu-3 human airway epithelial cells," *Journal of General Physiology*, vol. 113, no. 5, pp. 743–760, 1999.

[22] H. L. Winton, H. Wan, M. B. Cannell et al., "Cell lines of pulmonary and non-pulmonary origin as tools to study the effects of house dust mite proteinases on the regulation of epithelial permeability," *Clinical and Experimental Allergy*, vol. 28, no. 10, pp. 1273–1285, 1998.

[23] C. E. Stewart, E. E. Torr, N. H. Mohd Jamili, C. Bosquillon, and I. Sayers, "Evaluation of differentiated human bronchial epithelial cell culture systems for asthma research," *Journal of Allergy*, vol. 2012, Article ID 943982, 11 pages, 2012.

[24] P. B. R. Babu, A. Chidekel, and T. H. Shaffer, "Hyperoxia-induced changes in human airway epithelial cells: the protective effect of perflubron," *Pediatric Critical Care Medicine*, vol. 6, no. 2, pp. 188–194, 2005.

[25] Y. Zhu, T. L. Miller, C. J. Singhaus, T. H. Shaffer, and A. Chidekel, "Effects of oxygen concentration and exposure time on cultured human airway epithelial cells," *Pediatric Critical Care Medicine*, vol. 9, no. 2, pp. 224–229, 2008.

[26] K. A. Foster, M. L. Avery, M. Yazdanian, and K. L. Audus, "Characterization of the Calu-3 cell line as a tool to screen pulmonary drug delivery," *International Journal of Pharmaceutics*, vol. 208, no. 1-2, pp. 1–11, 2000.

[27] N. R. Mathias, J. Timoszyk, P. I. Stetsko, J. R. Megill, R. L. Smith, and D. A. Wall, "Permeability characteristics of Calu-3 human bronchial epithelial cells: in vitro-in vitro correlation to predict lung absorption in rats," *Journal of Drug Targeting*, vol. 10, no. 1, pp. 31–40, 2002.

[28] G. Y. Chang, C. A. Cox, and T. H. Shaffer, "Nasal cannula, CPAP, and high-flow nasal cannula: effect of flow on temperature, humidity, pressure, and resistance," *Biomedical Instrumentation and Technology*, vol. 45, no. 1, pp. 69–74, 2011.

[29] J. J. Coalson, "Pathology of new bronchopulmonary dysplasia," *Seminars in Neonatology*, vol. 8, no. 1, pp. 73–81, 2003.

[30] U. K. . Munshi, J. O. Niu, M. M. Siddiq, and L. A. Parton, "Elevation of interleukin-8 and interleukin-6 precedes the influx of neutrophils in tracheal aspirates from preterm infants who develop bronchopulmonary dysplasia," *Pediatric Pulmonology*, vol. 24, pp. 331–336, 1997.

[31] K. Tullus, G. W. Noack, L. G. Burman, R. Nilsson, B. Wretlind, and A. Brauner, "Elevated cytokine levels in tracheobronchial aspirate fluids from ventilator treated neonates with bronchopulmonary dysplasia," *European Journal of Pediatrics*, vol. 155, no. 2, pp. 112–116, 1996.

[32] M. F. Krause, T. Wiemann, A. Reisner, M. Orlowska-Volk, H. Köhler, and T. Ankermann, "Surfactant reduces extravascular lung water and invasion of polymorphonuclear leukocytes into the lung in a piglet model of airway lavage," *Pulmonary Pharmacology and Therapeutics*, vol. 18, no. 2, pp. 129–139, 2005.

[33] R. J. Baier, J. Loggins, and T. E. Kruger, "Monocyte chemoattractant protein-1 and interleukin-8 are increased in bronchopulmonary dysplasia: relation to isolation of ureaplasma urealyticum," *Journal of Investigative Medicine*, vol. 49, no. 4, pp. 362–369, 2001.

[34] R. J. Baier, J. Loggins, and T. E. Kruger, "Increased interleukin-8 and monocyte chemoattractant protein-1 concentrations in mechanically ventilated preterm infants with pulmonary hemorrhage," *Pediatric Pulmonology*, vol. 34, no. 2, pp. 131–137, 2002.

[35] A. Oshodi, K. Dysart, A. Cook et al., "Airway injury resulting from repeated endotracheal intubation: possible prevention strategies," *Pediatric Critical Care Medicine*, vol. 12, no. 1, pp. e34–e39, 2011.

[36] E. Chong, K. C. Dysart, A. Chidekel, R. Locke, T. H. Shaffer, and T. L. Miller, "Heat shock protein 70 secretion by neonatal tracheal tissue during mechanical ventilation: association with indices of tissue function and modeling," *Pediatric Research*, vol. 65, no. 4, pp. 387–391, 2009.

9

Do We Need Exercise Tests to Detect Gas Exchange Impairment in Fibrotic Idiopathic Interstitial Pneumonias?

Benoit Wallaert,[1] Lidwine Wemeau-Stervinou,[1] Julia Salleron,[2] Isabelle Tillie-Leblond,[1] and Thierry Perez[1, 3]

[1] Clinique des Maladies Respiratoires, Centre de Compétence des Maladies Pulmonaires Rares, Hopital Calmette,
 Lille 2 University Boulevard Leclercq, CHRU, 59037 Lille, France
[2] Unité de Biostatistiques, CHRU, 59037 Lille, France
[3] Service d'Explorations Fonctionnelles Respiratoires, Hopital Calmette, CHRU, 59037 Lille, France

Correspondence should be addressed to Benoit Wallaert, benoit.wallaert@chru-lille.fr

Academic Editor: Marc A. Judson

In patients with fibrotic idiopathic interstitial pneumonia (f-IIP), the diffusing capacity for carbon monoxide (DLCO) has been used to predict abnormal gas exchange in the lung. However, abnormal values for arterial blood gases during exercise are likely to be the most sensitive manifestations of lung disease. The aim of this study was to compare DLCO, resting PaO_2, $P(A-a)O_2$ at cardiopulmonary exercise testing peak, and oxygen desaturation during a 6-min walk test (6MWT). Results were obtained in 121 patients with idiopathic pulmonary fibrosis (IPF, $n = 88$) and fibrotic nonspecific interstitial pneumonias (NSIP, $n = 33$). All but 3 patients (97.5%) had low DLCO values (<LLN) whereas only 66.6% had low KCO; 42 patients (65%) exhibited resting hypoxemia (<75 mmHg); 112 patients (92.5%) exhibited a high $P[(A-a)O_2]$, peak (>35 mmHg) and 100 (83%) demonstrated significant oxygen desaturation during 6MWT (>4%). Interestingly 27 patients had low DLCO and normal $P(A-a)O_2$, peak and/or no desaturation during the 6MWT. The 3 patients with normal DLCO also had normal PaO_2, normal $P(A-a)O_2$, peak, and normal oxygen saturation during 6MWT. Our results demonstrate that in fibrotic IIP, DLCO better defines impairment of pulmonary gas exchange than resting PaO_2, exercise $P(A-a)O_2$, peak, or 6MWT SpO_2.

1. Introduction

According to the ATS/ERS statement, fibrotic interstitial idiopathic pneumonia (f-IIP) includes idiopathic pulmonary fibrosis (IPF) and fibrotic nonspecific interstitial pneumonia (f-NSIP) [1–4]. Although pathological abnormalities are quite different between these two diseases [5], alteration of gas exchange is a major abnormality which is thought to reflect the severity of fibrotic process [6].

Given the simplicity of pulmonary function testing, many investigators have examined the potential for simple resting physiologic measurements to stratify disease severity. The classic physiologic findings in the fibrotic IIP include a reduction in lung volumes (vital capacity; total lung capacity), a reduction in carbon monoxide diffusing capacity (DLCO), and hypoxemia that worsens with exercise [2].

Evaluation of gas exchange impairment can be performed in clinical practice by simple tests like DLCO, resting PaO_2, and $P(A-a)O_2$, measurement of SpO_2 during a 6-min walk test (6MWT) or PaO_2 and alveolar-arterial oxygen pressure difference $P(A-a)O_2$ during cardiopulmonary exercise testing (CPET).

Whereas DLCO is a valuable tool in the assessment of the efficiency of pulmonary gas exchange, the $P(A-a)O_2$, especially during exercise, is thought to better reflect the normality of respiratory gas exchange [8, 9]. In addition exercise-induced gas exchange can also be readily identified by simple testing such as the 6MWT [10].

To the best of our knowledge, comparison of all the various methods to detect pulmonary gas exchange abnormalities has never been performed. Previous studies compared DLCO and $P(A-a)O_2$ in a small number of IPF patients but did not include 6MWT [9, 11] or analysed 6MWT oxygen desaturation but did not include analysis of exercise PaO_2 or $P(A\text{-}a)O_2$ [12, 13]. With this in mind we performed a retrospective analysis of resting and exercise tests in 138 consecutive patients with IPF or f-NSIP.

2. Patients and Methods

One hundred and thirty eight caucasian patients with a diagnosis of IPF or f-NSIP were consecutively referred for evaluation of dyspnea and CPET at the time of diagnosis or during followup, over a period of six years. Inclusion criteria consisted of diagnosis of IPF according to the American Thoracic Society/European Respiratory Society guidelines and/or histopathological evidence for usual interstitial pneumonia, or diagnosis of f-NSIP (radiographic or histopathological diagnosis) [1, 2]. Patients were not included if they had another pulmonary disease (including obstructive disease), left heart failure or a history of pulmonary embolism. Connective tissue diseases were ruled out. No acute exacerbation was observed in the three months preceding inclusion. Seventeen patients were excluded from the study because CPET was not performed (arthrosis). Therefore 121 patients (31 females, 90 males) were included. In 44 out of the 88 IPF patients and 20 out of the 33 patients with f-NSIP, diagnosis was confirmed by histopathological examination of lung biopsy. At the time of inclusion in the study, a majority of patients (76%) were not treated, 19 patients received corticosteroids, 12 patient received azathioprine, and 3 patients received mycophenolate mofetil. Clinical data and results of pulmonary function tests, 6MWT, and of CPET were collected. Only initial data were recorded when the patient was seen several times. Approval for the use of these data was provided by the Institutional Review Board of the French learned society for respiratory medicine (CEPRO 2011-039).

3. Pulmonary Function Tests

Forced vital capacity (FVC), forced expiratory volume in 1 second (FEV_1), and total lung capacity (TLC) were measured by spirometry and plethysmography with a Jaeger-Master lab cabin. Single-breath diffusing capacity of the lung for carbon monoxide (DLCO: $mLCO \cdot min^{-1} \cdot mmHg^{-1}$) and carbon monoxide transfer coefficient (KCO = DLCO/alveolar volume) were measured. DLCO was corrected for hemoglobin concentration in $g \cdot dL^{-1}$, according to Cotes' equation: corrected (Hb) DLCO = DLCO $\times$ (10.2 + Hb)/(1.7 $\times$ Hb). Values were expressed as percentages of the predicted normal values calculated according to gender, weight, and age. Reference equations for spirometry were taken from ERS for lung volumes and DLCO [14, 15]. Following ATS/ERS 2005 guidelines, the lower limits of normal (LLN) were set at the level of 5th percentile (or predicted minus 1.64 SD) of each reference population [16]. Results were conventionally expressed as percent predicted.

The 6MWT was performed in accordance with international recommendations [17] and was designed to ensure an accurate assessment of oxygen desaturation Patients were instructed as follows: "The object of this test is to walk as quickly as you can for 6 minutes to cover as much ground as possible. You may slow down if necessary. If you stop we wish you to continue the walk again as soon as possible. Your goal is to walk as fast and as far as you can in 6 minutes." [18]. The pulse oximeter was lightweight, battery powered, and held in place by a "fanny pack" so that the patient does not have to hold or stabilize it. We evaluated the oxygen saturation at rest and the lowest saturation during the test. A desaturation $\geq 4\%$ was considered as significant [2].

CPET was carried out using a standardized protocol as previously described [19] and consisted of a triangular test, carried out on an ergometric bicycle (Ergoline-Ergometrics 800). Briefly the expired gases were determined in each cycle with an Ergocard. During exercise, heart rate (HR) was monitored continually by 12-lead ECG and arterial oxygen saturation (SpO_2) was measured by pulse oximetry with a Nellcor N-395 apparatus. Arterial blood samples were obtained from a small catheter placed in the radial artery under local anesthesia. Measurements of PaO_2 and $PaCO_2$ were performed on room air at rest and at peak exercise. Normal values for PaO_2 were derived from Sorbini et al. [20]. The alveolar-arterial gradient in oxygen [$P(A\text{-}a)O_2$] was calculated from the alveolar gas equation. According to ATS statement, [$P(A\text{-}a)O_2$], peak >35 mmHg was considered as abnormal [21]. Exercise pulmonary gas exchange variables were either related or not related to the metabolic demand (VO_2), that is, peak exercise-rest (Δ) [19, 22]. The modified Bohr equation was used to calculate dead space to tidal volume ratio (VD/VT). Predicted values were calculated from reference equations [22, 23]. Poor motivation was not a factor interfering with our analysis as suggested by the fact that all of the patients had one or more of the following criteria: breathing reserve less than 15%, peak HR more than 90% of predicted, peak lactate more than 7 mEq/L, peak exercise PaO_2 less than 55 mmHg or peak VE/VO_2 more than 35 or RER >1.15 [24, 25].

4. Statistical Analysis

After certification of normal distribution, data are reported as mean $\pm$ SD. Student's t-test was used to determine differences between IPF and f-NSIP. Differences in proportions were assessed by $\chi 2$ tests. Correlations were analysed using Spearman's rank correlation test. All statistical analysises were carried out with GraphPad Prism 4.0 software (San Diego, Calif, USA). Values of $P < 0.05$ were considered significant.

5. Results

Characteristics of the population are summarized in Table 1. The overall population consisted of 90 men and 31 women with a mean age of 63.6 $\pm$ 8.4 years: 88 patients had a diagnostic of IPF and 33 of f-NSIP. Pulmonary function tests results are shown in Tables 1 and 2. As expected, we observed a reduction in TLC, VC, and FEV_1, a reduced DLCO and

TABLE 1: Pulmonary function tests results.

	All patients $n = 121$	IPF $n = 88$	f-NSIP $n = 33$
Age	63.6 ± 8.4	64.3 ± 8.3	61.6 ± 8.5
BMI	28.4 ± 4.4	28.2 ± 4.1	29.1 ± 5.1
TLC (L)	4.35 ± 1	4.39 ± 1.01	4.23 ± 1
TLC (%)	70 ± 14.5	69.4 ± 14.6	73 ± 13.9
% with low TLC	76	82	62
FVC (L)	2.72 ± 0.74	2.77 ± 0.72	2.61 ± 0.8
FVC (%)	76 ± 16	75.5 ± 16.9	77.2 ± 13.6
% with low FVC	61	58	65
FEV_1 (L/sec)	2.24 ± 0.58	2.26 ± 0.57	2.12 ± 0.6
FEV_1 (%)	78.5 ± 16.4	78.4 ± 17.2	78.8 ± 14.1
% with low FEV_1	55	52	62
DLCO ($mLCO \cdot min^{-1} \cdot mmHg^{-1}$)	11.2 ± 4	11.17 ± 4.4	11.3 ± 3.2
DLCO (%)	42.9 ± 12.3	41.9 ± 12.5	45.6 ± 11.6
% with low DLCO	98	98	97
KCO ($mLCO \cdot min^{-1} \cdot mmHg^{-1}/L$)	2.99 ± 0.76	2.92 ± 0.77	3.2 ± 0.7
KCO (%)	71.3 ± 17	70.3 ± 17.7	74.2 ± 3.7
% with low KCO	66.6	70	56
PaO_2, rest (mmHg)	76.8 ± 12.6	75.9 ± 12.8	79.4 ± 12
% with low PaO_2	42	46	31
P(A-a) O_2, rest (mmHg)	30.8 ± 12.5	31.4 ± 12.6	29.2 ± 12.2
% with low P(A-a) O_2, rest	26	30	16

TABLE 2: Cardiopulmonary exercise testing and walking test results.

	All patients $n = 121$	IPF $n = 88$	f-NSIP $n = 33$
Workload, peak (Watts)	81.4 ± 24	82.5 ± 23.7	78.3 ± 25.9
Workload, peak (%)	71.3 ± 9.9	61.2 ± 18.8	67.2 ± 24.8
VO_2, peak (mL/Kg/min)	15.9 ± 3.9	15.9 ± 3.6	15.9 ± 4.6
VO_2, peak (%)	66.5 ± 15.7	66 ± 15	67.8 ± 17.7
% low VO2, peak (%)	84	87	80
PaO_2, peak (mmHg)	57.9 ± 13	56.6 ± 12.9	61.6 ± 12.6
ΔPaO_2 (mmHg)	18.9 ± 8.3	19.4 ± 8.5	17.6 ± 7.8
P(A-a)O_2, peak (mmHg)	58.1 ± 13	58.9 ± 13.2	61.7 ± 12.7
% with high P(A-a)O_2, peak	92.5	95	84
$\Delta P(A-a)O_2/\Delta VO_2$ (mmHg/L)	34.2 ± 16.9	34.4 ± 17.1	33.6 ± 16.7
% with high $\Delta P(A-a)O_2/\Delta VO_2$	83	82	84
VD/VT, peak	0.43 ± 0.09	0.44 ± 0.09	$0.39 \pm 0.08^*$
Walk test, distance (m)	388 ± 102	393 ± 98	375 ± 114
Walt test, nadir SaO_2 (%)	86 ± 5.7	85.6 ± 6	88.3 ± 4.6
Walk test, ΔSaO_2 (%)	9.2 ± 4.7	9.7 ± 5	7.9 ± 3.7
% with $\Delta SaO_2 \geq 4\%$	83	83	84

* Significantly different from IPF group ($P = 0.01$).

KCO. DLCO was reduced to a greater extent than the lung volumes: 45 out of 121 patients (37%) showed a normal FVC and 24% a normal TLC despite a low DLCO.

All but 3 Patients (97.5%) had low DLCO values (<LLN, corresponding to a mean $73 \pm 0.4\%$ predicted) whereas only 66.6% had a low KCO; 42% patients exhibited resting hypoxemia (<75 mmHg) and 26% a high resting P(A-a)O_2; 112 patients (92.5%) exhibited an increased P[(A-a)O_2],

peak, 83% a high $\Delta P(A-a)O_2/\Delta VO_2$ and 100 patients (83%) demonstrated significant O_2 desaturation during 6MWT. There was no significant difference between IPF and f-NSIP for all parameters except VD/VT peak which was higher in IPF ($P = 0.01$).

DLCO was severely reduced in the 79 patients with normal resting PaO_2. Interestingly 27 patients had low DLCO and normal P(A-a)O_2, peak and/or no desaturation during

TABLE 3: Correlation between percent-predicted DLco and other measures.

Variable	coefficient	P value
FVC	0.56	<0.0001
TLC	0.437	<0.0001
FEV$_1$	0.508	<0.0001
Kco	0.56	<0.0001
Resting PaO$_2$	0.525	<0.0001
P(A-a)O$_2$, peak (mmHg)	−0.465	<0.0001
ΔP(A-a)O$_2$/ ΔVO$_2$ (mmHg/L)	−0.534	<0.0001
6MWT, nadir SpO$_2$ (%)	0.511	<0.0001
6MWT, ΔSpO$_2$ (%)	−0.47	<0.0001
VD/VT, peak	−0.404	<0.0001

the 6MWT. Nine patients had normal P(A-a)O$_2$, peak: 6 out of 9 did not show significant desaturation during walk test. Conversely among the 21 patients with low DLCO and without significant desaturation at the 6MWT, all had abnormal P(A-a)O$_2$, peak. The 3 patients with normal DLCO also had normal PaO$_2$, normal P(A-a)O$_2$, peak, and normal oxygen saturation during 6MWT.

We found a very good correlation between DLCO and lung volumes and other measures of gas exchange (Table 3 and Figure 1). Interestingly we also found a good correlation between DLCO and VD/VT.

Resting parameters and indexes of gas exchange were more severely altered according to disease severity as judged on alteration of DLCO (Table 4).

6. Discussion

There were three main findings in this study: first, abnormal gas exchange is present in patients with normal lung volumes; second, a low DLCO was found in 97.5% patients with f-IIP whereas resting PaO$_2$, 6MWT oxygen desaturation and P(A-a)O$_2$, peak were abnormal, respectively, in 42%, 83%, and 92.5%; and third, no patient had normal DLCO and abnormal PaO$_2$, 6MWT oxygen desaturation, or increased P(A-a)O$_2$, peak. As a consequence, DLCO is more sensitive for demonstrating gas exchange abnormality in fibrotic IIP than resting PaO$_2$, exercise P(A-a)O$_2$, peak, or 6MWT SpO$_2$.

Clearly, DLCO is reduced in a greater extent than lung volumes in f-IIP and therefore abnormal DLCO is a frequent finding in patients with normal lung volumes. This has been demonstrated in previous studies [26, 27], both in IPF and f-NSIP [28–39]. Along this line, Gaensler and coworkers noted a fair correlation between histologic severity and physiologic indices [38]. Crystal and colleagues reported a poor correlation with spirometry, lung volumes, DLCO, and resting gas exchange in IPF [39]. In 14 untreated patients with IPF, DLCO, and lung volumes correlated with the extent of fibrosis and cellular infiltration; both of these correlated more strongly than gas exchange with exercise [6].

In patients with f-IIP, the DLCO has been widely used to predict abnormal gas exchange in the lung. Resting PaO$_2$ correlates poorly with disease severity. In our studies, resting PaO$_2$ was in the normal range in 58% cases. In contrast, abnormal values for arterial blood gases during exercise are more sensitive than resting PaO$_2$. However our study in a large group of patients demonstrated that patients with abnormal gas exchange during exercise always exhibited abnormal DLCO and that, in contrast, abnormal DLCO was found in patients with normal gas exchange during exercise. A significant 6MWT oxygen desaturation and/or an increased P(A-a)O$_2$ was never observed in f-IIP patients with normal DLCO whereas this has been previously reported in sarcoidosis [40, 41].

Our 6MWT results are in agreement with the results of Lama and coworkers [18] who reported 6MWT oxygen desaturation results in IPF and NSIP: in this study, 80% IPF patients and 64% NSIP patients exhibited an oxygen desaturation ≥4% during 6MWT. The 6MWT is a noninvasive, cheap, and simple field test to carry out and interpret. However despite these advantages, some variabilities in the results obtained are observed [42] and an increased ventilatory response during 6MWT might be responsible for higher PAO$_2$ minimizing the decrease in SaO$_2$.

Factors that contribute to reduction in DLCO include abnormal thickness of the alveolar capillary membrane and reduced pulmonary capillary blood volume. Thus, DLCO is highly dependent on pulmonary vascular blood volume. We recently reported in patients with f-IIP that the Vc component of the DLCO was significantly decreased in addition to the already lowered Dm, CO component as a consequence of the thickened membranes [43]. The correlation between DLCO and VD/VT, peak is in agreement with the findings by Agusti and coworkers [8] and supports the concept that the abnormalities of the pulmonary vasculature are important to modulate gas exchange in IPF during exercise.

It was not the scope of our study to evaluate the prognostic value of each test. Several studies found that distance or desaturation during a 6MWT was a strong predictor of mortality [18]. Mortality rate is higher among patients with DLCO <30% to 45% predicted [33, 44–46], but it is clear that the prognostic value of any pulmonary functional parameter at one point is limited.

In conclusion, DLCO appears as the best physiologic index to evaluate gas exchange abnormalities in fibrotic IIP and could take the place of formal exercise testing with arterial blood gas to evaluate the severity of gas exchange in patients with fibrotic IIP.

Author's Contribution

Benoit Wallaert and LidwineWemeau-Stervinou were responsible for Conception and design; Benoit Wallaert, LidwineWemeau-Stervinou, Julia Salleron, Isabelle Tillie-Leblond, and Thierry Perez were responsible for analysis and interpretation; BenoitWallaert, LidwineWemeau-Stervinou, Isabelle Tillie-Leblond, and Thierry Perez were responsible for drafting the paper for important intellectual content.

TABLE 4: Rest and exercise parameters as a function of disease severity defined by DLco%: mild: DLco $\geq$ 60%, moderate: DLco < 60% and $\geq$40% and severe (advanced disease): DLco < 40% [7].

Disease severity	Mild	Moderate	Severe
Parameter	Dlco $\geq$ 60%	40% $\leq$ DLco < 60%	DLco < 40%
	$n = 10$	$n = 65$	$n = 46$
FVC	99 ± 20	77 ± 11*	69 ± 16$^{\$**}$
FEV1	99 ± 19	81 ± 12*	70 ± 16$^{\$£}$
TLC	89 ± 13	70 ± 11*	66 ± 16$^{\$}$
PaO$_2$, rest (mmHg)	89 ± 6.4	80 ± 9*	69 ± 13.7$^{\$**}$
PaO$_2$, peak (mmHg)	78.7 ± 9	59 ± 10*	51 ± 11$^{\$**}$
P(A-a)O$_2$, rest (mmHg)	22 ± 9	27 ± 9.8	38 ± 13$^{\$**}$
P(A-a)O$_2$, peak (mmHg)	40 ± 7	57 ± 12*	64 ± 12$^{\$£}$
ΔP(A-a)O$_2$/ΔVO$_2$ (mmHg/L)	14.8 ± 11	31 ± 12.5*	44 ± 18$^{\$**}$
Walt test, nadir SaO$_2$ (%)	92 ± 3	87 ± 4*	83 ± 6$^{\$**}$
Walk test, ΔSaO$_2$ (%)	4.3 ± 2.4	8.4 ± 3.8*	11.5 ± 5.2$^{\$**}$

Significantly different from group moderate $^{£}P$ < 0.001, $^{**}P$ < 0.01.
Significantly different from group mild $^{\$}P$ < 0.001, $^{*}P$ < 0.01.

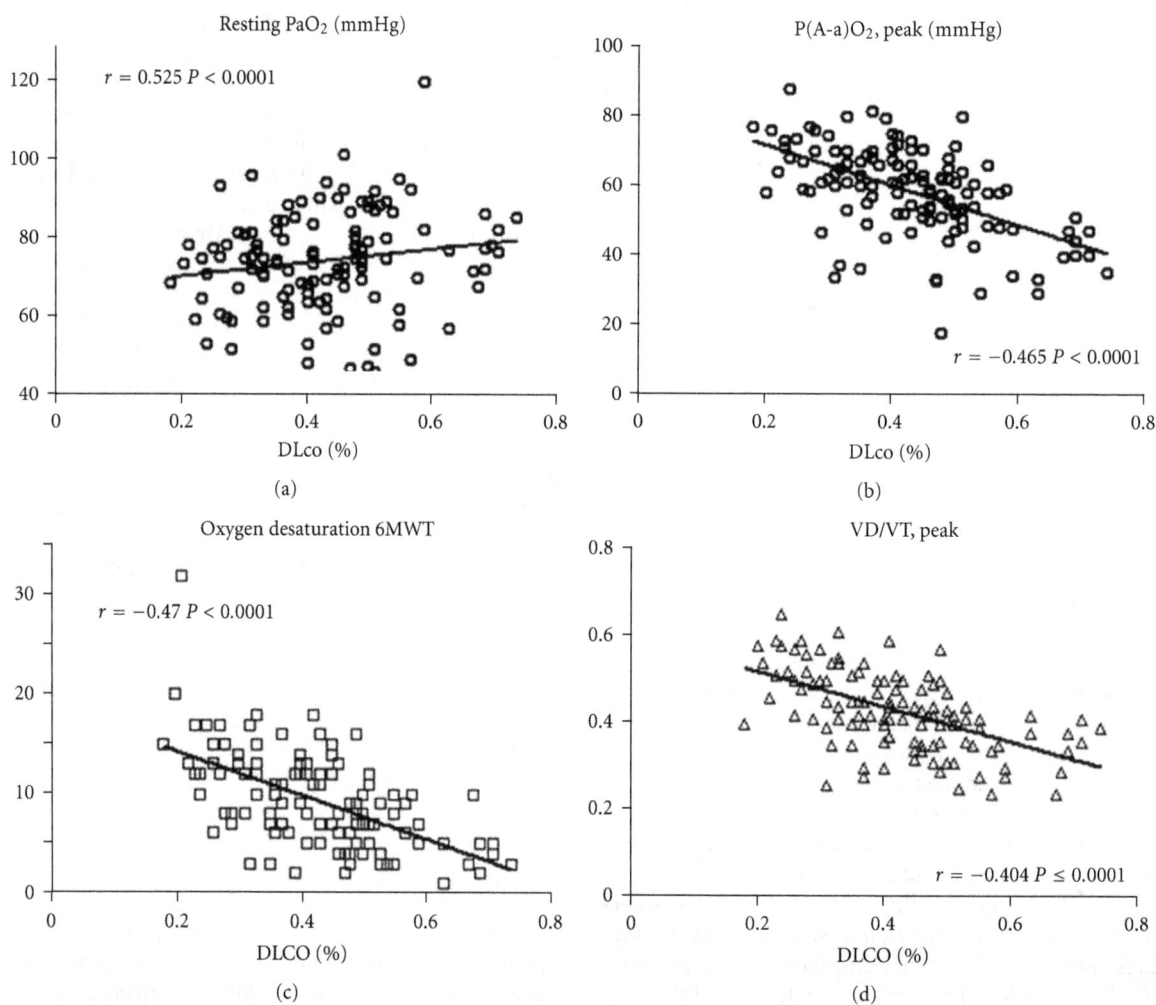

FIGURE 1: Correlation between DLCO (percent predicted) and resting PaO$_2$, P(A-a)O$_2$, peak, oxygen desaturation during 6MWT and VD/VT, peak in fibrotic IIP.

Conflict of Interests

For each author, no significant conflict of interest exist with any companies/organizations whose products or services may be discussed in this paper.

References

[1] American Thoracic Society and European Respiratory Society, "American Thoracic Society/European Respiratory Society International Multidisciplinary Consensus Classification of the Idiopathic Interstitial Pneumonias. This joint statement of the American Thoracic Society (ATS), and the European Respiratory Society (ERS) was adopted by the ATS board of directors, June 2001 and by the ERS Executive Committee," *American Journal of Respiratory and Critical Care Medicine*, vol. 165, no. 2, pp. 277–304, 2002.

[2] American Thoracic Society, "Idiopathic pulmonary fibrosis: diagnosis and treatment. International consensus statement. American Thoracic Society (ATS), and the European Respiratory Society (ERS)," *American Journal of Respiratory and Critical Care Medicine*, vol. 161, no. 2, part 1, pp. 646–664, 2000.

[3] B. Bradley, H. M. Branley, and J. J. Egan, "Interstitial lung disease guideline: the British Thoracic Society in collaboration with the Thoracic Society of Australia and New Zealand and the Irish Thoracic Society," *Thorax*, vol. 63, no. 5, pp. v1–v58, 2008.

[4] G. Raghu, H. R. Collard, J. J. Egan et al., "An Official ATS/ERS/JRS/ALAT Statement: idiopathic pulmonary fibrosis: evidence-based guidelines for diagnosis and management," *American Journal of Respiratory and Critical Care Medicine*, vol. 183, no. 6, pp. 788–824, 2011.

[5] A. L. Katzenstein, "Idiopathic interstitial pneumonia: classification and diagnosis," *Monographs in Pathology*, pp. 1–31, 1993.

[6] J. D. Fulmer, W. C. Roberts, E. R. von Gal, and R. G. Crystal, "Morphologic-physiologic correlates of the severity of fibrosis and degree of cellularity in idiopathic pulmonary fibrosis," *Journal of Clinical Investigation*, vol. 63, no. 4, pp. 665–676, 1979.

[7] J. J. Egan, F. J. Martinez, A. U. Wells, and T. Williams, "Lung function estimates in idiopathic pulmonary fibrosis: the potential for a simple classification," *Thorax*, vol. 60, no. 4, pp. 270–273, 2005.

[8] A. G. N. Agusti, J. Roca, J. Gea, P. D. Wagner, A. Xaubet, and R. Rodriguez-Roisin, "Mechanisms of gas-exchange impairment in idiopathic pulmonary fibrosis," *American Review of Respiratory Disease*, vol. 143, no. 2, pp. 219–225, 1991.

[9] C. Risk, G. R. Epler, and E. A. Gaensler, "Exercise alveolar-arterial oxygen pressure difference in interstitial lung disease," *Chest*, vol. 85, no. 1, pp. 69–74, 1984.

[10] T. S. Hallstrand, L. J. Boitano, W. C. Johnson, C. A. Spada, J. G. Hayes, and G. Raghu, "The timed walk test as a measure of severity and survival in idiopathic pulmonary fibrosis," *European Respiratory Journal*, vol. 25, no. 1, pp. 96–103, 2005.

[11] C. Agusti, A. Xaubet, A. G. N. Agusti, J. Roca, J. Ramirez, and R. Rodriguez-Roisin, "Clinical and functional assessment of patients with idiopathic pulmonary fibrosis: results of a 3 year follow-up," *European Respiratory Journal*, vol. 7, no. 4, pp. 643–650, 1994.

[12] R. M. Cherniack, T. V. Colby, A. Flint et al., "Correlation of structure and function in idiopathic pulmonary fibrosis," *American Journal of Respiratory and Critical Care Medicine*, vol. 151, no. 4, pp. 1180–1188, 1995.

[13] A. Xaubet, C. Agustí, P. Luburich et al., "Pulmonary function tests and CT scan in the management of idiopathic pulmonary fibrosis," *American Journal of Respiratory and Critical Care Medicine*, vol. 158, no. 2, pp. 431–436, 1998.

[14] J. Stocks and P. H. Quanjer, "Reference values for residual volume, functional residual capacity and total lung capacity: ATS Workshop on Lung Volume Measurements Official Statement of the European Respiratory Society," *European Respiratory Journal*, vol. 8, no. 3, pp. 492–506, 1995.

[15] "Standardized lung function testing. Official statement of the European Respiratory Society," *The European Respiratory Journal. Supplement*, vol. 16, pp. 1–100, 1993.

[16] R. Pellegrino, G. Viegi, V. Brusasco et al., "Interpretative strategies for lung function tests," *European Respiratory Journal*, vol. 26, no. 5, pp. 948–968, 2005.

[17] "ATS statement: guidelines for the six-minute walk test," *American Journal of Respiratory and Critical Care Medicine*, vol. 1, no. 166, pp. 111–117, 2002.

[18] V. N. Lama, K. R. Flaherty, G. B. Toews et al., "Prognostic value of desaturation during a 6 minute walk test in idiopathic interstitial pneumonia," *American Journal of Respiratory and Critical Care Medicine*, vol. 168, no. 9, pp. 1084–1090, 2003.

[19] B. Wallaert, C. Talleu, L. Wemeau-Stervinou, A. Duhamel, S. Robin, and B. Aguilaniu, "Reduction of maximal oxygen uptake in sarcoidosis: relationship with disease severity," *Respiration*, vol. 82, pp. 501–508, 2011.

[20] C. A. Sorbini, V. Grassi, E. Solinas, and G. Muiesan, "Arterial oxygen tension in relation to age in healthy subjects," *Respiration*, vol. 25, no. 1, pp. 3–13, 1968.

[21] "ATS/ACCP Statement on cardiopulmonary exercise testing," *American Journal of Respiratory and Critical Care Medicine*, vol. 167, pp. 211–277, 2003.

[22] C. Cooper and T. Storer, *Exercise Testing and Interpretation. A Practical Approach*, Cambridge, UK, 2001.

[23] N. L. Jones, *Clinical Exercise Testing*, WB Saunders, Philadelphia, Pa, USA, 1997.

[24] K. Wasserman, J. E. Hansen, D. Y. Sue, R. Casaburi, and B. J. Whipp, *Principles of Exercise Testing and Interpretation*, 3rd edition, 1999.

[25] B. Aguilaniu, R. Richard, F. Costes et al., "Cardiopulmonary exercise testing," *Revue des Maladies Respiratoires*, vol. 24, no. 3, part 2, pp. 2S111–2S160, 2007.

[26] T. L. Dunn, L. C. Watters, C. Hendrix, R. M. Cherniack, M. I. Schwarz, and T. E. King, "Gas exchange at a given degree of volume restriction is different in sarcoidosis and idiopathic pulmonary fibrosis," *American Journal of Medicine*, vol. 85, no. 2, pp. 221–224, 1988.

[27] B. A. Keogh, E. Lakatos, D. Price, and R. G. Crystal, "Importance of the lower respiratory tract in oxygen transfer. Exercise testing in patients with interstitial and destructive lung disease," *American Review of Respiratory Disease*, vol. 129, no. 2, pp. S76–S80, 1984.

[28] R. Erbes, T. Schaberg, and R. Loddenkemper, "Lung function tests in patients with idiopathic pulmonary fibrosis: are they helpful for predicting outcome?" *Chest*, vol. 111, no. 1, pp. 51–57, 1997.

[29] S. Nagai, M. Kitaichi, H. Itoh, K. Nishimura, T. Izumi, and T. V. Colby, "Idiopathic nonspecific interstitial pneumonia/fibrosis: comparison with idiopathic pulmonary fibrosis and BOOP," *European Respiratory Journal*, vol. 12, no. 3, pp. 1010–1019, 1998.

[30] J. A. Bjoraker, J. H. Ryu, M. K. Edwin et al., "Prognostic sig-nificance of histopathologic subsets in idiopathic pulmonary fibrosis," *American Journal of Respiratory and Critical Care Medicine*, vol. 157, no. 1, pp. 199–203, 1998.

[31] Z. D. Daniil, F. C. Gilchrist, A. G. Nicholson et al., "A histologic pattern of nonspecific interstitial pneumonia is associated with a better prognosis than usual interstitial pneumonia in patients with cryptogenic fibrosing alveolitis," *American Journal of Respiratory and Critical Care Medicine*, vol. 160, no. 3, pp. 899–905, 1999.

[32] A. G. Nicholson, T. V. Colby, R. M. Dubois, D. M. Hansell, and A. U. Wells, "The prognostic significance of the histologic pattern of interstitial pneumonia in patients presenting with the clinical entity of cryptogenic fibrosing alveolitis," *American Journal of Respiratory and Critical Care Medicine*, vol. 162, no. 6, pp. 2213–2217, 2000.

[33] N. Mogulkoc, M. H. Brutsche, P. W. Bishop, S. M. Greaves, A. W. Horrocks, and J. J. Egan, "Pulmonary function in idiopathic pulmonary fibrosis and referral for lung trans-plantation," *American Journal of Respiratory and Critical Care Medicine*, vol. 164, no. 1, pp. 103–108, 2001.

[34] P. I. Latsi, R. M. Du Bois, A. G. Nicholson et al., "Fibrotic idiopathic interstitial pneumonia: the prognostic value of lon-gitudinal functional trends," *American Journal of Respiratory and Critical Care Medicine*, vol. 168, no. 5, pp. 531–537, 2003.

[35] H. R. Collard, T. E. King, B. B. Bartelson, J. S. Vourlekis, M. I. Schwarz, and K. K. Brown, "Changes in clinical and physiologic variables predict survival in idiopathic pulmonary fibrosis," *American Journal of Respiratory and Critical Care Medicine*, vol. 168, no. 5, pp. 538–542, 2003.

[36] K. R. Flaherty, J. A. Mumford, S. Murray et al., "Prognostic implications of physiologic and radiographic changes in idio-pathic interstitial pneumonia," *American Journal of Respiratory and Critical Care Medicine*, vol. 168, no. 5, pp. 543–548, 2003.

[37] Y. Jegal, S. K. Dong, S. S. Tae et al., "Physiology is a stronger predictor of survival than pathology in fibrotic interstitial pneumonia," *American Journal of Respiratory and Critical Care Medicine*, vol. 171, no. 6, pp. 639–644, 2005.

[38] E. A. Gaensler and C. B. Carrington, "Open biopsy for chronic diffuse infiltrative lung disease: clinical, roentgenographic, and physiological correlations in 502 patients," *The Annals of Thoracic Surgery*, vol. 30, no. 5, pp. 411–426, 1980.

[39] R. G. Crystal, J. D. Fulmer, W. C. Roberts, M. L. Moss, B. R. Line, and H. Y. Reynolds, "Idiopathic pulmonary fibrosis. Clinical, histologic, radiographic, physiologic, scinti-graphic, cytologic, and biochemical aspects," *Annals of Internal Medicine*, vol. 85, no. 6, pp. 769–788, 1976.

[40] A. Miller, L. K. Brown, M. F. Sloane, A. Bhuptani, and A. S. Teirstein, "Cardiorespiratory responses to incremental exercise in sarcoidosis patients with normal spirometry," *Chest*, vol. 107, no. 2, pp. 323–329, 1995.

[41] M. Karetzky and M. McDonough, "Exercise and resting pulmonary function in sarcoidosis," *Sarcoidosis Vasculitis and Diffuse Lung Disease*, vol. 13, no. 1, pp. 43–49, 1996.

[42] E. H. Elpern, D. Stevens, and S. Kesten, "Variability in performance of timed walk tests in pulmonary rehabilitation programs," *Chest*, vol. 118, no. 1, pp. 98–105, 2000.

[43] L. Wémeau-Stervinou, T. Perez, C. Murphy, A.-S. Polge, and B. Wallaert, "Lung capillary blood volume and membrane diffusion in idiopathic interstitial pneumonia," *Respiratory Medicine*, vol. 106, pp. 564–570, 2012.

[44] T. E. King Jr., S. Safrin, K. M. Starko et al., "Analyses of efficacy end points in a controlled trial of interferon-γ1b for idiopathic pulmonary fibrosis," *Chest*, vol. 127, no. 1, pp. 171–177, 2005.

[45] D. A. Lynch, J. D. Godwin, S. Safrin et al., "High-resolution computed tomography in idiopathic pulmonary fibrosis: diagnosis and prognosis," *American Journal of Respiratory and Critical Care Medicine*, vol. 172, no. 4, pp. 488–493, 2005.

[46] G. Raghu, K. K. Brown, W. Z. Bradford et al., "A placebo-controlled trial of interferon Gamma-1b in patients with idiopathic pulmonary fibrosis," *The New England Journal of Medicine*, vol. 350, no. 2, pp. 125–133, 2004.

10

Intravascular Talcosis due to Intravenous Drug Use Is an Underrecognized Cause of Pulmonary Hypertension

Christopher C. Griffith,[1] Jay S. Raval,[1,2] and Larry Nichols[1]

[1] Department of Pathology, University of Pittsburgh Medical Center, Pittsburgh, PA 15213, USA
[2] The Institute for Transfusion Medicine, Pittsburgh, PA 15220, USA

Correspondence should be addressed to Christopher C. Griffith, griffithc@upmc.edu

Academic Editor: Kewal Asosingh

Intravenous injection of illegal drugs or medications meant for oral administration can cause granulomatous disease of the lung. This intravascular talcosis results in pulmonary fibrosis and pulmonary hypertension. Nine cases of histologically confirmed intravascular talcosis were reviewed with specific attention given to the clinical histories in these patients. Five autopsy cases were included in this series with detailed investigation in the anatomic features associated with intravascular talcosis and pulmonary hypertension. All nine patients showed perivascular and/or intravascular deposition of polarizable foreign material in their lungs. Intravascular talcosis as a result of previous intravenous drug use was not clinically suspected in any patient despite clinically diagnosed pulmonary hypertension in five. All patients showed dilatation of the right and left heart, but none had dilatation of the aortic valve. Congestive heart failure with hepatosplenomegaly was also common. We conclude that intravascular talcosis is an underdiagnosed cause of pulmonary hypertension in patients with known history of intravenous drug use.

1. Introduction

Pulmonary disease as a result of talc exposure has been well documented and can have multiple etiologies [1]. Inhalational talc exposure causes talc pneumoconiosis, while intravenous talc exposure causes intravascular talcosis. The disease symptoms and gross anatomic findings in these two different etiologies are essentially identical, and the histology of these two forms of talc-related lung diseases are also quite similar. Pulmonary deposition of insoluble microscopic foreign material results in a foreign body giant cell reaction within the lung parenchyma. Over time and continued exposure this process results in pulmonary fibrosis, in some cases extensively. The differentiating feature between these two diseases is the location of the foreign material. Inhalational talc pneumoconiosis results in an alveolar distribution, and intravascular talcosis leads to a perivascular pattern of deposition. In acute settings it is also possible to identify polarizable foreign material within intravascular spaces.

The source of foreign material in intravascular talcosis is through the intravenous injection of drugs. Illegal street drugs commonly contain an adulterant to increase the mass, and this adulterant commonly contains microscopic insoluble material. Another common source is the injection of prescription medications meant for oral use. In these medications which are ground for intravenous injection, there are fillers and binders added to the medications. In fact the term intravascular talcosis is a misnomer as talc is only one of several possible materials used as excipients that also include methylcellulose and crospovidone [2]. Special stains have been shown to have the ability to differentiate the composition of intravascular foreign material in diagnostically difficult situations [3].

With the intravenous injection of foreign material, the lungs represent the first capillary bed to serve as a filter to remove this material. Due to the size of much of this material it usually becomes lodged in the pulmonary vasculature. This results in acute small embolization of vessels. Over time the foreign material is deposited in perivascular tissues, and foreign body giant cell reaction occurs with associated fibrosis. This fibrosis of the lung parenchyma in turn results in the development of pulmonary hypertension in some patients.

Intravascular talcosis as a cause of pulmonary hypertension has been well documented since the early description of this disease in the 1960s although the term intravascular talcosis has not been commonly used in the past [4, 5].

The diagnosis of intravascular talcosis has important social and medical treatment implications but is not commonly suspected in many patients even in the presence of known intravenous drug abuse [6]. Here we present nine cases of intravascular talcosis on biopsy and autopsy cases that were not clinically suspected. We give a detailed review of the patient histories. In five autopsy cases we also include detailed analysis of the pulmonary and cardiac disease relating to intravascular talcosis. The goal of this study is to increase awareness of intravascular talcosis as a cause for pulmonary hypertension and to present clinical and anatomic features that can suggest the diagnosis.

2. Materials and Methods

Cases of intravascular talcosis were identified through a natural language search for "talc" in our electronic laboratory information system over an eleven-year-period spanning 1/2000–12/2010. Surgical specimens and autopsy cases were included in the search. Final diagnoses were reviewed to select cases of intravascular talcosis, and slides were reviewed by the authors to confirm the diagnosis. Cases were excluded if slides or blocks were not available for review or the diagnosis was not confirmed. In autopsy cases, all slides were pulled and examined for the presence of polarizable foreign material in association with histocytic infiltration. The clinical histories of patients with confirmed intravascular talcosis were abstracted for relevant clinical data. This study was approved by the UPMC Institutional Review Board (IRB no. PRO11020060).

2.1. Definition of Normal Metrics. Left ventricular hypertrophy was defined as wall thickness greater than 1.5 cm and right ventricular hypertrophy as wall thickness greater than 0.5 cm. Mitral valve dilation was defined as valve circumference greater than 9.9 cm in males and 9.1 cm in females, aortic valve dilation as valve circumference greater than 8.5 cm in males and 7.9 cm in females, tricuspid valve dilation as valve circumference greater than 11.8 cm in males and 11.1 cm in females, and pulmonic valve dilation as valve circumference greater than 7.5 cm in males and 7.4 cm in females [7]. Cardiomegaly was determined as a function of sex and body mass using the report by Kitzman et al. [7]. Splenomegaly was defined as spleen weight greater than 245 grams in males and greater than 190 grams in females. Hepatomegaly was defined as liver weight greater than 2000 grams in males and greater than 1800 grams in females. Increased lung weight was defined as combined lung weight greater than 1050 grams.

3. Results

3.1. Clinical Features of Intravascular Talcosis. A total of nine cases of intravascular talcosis are included in this study—five autopsy cases and four lung biopsy cases. Demographics for

these patients are summarized in Table 1. The average age for all patients was 44 years. Three cases were diagnosed in patients with admitted drug use that was not recent, and these patients had a higher average age at 56 years. There was a predominance of males with only one female in the nine patients.

The clinical histories of the patients were variable and are briefly described herein. Case 1 had a history of intravenous drug use and IgA nephropathy and was admitted for dyspnea and chest pain. Case 2 had a history of intravenous drug use and coronary artery disease and presented with acute chest pain. Case 3 had a history of remote intravenous drug use and history of stroke and was found unresponsive at his skilled nursing facility. Case 4 had a history of remote intravenous drug use, chronic obstructive pulmonary disease, and multiple pneumothoraces and was admitted for new pneumothorax and possible lung transplant evaluation. Case 5 had a history of intravenous drug use, chronic obstructive pulmonary disease, and chronic back pain requiring multiple surgeries and presented with a new episode of severe back pain. Case 6 had a history of remote intravenous drug use and right lung transplantation for talcosis and presented with increased work of breathing. Case 7 presented in the trauma suite with multiple traumatic penetrating chest injuries; a pneumonectomy was performed, but the patient did not survive. No history is available for this patient. Case 8 had a history of deteriorating lung function due to severe emphysema and presented for double lung transplantation. Case 9 had a history of multiple spine surgeries and presented with an enlarged periaortic lymph node and pulmonary infiltrate. While the majority of patients (6 of 8) with histologically confirmed intravascular talcosis had admitted intravenous drug abuse, two denied intravenous drug use. Other common clinical features were hepatitis C seropositivity (7 of 8 tested) and tobacco use (6 of 8 with history).

Pulmonary hypertension was clinically diagnosed in five of the nine patients based on clinical features, cardiac catheterization, and echocardiography. Four patients had cardiac catheterization data available for review with all having elevated peak pulmonary artery pressures with an average of 43 mmHg (range 37–50 mmHg). End diastolic pulmonary artery pressures were increased in only two patients (average 15.25 mmHg, range 4–22 mmHg). Mean pulmonary artery pressures reported were elevated in two patients (average 25.25 mmHg, range 20–32 mmHg). Echocardiography (either transthoracic or transesophageal) studies were performed in six patients. Two patients had completely normal studies. Four patients had abnormal findings: mild right atrial dilatation (2), moderate-to-severe right ventricular dilatation (3), moderate pulmonary artery dilatation (2), moderate pulmonary hypertension (3; peak pulmonary systolic pressures 52–70 mmHg), moderate left atrial dilatation (2), mild left ventricular hypertrophy (1), severe left ventricular hypertrophy (1), and mildly decreased left ventricular ejection fraction (3).

Five patients had chest computed tomography performed prior to pathological examination. Three showed emphysematous changes, one showed centrilobular and interstitial nodules, and one showed bibasilar atelectasis versus

TABLE 1: Demographics for cases of talc granulomatosis.

Case	Specimen	Sex	Age (years)	Admitted IVDU	Hep C	Tobacco smoking	Pulmonary symptoms/diagnoses
1	Autopsy	M	37	Yes	Negative	no	Dyspnea Pulmonary HTN
2	Autopsy	M	40	Yes	Positive	yes	
3	Autopsy	M	62	Yes, remote	Positive	no	
4	Autopsy	M	55	Yes, remote	Positive	yes	IPF Pulmonary HTN Recurrent pneumothoraces
5	Autopsy	F	44	Yes	Positive	yes	COPD
6	Transbronchial biopsy	M	51	Yes, remote	Positive	yes	Dyspnea Pulmonary HTN s/p R lung transplant for talc exposure*
7	Pneumonectomy due to trauma	M	20	NA	NA	NA	
8	Double lung transplant native lungs	M	53	No	Positive	yes	Dyspnea Mild pulmonary HTN
9	Wedge resection	M	31	No	NA	yes	Dyspnea Pleuritic chest pain Pulmonary HTN

*Initially diagnosed with talc pneumoconiosis.
Abbreviations: HTN: hypertension, IPF: idiopathic pulmonary fibrosis, COPD: chronic obstructive pulmonary disease, s/p: status post, NA: not available.

pneumonia. In one patient with severe panlobular emphysema, diffuse fibrosis was also evident.

Pulmonary function testing was performed in four patients, and the following parameters were noted to be abnormal: forced vital capacity (FVC) (4 patients; 26–72% of predicted), forced expiratory volume in 1 second (FEV1) (4; 22–65% of predicted), diffusing capacity of the lung for carbon monoxide (DLCO) (4 patients; 1 with 62% of predicted and 3 others that were unattainable due to low lung volumes), and vital capacity (VC) (4 patients; 36 and 73% of predicted in 2 patients, and unattainable in 2 patients).

Regarding relevant medical comorbidities, seven out of eight patients with known baseline status had a past medical history significant for hypertension that required medical management. Three patients had a history of chronic renal insufficiency (one of whom had IgA nephropathy and eventually required hemodialysis), and one patient developed acute renal failure prior to death.

At the time of initial pathological diagnosis, no patients were clinically suspected of having intravascular talcosis. One patient had previously been diagnosed with inhalational talc pneumoconiosis at an outside institution based on biopsy. Following this diagnosis the patient had a single-sided lung transplant, and a later biopsy at our institution of the nontransplanted native lung was diagnostic of intravascular talcosis. This patient had a history of remote intravenous drug use. Another patient experienced multiple bilateral spontaneous pneumothoraces and was diagnosed with idiopathic pulmonary fibrosis; however, histological examination of the patient's lungs at autopsy demonstrated intravascular talcosis as a cause for his pulmonary fibrosis.

3.2. Histologic Features of Intravascular Talcosis. The low power microscopic appearance in histologic sections of the lungs varied from focal areas of foreign body reaction and fibrosis to cases with extensive areas of fibrosis (Figure 1). The common finding in all cases was the diagnostic feature of a perivascular localization of foreign material deposition and fibrosis (Figure 2). In cases with extensive fibrosis the perivascular deposition could still be seen in areas with residual alveolated lung. The morphology of the foreign material itself varied with some showing more plate-like material and others more needle-like material (Figures 3(a) and 3(b)). Occasional asteroid bodies were found in some cases (Figure 3(c)). The histologic sections from autopsy cases and two of the four surgical pathology specimens showed some classical features associated with pulmonary hypertension [8]. Many medium caliber arteries showed hypertrophy of the muscular walls and larger arteries, when seen on sections, showed intimal proliferation similar to that seen in atherosclerosis. Many of the smaller caliber vessels failed to show these changes, and no plexiform vascular lesions were seen.

3.3. Anatomic Findings in Intravascular Talcosis Seen at Autopsy. Anatomic findings in the five patients having autopsy can be seen in Table 2. Causes of death included cardiac failure with pulmonary edema, cardiac arrhythmia secondary to pulmonary thromboembolus, multisystem organ failure secondary to sepsis, pulmonary fibrosis, and cardiopulmonary decompensation from pulmonary hypertension. All five patients had increased lung weights with an average of 1,894 grams. Cardiomegaly was present in three

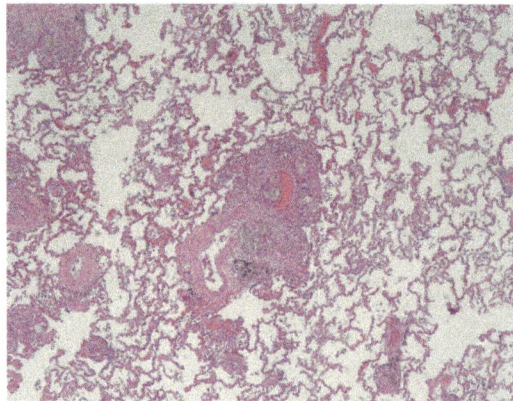

(a)

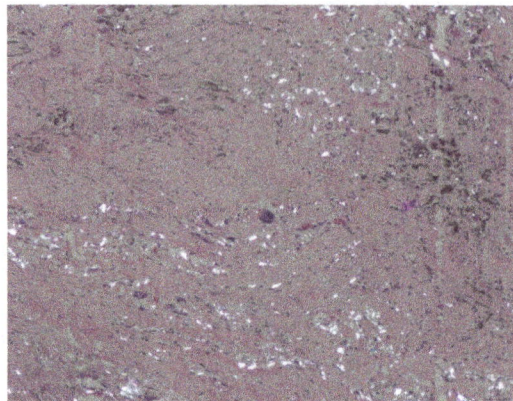

(b)

FIGURE 1: Low-power magnification of two cases of intravascular talcosis. The degree of fibrosis ranged from focal fibrosis in perivascular areas (a) to diffuse areas of fibrosis (b). Foreign material can be seen within areas of fibrosis associated with a foreign body giant cell reaction. Polarization of the material is evident in (b).

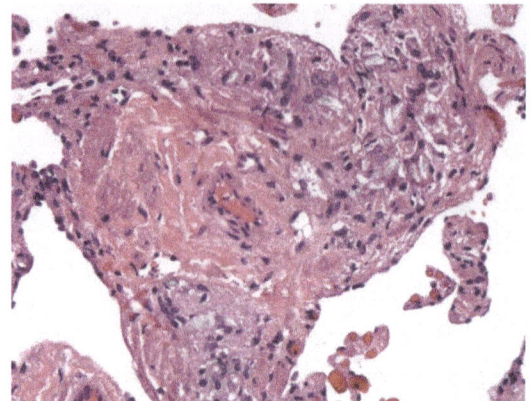

(a)

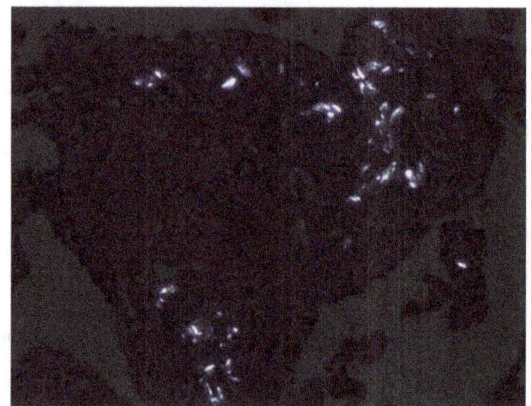

(b)

FIGURE 2: Higher magnification view of perivascular deposition of foreign material with foreign body giant cell reaction and fibrosis (a). The foreign material is highlighted under polarization (b).

TABLE 2: Anatomic features of intravascular talcosis.

Average organ weights (grams)		[range]
Lungs	(1894)	1490–2490
Heart	(600)	350–1030
Liver	(2421)	1300–4110
Spleen	(437)	80–860
Average heart valve circumference (cm)		
Mitral	(10.9)	10.5–11.5
Aortic	(7.2)	6.5–8
Tricuspid	(13.5)	12–15.5
Pulmonic	(8.5)	7–10

of five patients with an average heart weight of 600.4 grams. All five patients showed dilation of both right and left heart. The mitral and tricuspid valves were dilated in all 5 patients, average circumference of 10.9 cm and 13.5 cm, respectively. The pulmonic valve was dilated in 4 of 5 with an average circumference of 8.5 cm. None of the 5 patients had dilation of the aortic valve, average circumference 7.2 cm. Hepatomegaly was present in three of five and splenomegaly

in four of five patients. The presence of polarizable foreign material was also present in extrapulmonary tissues in each of the five patients—bone marrow (3), lymph nodes (2), kidneys (2), spleen (2), liver (2), myocardium (2), thyroid (1), venous thrombus (1), and right ventricular thrombus (1) (Figure 4). One patient that is not deceased had prior biopsies of the liver and retina which showed similar polarizable foreign material. In each of the extrapulmonary tissues, the foreign material was intra-or perivascular, showed smaller particles than in the lungs, and lacked significant giant cell reaction. In one patient with transbronchial lung biopsy, previous biopsies of the retina and liver were reported to show polarizable foreign material. Four patients had evidence of moderate-to-severe coronary artery atherosclerosis, and three had histologic evidence of subendocardial and/or myometrial ischemia.

4. Discussion

The finding of perivascular or intravascular polarizable foreign material in the lungs is essentially diagnostic of intravascular talcosis due to intravenous injection of illegal drugs. The most important differential to establish is

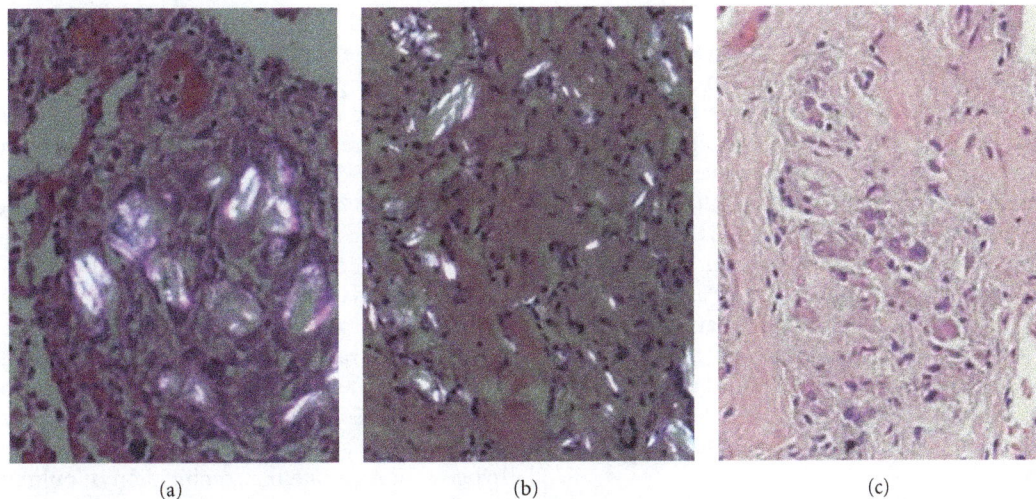

FIGURE 3: The foreign material deposits of intravascular talcosis have varying morphologies. Some cases showed more plate-like polarizable material (a) while other cases showed more needle-like morphology (b). Asteroid bodies are a common finding in intravascular talcosis (c).

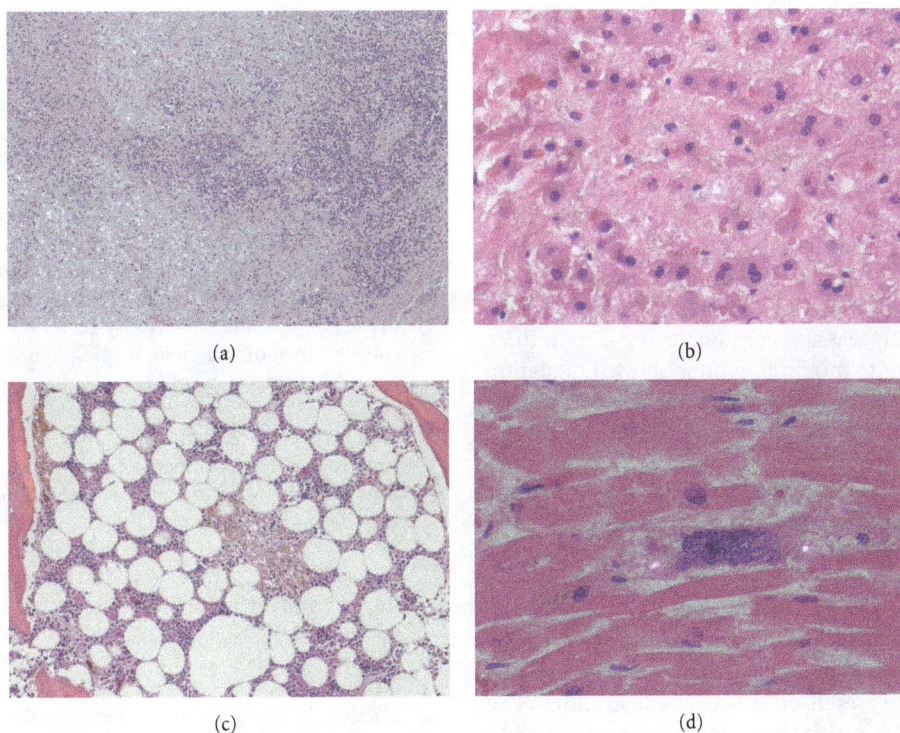

FIGURE 4: Systemic sites of foreign material are an important feature seen in intravascular talcosis. This material is smaller than seen in the lungs and only rarely incites a foreign body giant cell reaction. Representative figures show deposition in lymph node (a), liver (b), bone marrow (c), and heart (d).

between intravascular talcosis and talc pneumoconiosis due to inhalation of microscopic dust. The differentiation of these two etiologies in foreign material associated granulomatous lung disease can be challenging as perivascular location in some ways includes the entire lung parenchyma.

In this paper we searched for and selected cases of intravascular talcosis based on the histological location of the polarizable foreign material in perivascular or intravascular locations. Our findings show that none of the nine patients included in this study were clinically suspected of having intravascular talcosis due to intravenous drug abuse. This is despite the fact that five had clinically diagnosed pulmonary hypertension and six had admitted history of intravenous drug abuse.

While the effects of intravascularly injected talc had an adverse impact on these patients' hemodynamic profiles as described in the current study, it is interesting to note that many of the histologic specimens demonstrated talc that was found to be distributed in the perivascular area and not intravascularly. While a definitive answer to explain this is elusive, one plausible hypothesis is that small talc particles are extravasated from the vascular space over time by the hydrostatic pressure within the vessels. The fact that a majority of patients in the current analysis had systemic hypertension would also facilitate this movement. With time, macrophages (and resulting giant cells) may also contribute to the movement of this foreign material farther from the intravascular space. Ultimately, fibrosis of this milieu of talc, immune cells, and perivascular stroma around the pulmonary vessels would, in addition to any remaining intravascular talc, contribute to the increased pulmonary artery pressures.

Fibrosis and occlusion of small vessels within the lungs of these patients due to the intravascular and/or perivascular deposition of insoluble foreign material is the most probable cause of pulmonary hypertension in light of the clinical history and anatomic findings; however, contributions from other aspects of the patients' comorbidities, such as emphysema and fibrosis of other etiologies, cannot be completely excluded. The anatomic findings in the five patients undergoing autopsy were all likely related to the pulmonary hypertension in these patients. While the phenomenon of pulmonary hypertension in patients with intravenous drug use is well documented this is the first report to our knowledge to carefully examine the changes to the heart related to the disease. In the cases presented here all patients had dilatation of the left and right heart as determined by enlarged valve circumference. Cardiomegaly was also common being seen in three of five patients. Despite this finding none showed dilatation of the aortic valve. The reason for this is not known. Features of left sided congestive heart failure with hepatomegaly and splenomegaly were also common.

The additional evidence to support the diagnosis in these patients was the common finding of fine birefringent material in systemic locations in these patients. This feature has been previously reported in patient with intravascular talcosis [9]. This finding should suggest the diagnosis of intravascular talcosis rather than talc pneumoconiosis in patients with pulmonary granulomas as inhalation of talc and related material should not result in systemic deposition. The smaller size of the material in the systemic sites compared to the lung parenchyma suggests that this material was small enough to escape the pulmonary capillary bed.

Our analysis yielded findings from non-invasive testing which may increase suspicion for this disease in high risk individuals. Right-sided cardiac dilatation and pulmonary artery dilatation/hypertension were each found in at least half of patients that underwent echocardiography. Additionally, all patients (4/4) who underwent pulmonary function testing had decreased FVC and FEV1, along with either decreased or unattainable (due to low lung volumes) VC and DLCO.

In the current study, hypertension requiring medical treatment was present in 7 out of 8 patients that were assessed. Only three patients had chronic kidney insufficiency

(an additional patient had acute renal failure prior to death), and one of these required hemodialysis. Additionally, autopsy findings demonstrated either moderate-to-severe atherosclerotic disease or cardiac ischemia. These relevant cardiac and renal co-morbidities may have contributed to the observed cardiac findings, and while intravascular talcosis and its hemodynamic impacts may have exacerbated these conditions, their definitive relationship to intravascular talcosis is unknown.

Intravascular talcosis as a result of intravenous injection of drugs is not an uncommon finding but is not universally seen in all intravenous drug users, and the finding of pulmonary hypertension has been previously reported in these patients [5]. The current study demonstrates that intravascular talcosis is an underrecognized cause of pulmonary hypertension despite the combination of pulmonary hypertension and a history of intravenous drug use in many of our patients. Patients with risk factors and findings identified herein may benefit from further clinical evaluation for intravascular talcosis.

References

[1] S. Mukhopadhyay and A. A. Gal, "Granulomatous lung disease: an approach to the differential diagnosis," *Archives of Pathology and Laboratory Medicine*, vol. 134, no. 5, pp. 667–690, 2010.

[2] S. Ganesan, J. Felo, M. Saldana, V. F. Kalasinsky, M. R. Lewin-Smith, and J. F. Tomashefski, "Embolized crospovidone (poly[N-vinyl-2-pyrrolidone]) in the lungs of intravenous drug users," *Modern Pathology*, vol. 16, no. 4, pp. 286–292, 2003.

[3] V. M. Walley, W. A. Stinson, C. Upton et al., "Foreign materials found in the cardiovascular system after instrumentation or surgery (Including a guide to their light microscopic identification)," *Cardiovascular Pathology*, vol. 2, no. 3, pp. 157–185, 1993.

[4] E. N. Arnett, W. E. Battle, J. V. Russo, and W. C. Roberts, "Intravenous injection of talc containing drugs intended for oral use. A cause of pulmonary granulomatosis and pulmonary hypertension," *American Journal of Medicine*, vol. 60, no. 5, pp. 711–718, 1976.

[5] W. C. Roberts, "Pulmonary talc granulomas, pulmonary fibrosis, and pulmonary hypertension resulting from intravenous injection of talc-containing drugs intended for oral use," *Baylor University Medical Center Proceedings*, vol. 15, pp. 260–261, 2002.

[6] J. Kahn, "A cloud of smoke: The complicated death of a 9/11 hero," *The New Yorker*, 2008.

[7] D. W. Kitzman, D. G. Scholz, P. T. Hagen, D. M. Ilstrup, and W. D. Edwards, "Age-related changes in normal human hearts during the first 10 decades of life—part II (maturity): a quantitative anatomic study of 765 specimens from subjects 20 to 99 years old," *Mayo Clinic Proceedings*, vol. 63, no. 2, pp. 137–146, 1988.

[8] A. L. Katzenstein, *Katzenstein and Askin's Surgical Pathology of Non-Neoplastic Lung Disease*, W. B. Saunder, 4th edition, 2006.

[9] B. Kringsholm and P. Christoffersen, "The nature and the occurrence of birefringent material in different organs in fatal drug addiction," *Forensic Science International*, vol. 34, no. 1-2, pp. 53–62, 1987.

11

Clinical Outcomes of Stereotactic Body Radiotherapy for Patients with Lung Tumors in the State of Oligo-Recurrence

Tetsuya Inoue, Norio Katoh, Rikiya Onimaru, and Hiroki Shirato

Department of Radiology, Hokkaido University Graduate School of Medicine, North 15 West 7, Kita-ku, Sapporo 060-8638, Japan

Correspondence should be addressed to Tetsuya Inoue, t-inoue@med.hokudai.ac.jp

Academic Editor: Yuzuru Niibe

We retrospectively evaluated the clinical outcomes of patients with oligometastatic lung tumors who underwent stereotactic body radiotherapy (SBRT). Twenty-two patients with one or two oligometastatic lung tumors were treated with SBRT at our institution between 1999 and 2009. With a median follow-up period of 25 months from the date of SBRT to the detection of oligometastatic lung tumors, the patients' 3- and 5-year overall survival (OS) and progression-free survival (PFS) rates were 72% and 54%, respectively. The median disease-free interval (DFI) between the treatment of the primary site and SBRT to oligometastatic lung tumors was 41 months. The OS of patients with a DFI $\geq$ 36 months was significantly longer than that of the patients with a DFI < 36 months by the log-rank test ($P = 0.02$). For patients with a DFI $\geq$ 36 months, the 3- and 5-year OS rates were both 88%, compared to 50% for the patients with a DFI < 36 months. The primary tumor of all patients was locally controlled when SBRT to oligometastatic lung tumors was performed, and thus they were in the state of "oligo-recurrence." Patients with oligometastatic lung lesions treated by SBRT had good prognoses. This was especially true of the patients with a long DFI and in the state of "oligo-recurrence."

1. Introduction

Most patients who have had any recurrent or metastatic sites of cancer are considered to be in their last stage of life. However, new notions of oligometastases and oligo-recurrence have been proposed [1–9]. Oligometastases is the state in which the patient shows distant recurrence in only a limited number of regions. The clinical state of oligometastatic dise-ase was proposed in 1995 by Hellman and Weichselbaum [1], who hypothesized that local control of oligometastases may yield improved systemic control and prolonged survival. Niibe et al. also discussed the state of oligo-recurrence [2–4]; they defined it as oligometastases with a controlled primary cancer site.

Stereotactic body radiotherapy (SBRT) with a high local dose has been applied to extracranial diseases such as peripheral stage I nonsmall cell lung cancer (NSCLC), and it has been reported to provide excellent local control and survival compatible with surgery [10, 11]. SBRT has also been used in Japan for patients with fewer than three lung metastases ≤ 5 cm in diameter. In the present study, we retrospectively analyzed our experience with SBRT for patients with oligometastatic lung tumors.

2. Methods and Materials

2.1. Patient Characteristics. A database of patients who received SBRT for metastatic lung tumors at our institution was used for the patient selection. There were 22 patients who had one or two oligometastatic lung tumors at the time of SBRT and had been treated with SBRT between 1999 and 2009. The diagnosis of the oligometastatic lung tumors was based on whole-body computed tomography (CT). Fluoro-deoxy-glucose (FDG)-positron emission tomography (PET) was performed as needed. The primary tumor of all patients was locally controlled when SBRT to the oligometastatic lung tumors was performed. The treatment methods for the primary sites were surgery in 13 patients and definitive radiotherapy in nine. Definitive radiotherapy consisted of conventional radiotherapy in one patient, brachytherapy in one patient, and SBRT in seven.

We labeled the treatment interval time from the primary sites to oligometastatic lung tumors as the disease-free interval (DFI). In this study, all analyses started from the day of SBRT to oligometastatic lung tumors.

The patient characteristics are given in Table 1. There were 8 men and 14 women, and the median age was 67 years (range 30–84 years). The primary cancers consisted of lung cancer ($n = 9$), head and neck cancer ($n = 4$), breast cancer ($n = 3$), colorectal cancer ($n = 2$), genitourinary cancer ($n = 2$), thymic cancer ($n = 1$), and skin cancer ($n = 1$). The primary histology consisted of adenocarcinoma ($n = 13$), squamous cell carcinoma ($n = 4$), renal cell carcinoma ($n = 1$), transitional cell carcinoma ($n = 1$), large-cell carcinoma ($n = 1$), malignant melanoma ($n = 1$), and apocrine gland carcinoma ($n = 1$). There were 13 patients who had only one oligometastatic lung tumor and nine patients who had two oligometastatic lung tumors. The median tumor size was 15 mm (range 8–47 mm). No chemotherapy was allowed until tumor progression.

2.2. SBRT Technique.
All patients received SBRT to oligometastatic lung tumors as the definitive radiotherapy. Nine patients received SBRT using a real-time tumor-tracking radiotherapy (RTRT) system, and 13 patients received SBRT without RTRT.

The RTRT system has been described in detail elsewhere [12, 13]. In brief, 1.5 to 2.0 mm gold markers were implanted near the tumor by means of image-guided procedures. CT scans were taken with the patients holding their breath at the end of normal expiration. The gross tumor volume (GTV) was contoured in axial CT images. The clinical target volume (CTV) was defined three-dimensionally as the GTV on CT with a 5 mm margin for metastatic lung tumors and was considered to be equal to the internal target volume (ITV). The planning target volume (PTV) was three-dimensionally defined as the CTV plus a 5 mm margin with optimal reduction near the organ at risk (OAR).

SBRT without RTRT was described as follows. To determine the ITV margin, CT scans were performed three times, with breath holding at the expiratory and inspiratory phases and with free breathing. The three GTVs on CT at three phases were superimposed on the radiation treatment system to represent GTV + ITV. The CTV was defined three-dimensionally as the GTV + ITV on CT with a 5 mm margin. The PTV was three-dimensionally defined as the CTV plus a 5 mm margin with optimal reduction near the OAR.

We administered 48 Gy in four fractions at the isocenter calculated by Clarkson algorism or 40 Gy in four fractions to the 95% volume of PTV by superposition algorism with a treatment period of 4 to 7 days. Patients were treated with 4- or 6-MV photons. SBRT was delivered using multiple non-coplanar static ports.

2.3. Followup after SBRT.
Follow-up visits were usually every 3 months after SBRT. CT scans were usually performed every 3–6 months after SBRT. Local progression was diagnosed on the basis of histologic confirmation or enlargement of the local tumor on CT that continued for at least 6 months.

TABLE 1: Patient characteristics (22 patients).

Characteristics	Value
Age (years)	
Median	67
Range	30–84
Gender (n)	
Male	8
Female	14
Primary cancer (n)	
Lung	9
Head and neck	4
Breast	3
Colorectal	2
Genitourinary	2
Thymic	1
Apocrine gland	1
Primary histology (n)	
Adenocarcinoma	13
Squamous cell carcinoma	4
Others	5
Treatment for primary cancer (n)	
Resection	13
SBRT	7
Conventional radiation therapy	1
Brachytherapy	1
Number of oligometastatic tumors (n)	
1	13
2	9
Tumor diameter (n)	
<20 mm	25
21–30 mm	4
>30 mm	2

SBRT: stereotactic body radiotherapy.

FDG-PET was recommended when local recurrence was suspected, but this was not mandatory.

2.4. Ethical Considerations.
Written informed consent to receive SBRT was obtained from all patients. This retrospective study was performed in accordance with the 1975 Declaration of Helsinki, as revised in 2000.

2.5. Statistical Analysis.
The overall survival (OS) and progression-free survival (PFS) rates were calculated from the date of SBRT to oligometastatic lung tumors using the Kaplan-Meier method. The log-rank test was used to identify significant differences. R version 2.14.2 with the survival packages (R project for statistical computing, Vienna, Austria) was used for the statistical analyses. A value of $P < 0.05$ was considered significant.

TABLE 2: Patterns of disease progression (9 patients).

Pattern	n
New pulmonary metastases	4
Liver metastases	1
Bone metastases	1
Multiple metastases	3

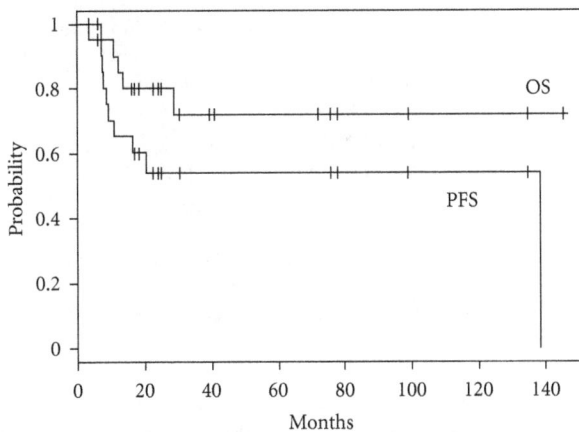

FIGURE 1: Kaplan-Meier actuarial overall survival (OS) and progression-free survival (PFS) rates.

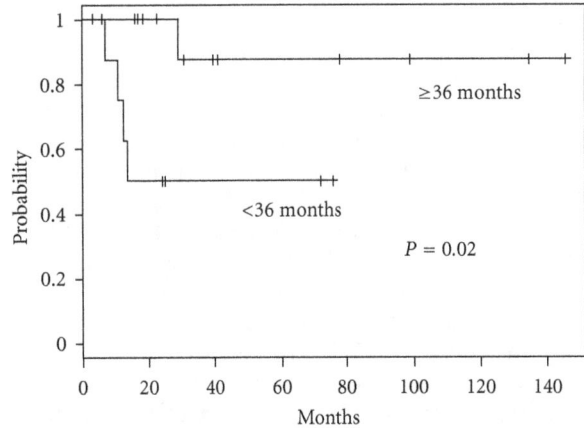

FIGURE 2: Kaplan-Meier curve of overall survival rates for patients with a disease-free interval (DFI) <36 months ($n = 9$) or ≥36 months ($n = 13$). The groups' survival rates differed significantly ($P = 0.02$).

3. Results

3.1. Survival. With a median follow-up period of 25 months (range 4–146 months) from the day of SBRT to oligometastatic lung tumors, the 3- and 5-year overall survival and progression-free survival rates were 72% and 54% (Figure 1). The median DFI between the treatment of the primary site and SBRT to oligometastatic lung tumors was 41 months. The primary tumor of all patients was locally controlled when SBRT to oligometastatic lung tumors was performed; the patients were thus in the state of "oligo-recurrence."

3.2. Patterns of Failure. Disease progression was observed in nine patients (Table 2). All irradiated lesions by SBRT were controlled. New intrapulmonary metastases were observed in four patients, bone metastases were observed in one patient, and liver metastases were observed in one patient. Multiple metastatic lesions including regional lymph node, brain, bone and/or liver were observed in three patients.

3.3. Toxicities. Adverse effects were graded according to the Common Toxicity Criteria for Adverse Events, version 3.0. Grade 2. Intercostal neuralgia occurred in one patient. No radiation pneumonitis of grade 3 or more was observed.

3.4. Prognostic Factors. We also analyzed the survival differences stratified by DFI duration. DFI duration was divided into <36 or ≥36 months. The OS of patients with a DFI ≥ 36 months ($n = 13$) was significantly longer than the OS of

those with a DFI < 36 months ($n = 9$) ($P = 0.02$). For patients with a DFI ≥ 36 months, the 3- and 5-year OS rates were both 88%, compared to 50% for patients with a DFI < 36 months (Figure 2).

4. Discussion

In this patient population, the 3- and 5-year overall survival and progression-free survival rates were 72% and 54%, respectively, which was equivalent to or better than those in previous studies of oligometastatic lung tumors as follows. Norihisa et al. reported the results of SBRT for oligometastatic lung tumors [14]. The OS rate and PFS rates at 2 years were 84.3% and 34.8%. Rusthoven et al. recently reported the results of multi-institutional phase I/II trials of SBRT for lung metastases [15]. The actual local control rates at 1 and 2 years after SBRT for oligometastatic lung tumors were 100% and 96%, respectively, and the median survival time was 19 months.

A landmark study of more than 5,000 patients by the International Registry of Lung Metastases (IRLM) demonstrated that long-term survival can be achieved in a proportion of patients with lung metastases treated with metastasectomy [16]. The actuarial survival after complete metastasectomy was 36% at 5 years. With the exclusion of the apparently favorable tumors, the survival outcome at 2 years was approximate 70%.

We previously reported the clinical outcomes of stereotactic brain and/or body radiotherapy for patients with oligometastatic lesions. The organs affected by oligometastatic lesions were the brain, lung, and/or adrenal gland [17]. For patients with oligometastatic lung disease, the 3- and 5-year OS rates were both 63%, significantly better than the 22% and 14% of those with brain/adrenal metastases.

In the present study, the DFI between the treatment of primary site and SBRT to oligometastatic lung tumors was the prognostic factor. Norihisa et al. also reported that patients with a longer DFI had a greater overall survival rate

[14]. Patients with a DFI ≥ 36 months had significantly greater OS compared to those with a DFI < 36 months. In the IRLM study, a multivariate analysis revealed that a DFI longer than 36 months is a factor associated with improved survival [15]. In our previous study, we also found that patients with a DFI ≥ 12 months had significantly greater OS compared to those with a DFI < 12 months [17].

The IRLM study and multi-institutional phase I/II trials by Rusthoven et al. included locally uncontrolled primary tumors, so-called oligometastases [15, 16]. However, in the present study, the primary tumor of all patients was locally controlled when SBRT to oligometastatic lung tumors was performed, that is, in the so-called state of "oligo-recurrence." Therefore, the present population's outcomes were equivalent or better than those in the previous study of oligo-metastatic lung tumors. We were also curious about survival differences between patients with and without oligo-recurrence, but all of the patients in this population were in the state of oligo-recurrence. Moreover, in the present study, the median DFI between the treatment of the primary site and the SBRT to oligometastatic lung tumors reached 41 months, a very long period compared with other studies. However, it was difficult in this study to distinguish second primary lung cancers from metastatic lung cancers, and oligometastatic lung tumors from NSCLC might be second primary lung cancers, which may have better prognoses than metastatic lung cancers.

One shortcoming of the present study is the retrospective nature of the analysis. Patients with sufficient medical conditions were probably selected beforehand to receive SBRT. The large number of patients who died within a short period may have masked the possible progression of the disease and local failure. However, it is notable that there was a definite group of patients treated with SBRT for oligometastatic tumors who experienced long survival even with distant metastasis. A large prospective trial is required to establish the precise benefits of SBRT for patients with oligometastatic lung tumors. Our findings suggest that the DFI should be included in the stratification criteria in a prospective randomized trial comparing treatment with and without SBRT.

In conclusion, patients with oligometastatic lung lesions treated by SBRT had good prognoses, especially the patients with a long DFI and in the state of "oligo-recurrence."

Acknowledgment

This study was supported in part by grants from The Funding Program for World-Leading Innovative R&D on Science and Technology (FIRST program).

References

[1] S. Hellman and R. R. Weichselbaum, "Oligometastases," *Journal of Clinical Oncology*, vol. 13, no. 1, pp. 8–10, 1995.

[2] Y. Niibe, T. Kazumoto, T. Toita et al., "Frequency and characteristics of isolated para-aortic lymph node recurrence in patients with uterine cervical carcinoma in Japan: a multi-institutional study," *Gynecologic Oncology*, vol. 103, no. 2, pp. 435–438, 2006.

[3] Y. Niibe, M. Kenjo, T. Kazumoto et al., "Multi-institutional study of radiation therapy for isolated para-aortic lymph node recurrence in uterine cervical carcinoma: 84 subjects of a population of more than 5,000," *International Journal of Radiation Oncology Biology Physics*, vol. 66, no. 5, pp. 1366–1369, 2006.

[4] Y. Niibe, M. Kuranami, K. Matsunaga et al., "Value of high-dose radiation therapy for isolated osseous metastasis in breast cancer in terms of oligo-recurrence," *Anticancer Research*, vol. 28, no. 6 B, pp. 3929–3931, 2008.

[5] J. K. Salama, S. J. Chmura, N. Mehta et al., "An initial report of a radiation dose-escalation trial in patients with one to five sites of metastatic disease," *Clinical Cancer Research*, vol. 14, no. 16, pp. 5255–5259, 2008.

[6] M. T. Milano, A. W. Katz, A. G. Muhs et al., "A prospective pilot study of curative-intent stereotactic body radiation therapy in patients with 5 or fewer oligometastatic lesions," *Cancer*, vol. 112, no. 3, pp. 650–658, 2008.

[7] T. W. Flannery, M. Suntharalingam, W. F. Regine et al., "Long-term survival in patients with synchronous, solitary brain metastasis from non-small-cell lung cancer treated with radiosurgery," *International Journal of Radiation Oncology Biology Physics*, vol. 72, no. 1, pp. 19–23, 2008.

[8] M. T. Milano, H. Zhang, S. K. Metcalfe, A. G. Muhs, and P. Okunieff, "Oligometastatic breast cancer treated with curative-intent stereotactic body radiation therapy," *Breast Cancer Research and Treatment*, vol. 115, no. 3, pp. 601–608, 2009.

[9] A. J. Khan, P. S. Mehta, T. W. Zusag et al., "Long term disease-free survival resulting from combined modality management of patients presenting with oligometastatic, non-small cell lung carcinoma (NSCLC)," *Radiotherapy and Oncology*, vol. 81, no. 2, pp. 163–167, 2006.

[10] H. Onishi, H. Shirato, Y. Nagata et al., "Hypofractionated stereotactic radiotherapy (HypoFXSRT) for stage I non-small cell lung cancer: updated results of 257 patients in a Japanese multi-institutional study," *Journal of Thoracic Oncology*, vol. 2, supplement 7, pp. S94–S100, 2007.

[11] P. Baumann, J. Nyman, M. Hoyer et al., "Outcome in a prospective phase II trial of medically inoperable stage I non-small-cell lung cancer patients treated with stereotactic body radiotherapy," *Journal of Clinical Oncology*, vol. 27, no. 20, pp. 3290–3296, 2009.

[12] H. Shirato, S. Shimizu, T. Kunieda et al., "Physical aspects of a real-time tumor-tracking system for gated radiotherapy," *International Journal of Radiation Oncology Biology Physics*, vol. 48, no. 4, pp. 1187–1195, 2000.

[13] H. Shirato, S. Shimizu, K. Kitamura et al., "Four-dimensional treatment planning and fluoroscopic real-time tumor tracking radiotherapy for moving tumor," *International Journal of Radiation Oncology Biology Physics*, vol. 48, no. 2, pp. 435–442, 2000.

[14] Y. Norihisa, Y. Nagata, K. Takayama et al., "Stereotactic body radiotherapy for oligometastatic lung tumors," *International Journal of Radiation Oncology Biology Physics*, vol. 72, no. 2, pp. 398–403, 2008.

[15] K. E. Rusthoven, B. D. Kavanagh, S. H. Burri et al., "Multi-institutional phase I/II trial of stereotactic body radiation therapy for lung metastases," *Journal of Clinical Oncology*, vol. 27, no. 10, pp. 1579–1584, 2009.

[16] The International Registry of Lung Metastases, "Long-term results of lung metastasectomy: prognostic analyses based on

5206 cases," *Journal of Thoracic and Cardiovascular Surgery*, vol. 113, no. 1, pp. 37–49, 1997.

[17] T. Inoue, N. Katoh, H. Aoyama et al., "Clinical outcomes of stereotactic brain and/or body radiotherapy for patients with oligometastatic lesions," *Japanese Journal of Clinical Oncology*, vol. 40, no. 8, pp. 788–794, 2010.

12

Cigarette-Smoking Intensity and Interferon-Gamma Release Assay Conversion among Persons Who Inject Drugs: A Cohort Study

Sanghyuk S. Shin,[1,2] Manuel Gallardo,[3] Remedios Lozada,[3] Daniela Abramovitz,[2]
Jose Luis Burgos,[2] Rafael Laniado-Laborin,[4] Timothy C. Rodwell,[2] Thomas E. Novotny,[1]
Steffanie A. Strathdee,[2] and Richard S. Garfein[2]

[1] San Diego State University, 5500 Campanile Drive, San Diego, CA 92182-4162, USA
[2] Division of Global Public Health, Department of Medicine, School of Medicine, University of California San Diego,
  9500 Gilman Drive, MC-0507, San Diego, CA 92093-0507, USA
[3] Patronato Pro-COMUSIDA, Ninos Heroes No. 697, Zona Centro, Tijuana, BC, Mexico
[4] Parque Industrial Internacional, Universidad Autonoma de Baja California, Calzada Universidad 14418, Tijuana, BC, Mexico

Correspondence should be addressed to Richard S. Garfein, rgarfein@ucsd.edu

Academic Editor: Jonathan Golub

We analyzed data from a longitudinal cohort study of persons who inject drugs (PWID) in Tijuana, Mexico, to explore whether cigarette smoking increases the risk of interferon gamma release assay (IGRA) conversion. PWID were recruited using respondent driven sampling (RDS). QuantiFERON-TB Gold In-Tube (QFT) assay conversion was defined as interferon-gamma concentrations <0.35 IU/mL at baseline and ≥0.7 IU/mL at 18 months. We used multivariable Poisson regression adjusted for RDS weights to estimate risk ratios (RRs). Of 129 eligible participants, 125 (96.9%) smoked at least one cigarette during followup with a median of 11 cigarettes smoked daily, and 52 (40.3%) had QFT conversion. In bivariate analysis, QFT conversion was not associated with the number of cigarettes smoked daily ($P = 0.716$). Controlling for age, gender, education, and alcohol use, the RRs of QFT conversion for smoking 6–10, 11–15, and ≥16 cigarettes daily compared to smoking 0–5 cigarettes daily were 0.9 (95% confidence interval (CI), 0.5–1.6), 0.5 (95% CI, 0.3–1.2), and 0.7 (95% CI, 0.3–1.6), respectively. Although this study did not find an association between self-reported smoking intensity and QFT conversion, it was not powered sufficiently to negate such an association. Larger longitudinal studies are needed to fully explore this relationship.

1. Introduction

Evidence has accumulated over the years which demonstrates a causal relationship between tobacco use and increased tuberculosis (TB) morbidity and mortality [1–6]. However, the strength of evidence for this relationship varies by TB outcome [3]. For example, while high-quality longitudinal cohort studies provide strong evidence that tobacco use increases the risk of TB disease, the evidence for the relationship between tobacco use and the risk of *Mycobacterium tuberculosis* infection is relatively weak [3, 7, 8]. Previous studies exploring this relationship utilized cross-sectional or case-control methodologies to determine the association between "ever" or "current" smoking and lifetime infection with *M. tuberculosis* as determined by a single tuberculin skin test (TST) result [9–14]. Therefore, these studies were not able to assess the temporality between tobacco use and *M. tuberculosis* infection. For example, a participant infected with *M. tuberculosis* as a child who subsequently began smoking years later would contribute to the positive association between smoking and TST positivity.

An improved understanding of the relationship between cigarette smoking and *M. tuberculosis* infection would help inform the implementation of tobacco control efforts as a part of global TB interventions. However, due to the low incidence of *M. tuberculosis* infection in most populations, conducting longitudinal cohort studies to strengthen the evidence regarding this relationship would necessitate the enrollment and long-term followup of a large number of participants. Furthermore, while interferon gamma release assays (IGRAs) have been shown to have higher specificity than TSTs for the diagnosis of latent TB infection (LTBI), no study has explored the effect of tobacco use on serial IGRA test results [15, 16].

The objective of the present study was to investigate the association between level of cigarette smoking and IGRA conversion among persons who inject drugs (PWID) in Tijuana, Mexico, a population at high risk for *M. tuberculosis* infection. Previous studies using this cohort showed a high baseline LTBI prevalence LTBI of 67% and an 18-month IGRA conversion rate of 28.7% to 51.9%, depending on the definition of conversion used [17, 18]. We hypothesized that higher levels of cigarette smoking in this population would be associated with increased risk for IGRA conversion in a dose-response relationship.

2. Materials and Methods

2.1. Study Design and Population. We analyzed data from a longitudinal cohort study of PWID in Tijuana, Mexico that sought to determine risk factors for incident HIV, TB, and syphilis [19]. Study recruitment and data collection methods have been described in detail previously [19]. Briefly, eligible study participants were ages 18 years or older, had injected illicit drugs within the previous month, and had no plans to move from Tijuana during the followup period. Participants were recruited through respondent-driven sampling (RDS), which relies on recruiting participants through referrals from previously enrolled participants [20, 21]. RDS allows for the derivation of population-representative estimates of prevalence and risk factors by adjusting for the information collected on the participants' social networks during analysis [20, 21]. Enrolled participants made study visits at baseline and at 6, 12, and 18 months. To increase retention, community outreach workers actively contacted participants to remind them of their followup appointments. Participants were also provided with $10 at baseline and $5 at followup visits as compensation for their time and travel expenses. Only participants who tested IGRA negative at baseline and who had IGRA results available at 18 months were included in the present analysis. Institutional Review Boards at University of California, San Diego and the Tijuana General Hospital reviewed and approved the study protocol, and informed consent was obtained from all participants.

2.2. Measures. An in-depth questionnaire was administered via person-to-person interview at each visit. The questionnaire contained items on demographic characteristics and substance use behavior, including injection and noninjection use of illicit drugs, alcohol consumption, and cigarette smoking. Cigarette smoking was ascertained by first asking,

"Have you smoked cigarettes in the past 6 months?" Participants who responded "Yes" were asked, "In the past 6 months, how many cigarettes did you usually smoke per day?" Based on preliminary analysis, we anticipated a high prevalence of cigarette smoking in this population and, consequently, insufficient number of nonsmokers for categorization. Therefore, we used the average number of cigarettes smoked daily during the 18-month study period as the exposure of interest. This exposure was stratified into quartiles (0–5, 6–10, 11–15, and ≥16 cigarettes) for the primary analysis.

IGRA conversion at 18 months was ascertained using QuantiFERON-TB Gold In-Tube ((QFT) Cellestis, VIC, Australia). For this test, whole blood samples were collected in three separate tubes: a Nil Control tube, TB Antigen tube, and a Mitogen Control tube. The tubes were incubated at 37°C for 16 to 24 hours and centrifuged. The interferon-gamma (IFN-γ) released in the Nil Control tube was then measured using enzyme-linked immunosorbent assay (ELISA) and subtracted from that found in the TB Antigen Tube. QFT was administered at baseline for all participants. However, because of an unexpected delay in procuring the supplies necessary for specimen collection and testing, only a subset of the participants who were QFT negative using the manufacturer recommended cutoff of <0.35 IU/mL at baseline were retested at 18 months. For the primary analysis, we used a previously published conservative definition of QFT conversion (i.e., baseline IFN-γ < 0.35 IU/mL and IFN-γ ≥ 0.70 IU/mL at followup), which reduces false positive conversions that could potentially arise due to within-subject variability observed in serial QFT tests [22]. In a secondary sensitivity analysis, we used the cutoff of 0.35 IU/mL at 18 months to define conversion.

2.3. Statistical Analysis. The Pearson's χ^2 test was used for comparisons involving categorical variables, and the Wilcoxon rank-sum and the Kruskal-Wallis tests were used for continuous variables. We considered statistical tests to be significant at α of 0.05. We constructed Poisson regression models with robust variance estimation, via generalized estimating equation (GEE), to determine risk ratios (RRs) for QFT conversion for participants in each smoking exposure quartile compared to those in the first quartile [23, 24]. The models were weighted by inverse probability weights derived using the RDS Analytical Tool [25]. The GEE algorithm also accounted for clustering by recruiter assuming an exchangeable correlation structure.

The base model included covariates representing established risk factors for *M. tuberculosis* infection, including age, gender, education, and alcohol use, regardless of their association with QFT conversion in our study population. We also evaluated the effect of drug use behavior using the "change-in-estimate" approach; drug use variables were added to the base model only if their inclusion changed the RRs between smoking and QFT by >10% [26]. Drug use variables evaluated included frequency and duration of heroin, methamphetamine, cocaine and marijuana use, including smoking of these substances. To account for the

TABLE 1: Demographic and behavioral characteristics of participants with negative QFT results (IFN-γ < 0.35 IU/mL) at baseline, included versus not included in the analysis; Tijuana, Mexico, 2006–2008.

Characteristic	Included N = 129 n (%)	Not included N = 212 n (%)	P value*
Gender			0.806
Male	107 (82.9)	178 (84.0)	
Female	22 (17.1)	34 (16.0)	
Age, median (IQR)	38 (32–43)	37 (30–42)	0.247
Education			0.389
Up to primary	39 (30.2)	76 (35.8)	
Primary to middle	60 (46.5)	83 (39.2)	
High school and higher	30 (23.3)	53 (25.0)	
Unstable housing			0.357
No	113 (87.6)	178 (84.0)	
Yes	16 (12.4)	34 (16.0)	
History of incarceration			0.719
No	78 (60.5)	124 (58.5)	
Yes	51 (39.5)	88 (41.5)	
HIV infection			0.366
No	123 (95.3)	197 (92.9)	
Yes	6 (4.7)	15 (7.1)	
Alcohol			0.154
None	76 (58.9)	134 (63.2)	
Less than twice per week	31 (24.0)	57 (26.9)	
Twice per week or more	22 (17.1)	21 (9.9)	
Smoked cigarette during study periods (18 months)			0.919
No	4 (3.1)	7 (3.3)	
Yes	125 (96.9)	205 (96.7)	
Number of cigarettes smoked daily, median (IQR)	10.5 (6–15)	12.5 (7–19)	0.023
Number of cigarettes smoked daily (quartiles)			0.058
0–5	30 (23.3)	41 (19.3)	
6–10	36 (27.9)	50 (23.6)	
11–15	37 (28.7)	49 (23.1)	
16+	26 (20.2)	72 (34.0)	
QFT conversion at 18 mos (IFN-γ ≥ 0.70 IU/mL)			
No	77 (59.7)	—	
Yes	52 (40.3)	—	

* P values for the difference between included versus excluded participants were generated using the Pearson's χ^2 test for categorical variables and the Wilcoxon rank sum for continuous variables.
IFN-γ: interferon-gamma; QFT: QuantiFERON-TB Gold In-Tube; IQR: interquartile range.

possible loss of statistical power due to overfitting the final model with covariates, we also constructed a reduced model that included the stratified smoking exposure variable and only the covariates that were statistically significant predictors of QFT conversion. For the final model, we calculated tolerance and condition index statistics to assess multicollinearity, and Pearson residuals, Cook's distance, and leverage statistics to identify outlier observations [27]. SAS 9.3 (Cary, North Carolina) was used for all analyses.

3. Results

Of the 1056 participants enrolled during April 2006–April 2007, 341 had negative QFT (IFN-γ < 0.35 IU/mL) at baseline. Of these, 129 (37.8%) who had QFT results available at 18 months were included in the analysis. Among included participants, the median age was 38 (interquartile range (IQR) = 32–43), 107 (82.9%) were male, and 99 (76.7%) had obtained middle school education or less (Table 1). Nearly

TABLE 2: QFT conversion (IFN-$\gamma \geq$ 0.70 IU/mL) at 18 months by quartiles of number of cigarettes smoked among persons who inject drugs in Tijuana, Mexico, 2006–2008.

Number of cigarettes smoked daily (quartiles)	QFT conversion	P value
0–5	13/30 (43.3)	
6–10	16/36 (44.4)	0.716
11–15	15/37 (40.5)	
16+	8/26 (30.8)	

*P value for the difference in QFT conversion at 18 months across quartiles was generated using the Pearson's χ^2 test.
IFN-γ: interferon-gamma; QFT: QuantiFERON-TB Gold In-Tube.

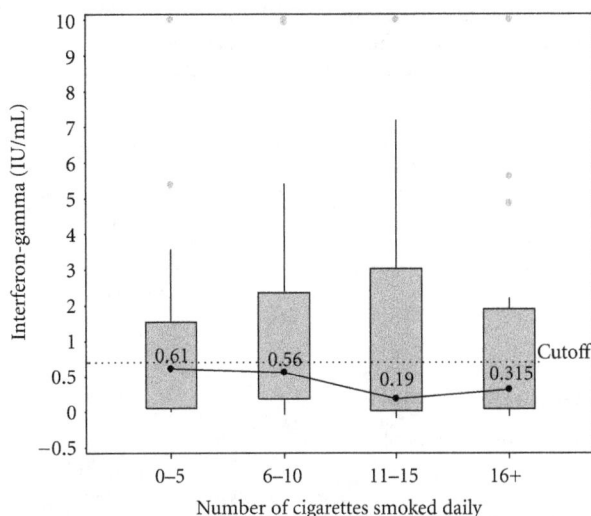

FIGURE 1: Median IFN-γ and interquartile range at 18 months by quartiles of number of cigarettes smoked. IFN-γ > 10 IU/mL were set to 10 IU/mL due to imprecision at high concentration levels. The dotted line represents the 0.70 IU/mL cutoff which was used to define QFT conversion. IFN-γ: interferon-gamma. QFT: QuantiFERON-TB Gold In-Tube.

all of the included participants (96.9%) reported smoking at least one cigarette during the followup period. On average, participants included in the analysis smoked fewer cigarettes per day compared to the 212 participants who were excluded due to missing QFT results at 18 months (median of 10.5 [IQR = 6–15] versus 12.5 [IQR = 7–19] cigarettes per day, resp., $P = 0.023$). None of the other characteristics differed between included and excluded participants (Table 1). At 18 months, 52 (40.3%) participants met the primary QFT conversion definition.

Across quartiles of self-reported daily cigarettes smoked, the median IFN-γ concentrations were 0.61, 0.56, 0.19, and 0.315 IU/mL, respectively (Figure 1), and the proportion of participants with QFT conversion was 43.4%, 44.4%, 40.5%, and 30.8%, respectively (Table 2). There was no association between IFN-γ distribution or QFT conversion across quartile levels of daily cigarettes smoked ($P = 0.523$ and $P = 0.716$, resp.). In the bivariate model adjusted for RDS weights, which included only the smoking quartiles as the independent variable, the RRs for QFT conversion for each quartile of daily number of cigarettes smoked compared to the lowest exposure quartile were 0.75 (95% confidence interval [CI] 0.37–1.55), 0.53 (95% CI 0.23–1.20), and 0.59 (95% CI 0.24–1.43), respectively (Table 3).

In multivariable analysis adjusted for RDS, inclusion of drug use variables to the base model did not change the association between cigarette smoking quartiles and QFT conversion. Therefore, the final model consisted of daily cigarette smoking quartiles, age, gender, education, and alcohol use as independent variables (Table 3). The adjusted RRs for QFT conversion for each quartile of daily number of cigarettes smoked compared to the lowest exposure quartile were 0.86 (95% CI 0.46–1.63), 0.54 (95% CI 0.25–1.17), and 0.74 (95% CI 0.33–1.64), respectively (Table 3; Figure 2). There was no statistically significant difference in the risk of QFT conversion at any of the quartiles of daily cigarettes smoked compared with that of the lowest exposure quartile. Furthermore, age, gender, education, and alcohol use were not statistically significant predictors of QFT conversion. In the reduced model that included the smoking variables and educational attainment only, having attained less than high school education compared with higher education was found to increase the risk of QFT conversion (RR = 2.83; 95% CI 1.08–7.42). As with the full model, higher levels of daily

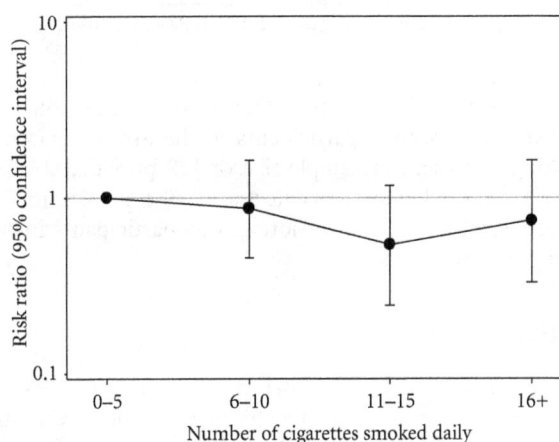

FIGURE 2: Adjusted risk ratios for QFT conversion (IFN-$\gamma \geq$ 0.70 IU/mL) at 18 months based on the final multivariable Poisson regression model with robust variance which included the following covariates: quartiles of the number of cigarettes smoked daily, education, age, gender, and alcohol use. IFN-γ: interferon-gamma. QFT: QuantiFERON-TB Gold In-Tube.

cigarette smoking exposure quartiles were not associated with QFT conversion risk in this model (Table 3).

All tolerance estimates were greater than 0.10, and the highest condition index was 11.8 in the final model, indicating that multicollinearity did not affect our findings. We found five potential outliers based on residual and influence statistics, but removing these had no effect on our findings. Additionally, using a cutoff of 0.35 IU/mL instead of 0.70 IU/mL at 18 months to define conversion and fitting the final model with daily number of cigarettes smoked as a continuous variable did not alter our findings. In post

TABLE 3: Adjusted risk ratios for QFT conversion (IFN-$\gamma \geq 0.70$ IU/mL) at 18 months based on multivariable Poisson regression models with robust variance; Tijuana, Mexico, 2006–2008.

Variable	Risk Ratio (95% Confidence Interval)		
	Bivariate Model	Reduced Model	Final Model
Number of cigarettes smoked daily (quartiles)			
0–5	1.00	1.00	1.00
6–10	0.75 (0.37–1.55)	1.04 (0.53–2.04)	0.86 (0.46–1.63)
11–15	0.53 (0.23–1.20)	0.73 (0.36–1.51)	0.54 (0.25–1.17)
≥16	0.59 (0.24–1.43)	0.79 (0.34–1.83)	0.74 (0.33–1.64)
Education			
High school or higher		1.00	1.00
Less than high school		2.83 (1.08–7.42)	2.60 (0.96–7.03)
Age			
+10 years			1.25 (0.80–1.94)
Gender			
Male			1.00
Female			0.81 (0.34–1.93)
Alcohol use			
<2x per week			1.00
≥2x per week			1.04 (0.52–2.08)

IFN-γ: interferon-gamma; QFT: QuantiFERON-TB Gold In-Tube.

hoc power analysis, assuming 43.3% QFT conversion risk that we found among participants in the lowest cigarette-smoking quartile, our sample size of 129 provided 28.1%, 55.6%, and 82.6% power to detect a RR of 1.4, 1.6, and 1.8, respectively, for QFT conversion among participants in the highest exposure quartile.

4. Discussion

In our analysis of longitudinal cohort data from PWID in Tijuana, we were not able to detect a dose-response relationship between the number of cigarettes smoked per day and QFT conversion. Previous studies evaluating dose-response relationships between cigarette-smoking and *M. tuberculosis* infection have shown mixed results for this putative association. A study of population survey data in South Africa found no evidence of a dose-response relationship between pack-years and TST positivity [9]. Likewise, a study of people with silicosis in Hong Kong found no relationship between the number of cigarettes smoked per day or cigarette pack-years and TST positivity [10]. In contrast, a study of prisoners in Pakistan found that TST prevalence increased with number of cigarettes smoked per day [11]. However, these previous studies employed cross-sectional or case-control study designs, which limit their ability to evaluate temporality between cigarette-smoking exposures and *M. tuberculosis* infection.

Cigarette smoking has been hypothesized to increase the risk of *M. tuberculosis* infection by adversely affecting the innate immune system of the host and/or causing structural damage to the respiratory tract [28]. First, expo-

sure to cigarette smoke might impair the ability of alveolar macrophages to clear the *M. tuberculosis* bacilli before T cells are primed for adaptive immunity. Under this model, increased exposure to cigarette smoke in the lungs would result in increased acute susceptibility to *M. tuberculosis* infection. We were unable to generate evidence to support this model in our study. Smoking also impairs the mucociliary clearance of pathogens and causes other changes to the respiratory tract that could increase the risk for *M. tuberculosis* infection over time [28–30]. Because we did not collect information regarding lifetime history of smoking, we were not able to evaluate the long-term effect of cigarette smoking on *M. tuberculosis* infection.

Our findings should be interpreted with consideration of the following limitations. First, we were not able to compare QFT conversion risk between smokers and nonsmokers because nearly all of our study participants reported smoking during the study followup period. If even low levels of cigarette smoking increase IGRA conversion substantially, there might have been minimal increased risk for higher frequency smokers, and our study might not have had sufficient power to detect a dose-response relationship. While we had adequate sample size to detect a RR of 1.8 or greater for QFT conversion between participants in the lowest and highest smoking exposure quartiles, the study was under-powered to conclude that there is no association between smoking and QFT conversion. We were also unable to control for history of exposure to persons with TB disease, which is a necessary causal factor for incident *M. tuberculosis* infection. The inclusion of participants who were not exposed to persons with TB disease in our analysis could have biased our results towards the null. However, controlling for a proxy variable "Have you ever known someone who had TB?" did not alter our findings (data not shown). Future longitudinal studies should investigate the risk of cigarette smoking on *M. tuberculosis* infection among study participants recruited from persons with known history of exposure to someone with TB disease.

It is also possible that our study participants were already at high risk for *M. tuberculosis* infection due to other risk factors, which might have overshadowed an incremental increase in risk due to cigarette smoking. In addition, as with TSTs, QFT assays have significant within-subject variability such that conversions and reversions often occur around the 0.35 IU/mL cutoff during serial testing even among persons who are at low risk for *M. tuberculosis* infection [31, 32]. While we used a conservative definition of QFT conversion to minimize misclassification in our analysis, the conversions observed in our study might not represent incident *M. tuberculosis* infection. Furthermore, since the recommended QFT cutoff of 0.35 IU/mL was derived to maximize specificity for *M. tuberculosis* infection, the use of this cutoff as an inclusion criterion could have resulted in the inclusion of some participants who were already infected with *M. tuberculosis* at baseline. However, restricting the analysis to only those participants with baseline QFT of <0.20 did not alter our findings (data not shown). Participants included in our study smoked fewer cigarettes than the participants who were excluded due to unavailable QFT results at 18 months. Therefore, our findings might not be generalizable to all PWID at risk for *M. tuberculosis* infection. Smoking levels were ascertained by self-report, which might have insufficient precision to evaluate a dose-response relationship. Lastly, we did not collect information regarding secondhand smoke exposure, which has been shown to be associated with *M. tuberculosis* infection among children [33].

5. Conclusions

The present study is the first longitudinal cohort study to explore the relationship between cigarette-smoking intensity and *M. tuberculosis* infection, and the first to use IGRA conversion as the outcome. Given our findings and the limitations of previous research on this topic, additional research is needed to determine whether there is a causal relationship between smoking and *M. tuberculosis* infection. For example, a recent mathematical modeling study concluded that intensified tobacco control efforts could prevent 27 million TB-related deaths by 2050 [34]. However, the authors of that study assumed a RR of 2.0 for the effect of smoking on *M. tuberculosis* infection in their model to arrive at this conclusion. Stronger evidence from larger longitudinal studies is needed to justify such assumptions. Ideally, such a study would be conducted among persons at high risk for *M. tuberculosis* infection, such as those with household exposure to persons with TB disease, and consists of sufficient numbers of smokers and nonsmokers. While the evidence of a causal relationship between smoking and

M. tuberculosis infection is weak, substantial evidence exists that implicates smoking as an independent risk factor for the development of TB disease [1–8]. Therefore, integration of tobacco and TB control interventions remains a high priority for global health [1].

Acknowledgments

The authors wish to thank the study participants and the staff at Pro-COMUSIDA who assisted with data collection. The parent study was supported by U.S. National Institute on Drug Abuse (NIDA; R37DA019829). S. S. Shin received support from NIDA Dissertation Grant 1R36DA033152. Rodwell received support from a NIAID Career Development Award K01AI083784. Garfein received support from a NIDA grant (R01DA031074).

References

[1] WHO & The Union, *Monograph on TB and Tobacco Control: Joining Efforts to Control Two Related Global Epidemics*, World Health Organization & International Union Against Tuberculosis and Lung Disease, Geneva, Switzerland, 2007.

[2] H. H. Lin, M. Ezzati, and M. Murray, "Tobacco smoke, indoor air pollution and tuberculosis: a systematic review and meta-analysis," *PLoS Medicine*, vol. 4, article e20, 2007.

[3] K. Slama, C. Y. Chiang, D. A. Enarson et al., "Tobacco and tuberculosis: a qualitative systematic review and meta-analysis," *International Journal of Tuberculosis and Lung Disease*, vol. 11, no. 10, pp. 1049–1061, 2007.

[4] M. N. Bates, A. Khalakdina, M. Pai, L. Chang, F. Lessa, and K. R. Smith, "Risk of tuberculosis from exposure to tobacco smoke: a systematic review and meta-analysis," *Archives of Internal Medicine*, vol. 167, no. 4, pp. 335–342, 2007.

[5] R. N. Van Zyl Smit, M. Pai, W. W. Yew et al., "Global lung health: the colliding epidemics of tuberculosis, tobacco smoking, HIV and COPD," *European Respiratory Journal*, vol. 35, no. 1, pp. 27–33, 2010.

[6] N. K. Schneider and T. E. Novotny, "Addressing smoking cessation in tuberculosis control," *Bulletin of the World Health Organization*, vol. 85, no. 10, pp. 820–821, 2007.

[7] S. H. Jee, J. E. Golub, J. Jo, I. S. Park, H. Ohrr, and J. M. Samet, "Smoking and risk of tuberculosis incidence, mortality, and recurrence in South Korean men and women," *American Journal of Epidemiology*, vol. 170, no. 12, pp. 1478–1485, 2009.

[8] H. H. Lin, M. Ezzati, H. Y. Chang, and M. Murray, "Association between tobacco smoking and active tuberculosis in Taiwan: prospective cohort study," *American Journal of Respiratory and Critical Care Medicine*, vol. 180, no. 5, pp. 475–480, 2009.

[9] S. Den Boon, S. W. P. Van Lill, M. W. Borgdorff et al., "Association between smoking and tuberculosis infection: a population survey in a high tuberculosis incidence area," *Thorax*, vol. 60, no. 7, pp. 555–557, 2005.

[10] C. C. Leung, W. W. Yew, W. S. Law et al., "Smoking and tuberculosis among silicotic patients," *European Respiratory Journal*, vol. 29, no. 4, pp. 745–750, 2007.

[11] H. Hussain, S. Akhtar, and D. Nanan, "Prevalence of and risk factors associated with Mycobacterium tuberculosis infection in prisoners, North West Frontier Province, Pakistan," *International Journal of Epidemiology*, vol. 32, no. 5, pp. 794–799, 2003.

[12] A. J. Plant, R. E. Watkins, B. Gushulak et al., "Predictors of tuberculin reactivity among prospective Vietnamese migrants: the effect of smoking," *Epidemiology and Infection*, vol. 128, no. 1, pp. 37–45, 2002.

[13] S. A. McCurdy, D. S. Arretz, and R. O. Bates, "Tuberculin reactivity among California Hispanic migrant farm workers," *American Journal of Industrial Medicine*, vol. 32, pp. 600–605, 1997.

[14] M. Nisar, C. S. D. Williams, D. Ashby, and P. D. O. Davies, "Tuberculin testing in residential homes for the elderly," *Thorax*, vol. 48, no. 12, pp. 1257–1260, 1993.

[15] M. Pai, "Spectrum of latent tuberculosis existing tests cannot resolve the underlying phenotypes," *Nature Reviews Microbiology*, vol. 8, article 242, 2010.

[16] P. A. Lobue and K. G. Castro, "Is it time to replace the tuberculin skin test with a blood test?" *The Journal of The American Medical Association*, vol. 308, pp. 241–242, 2012.

[17] R. S. Garfein, R. Lozada, L. Liu et al., "High prevalence of latent tuberculosis infection among injection drug users in Tijuana, Mexico," *International Journal of Tuberculosis and Lung Disease*, vol. 13, no. 5, pp. 626–632, 2009.

[18] R. S. Garfein, "Serial testing using QuantiFERON TB Gold In-tube assay in a high-risk population," in *Proceedings of the 3rd Annual Symposium on Interferon Gamma Release Assays*, Waikoloa, Hawaii, USA, 2012.

[19] S. A. Strathdee, R. Lozada, R. A. Pollini et al., "Individual, social, and environmental influences associated with HIV infection among injection drug users in Tijuana, Mexico," *Journal of Acquired Immune Deficiency Syndromes*, vol. 47, no. 3, pp. 369–376, 2008.

[20] D. D. Heckathorn, "Respondent-driven sampling II: deriving valid population estimates from chain-referral samples of hidden populations," *Social Problems*, vol. 49, no. 1, pp. 11–34, 2002.

[21] M. J. Salganik, "Respondent-driven sampling in the real world," *Epidemiology*, vol. 23, pp. 148–150, 2012.

[22] M. Pai, R. Joshi, S. Dogra et al., "Serial testing of health care workers for tuberculosis using interferon-γ assay," *American Journal of Respiratory and Critical Care Medicine*, vol. 174, no. 3, pp. 349–355, 2006.

[23] L. A. McNutt, C. Wu, X. Xue, and J. P. Hafner, "Estimating the relative risk in cohort studies and clinical trials of common outcomes," *American Journal of Epidemiology*, vol. 157, no. 10, pp. 940–943, 2003.

[24] D. Spiegelman and E. Hertzmark, "Easy SAS calculations for risk or prevalence ratios and differences," *American Journal of Epidemiology*, vol. 162, no. 3, pp. 199–200, 2005.

[25] D. Abramovitz, E. M. Volz, S. A. Strathdee, T. L. Patterson, A. Vera, and S. D. W. Frost, "Using respondent-driven sampling in a hidden population at risk of HIV infection: who do HIV-positive recruiters recruit?" *Sexually Transmitted Diseases*, vol. 36, no. 12, pp. 750–756, 2009.

[26] S. Greenland, "Modeling and variable selection in epidemiologic analysis," *American Journal of Public Health*, vol. 79, no. 3, pp. 340–349, 1989.

[27] D. G. Kleinbaum, L. L. Kupper, K. E. Muller, and N. Azhar, *Applied Regression Analysis and Other Multivariable Methods*, Duxbury Press, North Scituate, Mass, USA, 4th edition, 2008.

[28] L. Arcavi and N. L. Benowitz, "Cigarette smoking and infection," *Archives of Internal Medicine*, vol. 164, no. 20, pp. 2206–2216, 2004.

[29] J. Garmendia, P. Morey, and B. J. Antonio, "Impact of cigarette smoke exposure on host-bacterial pathogen interactions," *European Respiratory Journal*, vol. 39, no. 2, pp. 467–477, 2012.

[30] R. H. Anderson, F. S. Sy, S. Thompson, and C. Addy, "Cigarette smoking and tuberculin skin test conversion among incarcerated adults," *American Journal of Preventive Medicine*, vol. 13, no. 3, pp. 175–181, 1997.

[31] R. N. van Zyl-Smit, A. Zwerling, K. Dheda, and M. Pai, "Within-subject variability of interferon-g assay results for tuberculosis and boosting effect of tuberculin skin testing: a systematic review," *PLoS ONE*, vol. 4, no. 12, Article ID e8517, 2009.

[32] A. Zwerling, S. van den Hof, J. Scholten, F. Cobelens, D. Menzies, and M. Pai, "Interferon-gamma release assays for tuberculosis screening of healthcare workers: a systematic review," *Thorax*, vol. 67, pp. 62–70, 2012.

[33] S. Den Boon, S. Verver, B. J. Marais et al., "Association between passive smoking and infection with Mycobacterium tuberculosis in children," *Pediatrics*, vol. 119, no. 4, pp. 734–739, 2007.

[34] S. Basu, D. Stuckler, A. Bitton, and S. A. Glantz, "Projected effects of tobacco smoking on worldwide tuberculosis control: mathematical modelling analysis," *British Medical Journal*, vol. 343, article d5506, 2011.

13

Concave Pattern of a Maximal Expiratory Flow-Volume Curve: A Sign of Airflow Limitation in Adult Bronchial Asthma

Akihiko Ohwada[1, 2] and Kazuhisa Takahashi[2]

[1] Ohwada Clinic, 4-7-13 Minamiyawata, Ichikawa, Chiba 272-0023, Japan
[2] Department of Respiratory Medicine, Juntendo University School of Medicine, Tokyo 113-8421, Japan

Correspondence should be addressed to Akihiko Ohwada, aohwada@hotmail.co.jp

Academic Editor: Roberto Walter Dal Negro

Background. In patients with bronchial asthma, spirometry could identify the airflow limitation of small airways by evaluating the concave shape of the maximal expiratory flow-volume (MEFV) curve. As the concave shape of the MEFV curve is not well documented, we reevaluated the importance of this curve in adult asthmatic patients. *Methods.* We evaluated spirometric parameters, the MEFV curve, and its concave shape (scoop between the peak and endpoint of expiration) in 27 nonsmoking asthmatic patients with physician-confirmed wheeze and positive bronchial reversibility after a short-acting β2-agonist inhalation. We also calculated angle β and shape factors ($SF_{25\%}$ and $SF_{50\%}$) to quantitate the curvilinearity of the MEFV curve. *Results.* The MEFV curve was concave in all patients. Along with improvements in standard spirometric parameters, curvilinear parameters, angle β, $SF_{25\%}$, and $SF_{50\%}$ were significantly improved after bronchodilator inhalation. There were significant correlations between improvements in angle β, and $FEF_{50\%}$, and $FEF_{25-75\%}$, and between improvements in $SF_{25\%}$, and $SF_{50\%}$, and $FEF_{75\%}$. *Conclusions.* The bronchodilator greatly affected the concave shape of the MEFV curve, correlating with spirometric parameters of small airway obstructions ($FEF_{50\%}$, $FEF_{75\%}$, and $FEF_{25-75\%}$). Thus, the concave shape of the MEFV curve is an important indicator of airflow limitation in adult asthmatic patients.

1. Introduction

Evaluation of airflow limitation is crucial for diagnosis of bronchial asthma and chronic obstructive pulmonary diseases. Spirometry is a simple but important procedure to detect airflow limitation. Reductions of forced expiratory volume in 1 s (FEV_1), FEV_1/forced vital capacity (FVC) ratio, and peak expiratory flow (PEF) are proven signs [1].

In the 1970s and 80s, analysis of the configuration of maximal expiratory flow-volume (MEFV) curve concluded that the concave shape of the MEFV curve reflects the presence of small airway obstructions. Kraan et al. analyzed the changes in the MEFV curve in patients with bronchial asthma after treatment with inhaled steroids using indices of curvilinearity of the MEFV curve, shape factors (SFs), and slope ratio (SR) [2]. They revealed that the shape of the curve became less bowed toward the volume axis after inhaled corticosteroids and concluded that such a change in

the MEFV curve reflects a decrease in the inhomogeneous distribution of airflow narrowing. Kapp et al. defined a new parameter, angle β, to characterize the shape of the MEFV curve and revealed that patients with asthma, chronic bronchitis, dyspnea, and wheeze had significantly lower β angles than healthy individuals [3].

In 2005, the American Thoracic Society (ATS)/European Respiratory Society (ERS) task force noted that the earliest changes associated with airflow obstruction in small airways are thought to be slowing in the terminal portion of the spirogram, even when the initial part of the spirogram is barely affected. This slowing of expiratory flow is most obviously reflected in the concave shape on the MEFV curve. It is reflected quantitatively in a reduced force expiratory flow (FEF) at 75% of FVC expired ($FEF_{75\%}$) or FEF between 25 and 75% of VC ($FEF_{25-75\%}$) [4]. However, abnormalities in these midrange flow measurements during forced exhalation are not specific for some cases of small airway diseases. It is thus still unclear whether the concave shape of the MEFV curve is an indicator of airflow limitation.

In this study, we analyzed the shape of the MEFV curve in patients with bronchial asthma with both physician-confirmed wheeze and positive bronchial reversibility and reevaluated the importance of the concave shape of the curve in diagnosis of bronchial asthma.

2. Methods

Subjects with physician-confirmed wheeze auscultated at their initial visit were enrolled from among nonsmoking asthmatic patients who complained of cough and dyspnea. Patients with obvious acute respiratory infection were excluded. None of the patients had taken inhaled steroids or $\beta2$ agonists for at least 3 months before the visit.

Spirometry was performed with a Microspiro HI-801 (Chest Inc., Japan) following the instructions in the ATS/ERS statements, and the highest FVC, FEV_1, FEV_1/FVC ratio, and PEF values of the technically acceptable recordings were taken (4,5). FEF at 25%, 50%, and 75% of FVC expired ($FEF_{75\%}$, $FEF_{50\%}$, and $FEF_{25\%}$, resp.); $FEF_{25-75\%}$ were measured from the recording that had the largest sum of FEV_1 and FVC [4, 5]. These parameters are presented as absolute values and percentiles of the predicted values (% predicted). The spirometric reference values used have been reported by the Japanese Respiratory Society for FVC, FEV_1, FEV_1/FVC ratio, $FEF_{75\%}$, and $FEF_{50\%}$ [6] and elsewhere for PEF [7], $FEF_{25-75\%}$ [7], and $FEF_{75\%}$ [8].

Reversibility of airflow limitation was evaluated with FEV_1 at 15 min after the inhalation of salbutamol 200 μg using a spacer following ATS/ERS standardization [5]. Bronchial reversibility is defined as a SABA-induced increase in FEV_1 of ≥ 0.20 L and $\geq 12\%$ of baseline [1].

Several ways to quantify the shape of the MEFV curve have been proposed. To characterize the shape of the MEFV curve using angle β the residual volume (RV) point of the MEFV curve was joined to the flow point at midvolume and then the flow point at midvolume to a point at the level of the total lung capacity (TLC) at the height of the peak flow above the x-axis. Although angle β could obtain graphically by tracing angle β as in Figure 1(d), Kapp et al. validated the use of angle β with the following equation: $\beta = 180° - \beta' + \beta'' = 180° - \tan^{-1}(PEF - FEF_{50\%}/0.5 \times FVC) + \tan^{-1}(FEF_{50\%}/0.5 \times FVC)$ (all $\tan^{-1}$ values were calculated in degrees) to obtain results similar to manual tracing [3]. Hence, we calculated the angle from obtained spirometric parameters. Values of $\beta < 180°$ correspond to the concavity of MEFV [3].

Shape factors (SFs) were other indices of curvilinearity of the MEFV curve. $SF_{50\%}$ and $SF_{25\%}$ were obtained from the respective equations: $1/2 \times FEF_{50\%}/FEF_{75\%}$ and $1/3 \times FEF_{25\%}/FEF_{75\%}$ [2]. To calculate SFs, % predicted values were applied to $FEF_{75\%}$, $FEF_{50\%}$, and $FEF_{25\%}$. A value of $SF_{50\%}$ or $SF_{25\%}$ larger than 1 indicated a concave pattern of the MEFV curve. Percent change (from baseline) was also calculated for the spirometric parameters other than FEV_1, angle β, $SF_{25\%}$,

and $SF_{50\%}$. All patients provided an informed consent and the study was approved by the institutional review board.

2.1. Statistical Analysis. Data are presented as means ± SD. Baseline spirometric parameters were compared to those after SABA inhalation by paired t test. Correlation coefficients for angle β, $SF_{25\%}$, and $SF_{50\%}$ with other spirometric parameters were calculated for % change by the non-parametric Spearman method using Graphpad Prism (Graphpad Software, Inc., San Diego, CA). $P < 0.05$ was considered to indicate a significant difference.

3. Results

Among 1020 nonsmoking asthmatic patients over a 20-month period, 51 (5.2%) had physician-confirmed wheeze by auscultation at their first visit. Consecutively, we evaluated bronchial reversibility in these 51 patients. Of these, 27 (51%), aged 18–68 years had bronchial reversibility. All 27 included subjects were Japanese (10 males and 17 females) and had symptoms of cough and dyspnea at their first visit. Eight patients had a past history of childhood bronchial asthma, 5 had been diagnosed adult-onset asthma prior to their visits, and 8 had a family history of asthma. Fifteen of the patients had allergic rhinitis, allergic eczema, or were positive on an allergic blood test.

The baseline values of the spirometric parameters were shown in Table 1.

The concave shape of the MEFV curve was defined as a curve with a scoop between the peak of the curve and the endpoint of expiration (Figure 1). All patients had a concave flow-volume curve. Two (7.4%) of the 27 patients had normal values for FEV_1 ($\geq 80\%$ of predicted value), FEV_1/FVC ratio ($\geq 70\%$), and PEF ($\geq 80\%$).

The baseline angle β was 172 ± 21°. Twenty (74%) of the 27 patients had angle $\beta < 180°$, indicating the concavity of the MEFV curve. The baseline values of $SF_{25\%}$ and $SF_{50\%}$ were 0.62 ± 0.34 and 0.61 ± 0.19, respectively. $SF_{25\%}$ and $SF_{50\%}$ values <1 were found in three (11%) and two (7.4%) patients, respectively.

The change in FEV_1 from baseline after SABA inhalation was in Table 1. 0.61 ± 0.56 L (range: 0.20–2.67 L), with 25.4 ± 25.0% change (12.4–127.7%).

The values of the spirometric parameters after SABA inhalation were demonstrated in Table 1. All values after SABA inhalation were significantly higher than baseline values. The values of angle β, $SF_{25\%}$, and $SF_{50\%}$ after SABA inhalation were 188 ± 20°, 0.19 ± 0.07, 0.25 ± 0.13, respectively (Table 1). Angle β after SABA inhalation was increased in all patients except for one (data not shown). Both $SF_{25\%}$ and $SF_{50\%}$ were decreased after SABA inhalation in all but one. These changes indicated that the concavity of the MEFV curve improved after bronchodilating treatment.

To explore the factors that influence the changes in angle β, $SF_{25\%}$, and $SF_{50\%}$ after SABA inhalation, correlations were examined between their % changes and the % changes of the standard spirometric parameters (Table 2).

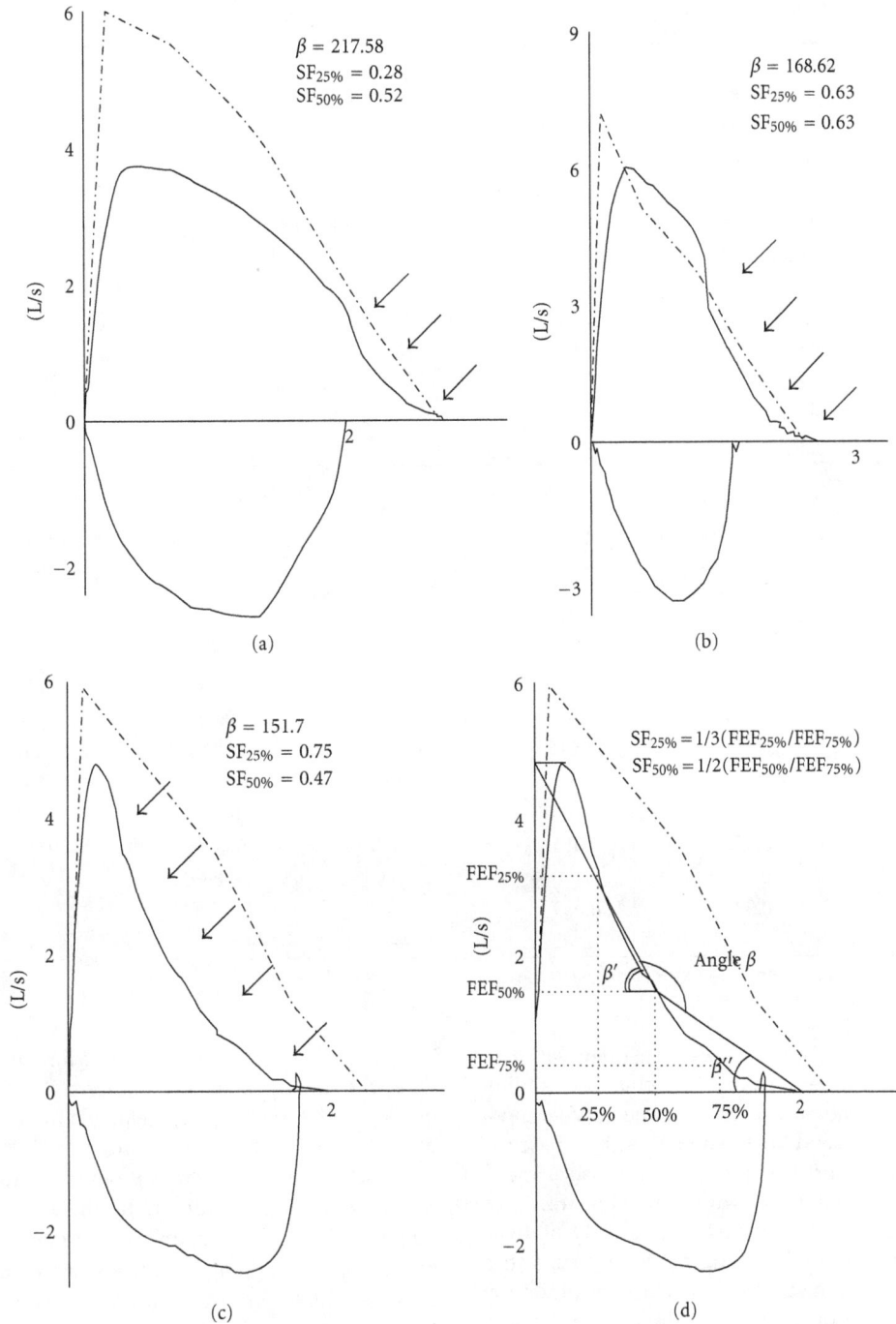

FIGURE 1: (a–c) Representative cases of various patterns of concave maximal expiratory flow-volume curves in the subjects analyzed in this study. Arrows indicate the concave region of the curve. (d) Calculation of angle β and shape factors ($SF_{25\%}$ and $SF_{50\%}$) from standard spirometric parameters.

Improvement in angle β was significantly correlated with improvements in $FEF_{50\%}$ ($r = 0.71$, $P < 0.0001$) and $FEF_{25-75\%}$ ($r = 0.57$, $P = 0.0017$). Improvements (decrease in values) in $SF_{25\%}$ and $SF_{50\%}$ were strongly linked with each other ($r = 0.9$, $P < 0.0001$) and significantly correlated with improvement in $FEF_{75\%}$ ($r = 0.53$, $P = 0.0046$ for $SF_{25\%}$; $r = 0.54$, $P = 0.0041$ for $SF_{50\%}$) after SABA inhalation.

4. Discussion

The prevalence of current wheeze in asthmatic children varied among countries ranged from 0.8% to 32.6% in the 13-14-year olds and ranged from 2.4% to 37.6% in the 6-7-years olds [9]. The prevalence of patient-recognized wheeze in adult asthmatic subjects would also vary widely and be

TABLE 1: Spirometric parameters in patients with wheeze and bronchial reversibility.

	Baseline		After SABA inhalation		P
	Absolute	% predict	Absolute	% predict	
FCV (L)	3.18 ± 1.05	84.4 ± 18.0	3.51 ± 1.05	93.0 ± 15.6	0.0003
FEV_1/FCV (%)	70.7 ± 10.2		78.4 ± 10.4		<0.0001
FEV_1 (L)	2.24 ± 0.74	72.9 ± 18.1	2.76 ± 0.92	89.1 ± 18.1	<0.0001
PEF (L/s)	4.90 ± 1.88	59.6 ± 16.5	5.64 ± 2.06	68.2 ± 17.1	0.0022
$FEF_{25-75\%}$ (L/s)	1.85 ± 0.92	48.1 ± 23.7	2.66 ± 1.38	67.4 ± 29.7	<0.0001
$FEF_{25\%}$ (L/s)	3.82 ± 1.52	63.0 ± 22.1	5.15 ± 1.99	84.2 ± 27.0	0.0034
$FEF_{50\%}$ (L/s)	2.04 ± 1.02	47.3 ± 23.6	3.20 ± 1.63	72.4 ± 31.0	<0.0001
$FEF_{75\%}$ (L/s)	0.81 ± 0.49	43.4 ± 28.0	1.22 ± 0.74	63.6 ± 36.3	<0.0001
Angle β	172 ± 21		188 ± 20		<0.0001
$SF_{25\%}$	0.62 ± 0.34		0.19 ± 0.07		<0.0001
$SF_{50\%}$	0.61 ± 0.19		0.25 ± 0.13		<0.0001

Each value is shown as the mean ± SD.

TABLE 2: Correlation between % changes of angle β, $SF_{25\%}$, and $SF_{50\%}$ and % changes of spirometric parameters after SABA inhalation.

	Angle β versus		$SF_{25\%}$ versus		$SF_{50\%}$ versus	
	r	P	r	P	r	P
FVC (% change)	0.0043	0.98	−0.085	0.57	−0.32	0.11
FEV_1 (% change)	0.32	0.1	−0.23	0.24	−0.32	0.1
PEF (% change)	−0.15	0.47	0.096	0.63	0.0067	0.97
$FEF_{25-75\%}$ (% change)	0.57	**0.0017**	−0.43	**0.024**	−0.31	0.12
$FEF_{25\%}$ (% change)	0.075	0.71	−0.12	0.54	−0.35	0.074
$FEF_{50\%}$ (% change)	0.71	**<0.0001**	−0.35	0.078	−0.25	0.21
$FEF_{75\%}$ (% change)	0.47	**0.013**	−0.53	**0.0046**	−0.54	**0.0041**
$SF_{50\%}$ (% change)	0.12	0.54	−0.9	**<0.0001**	—	—
$SF_{25\%}$ (% change)	0.33	0.089	—	—	—	—
Angle β (% change)	—	—	—	—	—	—

Bold text indicates significant correlation between the parameters.

reported as 5.4% in Japan; that rate was consistent with our observation [10]. Moreover, positive bronchial reversibility is thought to be dependent on the baseline FEV_1 values. Yancey and Ortega showed that patients with a baseline FEV_1 of 40% to <50% predicted at screening had a mean reversibility of 42%, and those with a baseline FEV_1 of 90% to <100% predicted had a mean reversibility of 18%, suggesting that a lower baseline lung function results in a higher reversibility [11]. In our previous study, we randomly enrolled 45 patients with bronchial asthma with a mean FEV_1 value of 88.96% predicted in outpatient clinic and found that 9 (20%) of them were positive for bronchial reversibility [12]. In this study, the positive rate of bronchial reversibility was higher (51%) than that expected for patients with physician-confirmed wheeze (mean baseline FEV_1; 72.9% predicted). Although patients with bronchial asthma are heterogeneous in respect to bronchial responsiveness to bronchodilator treatment [11], our result indicates that the patients with wheeze are well responders for bronchodilators. Hence, we chose in this study only asthmatic patients with both physician-confirmed wheeze and positive bronchial reversibility to reduce the divergence of the SABA response. Thus, our cohort was small in this outpatient clinical setting.

We recognized the presence of some limitations in this study. One was small numbers of subjects. Another was whether our selected patients group belonged to peculiar or ordinary phenotype of adult asthma. Interestingly recent analysis of the Severe Asthma Research Program (SARP) revealed that severe asthma was peculiar to be characterized by abnormal lung function that is responsive to bronchodilators [13] and prominent air trapping (detected as increased RV/TLC ratio) over the entire range of airflow obstruction severity and that nonsevere asthmatic patients did not exhibit significant air trapping even at the more severe stages of airflow limitation expressed as FEV_1/FVC ratio [14].

Mead developed the slope ratio (SR), defined as tangent slope $(d\dot{V}/dV)$ divided by the chord $\dot{V}/(FVC-V)$, as an index of the curvilinearity of the MEFV curve [15]. However, special values of FEF are needed, for example, at 87.5%, 62.5%, 37.5%, and 12.5% of FVC expired, to obtain SRs at 75%, 50%, and 25%, or the values need to be directly measured from the plotted MEFV curve [15, 16]. As it is impractical to use SRs in a standard pulmonary function test, we used angle β, $SF_{25\%}$, and $SF_{50\%}$ to quantify the concave pattern of the MEFV curve.

The concave shape of the MEFV curve was confirmed in 74% of the patients based on the baseline angle β ($<180°$), in 11% based on baseline $SF_{25\%}$ (<1.0), and in 7% based on baseline $SF_{50\%}$ (<1.0). One reason of rather poor concordance of these three indexes with curve shape might be due to inappropriate threshold values to classify the curve. For angle β, Kapp et al. demonstrated that the values for adult male and female individuals with no impairment of FEV_1 were $190.5 \pm 17.7°$, $198.8 \pm 17.9°$, respectively [3]. Normal value of angle β is probably larger than $180°$ and is influenced with age and gender [3]. For SFs, there is no additional study found. In our study, both $SF_{25\%}$ and $SF_{50\%}$ were significantly improved along with angle β and other standard spirometric parameters after SABA inhalation (Table 1). This finding indicates that the values of SFs also respond to the effects of the bronchodilator. Hence we are unable to easily discard SF indexes due to poor discriminatory power in this small-scaled evaluation. Further analysis of concordance/disagreement of these three indexes with or without regard to the FEF values should be necessary. It must also apply to evaluate with the spirometric values after bronchodilating treatment.

Next, we evaluated which spirometric parameters were related to the improvements in angle β, $SF_{25\%}$, and $SF_{50\%}$ after SABA inhalation by analyzing correlation coefficients (Table 2). We revealed that % changes from baseline values of angle β, $SF_{25\%}$, and $SF_{50\%}$ were related to % changes of $FEF_{50\%}$, $FEF_{75\%}$ and $FEF_{25-75\%}$, the parameters of airflow limitation in small airways [4, 17]. Thus, we considered that the concave shape of the MEFV curve reflected the airflow limitation in small airways.

A concave flow-volume curve has been described in a few studies of childhood asthma [18, 19]. It was suggested that the severity of asthma in school-aged children could be predicted at the first visit based on a concave flow-volume curve and the past frequency of symptoms [18]. Ethnic differences may also play a role in pulmonary function in child asthma. Hispanic girls with asthma have a larger flow deficit than non-Hispanic girls and have larger reductions in $FEF_{75\%}$, FEV_1, and PEF [19]. Further investigations are needed to evaluate ethnic differences in the concave pattern of the MEFV curve in adult patients with bronchial asthma. Recently it was demonstrated that children with wheezing disorders had lower angle β than healthy children [20].

After several years of debate surrounding this topic, the contribution of small airway abnormalities in asthma pathobiology remains mainly unanswered. It is likely that a combination of techniques, including lung function tests such as evaluation of lung volumes through spirometry and/or the single-breath nitrogen washout, possibly associated with imaging, could be the most suitable approach. Once defined and accepted, these techniques would have to be used in a properly designed clinical study aimed at assessing the impact of treatments targeting the distal lung and possibly at establishing a correlation between the modification of distal lung parameters and improvement in the clinical status of the patient [21, 22].

In our analysis, angle β proposed by Kapp et al. reflected the configuration of the MEFV curve. Based on our definition of the concave shape, direct observation of the curve is simple. Even a patient with the curve seen in Figure 1(a) has wheeze and positive bronchial reversibility. Of note, two patients (7.4%) with wheeze and positive bronchial reversibility had normal values of FEV_1, FEV_1/FVC, and PEF, but showed a concave shape in their MEFV curves.

Here, we emphasize the importance of the shape of the MEFV curve as a simple indicator of airflow limitation, even in patients with normal values of FEV_1, PEF, and FEV_1/FVC.

Conflict of Interests

There are no financial or other potential conflicts of interest of relevance to this article.

Acknowledgments

The authors are grateful to the colleagues of the Department of Respiratory Medicine, Juntendo University for their helpful discussion and advice.

References

[1] Global Initiative for Asthma (GINA), "Global strategy for asthma management and prevention," NHLBI/WHO Workshop Report, National Institutes of Health, National Heart, Lung and Blood Institute, Bethesda, Md, USA, 2009.

[2] J. Kraan, T. W. van der Mark, and G. H. Koeter, "Changes in maximum expiratory flow-volume curve configuration after treatment with inhaled corticosteroids," Thorax, vol. 44, no. 12, pp. 1015–1021, 1989.

[3] M. C. Kapp, E. N. Schachter, G. J. Beck, L. R. Maunder, and T. J. Witek, "The shape of the maximum expiratory flow volume curve," Chest, vol. 94, no. 4, pp. 799–806, 1988.

[4] R. Pellegrino, G. Viegi, V. Brusasco et al., "Interpretative strategies for lung function tests," European Respiratory Journal, vol. 26, no. 5, pp. 948–968, 2005.

[5] M. R. Miller, J. Hankinson, V. Brusasco et al., "Standardisation of spirometry," European Respiratory Journal, vol. 26, no. 2, pp. 319–338, 2005.

[6] Japanese Respiratory Society, "Standard reference values of spirometric parameters and arterial blood gas analysis," (Author translated) in Japanese, The Japanese Respiratory Society Journal http://www.jrs.or.jp/quicklink/glsm/guideline/nopass_pdf/spirogram.pdf, 2004.

[7] J. L. Hankinson, J. R. Odencrantz, and K. B. Fedan, "Spirometric reference values from a sample of the general U.S. population," American Journal of Respiratory and Critical Care Medicine, vol. 159, no. 1, pp. 179–187, 1999.

[8] A. Bouhuys, "Pulmonary function measurements in epidemiological studies," Bull Eur Physiopathol Respir, vol. 6, no. 3, pp. 561–578, 1970.

[9] C. K. W. Lai, R. Beasley, J. Crane et al., "Global variation in the prevalence and severity of asthma symptoms: phase three of the International Study of Asthma and Allergies in Childhood (ISAAC)," Thorax, vol. 64, no. 6, pp. 476–483, 2009.

[10] Y. Fukutomi, M. Taniguchi, J. Watanabe et al., "Time trend in the prevalence of adult asthma in Japan: findings from population-based surveys in Fujieda City in 1985, 1999, and

2006," *Allergology International*, vol. 60, no. 4, pp. 443–448, 2011.

[11] S. W. Yancey and H. G. Ortega, "Retrospective characterization of airway reversibility in patients with asthma responsive to bronchodilators," *Current Medical Research and Opinion*, vol. 23, no. 12, pp. 3205–3207, 2007.

[12] A. Ohwada, K. Inami, E. Onuma, M. Matsumoto-Yamazaki, R. Atsuta, and K. Takahashi, "Bronchial reversibility with a short-acting β2-agonist predicts the FEV1 response to administration of a long-acting β2-agonist with inhaled corticosteroids in patients with bronchial asthma," *Experimental and Therapeutic Medicine*, vol. 2, no. 4, pp. 619–623, 2011.

[13] W. C. Moore, E. R. Bleecker, D. Curran-Everett et al., "Characterization of the severe asthma phenotype by the National Heart, Lung, and Blood Institute's Severe Asthma Research Program," *Journal of Allergy and Clinical Immunology*, vol. 119, no. 2, pp. 405–413, 2007.

[14] R. L. Sorkness, E. R. Bleecker, W. W. Busse et al., "Lung function in adults with stable but severe asthma: air trapping and incomplete reversal of obstruction with bronchodilation," *Journal of Applied Physiology*, vol. 104, no. 2, pp. 394–403, 2008.

[15] J. Mead, "Analysis of the configuration of maximum expiratory flow-volume curves," *Journal of Applied Physiology Respiratory Environmental and Exercise Physiology*, vol. 44, no. 2, pp. 156–165, 1978.

[16] O. Omland, T. Sigsgaard, O. F. Pedersen, and M. R. Miller, "The shape of the maximum expiratory flow-volume curve reflects exposure in farming," *Annals of Agricultural and Environmental Medicine*, vol. 7, no. 2, pp. 71–78, 2000.

[17] R. Drewek, E. Garber, S. Stanclik, P. Simpson, M. Nugent, and W. Gershan, "The FEF_{25-75} and its decline as a predictor of methacholine responsiveness in children," *Journal of Asthma*, vol. 46, no. 4, pp. 375–381, 2009.

[18] O. Linna, "A doctor's ability to assess the severity of childhood asthma by simple clinical features," *Acta Paediatrica*, vol. 94, no. 5, pp. 559–563, 2005.

[19] Y. Zhang, R. McConnell, F. Gilliland, and K. Berhane, "Ethnic differences in the effect of asthma on pulmonary function in children," *American Journal of Respiratory and Critical Care Medicine*, vol. 183, no. 5, pp. 596–603, 2011.

[20] V. Nève, R. Matran, G. Baquet et al., "Quantification of shape of flow-volume loop of healthy preschool children and preschool children with wheezing disorders," *Pediatric Pulmonology*, vol. 47, no. 9, pp. 884–894, 2012.

[21] M. Contoli, J. Bousquet, L. M. Fabbri et al., "The small airways and distal lung compartment in asthma and COPD: a time for reappraisal," *Allergy*, vol. 65, no. 2, pp. 141–151, 2010.

[22] M. Contoli, M. Kraft, Q. Hamid et al., "Do small airway abnormalities characterize asthma phenotypes? In search of proof," *Clinical & Experimental Allergy*, vol. 42, no. 8, pp. 1150–1160, 2012.

14

Flow-Volume Parameters in COPD Related to Extended Measurements of Lung Volume, Diffusion, and Resistance

Linnea Jarenbäck, Jaro Ankerst, Leif Bjermer, and Ellen Tufvesson

Department of Clinical Sciences, Respiratory Medicine and Allergology, Lund University, 221 84 Lund, Sweden

Correspondence should be addressed to Leif Bjermer; leif.bjermer@med.lu.se

Academic Editor: S. L. Johnston

Classification of COPD into different GOLD stages is based on forced expiratory volume in 1 s (FEV_1) and forced vital capacity (FVC) but has shown to be of limited value. The aim of the study was to relate spirometry values to more advanced measures of lung function in COPD patients compared to healthy smokers. The lung function of 65 COPD patients and 34 healthy smokers was investigated using flow-volume spirometry, body plethysmography, single breath helium dilution with CO-diffusion, and impulse oscillometry. All lung function parameters, measured by body plethysmography, CO-diffusion, and impulse oscillometry, were increasingly affected through increasing GOLD stage but did not correlate with FEV_1 within any GOLD stage. In contrast, they correlated fairly well with FVC%p, FEV_1/FVC, and inspiratory capacity. Residual volume (RV) measured by body plethysmography increased through GOLD stages, while RV measured by helium dilution decreased. The difference between these RV provided valuable additional information and correlated with most other lung function parameters measured by body plethysmography and CO-diffusion. Airway resistance measured by body plethysmography and impulse oscillometry correlated within COPD stages. Different lung function parameters are of importance in COPD, and a thorough patient characterization is important to understand the disease.

1. Introduction

Spirometry and body plethysmography are the most commonly used methods to diagnose, characterize, and assess chronic pulmonary obstructive disease (COPD). The global initiative of obstructive lung diseases (GOLD) classification of COPD [1] is acknowledged around the globe and is recommended both by the American Thoracic Society and the European Respiratory Society. It has long been based on spirometry and health status alone. However, a new version from 2011 proposes the importance of considering exacerbation frequency and assessing the severity of breathlessness, using the modified Medical Research Council Questionnaire (mMRC), in the classification of COPD. For practical purposes, flow-volume spirometry is used to characterize lung function in COPD patients. It is easily used, and the measurements derive reproducible data. Forced expiratory volume in 1 s (FEV_1) is most commonly used but is of limited value in relation to functional ability and quality of life when used

alone [2, 3]. On the other hand, spirometry also provides data of forced vital capacity (FVC) and inspiratory capacity (IC) which are the tools of choice for most population surveys.

It has long been known that spirometry measures mostly the proximal parts of the airway, while COPD is mostly a disease of the distal airways [4]. Akamatsu et al. screened patients from a nonrespiratory section of the hospital, including smokers, former smokers, and never-smokers [5]. They found that 25 out of 288 patients had COPD according to the GOLD standard (21 patients GOLD1, 4 patients GOLD2), but 52% of these patients still claimed to have no respiratory symptoms at all. This suggests that the symptoms of COPD can develop later in the disease stage. It is important to diagnose the patients at an early stage since the disease is progressive and irreversible. Since no treatment is available to stop the progression in the early stage, it is of great importance to identify patients in this stage to evaluate novel therapies for disease progression.

It is therefore important to use plausible lung function measurements for a satisfactory diagnosis and monitoring of COPD. Body plethysmography and single breath helium dilution with carbon monoxide- (CO-) diffusion are two commonly used techniques to evaluate lung volumes in order to look at hyperinflation that is not reflected by spirometry. However, the helium dilution method is known to underestimate lung volumes, while body plethysmography measures increased lung volumes in obstructive patients [6]. After administration of tiotropium for two weeks in obstructive patients with hyperinflation, lung volumes such as residual volume (RV) and functional residual capacity (FRC) measured with body plethysmography decreased, while RV and FRC measured by helium dilution method increased [7].

Impulse oscillometry (IOS) can detect distal airway malfunctions that are not measured with normal spirometry. COPD patients have a higher total resistance (R5), and peripheral resistance (R5–R20), and a more negative reactance at 5 Hz (X5) than healthy never-smokers [8]. Increased effect on R5, R5–R20, and X5 was seen with increased disease severity. However, none of the IOS parameters could separate healthy never-smokers from GOLD1 [8]. Interestingly, subgroups of COPD patients showed normal IOS values, as some patients with low reactance area (AX) displayed low FEV_1, and patients with abnormal R5 showed less emphysema [9]. Several studies have shown a correlation between several IOS parameters and FEV_1 [8, 10, 11], CT scans, dyspnea, and health status [12]. Frantz et al. recently showed that patients with self-reported chronic bronchitis, emphysema, or COPD have higher resistance and lower reactance than patients without self-reported disease independent of spirometry-based diagnosis [13]. This suggests that IOS could be used to detect pathological changes in COPD earlier than spirometry. In contrast, it has been shown that commonly used pulmonary function tests were more sensitive in detecting COPD than was IOS but had the same specificity in excluding COPD [14].

The aim of the present study was to relate established flow-volume spirometry values to other more advanced measures of lung function using body plethysmography, single breath helium dilution with CO-diffusion and IOS in COPD patients in different stages, and healthy smokers that have not developed COPD. A secondary aim was to evaluate better characterization of lung function impairment of importance in different degrees of COPD. We hope to expand characterization of COPD patients using other parameters than from normally used flow-volume measurements to get an extended picture of the lung physiology in different COPD phenotypes.

2. Methods

2.1. Subjects. Ninety-nine volunteers were screened with spirometry; 65 were classified as COPD patients (FEV_1/FVC < 0.7) and 34 as healthy smokers ($FEV_1 \geq$ 80%, FEV_1/FVC $\geq$ 0.7) (Table 1). The COPD patients were diagnosed and categorized into GOLD stages according to GOLD standards (http://www.goldcopd.org/ version 2011 [1]). Thirteen GOLD1 ($FEV_1 \geq$ 80% of predicted normal), 22 GOLD2 (50 $\geq$

FEV_1 < 80% of predicted normal), 15 GOLD3 (30 $\geq$ FEV_1 < 50% of predicted normal) and 15 GOLD4 (FEV_1 < 30% of predicted normal) were included. Study participants had no history of lung cancer, asthma, or cardiorespiratory diseases and had a history as smokers or former smokers with $\geq$ 15 pack years. Neither exacerbation nor respiratory infection was allowed within the last 3 weeks. All lung function measurements were done after receiving 400 μg short-acting beta-2 agonist (salbutamol, Buventol Easyhaler) according to the GOLD classification system. Three patients with GOLD3 and eight patients with GOLD4 had also inhaled long-acting muscarinic antagonists (18 μg tiotropium, Spiriva).

2.2. Study Design. The study was approved by the Regional Ethical Review Board in Lund (431/2008), and all study participants signed written informed consent. A physical examination was performed before the start of the study. All subjects performed IOS (Jaeger MasterScreen, Erich Jaeger GmbH, Würzburg, Germany), body plethysmography together with flow-volume spirometry (MasterScreen Body Jaeger) and single breath helium dilution with CO-diffusion test (MasterScreen Diffusion Jaeger) in given order. FEV_1 and FVC were measured using established flow-volume spirometry, and FEV_1/FVC was calculated. From body plethysmography (BP) inspiratory resistance (R_{in}), expiratory resistance (R_{ex}), IC, RV_{BP}, total lung capacity ($TLC)_{BP}$, and FRC_{BP} were recorded. The technique of single breath helium dilution with CO-diffusion tests (SB) estimates lung volumes, such as RV_{SB}, TLC_{SB}, and FRC_{SB}, diffusing capacity of the lung for carbon monoxide (DLCO) and alveolar volume (VA) was measured, and DLCO/VA was calculated. Resistance at 5 HZ (R5; total resistance) and 20 Hz (R20; central resistance), Resonance frequency (Fres), Reactance at 5 Hz (X5), and Reactance area (AX) were measured by IOS, and R5–R20 (peripheral resistance) was subsequently calculated. All lung function measurements were made according to ERS/ATS standardizations [15–17]. Reference values established by Crapo were used [18]. Information about COPD symptoms was documented in a self-filled in Clinical COPD Questionnaire (CCQ) [19].

2.3. Statistics. Nonparametric unpaired data were analyzed first using the Kruskal-Wallis test for trend analyses between several groups and thereafter the Mann-Whitney test between two groups (with correction for ties). Paired data were analyzed using the Wilcoxon test. Correlations were analyzed using Spearman's nonparametric correlation test. All statistical analyses were done using SPSS 20.0 for Windows (SPSS, Inc., Chicago, IL, USA), and a P value <0.05 was considered significant. All data were presented as median (interquartile range).

3. Results

3.1. Patient Characteristics. There were no significant differences in sex or body mass index between healthy smokers and COPD patients (Table 1). All subjects had matched age (except for patients with GOLD2 that were younger than

TABLE 1: Patient characteristics.

	Controls $n = 34$	GOLD1 $n = 13$	GOLD2 $n = 22$	GOLD3 $n = 15$	GOLD4 $n = 15$
Female/Male, n	16/18	6/7	10/12	7/8	9/6
Age, years	67 (66–70)	68 (66–69)	66 (61–68)**	65 (60–69)	66 (62–68)
Smoker/Former smoker, n	5/29	7/6	7/15	1/14	0/15
Packyears	27 (21–35)	27 (17–45)	31 (23–51)	40 (30–48)**	35 (28–40)
Body mass index	27 (24–28)	26 (25–28)	27 (24–30)	24 (21–27)	24 (21–27)
No inhaled medication	33	12	7	0	0
SABA use	0	0	7	6	3
LAMA use	0	1	13	15	15
LABA use	1	1	11	11	14
ICS use	1	1	12	13	14
O_2 use	0	0	0	2	5
CCQ-score	4.0 (1.8–7.0)	6.0 (2.0–10.0)	11.0 (4.0–17.3)***	14.2 (19.0–21.0)***†††‡	25 (24–30)**†
FEV_1 (L)	2.8 (2.3–3.4)	2.5 (2.2–3.4)	1.9 (1.6–2.2)***††	1.2 (1.0–1.4)***†††‡‡‡	0.7 (0.5–0.9)***†††‡‡‡###
FEV_1 (%)	95 (90–105)	90 (87–94)	61 (55–70)***†††	41 (33–49)***†††‡‡‡	27 (22–28)***†††‡‡‡###
FVC (L)	3.7 (3.0–4.3)	4.2 (3.3–4.8)	3.4 (2.9–4.1)	2.9 (2.2–3.4)**††‡	2.1 (1.1–3.0)***†††‡‡‡#
FVC (%)	96 (88–103)	106 (99–114)**	85 (73–94)**†††	76 (68–83)***†††‡	63 (35–73)***†††‡‡‡#
FEV_1/FVC	0.77 (0.74–0.80)	0.66 (0.63–0.70)***	0.58 (0.49–0.65)***††	0.39 (0.36–0.47)***†††‡‡‡	0.31 (0.30–0.46)***†††‡‡‡#

*Significant difference compared to healthy smokers, †significant difference compared to GOLD1, ‡significant difference compared to GOLD2, #significant difference compared to GOLD3, one symbol flagging $P < 0.05$, two symbols flagging $P < 0.01$ and three symbols flagging $P < 0.001$. SABA: short acting beta agonist, LAMA: long acting muscarinic agonist, LABA: long acting beta agonist, ICS: inhaled corticosteroids, O_2: oxygen therapy. All data are presented as median (interquartile range) or otherwise stated.

healthy controls), and pack years (except for patients with GOLD3 who had more pack years). CCQ value increased with increasing GOLD stage and was higher in GOLD stage 2–4 compared to healthy smokers (Table 1). One healthy smoker, three patients with GOLD2 and one patient with GOLD4 had low levels of alpha$_1$ antitrypsin (<0.86 g/L for men and <0.94 g/L for women). According to patient classification, FEV_1/FVC differed significantly between healthy smokers and GOLD1 but also continued to decrease with increasing GOLD stage. An interesting increase in FVC%p was seen in GOLD1 compared to healthy smokers, and thereafter FVC%p decreased with increasing GOLD stage.

3.2. Body Plethysmography.
The Kruskal-Wallis test showed an overall increasing trend among the groups for both R_{in} and R_{ex} ($P < 0.001$). Both the R_{in} and the R_{ex} measured with body plethysmography were increased in GOLD2–4 compared to healthy smokers (Figures 1(a) and 1(b)). IC was decreased, but only in later stages of the disease (GOLD3-4) (Table 2).

3.3. Increase in Lung Volume Measured by Body Plethysmography and Single Breath Helium Dilution with CO-Diffusion Already in GOLD1.
An increasing trend among all the groups was seen for TLC%p$_{BP}$ ($P < 0.01$), RV%p$_{BP}$ ($P < 0.001$), and for VA%p$_{SB}$ ($P < 0.001$) using the Kruskal-Wallis test. Interestingly, both TLC%p$_{BP}$ and FRC%p$_{BP}$ measured with body plethysmography were already significantly increased in GOLD1 (Table 2). In conjunction with this, the alveolar volume (VA%p) measured by single breath helium dilution with CO-diffusion was increased in GOLD1 and decreased in GOLD2–4 compared to healthy smokers (Figure 2).

3.4. Diffusing Capacity Decreased with Increasing GOLD Stage.
An overall difference between the groups regarding diffusion capacity was detected using Kruskal-Wallis. The diffusing capacity (DLCO%p) was decreased in GOLD2–4 compared to healthy smokers. When divided by the alveolar volume (DLCO/VA) a decrease was already seen from GOLD1, due to the early increase in VA%p seen in GOLD1, and extended to GOLD4 (Figure 2, Table 2).

3.5. Difference in RV and TLC Measured by Body Plethysmography and Single Breath Helium Dilution with CO-Diffusion.
RV measured with body plethysmography (RV%p$_{BP}$) was increased only in later stages of the disease (GOLD3-4, Table 2). In contrast, a parallel decrease in RV measured by single breath helium dilution with CO-diffusion (RV%p$_{SB}$) was seen (Figure 3(a)) and decreased by advancing GOLD stages. This indicates increased air trapping. To pronounce the outcome on individuals' RV, a difference in RV measured with body plethysmography and by single breath helium dilution with CO-diffusion was calculated (RV%p$_{BP-SB}$). A clear increasing pattern in RV%p$_{BP-SB}$ was seen with increasing GOLD stage (Figure 3(c)) already from GOLD2.

A similar pattern was seen for TLC, but not as pronounced as for RV. An increase in TLC%p$_{BP}$ was seen in GOLD3-4, together with a decrease in TLC%p$_{SB}$ (Figure 3(b)) in GOLD2–4. Individual differences in TLC%p (TLC%p$_{BP-SB}$) show a clear increasing pattern through the GOLD stages already from GOLD2 (Figure 3(d)).

3.6. IOS Parameters Increased with Increasing GOLD Stage.
Trends of difference between groups were detected by the

TABLE 2: Body plethysmography and single breath helium dilution with CO-diffusion (SB) parameters.

	Controls	GOLD1	GOLD2	GOLD3	GOLD4
Body plethysmography (BP)					
R_{in}, cmH$_2$O*s/L	2.0 (1.6–2.4)	2.0 (1.6–2.8)	3.0 (2.1–3.2)**	3.6 (2.8–5.3)***††††	35.4 (4.6–6.6)***†††††###
R_{ex}, cmH$_2$O*s/L	3.2 (2.4–3.7)	2.7 (2.3–4.4)	4.8 (3.2–6.8)***†††	13.2 (5.1–21.0)***†††††#	21.2 (14.1–33.1)***†††††‡‡
IC, L	3.2 (2.7–3.8)	3.0 (2.7–3.7)	2.7 (2.4–3.2)	2.3 (1.9–3.0)***††	1.4 (1.0–2.6)***†††
IC, %p	101 (88–108)	97 (88–108)	85 (73–98)†	77 (67–91)***††	52 (31.66)***†††##
RV_{BP}, L	2.5 (2.2–2.9)	2.5 (2.3–3.0)	2.8 (2.4–3.1)	3.6 (3.2–4.8)***†††††	4.5 (4.3–5.3)***†††††
RV_{BP}, %p	111 (98–120)	115 (105–124)	124 (100–144)	174 (148–187)***†††††	217 (193–245)***†††††
TLC_{BP}, L	6.4 (5.4–7.3)	6.7 (5.7–8.1)	6.2 (5.7–7.1)	7.3 (6.0–7.7)	7.0 (5.7–7.6)
TLC_{BP}, %p	105 (97–111)	108 (107–117)*	104 (88–123)	113 (107–126)**	121 (100–138)**‡
FRC_{BP}, L	3.1 (2.6–3.4)	3.4 (3.0–4.1)*	3.6 (3.2–4.0)**	4.4 (3.9–5.7)***†††	5.4 (4.6–5.8)***†††††
FRC_{BP}, %p	94 (88–108)	109 (102–120)**	106 (91–142)*	135 (123–152)***†††††	172 (161–203)***†††††###
Single breath helium dilution with carbon monoxide diffusion (SB)					
$DLCO_{SB}$, mmol/min/kPa	6.2 (5.3–7.1)	5.6 (4.5–7.7)	5.2 (4.6–6.3)**	3.0 (2.4–4.5)***†††††	1.8 (1.1–2.5)***†††††###
$DLCO_{SB}$, %p	75 (69–83)	75 (53–87)	63 (53–70)***	40 (32–46)***†††††	22 (15–29)***†††††###
VA, L	5.3 (4.7–5.3)	5.6 (4.9–5.6)	4.8 (4.2–5.7)†	4.4 (4.0–5.2)*††	3.7 (3.1–4.5)***†††††
VA, %p	90 (83–97)	96 (93–103)*	84 (74–89)*†††	78 (64–83)***†††	67 (58–77)***†††
$DLCO_{SB}$/VA, mmol/min/kPa/L	1.2 (1.1–1.3)	1.1 (0.9–1.2)*	1.1 (0.9–1.3)*	0.71 (0.64–0.83)***†††††	0.46 (0.35–0.56)***†††††###
$DLCO_{SB}$/VA, %p	89 (78–95)	73 (61–90)*	76 (64–93)	50 (45–60)***†††††	35 (23–41)***†††††###
RV_{SB}, L	1.9 (1.7–2.0)	2.0 (1.6–2.3)	1.7 (1.5–2.0)†	1.5 (1.3–1.9)**†	1.6 (1.3–1.8)*
RV_{SB}, %p	81 (72–87)	90 (77–96)	77 (64–89)	67 (59–79)**†	69 (58–95)
TLC_{SB}, L	5.5 (4.9–6.2)	5.8 (5.1–7.1)	5.0 (4.4–5.9)†	4.6 (4.1–5.3)*††	3.9 (3.3–4.7)***†††††
TLC_{SB}, %p	91 (85–97)	97 (93–103)*	85 (75–90)*†††	79 (65–84)***†††	68 (60–77)***†††
FRC_{SB}, L	2.5 (2.1–2.7)	3.0 (2.8–3.2)**	2.5 (2.1–2.8)†	2.1 (1.6–2.9)†	2.4 (1.8–2.9)†††††
FRC_{SB}, %p	75 (67–87)	93 (81–104)**	76 (66–91)††	71 (56–80)††	69 (61–102)†††††
Difference between BP and SB					
RV %p$_{BP-SB}$	28 (19–40)	33 (23–40)	43 (29–62)*†	95 (80–129)***†††††	149 (119–192)***†††††###
TLC %p$_{BP-SB}$	14 (11–18)	14 (11–18)	18 (13–27)*	35 (30–49)***†††††	57 (39–70)***†††††

* Significant difference compared to healthy smokers, † significant difference compared to GOLD1, ‡ significant difference compared to GOLD2, # significant difference compared to GOLD3, one symbol flagging $P < 0.05$, two symbols flagging $P < 0.01$ and three symbols flagging $P < 0.001$. All data are presented as median (interquartile range).

TABLE 3: Impulse oscillometry parameters.

	Controls	GOLD1	GOLD2	GOLD3	GOLD4
R_5, kPa*/L	0.27 (0.23–0.32)	0.29 (0.26–0.31)	0.37 (0.30–0.44)***†	0.50 (0.39–0.67)***†††‡‡	0.52 (0.41–0.70)***†††‡‡‡
R_5 %p	90 (68–91)	83 (74–97)	105 (90–120)***†	136 (121–195)***†††‡‡‡	134 (126–173)***†††‡‡‡
R_{20}, kPa*/L	0.21 (0.18–0.26)	0.22 (0.19–0.27)	0.26 (0.20–0.28)	0.30 (0.24–0.38)***†††‡	0.28 (0.25–0.34)**†
R_{20} %p	70 (62–89)	79 (64–86)	81 (73–96)*	104 (85–130)***†††‡‡	89 (79–99)**†
R_5–R_{20}, kPa*/L	0.04 (0.03–0.08)	0.07 (0.03–0.10)	0.12 (0.06–0.15)***†	0.17 (0.12–0.33)***†††‡‡	0.24 (0.17–0.36)***†††‡‡‡
R_5–R_{20} %p	100 (67–150)	167 (75–192)	250 (131–306)***†	388 (281–554)***†††‡‡	425 (367–650)***†††‡‡‡
AX, kPa*/L	0.18 (0.13–0.44)	0.16 (0.11–0.57)	0.69 (0.34–1.49)***††	1.64 (0.97–3.61)***†††‡	3.17 (1.46–3.54)***†††‡‡‡
F_{res}, Hz	10.5 (8.9–14.6)	12.5 (9.1–15.5)	16.4 (13.9–19.9)***††	20.4 (18.2–25.3)***†††‡	23.9 (21.3–27.7)***†††‡‡‡#
X5, kPa*/L	−0.09 (−0.11–−0.07)	−0.08 (−0.12–−0.06)	−0.14 (−0.22–−0.10)***††	−0.25 (−0.43–−0.16)***†††‡‡	−0.42 (−0.49–−0.23)***†††‡‡‡
X5 %p	199 (104–312)	175 (145–263)	389 (182 –541)***†	494 (447–795)***†††	677 (501–859)***†††‡‡

*Significant difference compared to healthy smokers, †significant difference compared to GOLD1, ‡significant difference compared to GOLD2, #significant difference compared to GOLD3, one symbol flagging $P < 0.05$, two symbols flagging $P < 0.01$ and three symbols flagging $P < 0.001$. All data are presented as median (interquartile range).

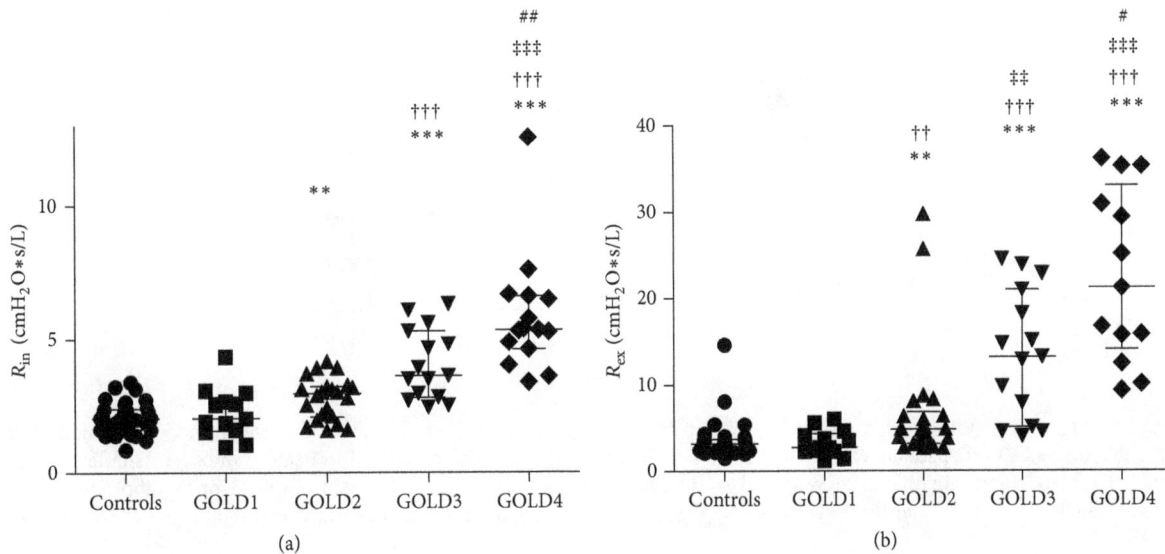

FIGURE 1: R_{in} (a) and R_{ex} (b) measured by body plethysmography in controls (healthy smokers) and COPD patients with GOLD stage 1–4. *Significant difference compared to healthy smokers, †significant difference compared to GOLD1, ‡significant difference compared to GOLD2, #significant difference compared to GOLD3, one symbol flagging $P < 0.05$, two symbols flagging $P < 0.01$, and three symbols flagging $P < 0.001$. Data are presented as individual dots together with median with interquartile range.

Kruskal-Wallis test, and all IOS parameters showed similar patterns, with no difference between healthy smokers and GOLD1, but increasing significantly from GOLD2 (except for R20) to GOLD4 (Figure 4, Table 3).

3.7. Established FEV_1%p Did Not Correlate with Extended Lung Volume and Diffusing Capacity Measurements.

Due to an increasing effect in all lung function parameters with increasing GOLD stage, there was also an evident overall correlation between all lung function parameters within all subjects (data not shown). When correlating the conventionally used parameter FEV_1%p within each GOLD stage, no correlation was seen with any parameters measured by body plethysmography, single breath helium dilution with CO-diffusion, or IOS. Correlations to a subset of the parameters (that differ most pronouncedly between the different GOLD

stages) are shown in Table 4. On the other hand, FVC%p and FEV_1/FVC correlated significantly with some lung function parameters, such as RV%p$_{BP-SB}$ and TLC%p$_{BP-SB}$.

The difference in RV%p (RV%p$_{BP-SB}$) strongly correlated with several lung volume and diffusing capacity parameters, such as IC %p, FRC%p, TLC%p, TLC%p$_{BP-SB}$, and DLCO/VA%p, within most GOLD stages. The difference in TLC%p (TLC%p$_{BP-SB}$) correlated in a similar way to IC %p, FRC%p, RV%p, RV%p$_{BP-SB}$, and DLCO/VA%p.

3.8. Correlations between Parameters of Resistance Measured by Body Plethysmography and IOS, but Not to Lung Volume or Diffusing Capacity Parameters.

An interesting finding was that resistance parameters measured by body plethysmography (R_{in} and R_{ex}) correlated significantly with several resistance and reactance parameters measured by IOS. R_{in}

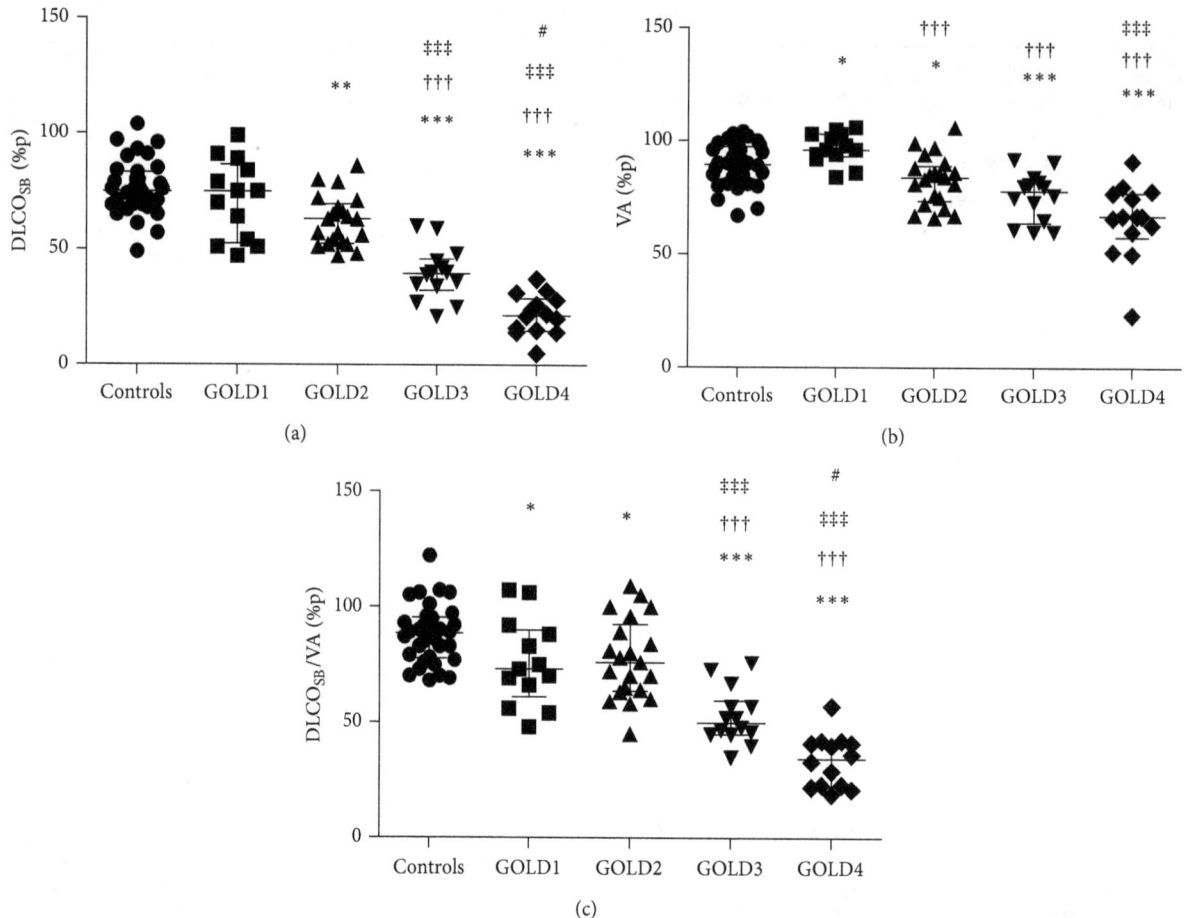

FIGURE 2: $DLCO_{SB}\%p$ (a), VA%p (b), and $DLCO_{SB}/VA\%p$ (c) measured by single breath helium dilution with CO-diffusion in controls (healthy smokers) and COPD patients with GOLD stage 1–4. *Significant difference compared to healthy smokers, †significant difference compared to GOLD1, ‡significant difference compared to GOLD2, #significant difference compared to GOLD3, one symbol flagging $P < 0.05$, two symbols flagging $P < 0.01$, and three symbols flagging $P < 0.001$. Data are presented as individual dots together with median with interquartile range.

and R_{ex} correlated with R5, R20, R5–R20, and Fres (Table 4) in most GOLD stages (and most pronouncedly in early GOLD stages) and AX and X5 in all GOLD stages. However, neither resistance parameters measured by body plethysmography nor IOS (except for R5–R20 in GOLD4) correlated with lung volume or diffusion parameters in any GOLD stage.

3.9. Dyspnea Did Not Correlate to Lung Function Parameters in Different GOLD Stages. The CCQ score increased with increasing GOLD stage (Table 1), and hence there was an apparent overall correlation with all lung function parameters. However, within the different GOLD stages there was no correlation between the CCQ score and any lung function parameter measured with spirometry, body plethysmography, and single breath helium dilution with CO-diffusion or IOS.

4. Discussion

The main finding of this study was that established flow-volume parameters, such as FEV_1, did not correlate with advanced measurements of lung volume, diffusing capacity, and resistance. This illustrates that FEV_1 alone is not a good parameter when used for diagnosis and monitoring of COPD since it does not represent the whole picture of the disease. An interesting parameter was, however, the difference in RV%p measured with body plethysmography and single breath helium dilution with CO-diffusion. The $RV\%p_{BP}$ measured with body plethysmography was increased in parallel with a decrease in $RV\%p_{SB}$ measured with single breath helium dilution with CO-diffusion with increasing COPD severity. When using the difference between the two RV ($RV\%p_{BP-SB}$), a clearer and more pronounced pattern appeared, and the effect on lung volume becomes apparent in an earlier disease stage. This provides a good opportunity to measure air trapping and degree of hyperinflation. $RV\%p_{BP-SB}$ also correlated with several lung volume parameters, such as IC%p, FRC%p, TLC%p, and DLCO/VA%p, showing this to be an important factor in COPD characterization. A similar parameter, with similar characteristics, was the difference between TLC%p measured with body plethysmography and single breath helium dilution with CO-diffusion. However, it was not as

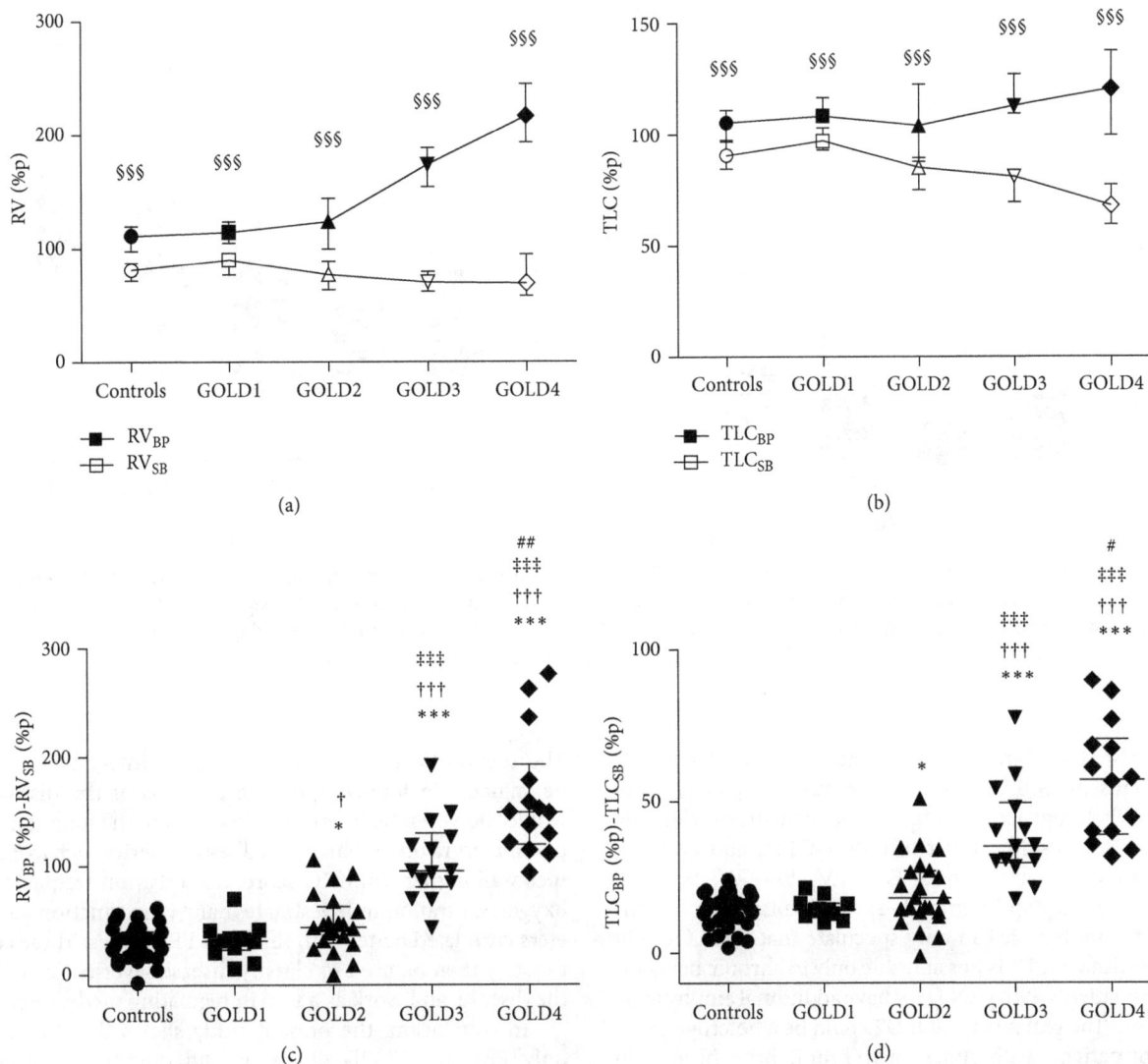

FIGURE 3: RV% (a) and TLC%p (b) measured by body plethysmography and single breath helium dilution with CO-diffusion. Difference in RV% (RV%p$_{BP-SB}$) (c) and TLC% (TLC%p$_{BP-SB}$) (d) measured by body plethysmography and single breath helium dilution with CO-diffusion in controls (healthy smokers) and COPD patients with GOLD stage 1–4. *Significant difference compared to healthy smokers, †significant difference compared to GOLD1, ‡significant difference compared to GOLD2, #significant difference compared to GOLD3; §significant difference between measurement from body plethysmography compared to single breath helium dilution with CO-diffusion, one symbol flagging $P < 0.05$, two symbols flagging $P < 0.01$, and three symbols flagging $P < 0.001$. Data are presented as median (IQR) in (a)-(b) and individual dots together with median with interquartile range (c)-(d).

pronounced as the difference in RV%p, and hence of less importance. When comparing RV and TLC from the different measurement methods, a significant difference was already seen in healthy smokers, and was most probably due to methodological dissimilarities (single breath helium dilution with CO-diffusion measuring only volume communicating with ventilated air space, while body plethysmography also measures trapped air space).

An important aim was to find a lung function parameter that may show early signs of COPD disease, since COPD is an irreversible progressive disease. When diagnosed with COPD today, the disease has already progressed to a partly irreversible limitation in airflow. It is therefore important to

identify patients at an earlier stage, so that novel therapies for earlier disease progression can be developed. It is thus also important to study the initial changes in COPD leading to severe stages. Interesting findings in the present study were increases in RV$_{BP}$%p, RV$_{SB}$%p, TLC$_{BP}$%p, TLC$_{SB}$%p, FRC%p, and VA%p already in GOLD1, with the increase in VA%p subsequently resulting in a parallel decrease in DLCO/VA %p. This could be the first signs of inadequate elasticity in GOLD1, resulting in increased lung volumes but sustained flow-volume parameters.

All lung function parameters were affected with an increasing pattern through GOLD1–4, but overall there are only minor differences between healthy smokers and GOLD1.

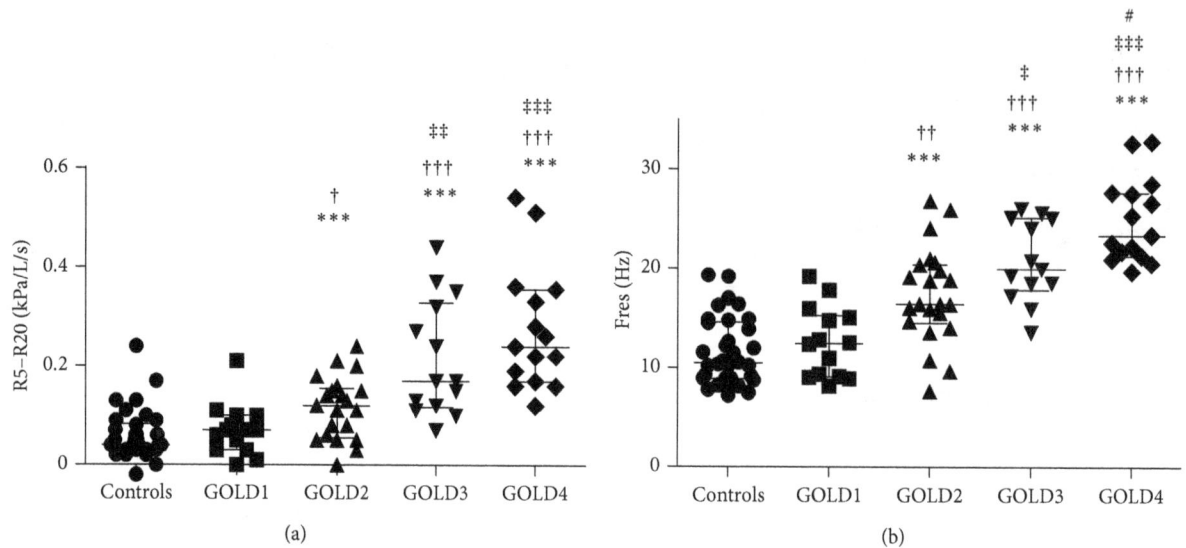

FIGURE 4: R5–R20 (a) and Fres (b) measured by impulse oscillometry in controls (healthy smokers) and COPD patients with GOLD stage 1–4. *significant difference compared to healthy smokers, †significant difference compared to GOLD1, ‡significant difference compared to GOLD2, #significant difference compared to GOLD3, one symbol flagging $P < 0.05$, two symbols flagging $P < 0.01$ and three symbols flagging $P < 0.001$. Data presented as individual dots together with median with interquartile range.

In contrast, there are marked effects in GOLD3-4, while the patients in GOLD2 show a more variable pattern, presenting a heterogeneous group of patient with overlapping lung function results similar to both GOLD1 and GOLD3. This was most clearly seen for Fres, $RV_{BP}\%p$–$RV_{SB}\%p$, and $TLC_{BP}\%p$–$TLC_{SB}\%p$ (Figures 3–4). The explanation for this is not known, but we can only speculate that the COPD in patients with GOLD1 is possibly due only to chronic bronchitis, while patients with GOLD3-4 have additional emphysema formation. The patients in GOLD2 could be a heterogeneous group of patients with either only chronic bronchitis or in combination with additional emphysema. We aim to investigate this hypothesis further because of the importance to categorize the disease not only by severity but also by disease pattern and phenotype in order to develop more specific therapies.

Another interesting findings were the correlations between several resistance parameters measured by body plethysmography and IOS. These resistance parameters did not relate to lung volume and diffusing capacity parameters suggesting different pathological entities and thereby different COPD phenotypes. Although IOS is an easy method to use, it may not replace spirometry but could be used as a complement or in cases when spirometry cannot be performed. These findings are in accordance with previous speculations on lung diseases overall [20].

The use of a self-filled in quality of life questionnaire is a subjective measure and is questionable as a valuable tool in diagnosing COPD [21]. In the present study there was an increase in CCQ with increasing GOLD stage, and subsequently an overall correlation to all lung function parameters. However, subgrouped within each GOLD stage, there was no correlation between CCQ and any lung function parameter, even though some of the groups were very heterogeneous.

The diagnostic use is hence of minor interest but could be valuable in following-up the progress of the disease. It would, however, be interesting to compare the lung function parameters to other markers of disease severity such as 6 minutes walking test, mMRC score, exacerbation frequency, or oxygen saturation to investigate if any lung function parameters correlated better with this than FEV_1 does. These could possibly then be used to classify disease severity, phenotype the disease, and work as a tool in regulating medication use.

In conclusion, the present study shows that the use of only FEV_1 in COPD diagnosis and monitoring gives an incomplete characterization of the patients. Extended lung function measurements using body plethysmography, single breath helium dilution with CO-diffusion and IOS show that there was no correlation between FEV_1, and more advanced lung volume, diffusing capacity, and resistance parameters within different COPD stages. However, other flow-volume parameters, FVC, FEV_1/FVC, and IC, are related to several more advanced lung function parameters. These parameters should be taken into consideration preferably when the access to more advanced equipment is limited. An interesting parameter is the difference in RV measured by body plethysmography and single breath helium dilution with CO-diffusion that gives a more pronounced measure of air trapping and hyperinflation. Different lung function parameters are of importance in different COPD stages, and a more thorough patient characterization is important for understanding the condition and giving better options for treatment in the future.

Abbreviations

BP: Body plethysmography
CCQ: Clinical COPD Questionnaire

TABLE 4: Correlations between established flow-volume parameters and extended volume and resistance parameters.

	Volume		Resistance			
	$RV\%p_{BP-SB}$	$TLC\%p_{BP-SB}$	R_{in}	R_{ex}	R_5-R_{20}	F_{res}
Flow-volume						
$FEV_1\%p$						
Controls	0.15	0.31	−0.01	0.06	−0.12	−0.21
GOLD1	0.50	−0.25	−0.18	−0.26	−0.27	−0.36
GOLD2	−0.37	−0.34	−0.19	−0.20	−0.26	−0.18
GOLD3	−0.21	0.12	−0.16	0.18	−0.3	−0.32
GOLD4	−0.33	−0.34	−0.14	−0.12	−0.14	−0.11
$FVC\%p$						
Controls	0.14	0.34	0.12	0.14	−0.05	−0.07
GOLD1	0.14	0.15	−0.19	−0.16	−0.22	−0.32
GOLD2	**0.59****	**0.60****	−0.35	−0.29	−0.29	−0.14
GOLD3	−0.14	0.01	−0.31	−0.05	−0.22	−0.2
GOLD4	**−0.55***	−0.21	−0.33	−0.45	−0.26	−0.11
FEV_1/FVC						
Controls	−0.02	−0.22	−0.26	−0.11	−0.19	−0.25
GOLD1	0.34	−0.07	−0.13	−0.29	−0.15	−0.13
GOLD2	**−0.71*****	**−0.71*****	0.12	0.09	0.15	0.08
GOLD3	−0.31	0.04	−0.08	0.35	−0.06	−0.14
GOLD4	**0.69****	0.37	0.32	**0.58***	0.24	0.05
$IC\%p$						
Controls	0.30	0.42*	0.07	−0.02	−0.06	−0.04
GOLD1	0.29	−0.04	**0.61***	**0.73****	−0.06	0.09
GOLD2	**0.66*****	**0.63****	0.06	0.29	0.11	0.10
GOLD3	0.11	0.46	−0.24	0.35	−0.3	−0.42
GOLD4	**0.72****	0.01	−0.36	**−0.61***	−0.61	−0.13
Resistance						
R_5-R_{20}						
Controls	−0.05	−0.12	**0.43****	**0.37***	—	**0.85*****
GOLD1	−0.26	0.00	0.44	0.21	—	**0.94*****
GOLD2	0.08	0.03	**0.80*****	**0.88*****	—	**0.87*****
GOLD3	0.04	0.22	**0.64***	0.44	—	**0.86*****
GOLD4	0.29	**0.54***	**0.71****	0.55	—	**0.69****
F_{res}						
Controls	−0.04	−0.2	**0.47****	**0.40***	**0.85*****	—
GOLD1	−0.28	0.27	**0.61***	0.4	**0.94*****	—
GOLD2	0.08	0.02	**0.63****	**0.77*****	**0.87*****	—
GOLD3	0.13	0.26	0.50	0.41	**0.86*****	—
GOLD4	−0.05	0.13	**0.61***	0.47	**0.69****	—

Data are presented as r-values. *$P < 0.05$, **$P < 0.01$ ***$P < 0.001$.

COPD: Chronic pulmonary obstructive disease
GOLD: Global initiative of obstructive lung dis-eases
FEV_1: Forced expiratory volume in 1 s
FRC: Functional residual capacity
FVC: Forced vital capacity
IC: Inspiratory capacity
R_{ex}: Expiratory resistance
R_{in}: Inspiratory resistance

RV: Residual volume
TLC: Total lung capacity
DLCO: Diffusing capacity of the lung for carbon monoxide
VA: Alveolar volume.

Conflict of Interests

The authors report no conflict of interests.

Authors' Contributions

Linnea Jarenbäck designed the study, tested the patients, analyzed and interpreted data, and co-wrote the paper. Jaro Ankerst included the patients, and revised the paper critically, Leif Bjermer designed the study, interpreted data, and revised the article critically, Ellen Tufvesson designed the study, analyzed and interpreted data and co-wrote the article.

Acknowledgments

This work was supported by Grants from the Swedish Heart and Lung foundation, Swedish Research Council, Evy and Gunnar Sandberg's Foundation, and the Royal Physiographic Society in Lund. The authors thank the staff at the Lung and Allergy Research Unit, Skåne University Hospital, for much appreciated help and support.

References

[1] R. Rodriguez-Roisin, J. Vestbo, S. S. Hurd et al., "Global strategy for the diagnosis, management and prevention of chronic obstructive pulmonary disease," Global Initiative for Chronic Obstructive Lung Disease, 2011, http://www.goldcopd.org/.

[2] B. D. L. Broekhuizen, A. P. E. Sachs, R. Oostvogels, A. W. Hoes, T. J. M. Verheij, and K. G. M. Moons, "The diagnostic value of history and physical examination for COPD in suspected or known cases: a systematic review," Family Practice, vol. 26, no. 4, pp. 260–268, 2009.

[3] B. D. L. Broekhuizen, A. P. E. Sachs, A. W. Hoes, T. J. M. Verheij, and K. G. M. Moons, "Diagnostic management of chronic obstructive pulmonary disease," The Netherlands Journal of Medicine, vol. 70, no. 1, pp. 6–11, 2012.

[4] J. C. Hogg, F. Chu, S. Utokaparch et al., "The nature of small-airway obstruction in chronic obstructive pulmonary disease," The New England Journal of Medicine, vol. 350, no. 26, pp. 2645–2653, 2004.

[5] K. Akamatsu, T. Yamagata, Y. Kida, H. Tanaka, H. Ueda, and M. Ichinose, "Poor sensitivity of symptoms in early detection of COPD," COPD: Journal of Chronic Obstructive Pulmonary Disease, vol. 5, no. 5, pp. 269–273, 2008.

[6] A. Deesomchok, K. A. Webb, L. Forkert et al., "Lung hyperinflation and its reversibility in patients with airway obstruction of varying severity," COPD: Journal of Chronic Obstructive Pulmonary Disease, vol. 7, no. 6, pp. 428–437, 2010.

[7] M. Cazzola, P. Rogliani, G. Curradi et al., "A pilot comparison of helium dilution and plethysmographic lung volumes to assess the impact of a long-acting bronchodilator on lung hyperinflation in COPD," Pulmonary Pharmacology and Therapeutics, vol. 22, no. 6, pp. 522–525, 2009.

[8] S. Kanda, K. Fujimoto, Y. Komatsu, M. Yasuo, M. Hanaoka, and K. Kubo, "Evaluation of respiratory impedance in asthma and COPD by an impulse oscillation system," Internal Medicine, vol. 49, no. 1, pp. 23–30, 2010.

[9] C. Crim, B. Celli, L. D. Edwards et al., "Respiratory system impedance with impulse oscillometry in healthy and COPD subjects: ECLIPSE baseline results," Respiratory Medicine, vol. 105, no. 7, pp. 1069–1078, 2011.

[10] U. Kolsum, Z. Borrill, K. Roy et al., "Impulse oscillometry in COPD: identification of measurements related to airway obstruction, airway conductance and lung volumes," Respiratory Medicine, vol. 103, no. 1, pp. 136–143, 2009.

[11] P. A. Williamson, K. Clearie, D. Menzies, S. Vaidyanathan, and B. J. Lipworth, "Assessment of small-airways disease using alveolar nitric oxide and impulse oscillometry in asthma and COPD," Lung, vol. 189, no. 2, pp. 121–129, 2011.

[12] A. Haruna, T. Oga, S. Muro et al., "Relationship between peripheral airway function and patient-reported outcomes in COPD: a cross-sectional study," BMC Pulmonary Medicine, vol. 10, article 10, 2010.

[13] S. Frantz, U. Nihlen, M. Dencker, G. Engstrom, C. G. Lofdahl, and P. Wollmer, "Impulse oscillometry may be of value in detecting early manifestations of COPD," Respiratory Medicine, vol. 106, no. 8, pp. 1116–2113.

[14] S. S. Al-Mutairi, P. N. Sharma, A. Al-Alawi, and J. S. Al-Deen, "Impulse oscillometry: an alternative modality to the conventional pulmonary function test to categorise obstructive pulmonary disorders," Clinical and Experimental Medicine, vol. 7, no. 2, pp. 56–64, 2007.

[15] N. MacIntyre, R. O. Crapo, G. Viegi et al., "Standardisation of the single-breath determination of carbon monoxide uptake in the lung," The European Respiratory Journal, vol. 26, no. 4, pp. 720–735, 2005.

[16] M. R. Miller, J. Hankinson, V. Brusasco et al., "Standardisation of spirometry," The European Respiratory Journal, vol. 26, no. 2, pp. 319–338, 2005.

[17] J. Wanger, J. L. Clausen, A. Coates et al., "Standardisation of the measurement of lung volumes," The European Respiratory Journal, vol. 26, no. 3, pp. 511–522, 2005.

[18] R. O. Crapo, A. H. Morris, and R. M. Gardner, "Reference spirometric values using techniques and equipment that meet ATS recommendations," The American Review of Respiratory Disease, vol. 123, no. 6, pp. 659–664, 1981.

[19] T. van der Molen, B. W. M. Willemse, S. Schokker, N. H. T. ten Hacken, D. S. Postma, and E. F. Juniper, "Development, validity and responsiveness of the clinical COPD questionnaire," Health and Quality of Life Outcomes, vol. 1, article 13, 2003.

[20] D. A. Kaminsky, "What does airway resistance tell us about lung function?" Respiratory Care, vol. 57, no. 1, pp. 85–99, 2012.

[21] L. M. Boer, G. M. Asijee, O. C. P. van Schayck, and T. R. J. Schermer, "How do dyspnoea scales compare with measurement of functional capacity in patients with COPD and at risk of COPD?" Primary Care Respiratory Journal, vol. 21, no. 2, pp. 202–207, 2012.

15

Persistent Pulmonary Hypertension of Non Cardiac Cause in a Neonatal Intensive Care Unit

Gustavo Rocha,[1] Maria João Baptista,[2] and Hercília Guimarães[1]

[1] *Division of Neonatology, Department of Pediatrics, Hospital de São João EPE, Faculty of Medicine of Porto University, 4202-451 Porto, Portugal*
[2] *Division of Pediatric Cardiology, Department of Pediatrics, Hospital de São João EPE, Faculty of Medicine of Porto University, 4202-451 Porto, Portugal*

Correspondence should be addressed to Gustavo Rocha, gusrocha@oninet.pt

Academic Editor: Despina Papakosta

Parenchymal lung diseases are the main cause of persistent pulmonary hypertension of the newborn (PPHN). We aimed to assess the non cardiac conditions associated to PPHN in the newborn and the survival rate over the last 15 years, at our center. A retrospective chart review of the neonates admitted for PPHN from 1996 to 2010 was performed. New therapies were introduced in 2003, and the survival rates between two periods (1996–2002 and 2003–2010) were compared. Out of 6750 newborns, 78 (1.1%) had the diagnosis of PPHN of non cardiac cause. The most prevalent causes were associated to pulmonary hypoplasia (30.7%), infection (24.3%), and aspiration syndromes (15.3%). Many other causes were identified in 33.3%. The overall survival rate was 68%. There was a significant difference on survival rates between the two periods (1996–2002 = 63.8% and 2003–2010 = 71.4%, $P = 0.04$). Our study showed a myriad of non cardiac aetiologies for PPHN of the newborn, most of them related to lung disease or lung hypoplasia. We observed an improvement in survival rate since 2003, which was associated to the use of new therapies.

1. Introduction

From the first clinical classification of pulmonary hypertension (PH), in Evian (France) in 1973, the knowledge about the disease significantly improved and recently, in 2008, that classification was updated at Dana Point (USA) [1]. This classification tries to include all possible causes of PH in children and adults; nevertheless, it is not a specific classification for PH presenting in the newborn.

PH presenting in the neonatal period may result from a myriad of causes [2]. Most commonly, it presents immediately after birth, a condition referred to as persistent pulmonary hypertension of the newborn (PPHN), when pulmonary vascular resistance fails to decrease at birth. This disease is recognized as arterial PH in the Dana Point classification of PH. Most cases of PPHN are associated with lung parenchymal diseases, such as meconium aspiration syndrome, and respiratory distress syndrome; however, some present without known lung disease as primary PPHN. Some infants who have PPHN have lethal causes of respiratory failure, such as alveolar-capillary dysplasia [3], genetic defects in surfactant synthesis [4], or severe lung hypoplasia secondary to oligohydramnios or congenital anomalies. Congenital heart diseases are also a possible cause of PH, but usually the prognosis and outcome are more related to the heart disease than to the pulmonary vascular involvement during the first weeks of life. In a new group of newborns, PH presents without known heart or lung disease, as primary PPHN.

Over the last decades, a timely referral to a tertiary centre, the use of new techniques of mechanical ventilation, extracorporeal membrane oxygenation, a better support therapy, the use of inhaled nitric oxide (iNO), and new pharmacological pulmonary vasodilators have ameliorated the prognosis of this clinical condition allowing a survival rate of about 90% in several referral centres [5].

The aims of this study were to review the non cardiac conditions associated to PPHN in the newborn and the survival rate of the affected patients over the last 15 years, at our centre.

2. Material and Methods

Neonates with the diagnosis of PPHN of non cardiac cause, admitted between 1996 and 2010, were identified from the database of our neonatal intensive care unit (NICU), a tertiary referral center for neonatal cardiac and pediatric surgery in the north of Portugal. Gestational data, demographic data, the cause of PPHN, treatment, days of NICU stay, neonatal outcome, and necropsy findings of the deceased neonates were retrieved from the clinical charts and retrospectively reviewed.

The diagnosis of PPHN was made on clinical grounds, chest X-ray, arterial blood gases analysis, and 2D-echocardiograhic findings. Pulmonary artery pressure estimation was based on the gradient between right ventricle and atrium, through tricuspid regurgitation, assuming the right atrium pressure as 15 mmHg (estimated pulmonary systolic artery pressure (PSAP) = right ventricle to right atrium gradient + 15 mmHg).

The diagnosis of PPHN was made on clinical grounds, chest X-ray, arterial blood gases analysis, and 2D-echocardiograhic findings. Pulmonary artery pressure estimation was based on the gradient between right ventricle and atrium, through tricuspid regurgitation, assuming the right atrium pressure as 10 mmHg (estimated pulmonary systolic artery pressure (PSAP) = right ventricle to right atrium gradient + 15 mmHg). Pulmonary hypertension was stratified as mild if estimated PSAP was less than 40 mmHg, moderate if between 40 and 60 mmHg, and severe if higher than 60 mmHg. Additionally, other parameters were evaluated to help in definition of the severity of PH: (i) shunt direction at ductus arteriosus or foramen ovale (left-to-right shunt was considered normal, bidireccional shunt was considered sign of mild to moderate PH and right to left shunt was considered sign of severe PH); (ii) orientation of ventricular septum (the normal orientation was considered left to right, septum rectification was indicative of mild-to-moderate PH, and when the septum budge from right-to-left a severe PH was likely), and (iii) systolic function of the left ventricle, through the left ventricular ejection fraction (in cases of moderate PH it was expected a hipercontractil left ventricle whilst in severe PH usually we found a decrease on left ventricle ejection fraction). All the parameters were evaluated routinely. Echocardiographic evaluation was also used to exclude or confirm any congenital heart disease.

Inhaled nitric oxide (iNO) (usually starting with 20 ppm) has been routinely used since 2003 after echocardiographic definition of severe PH and an oxygenation index (mean airway pressure × fraction of inspired oxygen × 100/partial arterial pressure of oxygen) over 20. Sildenafil has been used in infants with persistent pulmonary hypertension refractory to iNO. Since iNO and sildenafil have been used since 2003, a comparison of the survival rates between two epochs was made (1996–2002 and 2003–2010).

Since 2003, we have also routinely used a total daily water intake of 80 mL/kg (until start enteral feeds) along with a perfusion of dopamine 5 mcg/kg/min, in order to keep a systemic blood pressure over 40 mmHg, and a hematocrit of about 45% (haemoglobin ≥15 g/dL). A perfusion of

TABLE 1: Demographics ($n = 78$).

Gestational age (weeks), median (min–max)	39 (30–41)
Preterm (<37 weeks gestation)	16 (20.5%)
Birthweight (grams), median (min–max)	3080 (1450–4170)
Intrauterine growth restriction	4 (5%)
Gender	
male	53 (67.9%)
female	25 (32.1%)
C-section	51 (65.3%)
Outborn	34 (43.5%)

dobutamine (5 mcg/kg/min) is started if signs of myocardial dysfunction are present at echocardiographic evaluation. Higher doses of dopamine and dobutamine or epinephrine perfusion are used according to clinical criteria. Minimal stimulation as well as sedation and analgesia is usually performed with a perfusion of morphine (or fentanyl in the case of hypotension) and midazolam. Paralyzing agents as vecuronium are usually avoided; it is only used in selected cases as a rescue ventilation adjunt therapy. When mechanical ventilation is need, conventional ventilation is preferred to high-frequency oscillation ventilation, which is mainly used as rescue ventilation. The goals of mechanical ventilation are to maintain a PaO$_2$ of 60–90 mmHg and a PaCO$_2$ >30 mmHg (usually 35–50 mmHg), in order to avoid oxidative stress and hypocapnia.

ECMO treatment was not achievable in our country until 2010. Our centre, recently, started ECMO support to neonates and children.

Categorical variables were compared through Chi-square or the exact Fisher's test. The Mann-Whitney test was used to compare two independent samples.

This study has been approved by the ethics committee board of our institution.

3. Results

In the last 15 years, 6750 newborns were admitted to our unit. Seventy-eight (1.1%) had the diagnosis of PPHN of non cardiac cause. The demographics of the studied population are reported in Table 1, and the causes of PPHN are reported in Table 2. Twenty-five (32.0%) were deceased (13 males; 12 females). The median of death day was 7 (1–114). There were 34 outborns that were referred to our centre. Mortality rate in the outborn group was 32.3% (11/34), not different from the inborn group that was 31.8% (14/44) ($P = 0.967$). Pulmonary hypertension was classified as mild in 14 (17.9%) patients, moderate in 24 (30.7%), and severe in 40 (51.2%). Treatment aspects are reported in Table 3. The normalization of pulmonary hypertension occurred by day eight of life (2–160) in the survivors. The median of days of stay in the NICU was 12 days (1–167). The overall survival rate was 68%. There was a significant difference on survival rates between two periods (1996–2002 = 63.8% and 2003–2010 = 71.4%) ($P = 0.04$); see Table 4. Along with this increase in survival, days of NICU stay and of normalization of PH in the survivors accordingly increased.

TABLE 2: Causes of PPHN ($n = 78$).

Aspiration of bloody amniotic fluid, n (%)	1 (1.2)
Aspiration of blood from upper airways (traumatic intubation), n (%)	1 (1.2)
Meconium aspiration syndrome, n (%)	10 (12.8) (2[†])
Congenital pneumonia and sepsis, n (%)	19 (24.3) (4[†])
Severe hyaline membrane disease, n (%)	3 (3.8) (1[†])
Transient tachypnea of the newborn, n (%)	4 (5.1)
Intrauterine ductus arteriosus closure (indomethacin), n (%)	2 (2.5)
Congenital diaphragmatic hernia, n (%)	17 (21.7) (10[†])
Potter syndrome, n (%)	1 (1.2) (1[†])
Nephrourological malformation with oligoamnios, n (%)	1 (1.2)
Idiopathic hypoplastic lung, n (%)	2 (2.5) (1[†])
Idiopathic pulmonary arteriolar calcification, n (%)	1 (1.2) (1[†])
Pulmonary "arteriopathy", n (%)	1 (1.2) (1[†])
Arterial pulmonary thrombosis, n (%)	1 (1.2) (1[†])
Fetal tachyarrhythmia, n (%)	1 (1.2)
Maternal diabetes, n (%)	1 (1.2) (1[†])
Malformation of vein of Galeno, n (%)	2 (2.5) (2[†])
Perinatal asphyxia, n (%)	4 (5.1)
Unknown aetiology, n (%)	6 (7.6)

[†]: deceased.

TABLE 3: Treatment ($n = 78$).

Inhaled nitric oxide, n (%)	19 (24.3%)
Surfactant, n (%)	24 (30.7%)
Dopamine, n (%)	57 (73%)
Dobutamine, n (%)	35 (44.8%)
Epinephrine, n (%)	3 (3.8%)
Sildenafil, n (%)	12 (15.3%)
Diuretics, n (%)	33 (42.3%)
Sedation, n (%)	71 (91%)
Oxygen, n (%)	78 (100%)
Days of oxygen, median (min–max)	6 (1–114)
Mechanical ventilation, n (%)	71 (91%)
Days of mechanical ventilation, median (min–max)	7 (1–114)
Extracorporeal membrane oxygenation (ECMO), n (%)	1 (1.2%)
Days of ECMO	17

4. Discussion

Persistence of pulmonary hypertension leading to respiratory failure in the neonate has been recognized for 40 years since its original description by Gersony and colleagues in 1969 [6]. During the development of the pulmonary vasculature in the fetus, many structural and functional changes occur to prepare the lung for the transition to air breathing. The development of the pulmonary circulation is genetically controlled by an array of mitogenic factors in a temporospatial order. With advancing gestation, pulmonary vessels acquire increased vasoreactivity. The fetal pulmonary vasculature is exposed to a low oxygen tension environment that promotes high intrinsic myogenic tone and high vasocontractility. At birth, a dramatic reduction in pulmonary arterial pressure and resistance occurs with an increase in oxygen tension and blood flow. The striking hemodynamic differences in the pulmonary circulation of the fetus and newborn are regulated by various factors and vasoactive agents. Among them, nitric oxide, endothelin-1, and prostaglandin I(2) are mainly derived from endothelial cells and exert their effects via cGMP, cAMP, and Rho kinase signalling pathways. Alterations in these signalling pathways may lead to vascular remodelling, high vasocontractility, and PPHN [7, 8].

In this study we were able to document PPHN in 16 preterm neonates, including one with 30 weeks of gestational age with a congenital sepsis and pneumonia. It is already known that the mechanisms that could lead to PH are already present in the human fetus by 31 weeks of gestation [5, 9, 10]. In our patients we observed a high number of C-sections that are related to prenatal diagnosis of pulmonary hypoplasia, as congenital diaphragmatic hernias, Potter syndrome, or meconium-stained amniotic fluid.

The most common cause of PPHN in this study was pulmonary hypoplasia. Congenital diaphragmatic hernia was the most prevalent cause of pulmonary hypoplasia. Congenital diaphragmatic hernia and oligohydramnios secondary to renal anomalies or premature rupture of membranes leads to pulmonary hypoplasia. Pulmonary hypertension often occurs as a complication because of the decreased number of blood vessels and increased reactivity of the vessels in the hypoplastic lungs. PPHN is usually more chronic and less responsive to vasodilator therapy in these infants and their outcome is related to the degree of lung hypoplasia, associated anomalies, as well as lengt of pulmonary hypertension [11]. The outcome for neonates who have congenital diaphragmatic hernia has improved since gentle ventilation and permissive hypercapnia have been incorporated into the management, with many centers reporting 75% survival in recent years [11, 12]. The survival of patients with congenital diaphragmatic hernia has improved in our center since 2003, and is nowadys over 61% [13].

The second cause of PPHN in this study was congenital pneumonia and sepsis. PPHN can be a complication of pneumonia or sepsis secondary to common neonatal pathogens [14]. Bacterial endotoxin causes pulmonary hypertension from several mechanisms, including the release of thromboxane, endothelin, and several cytokines [15, 16]. Sepsis also leads to systemic hypotension from activation of inducible nitric oxide synthase with excess nitric oxide release in the systemic vascular beds, impaired myocardial function, and multiorgan failure. Addressing PH should be a component of the overall management of septic shock and prevention of multiorgan failure in the affected neonates.

Another significant group of causes of PPHN were the aspiration syndromes, mainly meconium aspiration syndrome, representing 12.8% of PPHN in this series. Although meconium staining of amniotic fluid occurs in 10% to 15% of pregnancies, meconium aspiration syndrome

Table 4: Survival rates between two periods.

| | 1996–2002 | 2003–2010 | P |
	n = 36	n = 42	
Gestational age, weeks, median (min–max)	41 (30–41)	39 (32–41)	0.032§
Preterm (<37 weeks of gestation), n (%)	8 (22)	8 (19)	0.081*
Birthweigt, g, median (min–max)	3100 (1450–4170)	3040 (1800–4070)	0.354§
Gender			
Male, n (%)	23 (64)	30 (71)	
Female, n (%)	13 (36)	12 (29)	0.456*
C-section, n (%)	23 (64)	28 (67)	0.657*
Outborn, n (%)	18 (50)	16 (38)	0.071*
NICU stay	10 (1–67)	16 (1–167)	0.034§
Time to normalization of PH	5 (2–25)	9 (2–160)	0.0391§
Survival, n (%)	23 (63.8)%	30 (71.4)	0.040**

§: Mann-Whitney test; *: Chi-Squared test; **: Fisher Exact test; NICU: neonatal intensive care unit; PH; pulmonary hypertension.

occurs infrequently, in up to 5% of neonates born through meconium stained fluid. The incidence of meconium aspiration syndrome has declined in recent years [17] with decreasing postterm pregnancies. This observation suggests that meconium aspiration syndrome is often a result of in utero stress with aspiration of meconium by a compromised fetus. Meconium can cause respiratory failure from several mechanisms. Meconium can cause mechanical obstruction to the airways, particularly during exhalation, resulting in air trapping, hyperinflation, and increased risk for pneumothorax. Meconium components also inactivate surfactant, [18] trigger an inflammatory response with release of cytokines, and increase the production of the vasoconstritors endothelin and thromboxane [19]. Recent advances in the management of PPHN have resulted in an excellent outcome for neonates who have meconium aspiration syndrome [20].

In this study PPHN occurred as a complication of hyaline membrane disease and transient tachypnea of the preterm newborn, often delivered by C-section, at 34–37 week's of gestation. The increasing reactivity of pulmonary arteries at this gestation period predisposes these neonates to PH when gas exchange is impaired because of surfactant deficiency [21].

The association of PPHN with maternal intake of nonsteroid anti-inflammatory drugs as indomethacin has been recognized in case reports since 1970 [22, 23]. A strong causal association is also suggested by the consistent reproduction of hemodynamic and structural features of PPHN by fetal ductal constriction [24, 25].

Maldevelopment of pulmonary arteries (pulmonary "arteriopathy" and idiopathic pulmonary arteriolar calcification) and thrombosis of pulmonary arteries (probably associated to coagulation disorders that were not assessed) were necropsy findings in three patients without any evident cause for the PH on clinical grounds. Maladaptation of the pulmonary vascular bed in asphyxia, maternal diabetes, and fetal tachyarrhythmia were also identified in this study, as well as in two patients with malformation of vein of Galeno and PPHN associated to high cardiac output failure from large arteriovenous malformations. These causes of PPHN have already been described [26]. The cases of PPHN

of unknown aetiology in this series were transient forms with a good outcome, suggesting transient maladaptation to extrauterine life.

Neonates who have PPHN require supportive care tailored to the degree of hypoxemia and physiologic instability. Oxygen is a potent vasodilator and was used in all patients, once hypoxemia is usually present. Mechanical ventilation facilitates alveolar recruitment and lung expansion, potentially improving the ventilation/perfusion (V/Q) match. In this study, mechanical ventilation was used in all, except in four cases of transient tachypnea of the newborn and three cases of PPHN of unknown aetiology with mild pulmonary hypertension. Surfactant has been shown to decrease the need for ECMO in full-term neonates with severe respiratory failure [27]. The beneficial effect of surfactant in this study was seen particularly in babies who had meconium aspiration syndrome and sepsis. Sedatives, although widely used to minimize fluctuations in oxygenation and facilitate ventilation, have not been tested in randomized trials [5]. We have used sedatives in all ventilated patients to ameliorate oxygenation and to decrease discomfort. We do not use for routine skeletal muscle relaxants. Inotropic and vasopressor support with dopamine, dobutamine, and epinephrine is used to optimize cardiac function, stabilize systemic blood pressure, and decrease right-to-left shunt. From 2003 we have used iNO and sildenafil, in selected cases of severe PPHN, mainly in congenital diaphragmatic hernia. Both the survival rate of congenital diaphragmatic hernia and all cases of PPHN showed a significant increase since 2003. ECMO has significantly improved the survival of neonates with severe but reversible lung disease [28, 29], but we do not have experience on that. We tried ECMO in a poor prognosis for of bilateral congenital diaphragmatic hernia with severe pulmonary hypoplasia and pulmonary hypertension, but the patient did not survive.

The overall survival rate described in the literature, including all causes of PPHN, is over 70–75% [30]. Our results are now according to these figures. There is, however, a marked difference depending on the underlying disease. There are also significant differences in long-term outcome according to the cause of PPHN.

This study is limited by the fact of being a single center retrospective analysis, including a small sample of some rare pulmonary disorders causing PH. Prospective studies with the objective of evaluating the different therapies in the various groups of underlying diseases, including a significant number of patients, will give much more information regarding therapeutic efficacy and survival.

Future research must address the different causes of PPHN and therapies separately, in large multicenter studies.

In conclusion, our study shows a myriad of non cardiac aetiologies for PPHN, most of them related to lung disease or lung hypoplasia. We observed an improvement in survival rate since 2003, and we believe that this is related to the use of new therapies. We hope that ECMO will offer additional advantages at our NICU for selected infants in the near future.

References

[1] G. Simonneau, I. M. Robbins, M. Beghetti et al., "Updated clinical classification of pulmonary hypertension," *Journal of the American College of Cardiology*, vol. 54, no. 1, pp. S43–S54, 2009.

[2] R. Rothstein, Y. Paris, and A. Quizon, "Pulmonary hypertension," *Pediatrics in Review*, vol. 30, no. 2, pp. 39–46, 2009.

[3] J. Alameh, A. Bachiri, L. Devisme et al., "Alveolar capillary dysplasia: a cause of persistent pulmonary hypertension of the newborn," *European Journal of Pediatrics*, vol. 161, no. 5, pp. 262–266, 2002.

[4] A. M. Kunig, T. A. Parker, L. M. Nogee, S. H. Abman, and J. P. Kinsella, "ABCA3 deficiency presenting as persistent pulmonary hypertension of the newborn," *Journal of Pediatrics*, vol. 151, no. 3, pp. 322–324, 2007.

[5] G. G. Konduri and U. O. Kim, "Advances in the diagnosis and management of persistent pulmonary hypertension of the newborn," *Pediatric Clinics of North America*, vol. 56, no. 3, pp. 579–600, 2009.

[6] W. M. Gersony, G. V. Duc, and J. C. Sinclair, "PFC syndrome," *Circulation*, vol. 40, supplement 3, p. 87, 1969.

[7] Y. Gao and J. U. Raj, "Regulation of the pulmonary circulation in the fetus and newborn," *Physiological Reviews*, vol. 90, no. 4, pp. 1291–1335, 2010.

[8] S. H. Abman, "Recent advances in the pathogenesis and treatment of persistent pulmonary hypertension of the newborn," *Neonatology*, vol. 91, no. 4, pp. 283–290, 2007.

[9] J. Rasanen, D. C. Wood, R. H. Debbs, J. Cohen, S. Weiner, and J. C. Huhta, "Reactivity of the human fetal pulmonary circulation to maternal hyperoxygenation increases during the second half of pregnancy: a randomized study," *Circulation*, vol. 97, no. 3, pp. 257–262, 1998.

[10] F. C. Morin, E. A. Egan, W. Ferguson, and C. E. G. Lundgren, "Development of pulmonary vascular response to oxygen," *American Journal of Physiology*, vol. 254, no. 3, pp. H542–H546, 1988.

[11] D. Bohn, "Congenital diaphragmatic hernia," *American Journal of Respiratory and Critical Care Medicine*, vol. 166, no. 7, pp. 911–915, 2002.

[12] J. Boloker, D. A. Bateman, J. T. Wung, and C. J. H. Stolar, "Congenital diaphragmatic hernia in 120 infants treated consecutively with permissive hypercapnea/spontaneous respiration/elective repair," *Journal of Pediatric Surgery*, vol. 37, no. 3, pp. 357–366, 2002.

[13] G. M. Rocha, R. F. Bianchi, M. Severo et al., "Congenital diaphragmatic hernia—the neonatal period (Part I)," *European Journal of Pediatric Surgery*, vol. 18, no. 4, pp. 219–223, 2008.

[14] S. Shankaran, Z. Q. Farooki, and R. Desai, "β-hemolytic streptococcal infection appearing as persistent fetal circulation," *American Journal of Diseases of Children*, vol. 136, no. 8, pp. 725–727, 1982.

[15] L. A. Shook, T. H. Pauly, S. L. Marple et al., "Group B streptococcus promotes oxygen radical-dependent thromboxane accumulation in young piglets," *Pediatric Research*, vol. 27, no. 4, pp. 349–352, 1990.

[16] C. T. Navarrete, C. Devia, A. C. Lessa et al., "The role of endothelin converting enzyme inhibition during group B Streptococcus-induced pulmonary hypertension in newborn piglets," *Pediatric Research*, vol. 54, no. 3, pp. 387–392, 2003.

[17] B. A. Yoder, E. A. Kirsch, W. H. Barth, and M. C. Gordon, "Changing obstetric practices associated with decreasing incidence of meconium aspiration syndrome," *Obstetrics and Gynecology*, vol. 99, no. 5, pp. 731–739, 2002.

[18] P. A. Dargaville, M. South, and P. N. McDougall, "Surfactant and surfactant inhibitors in meconium aspiration syndrome," *Journal of Pediatrics*, vol. 138, no. 1, pp. 113–115, 2001.

[19] H. Soukka, J. Jalonen, P. Kero, and P. Kääpä, "Endothelin-1, atrial natriuretic peptide and pathophysiology of pulmonary hypertension in porcine meconium aspiration," *Acta Paediatrica, International Journal of Paediatrics*, vol. 87, no. 4, pp. 424–428, 1998.

[20] R. S. Radhakrishnan, P. A. Lally, K. P. Lally, and C. S. Cox, "ECMO for meconium aspiration syndrome: support for relaxed entry criteria," *ASAIO Journal*, vol. 53, no. 4, pp. 489–491, 2007.

[21] C. K. Heritage and M. D. Cunningham, "Association of elective repeat cesarian delivery and persistent pulmonary hypertension of the newborn," *American Journal of Obstetrics & Gynecology*, vol. 152, pp. 627–629, 1985.

[22] I. F. Csaba, E. Sulyok, and T. Ertl, "Relationship of maternal treatment with indomethacin to persistence of fetal circulation syndrome," *Journal of Pediatrics*, vol. 92, no. 3, p. 484, 1978.

[23] F. F. Rubaltelli, M. L. Chiozza, V. Zanardo, and F. Cantarutti, "Effect on neonate of maternal treatment with indomethacin," *Journal of Pediatrics*, vol. 94, no. 1, p. 161, 1979.

[24] M. A. Alano, E. Ngougmna, E. M. Ostrea, and G. G. Konduri, "Analysis of nonsteroidal antiinflammatory drugs in meconium and its relation to persistent pulmonary hypertension of the newborn," *Pediatrics*, vol. 107, no. 3, pp. 519–523, 2001.

[25] S. H. Abman, P. F. Shanley, and F. J. Accurso, "Failure of postnatal adaptation of the pulmonary circulation after chronic intrauterine pulmonary hypertension in fetal lambs," *Journal of Clinical Investigation*, vol. 83, no. 6, pp. 1849–1858, 1989.

[26] S. A. Stayer and Y. Liu, "Pulmonary hypertension of the newborn," *Best Practice & Research. Clinical Anaesthesiology*, vol. 24, no. 3, pp. 375–386, 2010.

[27] A. Lotze, B. R. Mitchell, D. I. Bulas et al., "Multicenter study of surfactant (beractant) use in the treatment of term infants with severe respiratory failure," *Journal of Pediatrics*, vol. 132, no. 1, pp. 40–47, 1998.

[28] D. J. Field, C. Davis, D. Elbourne, A. Grant, A. Johnson, and D. Macrae, "UK collaborative randomised trial of neonatal extracorporeal membrane oxygenation," *Lancet*, vol. 348, no. 9020, pp. 75–82, 1996.

[29] M. Mugford, D. Elbourne, and D. Field, "Extracorporeal membrane oxygenation for severe respiratory failure in newborn infants," *Cochrane Database of Systematic Reviews*, no. 3, Article ID CD001340, 2008.

[30] G. Alpan, "Persistent pulmonary hypertension of the newborn," in *Neonatology—Management, Procedures, On-Call Problems, Diseases and Drugs*, T. L. Gomella, M. D. Cunningham, F. G. Eyal, and D. Tuttle, Eds., pp. 636–644, McGraw Hill, New York, NY, USA, 6th edition, 2009.

16

The Impact of Pulmonary Arterial Pressure on Exercise Capacity in Mild-to-Moderate Cystic Fibrosis: A Case Control Study

Katerina Manika,[1] **Georgia G. Pitsiou,**[2] **Afroditi K. Boutou,**[2] **Vassilis Tsaoussis,**[1]
Nikolaos Chavouzis,[2] **Marina Antoniou,**[1] **Maria Fotoulaki,**[3]
Ioannis Stanopoulos,[2] **and Ioannis Kioumis**[1]

[1] *Pulmonary Department, Aristotle University of Thessaloniki, "G. Papanikolaou" General Hospital, Exohi, 57010 Thessaloniki, Greece*
[2] *Respiratory Failure Unit, Aristotle University of Thessaloniki, "G. Papanikolaou" General Hospital, Exohi, 57010 Thessaloniki, Greece*
[3] *4th Department of Pediatrics, Aristotle University of Thessaloniki, "Papageorgiou" General Hospital, 56429 Thessaloniki, Greece*

Correspondence should be addressed to Georgia G. Pitsiou, gpitsiou@yahoo.gr

Academic Editor: Robert Naeije

Background. Pulmonary hypertension (PH) is an often complication of severe cystic fibrosis (CF); however, data on the presence and impact of pulmonary vasculopathy in adult CF patients with milder disease, is very limited. *Aim.* To investigate, for the first time, the impact of systolic pulmonary arterial pressure (PASP) on maximal exercise capacity in adults with mild-to-moderate cystic fibrosis, without PH at rest. *Methods.* This is a Case Control study. Seventeen adults with mild-to-moderate CF, without PH at rest (cases) and 10 healthy, nonsmoking, age, and height matched controls were studied. All subjects underwent maximal cardiopulmonary exercise testing and echocardiography before and within 1 minute after stopping exercise. *Results.* Exercise ventilation parameters were similar in the two groups; however, cases, compared to controls, had higher postexercise PASP and decreased exercise capacity, established with lower peak work rate, peak O_2 uptake, anaerobic threshold, and peak O_2 pulse. Furthermore, the change in PASP values before and after exercise was strongly correlated to the parameters of exercise capacity among cases but not among controls. *Conclusions.* CF adults with mild-to-moderate disease should be screened for the presence of pulmonary vasculopathy, since the elevation of PASP during exercise might contribute to impaired exercise capacity.

1. Introduction

Exercise impairment in cystic fibrosis (CF) is well established and a variety of determinants, such as pulmonary and nutritional factors, muscle dysfunction and deconditioning, have been studied in this direction [1–4]. It seems that the factors which are limiting exercise tend to vary across disease stages; ventilatory impairment is probably the major factor limiting exercise in severe disease, while nonpulmonary factors seem to be related to reduced exercise capacity in mild and moderate disease [4].

Pulmonary hypertension (PH), which is a common determinant of exercise capacity in patients with respiratory

disorders [5], is an often complication of CF. PH is observed in 20–65% of adult CF patients with severe disease [6–10], and it has been associated with increased mortality [6, 11]. However, data on its frequency and impact among patients with milder disease are limited. Although adult CF patients with mild-to-moderate disease achieve maximum exercise without generally reaching ventilatory limitation [4], the potential effect of pulmonary vasculopathy on exercise capacity, in this patient population, has not yet been clarified.

In this study we hypothesized that pulmonary vascular disease contributes to the exercise intolerance of adult CF patients with mild-to-moderate disease, without PH at rest. Under this scope we conducted a case-control study, utilizing maximal cardiopulmonary exercise testing (CPET), in order to investigate, for the first time in literature, the impact of post exercise PASP on this patient population.

2. Methods

2.1. Subjects. The study followed a case-control design. Seventeen adult CF patients with mild-to-moderate disease constituted the group of cases and 10 healthy nonsmoking volunteers matched for age and height, constituted the group of controls. All CF patients were regularly attending the outpatient CF clinic of "G. Papanikolaou" Hospital, were in stable clinical condition and were life-long nonsmokers. Mild pulmonary disease was defined by the presence of FEV_1 >65% of predicted, and moderate disease by the presence of ≤40% FEV_1 ≤65% of predicted [6]. Patients who presented with an exacerbation of the disease, that is increased sputum production, purulence, or dyspnea with or without systemic symptoms, combined with a 10% or more reduction in patient's forced expiratory volume in 1 second (FEV_1) usual value, were excluded from the study. Patients who were hospitalized or required per os antibiotics during the last 2 months prior to the study, received domiciliary oxygen therapy, or presented with any other condition affecting exercise capacity, were also excluded. Ethical approval for the study protocol was received from the "G. Papanikolaou" Hospital Scientific Committee and informed consent was provided by all participants.

2.2. Study Protocol. During the baseline visit, all CF patients were clinically assessed by the same physician, who documented their Schwachmann score (SS). An arterial blood sample was obtained for both cases and controls, while all participants underwent pulmonary function testing. Forced vital capacity (FVC) and FEV_1 were measured utilizing an electronic spirometer (Wright ventilometer, Clement Clarke International Ltd., England), according to the American Thoracic Society recommendations [12].

All participants visited again the CF clinic within one week and underwent a complete transthoracic echocardiographic study, including 2D, pulsed and continuous-wave Doppler and colour flow imaging using a HD7 cardiac ultrasound system (Philips medical system, Andover, MA, USA). Standard two-dimensional (2D) and colour flow Doppler images were obtained using the parasternal long and short axis and apical views. PASP was estimated by calculating the maximal velocity of the tricuspid regurgitant jet and by further using the Bernoulli equation and then adding to this value an estimated right atrial pressure based on both the size of the inferior vena cava and the change in diameter of this vessel during respiration. PH was defined as a PASP >35 mmHg at rest [13]. Left ventricular dimensions, ejection fraction, and cardiac index were obtained by previously recommended techniques [14].

A maximal exercise capacity test was then performed on a cycle ergometer (medical graphics), under continuous monitoring of heart rate (HR), oxygen saturation (SpO_2), and a 12-lead electrocardiogram, while blood pressure (BP)

measurements were obtained every two minutes using a standard-cuff mercury sphygmomanometer. A ramp protocol was used with an incremental rate of 20 Watts·min^{-1} for controls and of 10–20 Watts·min^{-1} for cases according to disease severity and estimated fitness, aiming for the test to last approximately 10–12 minutes [15]. Each test was preceded by 3 min of resting to enable subjects to achieve steady state conditions for HR, SpO_2, BP, and gas exchange variables, and of 2 min of unloaded cycling. Patients and controls were asked to score their sense of dyspnea and muscle fatigue using Borg scale, every 2 minutes during the test.

Gas exchange values and exercise parameters were collected breath-by-breath and computer-averaged over 10-second intervals. Anaerobic threshold was calculated by the V slope method, as previously described [15]. The following exercise parameters were recorded: maximal work rate (WR peak), peak oxygen uptake (VO_2 peak), oxygen uptake at anaerobic threshold (AT), peak oxygen pulse (VO_2 peak/HR), ventilatory equivalent for carbon dioxide at AT (VE/VCO_2), maximal ventilation VEmax, peak heart rate (HR), maximum minute ventilation to maximum voluntary ventilation ratio (VEmax/MVV), and breathing reserve (BR). The MVV was calculated as 40 × FEV_1 and the breathing reserve as MVV-VEmax. Ventilatory limitation was defined as (VEmax/MVV) × 100 > 85% or BR <11 lit [15, 16].

Within 1 minute after the completion of the exercise testing, a second echocardiogram was performed by the same investigator, following the same protocol and focusing on postexercise tricuspid regurgitation velocity.

2.3. Data Analysis. Data analysis was conducted using the Statistical Package for Social Sciences (SPSS) for Windows 2000XP, release 17.0. Normal predicted values for CPET parameters were calculated using standard equations [15, 16]. The Shapiro-Wilk test of normality was used to assess the normal or not distribution of data. Student's t-test for independent samples was used to compare CPET parameters between cases and controls, while the Mann-Whitney the U-test was applied to compare CPET parameters between CF patients with low (≤35 mmHg) and high (>35 mmHg) postexercise PASP. ΔSPAP was calculated as follows: PASP after exercise − PASP at rest. Pearson correlation coefficient (r) was used to assess potential correlations between ΔPASP and CPET parameters in cases and controls. A P value <0.05 was considered significant.

3. Results

Summary characteristics of cases and controls are shown in Tables 1 and 2. During rest, none of the CF patients suffered from PH and no difference was noted in PASP or any other echocardiographic measurement between the two groups. However, PASP immediately after exercise was significantly higher in the group of cases compared to controls (31.5 versus 25.8, $P = 0.041$).

Both cases and controls stopped exercise because of fatigue. At the end of exercise mean Borg scale for fatigue

TABLE 1: Demographic characteristics, pulmonary function variables and pulmonary artery pressure measurements in cases and controls.

	Cases	Controls	P value
Number (M/F)	17 (11/6)	10 (7/3)	
Age (years)	23.9 ± 3.5	26.8 ± 3.1	NS
BMI (kg/m^2)	21.3 ± 3.0	24.9 ± 4.1	NS
SS	72.3 ± 13.9	NA	
FEV$_1$ (% predicted)	66.3 ± 24.3	99.1 ± 5.4	0.004
FVC (% predicted)	78.4 ± 18.6	98.5 ± 6.1	0.007
pO$_2$ rest (mmHg)	75.7 ± 9.2	93.4 ± 9.2	0.008
SpO$_2$ rest (%)	95.4 ± 1.9	97.6 ± 1.4	NS
PASP rest (mmHg)	27.5 ± 6.4	24.6 ± 2.2	NS
PASP post ex. (mmHg)	31.5 ± 7.3	25.8 ± 1.3	0.041
ΔPASP (mmHg)	4.0 ± 3.1	1.2 ± 1.3	0.048

Data are presented as mean ± 1 standard deviation. NS: not significant, BMI: body mass index, SS: Schwachmann score, NA: not applicable, rest: at rest, post ex.: post exercise, FEV$_1$: forced expiratory volume in 1 second, FVC: forced vital capacity, pO$_2$: arterial oxygen partial pressure, SpO$_2$: oxygen saturation, PASP: right ventricular systolic pressure, ΔPASP: PASP post-PASP rest.

TABLE 2: Exercise parameters in cases and controls.

	Cases	Controls	P value
WR peak (% predicted)	66. ± 14.8	97.1 ± 5.3	0.002
VO$_2$ peak (mL/kg∗min)	28.5 ± 7.5	35.9 ± 4.8	0.026
VO$_2$ peak (% predicted)	73.7 ± 14.8	97.8 ± 5.9	0.002
AT (mL/kg∗min)	20.1 ± 5.4	27.1 ± 5.5	0.013
AT (% predicted)	48.8 ± 10.5	69.9 ± 12.3	0.008
VO$_2$/HR (mL/kg∗beats)	10.8 ± 3.4	15.9 ± 4.9	0.032
VO$_2$/HR (% predicted)	88 ± 17.2	98.1 ± 11.3	0.048
VE/VCO$_2$@AT	31.3 ± 3.7	25.1 ± 3.0	0.008
VEmax (lit)	69.8 ± 21	81.1 ± 30.5	NS
VEmax/MVV (%)	66.7 ± 21.5	53.4 ± 18.1	NS
MVV-VEmax (lit)	40.01 ± 36.3	79.96 ± 34.9	0.047
BR (lit)	40 ± 36.3	79.7 ± 34.7	0.045
RER	1.19 ± 0.7	1.21 ± 0.6	NS
SpO$_2$ peak (%)	93.9 ± 4	96 ± 1.9	NS
Borg scale fatigue (peak)	7.9 ± 1.4	8.2 ± 1.3	NS
Borg scale dyspnea (peak)	6.2 ± 2.9	5.9 ± 1.4	NS

Data are presented as mean ± 1 standard deviation. NS: not significant, WR peak: maximal work rate, VO$_2$ peak: maximal oxygen uptake, AT: oxygen uptake at anaerobic threshold, VO$_2$/HR: peak oxygen pulse, VE/VCO$_2$@AT: ventilatory equivalent for carbon dioxide at anaerobic threshold, VE max: minute ventilation at peak exercise, VEmax/MVV: minute ventilation at peak exercise to maximum voluntary ventilation ratio, BR: breathing reserve, RER: respiratory exchange ratio, SpO$_2$ peak: oxygen saturation at peak exercise.

was approximately 8 and mean Borg scale for dyspnea was 6 for both groups. Respiratory exchange ratio (RER) at peak exercise was >1.1 for all subjects. During maximal CPET, CF patients presented limited exercise capacity, compared to controls, as established by lower WR, VO$_2$ peak, AT, and oxygen pulse (Table 2). However, no participant presented with respiratory limitation. Although the absolute value of MVV-VEmax was higher among cases compared to controls, VEmax/MVV% predicted did not differ between the two groups and even though BR was significantly lower among cases (Table 2), it was higher than 11 liters in all participants. Oxygen saturation at peak exercise was also similar between the two groups (Table 2).

After exercise, 5 cases presented with PASP >35 mmHg and the rest 12 cases with PASP ≤35 mmHg, while all controls had PASP ≤35 mmHg. No difference was noted between the two CF patient groups with and without exercise-induced PH, regarding FEV$_1$% predicted and FVC% predicted values (data not shown). Those CF patients with post exercise PASP >35 mmHg exhibited lower WR peak% predicted, VO$_2$ peak% predicted, VO$_2$/HR% predicted, and SpO$_2$ peak, and a trend for higher VE/VCO$_2$@AT, compared to the rest of CF patients. However, none of the parameters indicative of ventilatory limitation during exercise, that is VEmax, VEmax/MVV and BR differed between CF patients with and without postexercise PH (Table 3).

In cases, but not in controls, ΔSPAP established an inverse, strong correlation to several parameters of exercise capacity, that is, WR peak (watts and % predicted), VO$_2$ peak (mL/kg∗min and % predicted), oxygen pulse (mL/kg∗beats and % predicted), and SpO$_2$ peak (Table 4). ΔSAP was also strongly correlated to Schwachman score (Spearman rho = −0.698, P = 0.002) in the group of cases. On the contrary, neither pulmonary function testing parameters, nor any variable indicative of ventilatory limitation during exercise

was correlated to ΔSPAP, in any of the groups (data not shown).

4. Discussion

The main findings of our study are (a) patients with mild-to-moderate CF without PH at rest, exhibit higher postexercise PASP and lower exercise capacity compared to controls, without reaching ventilatory limitation, (b) exercise impairment and dyspnea are probably more pronounced among CF patients with higher (≥35 mmHg) postexercise PASP, and (c) ΔPASP is inversely correlated with maximal work rate and oxygen uptake in cases, but not in controls.

The association of PH and exercise tolerance in mild-to-moderate CF is far from clear. Montgomery et al. have reported the case of a CF adult patient with severe lung disease and pulmonary hypertension that increased significantly after exercise and improved with sildenafil treatment [17]. Although recently published data demonstrate that CF patients suffer from endothelial dysfunction and defective dilatation of pulmonary vessels during exercise [18], in another study the estimated rest PASP was not correlated to submaximal exercise capacity among CF patients with both severe and moderate disease [19]. However, there is no data regarding the exercise-induced increase of pulmonary artery pressure and its possible impact on maximum exercise tolerance, in patients with less severe disease and no evident pulmonary vasculopathy at rest.

In this study, a group of mild-to-moderate CF patients without PH at rest exhibited a higher postexercise PASP,

TABLE 3: Exercise parameters in cystic fibrosis patients with postexercise PASP ≤35 mmHg and postexercise PASP >35 mmHg.

	PASP ≤35	PASP >35	P value
WR peak (watts)	135.7 ± 46.6	102.4 ± 30.1	NS
WR peak (% predicted)	73.6 ± 11.6	51.4 ± 7.5	0.008
VO$_2$ peak (mL/kg∗min)	30.1 ± 8.0	25.1 ± 5.5	NS
VO$_2$ peak (% predicted)	78.4 ± 15.4	63.4 ± 6.2	0.042
AT (mL/kg∗min)	20.3 ± 5.6	16.3 ± 1.6	NS
AT (% predicted)	51.9 ± 11.2	42.1 ± 4.6	NS
VO$_2$/HR (mL/kg∗beats)	11.4 ± 3.8	9.2 ± 2	NS
VO$_2$/HR (% predicted)	93.5 ± 17.6	75.9 ± 7.8	0.040
VE/VCO$_2$@AT	28.1 ± 4.1	32.8 ± 2.3	0.061
VEmax (lit)	63.3 ± 21.6	57.5 ± 18.7	NS
VEmax/MVV (%)	64.3 ± 23.8	70.5 ± 14.9	NS
MVV-VEmax (lit)	39.6 ± 35.1	42.1 ± 38.9	NS
BR (lit)	42.8 ± 40.7	31.7 ± 21.2	NS
RER	1.19 ± 0.7	1.19 ± 0.4	NS
SpO$_2$ peak (%)	95.4 ± 2.7	90.6 ± 4.7	0.016
Borg scale fatigue (peak)	7.9 ± 1.6	7.4 ± 0.6	NS
Borg scale dyspnea (peak)	5.9 ± 3.3	7.0 ± 2.2	0.046

Data are presented as mean ± 1 standard deviation. NS: not significant, WR peak: maximal work rate, VO$_2$ peak: maximal oxygen uptake, AT: oxygen uptake at anaerobic threshold, VO$_2$/HR: peak oxygen pulse, VE/VCO$_2$@AT: ventilatory equivalent for carbon dioxide at anaerobic threshold, VEmax: minute ventilation at peak exercise, VEmax/MVV: minute ventilation at peak exercise to maximum voluntary ventilation ratio, BR: breathing reserve, RER: respiratory exchange ratio, SpO$_2$ peak: oxygen saturation at peak exercise.

TABLE 4: Pearson correlations between ΔPASP and exercise variables in cases and controls.

	ΔPASP	
	Cases	Controls
WR peak (watts)	−0.539*	NS
WR peak (% predicted)	−0.764**	NS
VO$_2$ peak (mL/kg∗min)	−0.540*	NS
VO$_2$ peak (% predicted)	−0.714*	NS
AT (mL/kg∗min)	NS	NS
AT (% predicted)	NS	NS
VO$_2$/HR (mL/kg∗beats)	−0.530*	NS
VO$_2$/HR (% predicted)	−0.663**	NS
VE/VCO$_2$@AT	NS	NS
SpO$_2$ peak (%)	−0.701*	NS

ΔPASP: PASP (pulmonary artery systolic pressure) after exercise − PASP at rest, WR peak: maximal work rate, VO$_2$ peak: maximal oxygen uptake, AT: anaerobic threshold, VO$_2$/HR: peak oxygen pulse, VE/VCO$_2$@AT: ventilatory equivalent for carbon dioxide at anaerobic threshold, SpO$_2$ peak: oxygen saturation at peak exercise; *$P < 0.05$; **$P < 0.001$; NS: not significant.

a lower exercise capacity and a higher VE/VCO$_2$ ratio at anaerobic threshold compared to controls, although both groups terminated exercise due to fatigue, without presenting respiratory limitation. VE/VCO$_2$ is considered to be a noninvasive marker of pulmonary vascular resistance [20] and previous studies have reported a significant increase in

the VE/VCO$_2$ slope, during exercise, both in CF patients [1] and in patients with severe PH [21]. During maximal CPET, both dyspnea and exercise limitation were even more pronounced among patients with higher (>35 mmHg) postexercise PASP values, compared to the rest of the patients. Furthermore, ΔPASP values correlated to peak work rate, peak O$_2$ uptake, O$_2$ pulse and SpO$_2$ at peak exercise only in the group of cases, while no correlation was noted to any measurement of ventilation during exercise. These data indicate that in CF patients with less severe disease, pulmonary circulation could be defective, resulting to impaired exercise capacity, regardless of the patients' respiratory reserve.

As in several chronic respiratory diseases, exercise capacity in adult CF patients could also be influenced by suboptimal nutritional status and muscle dysfunction [22, 23]. Malnutrition results, through a loss of muscle mass, to a reduction in every day activities and to peripheral muscle deconditioning [23]. The current study was not designed to control for these confounders, so their specific impact on exercise limitation could not be assessed. However, patients and controls weighted the same, since they were height-matched and had the same BMI, which indicates that their nutritional status was similar. Moreover, there was no difference in peak Borg fatigue score neither between patients and controls, nor between patients with and without exercise induced PH, indicating a similar peripheral muscle effort. These results come to an agreement with a previous study where differences in Borg scores of muscle effort and lactic acid were noted only in the group of CF patients with severe respiratory limitation and not among those with mild and moderate disease [4]. Future studies are needed to assess the exact impact of pulmonary vasculopathy on exercise capacity in these patient group, independently of nutritional status and muscle dysfunction.

There are certain limitations in this study. The number of participants who were included was quite small. However, our findings regarding exercise performance are very similar to the ones from larger cohorts [2]. Moreover, although the "gold standard" for measurement of pulmonary artery pressure remains right heart catheterization, Doppler echocardiography has proved to be an easily accessible, noninvasive alternative in previous studies [24]. Another limitation is that PASP is very much affected by cardiac output, so a higher postexercise PASP might reflect not a pulmonary vascular disease but just a persistently higher cardiac index; however there is no sufficient explanation as to why this could be established in cases but not in controls. Furthermore, cardiac output and PASP rapidly recover after exercise in a variable and non-proportional rate [25] and Argiento et al. have previously reported that this could be a reason why post-exercise measurements may be problematic [26]. However, in the latter study, PASP was estimated 5 to 20 minutes after exercise, while in the current study all measurements were conducted within 60 seconds. Although the method adopted in our study may still estimate PASP values less accurately than echocardiography during exercise [25], it has been previously used in order to assess pulmonary hypertension among scleroderma patients and was found to correlate well with several parameters of exercise capacity [27, 28].

In conclusion, pulmonary vascular disease, as established by high post exercise PASP, might be added to the list of determinants of both exercise impairment and increased dyspnea among CF patients with mild-to-moderate disease. To our knowledge, this study is the first to directly investigate the potential association between estimated PASP and maximal exercise capacity in these patients. The limitation in physical functioning and the increased dyspnea are the two primary parameters which affect quality of life in CF patients [29]. Under this scope, further studies, including a larger number of patients with different stages of disease severity are needed, in order for the contribution of pulmonary vascular disease in the physical impairment of this population to be fully evaluated.

Conflict of Interests

The authors declare that they have no conflict of interests.

References

[1] C. Moser, P. Tirakitsoontorn, E. Nussbaum, R. Newcomb, and D. M. Cooper, "Muscle size and cardiorespiratory response to exercise in cystic fibrosis," *American Journal of Respiratory and Critical Care Medicine*, vol. 162, no. 5, pp. 1823–1827, 2000.

[2] A. R. Shah, D. Gozal, and T. G. Keens, "Determinants of aerobic and anaerobic exercise performance in cystic fibrosis," *American Journal of Respiratory and Critical Care Medicine*, vol. 157, no. 4, pp. 1145–1150, 1998.

[3] E. Pouliou, S. Nanas, A. Papamichalopoulos et al., "Prolonged oxygen kinetics during early recovery from maximal exercise in adult patients with cystic fibrosis," *Chest*, vol. 119, no. 4, pp. 1073–1078, 2001.

[4] A. J. Moorcroft, M. E. Dodd, J. Morris, and A. K. Webb, "Symptoms, lactate and exercise limitation at peak cycle ergometry in adults with cystic fibrosis," *European Respiratory Journal*, vol. 25, no. 6, pp. 1050–1056, 2005.

[5] A. K. Boutou, G. G. Pitsiou, I. Trigonis et al., "Exercise capacity in idiopathic pulmonary fibrosis: the effect of pulmonary hypertension," *Respirology*, vol. 16, no. 3, pp. 451–458, 2011.

[6] K. L. Fraser, D. E. Tullis, Z. Sasson, R. H. Hyland, K. S. Thornley, and P. J. Hanly, "Pulmonary hypertension and cardiac function in adult cystic fibrosis: role of hypoxemia," *Chest*, vol. 115, no. 5, pp. 1321–1328, 1999.

[7] P. M. E. Rovedder, B. Ziegler, A. F. F. Pinotti, S. S. M. Barreto, and P. D. T. R. Dalcin, "Prevalence of pulmonary hypertension evaluated by Doppler echocardiography in a population of adolescent and adult patients with cystic fibrosis," *Jornal Brasileiro de Pneumologia*, vol. 34, no. 2, pp. 83–90, 2008.

[8] V. G. Florea, N. D. Florea, R. Sharma et al., "Right ventricular dysfunction in adult severe cystic fibrosis," *Chest*, vol. 118, no. 4, pp. 1063–1068, 2000.

[9] C. D. Vizza, J. P. Lynch, L. L. Ochoa, G. Richardson, and E. P. Trulock, "Right and left ventricular dysfunction in patients with severe pulmonary disease," *Chest*, vol. 113, no. 3, pp. 576–583, 1998.

[10] A. A. Ionescu, N. Payne, I. Obieta-Fresnedo, A. G. Fraser, and D. J. Shale, "Subclinical right ventricular dysfunction in cystic fibrosis: a study using tissue Doppler echocardiography,"

[11] M. Eckles and P. Anderson, "Cor pulmonale in cystic fibrosis," *Seminars in Respiratory and Critical Care Medicine*, vol. 24, no. 3, pp. 323–330, 2003.

[12] American Thoracic Society, "Standardization of spirometry (1994 update)," *American Journal of Respiratory and Critical Care Medicine*, vol. 152, pp. 1107–1136, 1995.

[13] N. Galiè, M. M. Hoeper, M. Humbert et al., "Guidelines for the diagnosis and treatment of pulmonary hypertension," *European Respiratory Journal*, vol. 34, no. 6, pp. 1219–1263, 2009.

[14] N. B. Schiller, "Two-dimensional echocardiographic determination of left ventricular volume, systolic function, and mass. Summary and discussion of the 1989 recommendations of the American Society of Echocardiography," *Circulation*, vol. 84, no. 3, pp. I280–I287, 1991.

[15] K. Wasserman, J. E. Hansen, D. Y. Sue, W. W. Stringer, and B. J. Whipp, "Measurements during integrative cardiopulmonary exercise testing," in *Principles of Exercise-Testing and Interpretation*, K. Wasserman, J. E. Hansen, D. Y. Sue, W. W. Stringer, and B. J. Whipp, Eds., pp. 76–110, Lippincott Williams and Wilkins, Philadelphia, Pa, USA, 4th edition, 2005.

[16] American Thoracic Society/American College of Chest Physicians, "Statement on cardiopulmonary exercise testing," *American Journal of Respiratory and Critical Care Medicine*, vol. 167, pp. 211–277, 2001.

[17] G. S. Montgomery, S. D. Sagel, A. L. Taylor, and S. H. Abman, "Effects of sildenafil on pulmonary hypertension and exercise tolerance in severe cystic fibrosis-related lung disease," *Pediatric Pulmonology*, vol. 41, no. 4, pp. 383–385, 2006.

[18] P. Henno, C. Maurey, C. Danel et al., "Pulmonary vascular dysfunction in endstage cystic fibrosis: role of NF-κB and endothelin-1," *European Respiratory Journal*, vol. 34, no. 6, pp. 1329–1337, 2009.

[19] P. M. E. Rovedder, B. Ziegler, L. R. Pasin et al., "Doppler echocardiogram, oxygen saturation and submaximum capacity of exercise in patients with cystic fibrosis," *Journal of Cystic Fibrosis*, vol. 6, no. 4, pp. 277–283, 2007.

[20] H. Ting, X. G. Sun, M. L. Chuang, D. A. Lewis, J. E. Hansen, and K. Wasserman, "A noninvasive assessment of pulmonary perfusion abnormality in patients with primary pulmonary hypertension," *Chest*, vol. 119, no. 3, pp. 824–832, 2001.

[21] X. G. Sun, J. E. Hansen, R. J. Oudiz, and K. Wasserman, "Exercise pathophysiology in patients with primary pulmonary hypertension," *Circulation*, vol. 104, no. 4, pp. 429–435, 2001.

[22] J. Gea, C. Casadevall, S. Pascual, M. Orozco-Levi, and E. Barreiro, "Respiratory diseases and muscle dysfunction," *Expert Review of Respiratory Medicine*, vol. 6, no. 1, pp. 75–90, 2012.

[23] L. C. Lands, G. J. F. Heigenhauser, and N. L. Jones, "Analysis of factors limiting maximal exercise performance in cystic fibrosis," *Clinical Science*, vol. 83, no. 4, pp. 391–397, 1992.

[24] A. Homma, A. Anzueto, J. I. Peters et al., "Pulmonary artery systolic pressures estimated by echocardiogram vs cardiac catheterization in patients awaiting lung transplantation," *Journal of Heart and Lung Transplantation*, vol. 20, no. 8, pp. 833–839, 2001.

[25] R. Naeije, "In defence of exercise stress test for the diagnosis of pulmonary hypertension," *Heart*, vol. 97, no. 2, pp. 94–95, 2011.

[26] P. Argiento, N. Chesler, M. Mulè et al., "Exercise stress echocardiography for the study of the pulmonary circulation,"

European Respiratory Journal, vol. 35, no. 6, pp. 1273–1278, 2010.

[27] V. Steen, M. Chou, V. Shanmugam, M. Mathias, T. Kuru, and R. Morrissey, "Exercise-induced pulmonary arterial hypertension in patients with systemic sclerosis," *Chest*, vol. 134, no. 1, pp. 146–151, 2008.

[28] M. L. Alkotob, P. Soltani, M. A. Sheatt et al., "Reduced exercise capacity and stress-induced pulmonary hypertension in patients with scleroderma," *Chest*, vol. 130, no. 1, pp. 176–181, 2006.

[29] W. de Jong, A. A. Kaptein, C. P. van der Schans et al., "Quality of life in patients with cystic fibrosis," *Pediatric Pulmonology*, vol. 23, no. 2, pp. 95–100, 1997.

17

Relationship between Respiratory Load Perception and Perception of Nonrespiratory Sensory Modalities in Subjects with Life-Threatening Asthma

Kathleen L. Davenport,[1] Chien Hui Huang,[2] Matthew P. Davenport,[3] and Paul W. Davenport[4]

[1] Department of Rehabilitation Medicine, University of Washington, 1959 Northeast Pacific Street, P.O. Box 356490, Seattle, WA 98195, USA
[2] Department of Physical Therapy, Tzu Chi University, 701 Zhongyang Road, Section 3, Hualien 97004, Taiwan
[3] Department of Chemistry and Food Science, Framingham State University, 100 State Street, Framingham, MA 01701, USA
[4] Department of Physiological Sciences, University of Florida, P.O. Box 100144 HSC, Gainesville, FL 32610, USA

Correspondence should be addressed to Paul W. Davenport, pdavenpo@ufl.edu

Academic Editor: Dimitris Georgopoulos

Subjects with life-threatening asthma (LTA) have reported decreased sensitivity to inspiratory resistive (R) loads. It is unknown if decreased sensitivity is specific for inspiratory R loads, other types of respiratory loads, or a general deficit affecting sensory modalities. This study hypothesized that impairment is specific to respiratory stimuli. This study tested perceptual sensitivity of LTA, asthmatic (A), and nonasthmatic (NA) subjects to 4 sensory modalities: respiratory, somatosensory, auditory, visual. Perceptual sensitivity was measured with magnitude estimation (ME): respiratory loads ME, determined using inspiratory R and pressure threshold (PT) loads; somatosensory ME, determined using weight ranges of 2–20 kg; auditory ME, determined using graded magnitudes of 1 kHz tones delivered for 3 seconds bilaterally; visual ME, determined using gray-to-white disk intensity gradations on black background. ME for inspiratory R loads lessened for LTA over A and NA subjects. There was no significant difference between the 3 groups in ME for PT inspiratory loads, weight, sound, and visual trials. These results demonstrate that LTA subjects are poor perceivers of inspiratory R loads. This deficit in respiratory perception is specific to inspiratory R loads and is not due to perceptual deficits in other types of inspiratory loads, somatosensory, auditory, or visual sensory modalities.

1. Introduction

Asthma is a respiratory disease frequently diagnosed in childhood. To control and/or prevent an asthma attack, it is important for the patient to heed initial symptoms and to be compliant with their prescribed medication(s). Failure to recognize and self-manage of an asthma exacerbation is one cause of life-threatening asthma (LTA) [1–3]. Difficulty in perceiving asthma symptoms can be one of many factors causing the patient to fail to recognize the onset of an asthma attack [2, 4, 5]. A subpopulation of asthmatic patients with a history of LTA has been reported with reduced perception of both intrinsic and extrinsic respiratory loads [2, 4]. These LTA asthmatic patients have an increased threshold for detection of inspiratory resistive loads, a decreased ability to

scale the magnitude of inspiratory loads and a decreased perception of intrinsic bronchoconstriction [2, 4]. It has also been reported that the somatosensory cortex is not activated by inspiratory loads in these LTA subjects suggesting a sensory neural deficit in respiratory information processing in this subpopulation of asthmatic patients [1]. While it is evident that these LTA subjects have poor perception of respiratory mechanical loads, it is unknown if this is a specific deficit for respiratory mechanosensation or a general sensory perception deficit.

Perception of respiratory stimuli has been studied by asking patients to estimate various respiratory load magnitudes and types using the modified Borg scale, visual analog scale, or cross-modality matching [1–4, 6–24]. In order to successfully perform the load perception task, the subject must attend to the load, sense the magnitude of the load, and then provide an estimate of their sense of load magnitude using scaling techniques. These studies have shown that adults and children are capable of estimating inspiratory resistive load magnitudes [1–4, 6–24]. This load magnitude estimation (ME) technique has also been used in multiple sensory modalities to investigate the perceptual sensitivity in subjects to various stimuli such as light [25], sound [26–29], and weight [21, 30–32]. The perceptual sensitivity to respiratory loads is similar to other somatosensory stimuli [21] in normal subjects. However, it is unknown if subjects with poor perception of respiratory loads also have poor perception of other sensory modalities or if the load perception deficit is specific to respiratory information processing.

LTA patients have been shown to have a reduced detection and magnitude estimation of inspiratory resistive loads [2, 4]. It is unknown if this is specific to respiratory mechanosensation, specific to all somatosensation, or a general perceptual deficit. This study was designed to test the sensory perception of LTA subjects to respiratory, somatosensory, auditory, and visual stimuli. Respiratory perception was tested by two types in inspiratory mechanical loads, resistive loads, and pressure threshold loads. We reasoned that if LTA asthmatics have a general respiratory perception deficit, they would be poor perceivers of both types of loads. If LTA patients have a respiratory perception deficit that includes a somatosensory deficit, then they should have reduced perception of both respiratory and weight lifting magnitude estimation. If the LTA asthmatics have a respiratory perception deficit that includes a general sensory perception deficit, then they should have reduced perception of respiratory stimuli and arm weight, auditory, and visual stimuli would be expected. It was hypothesized that asthmatic patients with a history of LTA and a perception deficit of resistive respiratory stimuli exclusively will have unimpaired somatosensory, auditory, and visual perception. This hypothesis was tested in nonasthmatic, LTA asthmatics, and asthmatics without a history of LTA.

2. Methods

2.1. Subjects. Three groups of subjects were tested in this study: (1) subjects ($n = 7$) with life-threatening asthma (LTA), (2) subjects ($n = 10$) with stable asthma (A), and (3) nonasthmatic (NA) subjects ($n = 9$). The subject ages in all groups ranged between 11 and 25 years. Mean ages were 16.3 ± 3.0 years for the LTA group, 17.2 ± 3.0 years for the A group, and 19.0 ± 4.2 years for the NA group. All A and LTA subjects were followed at the Pediatric Pulmonary Clinic at Shands Hospital, University of Florida, Gainesville, FL. The diagnosis of asthma was made by a pediatric pulmonologist, based on the American Thoracic Society criteria [33]. The University of Florida, Health Science Center, Institutional Review Board reviewed and approved this study. All participation was voluntary, and all subjects and the parents of minor subjects received informed consent.

The LTA subjects were asymptomatic without exacerbation of their asthma within 4 weeks of the study. All LTA subjects had been admitted to the Pediatric Intensive Care unit with acute respiratory failure within the last four years. Following their life-threatening event, the LTA subjects were stabilized and maintained with inhaled corticosteroids and theophylline. The A subjects had moderate-to-severe asthma and were on daily maintenance treatment to control their asthma symptoms. However, they had never been admitted to an intensive care unit for respiratory failure. Both A and LTA groups used albuterol by metered dose inhaler (MDI) or by nebulizer as needed. The NA subjects were free of chronic respiratory disease. All subjects were free of any acute respiratory disease at least four weeks prior to the study. No subjects were hearing impaired or were visually impaired to the extent that contact lenses or glasses could not accurately correct their eye sight. Any subject requiring glasses or contact lenses wore them during all testing.

2.2. Pulmonary Function Tests. A pulmonary function test (PFT) was administered after consent was obtained and before testing began. FEV_1, FVC, FEV_1/FVC, and resistance by the forced oscillation method were measured. Any subject with a baseline FEV_1 less than 70% of predicted was eliminated from further participation in the study. No subject had a baseline FEV_1, FEV_1/FVC, or FVC lower than 70% of predicted, according to the American Thoracic Society standards.

2.3. Inspiratory Resistive Load Magnitude Estimation. Perception of extrinsic respiratory loads was determined using magnitude estimation of inspiratory resistive loads with a modified Borg scale [1, 9, 11]. The subject was seated conformably in a sound isolated chamber, separated from the investigator and the experimental apparatus. The subjects had their nose clamped and respired through a mouthpiece connected to a non-rebreathing valve (Hans Rudolph, Kansas City, MO). Care was taken to suspend the valve to eliminate the need for the subject to bite the mouthpiece yet maintain an airtight seal.

The resistive loads were sintered bronze disks placed in series in a loading manifold with stoppered ports between the disks [1]. The loading manifold was connected to a pneumotachograph by reinforced tubing to the inspiratory port of the non-rebreathing valve. The loading manifold was hidden from the subject's view. Mouth pressure (P_M) was recorded from a port in the center of the non-rebreathing valve. P_M was sensed with a differential pressure transducer and a signal conditioner. Inspiratory airflow (V'_I) was recorded with a differential pressure transducer and signal conditioner connected to the pneumotachograph. The V'_I was integrated to obtain the inspired volume (V_I). The P_M, V_I, and V'_I were recorded on a polygraph. The V'_I was also displayed on an oscilloscope placed in front of the subjects, which they used to target their breathing during the study. Resistances were selected by removing a stopper and allowing the subject a single inspiration through the selected port. They were monitored with a digital video camera throughout the study.

Before testing began, the peak V'_I during normal, tidal breathing was determined and displayed as a horizontal line on the oscilloscope. The subject was allowed to practice V_I' targeting prior to the load practice session. The load practice session consisted of a series of test loads, including a low and high load, presented with a verbal cue ("small" versus "large," resp.) to familiarize the subject with the range of loads.

Standard 10-point category Borg scale rating was the modality used by subjects to estimate magnitude of the external respiratory load. Subjects were asked to press a button on a battery-powered device that corresponded to the Borg scale rating for the test breath. The voltage from the device was displayed on the polygraph and calibrated to the corresponding Borg scale rating.

The presentation of the resistive loads for the magnitude estimation was divided into two experiment trials. Both trials consisted of six resistive load magnitudes (1.64, 2.48, 3.26, 6.95, 11.46, and 20.48 cm H_2O/L/s) and no-load presented five times each in randomized block order, as described previously [2]. Subjects were given a 5–10-minute break between each trial. Thus, each subject was exposed to each load magnitude a total of 10 times. Subjects were given a cue (red light) to signal that the next breath was a test breath, which the subject must estimate. The subject inspired to the target V_I' on each breath (control and test). The subject made the estimate immediately after the test breath using the Borg scale. Three to six unloaded breaths separated each test breath.

2.4. Inspiratory Pressure Threshold Load Magnitude Estimation.

Perception of pressure threshold (PT) loads was administered in the same fashion as the inspiratory resistive loads [16]. The same mouthpiece, Borg scale, and methods were used for this portion of the study. The only difference was the loading manifold, and therefore a theoretical difference in perception of the respiratory load. This loading manifold included spring-loaded pressure-threshold valves with stoppered ports over each valve. The valves would open when a calibrated, specific inspiratory pressure was achieved. The PT load magnitude was the inspiratory pressure required to open the valve allowing air to flow. There was a PT load practice session before this test to familiarize subjects with the respiratory loads. The PT load practice session consisted of a series of test loads, including a low and high load, presented after a verbal cue ("small" versus "large," resp.). The presentation of the PT loads for the ME was divided into two experiment trials. Both trials consisted of 7 PT load magnitudes (2.35, 4.12, 5.22, 10.27, 18.80, 23.14, and 27.45 cm H_2O) and no-load were presented five times each in a randomized block order. Thus, each subject was exposed to each PT load ten times. Subjects were given a 5–10-minute break in between each trial.

2.5. Weight Magnitude Estimation.

Subjects were seated conformably in a sound isolated chamber, separated from the investigator and the experimental apparatus. They placed the elbow of their dominant hand on an armrest of a chair. They placed their forearm vertically so their hands were raised in the air and grasped a handle which was attached to a rope. The rope was connected through a 2-pulley system to a bucket, where weights were added out of the subjects' view. Once subjects had gripped the handle comfortably, the rope was pulled taught so there was no slack in the rope.

Weights (5, 15, 30, 60, and 80 ounces) and no-weight were placed in the bucket out of view of the subjects. Subjects were then cued by a red light to lower their forearm directly down onto the armrest to sense the weight. Another investigator was seated in the room with the subjects during the experiment. After subjects pulled down once on the load and released it, they were asked to tell the researcher a modified Borg scale number that corresponded to the perceived heaviness of the weight. A practice trial, including heavy and light loads, was first administered with cues of "heavy" and "light," respectively, to familiarize subjects with the task. Then, the weights were presented to the subjects in three trials in a randomized block order. Each of the five weights was presented three times in the first two trials and twice in the third trial. Thus, each subject estimated each weight and no-weight 10 times. Subjects were given a 5–10-minute break between each trial.

2.6. Sound Magnitude Estimation.

Subjects were seated conformably in a sound isolated chamber and were given a set of headphones to wear. The headphones were connected to a laptop computer, which was hidden from the subjects' view. A single tone of 77, 81, 87, 92, and 96 decibels was used for sound magnitudes. The investigator was seated in the room with the subjects during the experiment. After the subjects were presented a tone, they were asked to tell the researcher a modified Borg scale number corresponding to the perceived tone loudness. A practice trial was first given with cues of "loud" and "soft" to familiarize subjects with the range of tone levels. Then, the tones were presented to the subjects in three trials in a randomized block order. Each magnitude of tone was presented three times in the first two trials and twice in the third trial. Thus, each subject estimated each sound a total of 10 times. Subjects were given a 2–5-minute break between each trial.

2.7. Light Magnitude Estimation.

Subjects were seated conformably in a sound isolated chamber and were asked to sit on the edge of the chair. A box fashioned into a wide, rectangular tube was used to block extraneous light from the room. One end of the box was placed around a computer monitor and the other end of the box was placed around the subjects' head and on the subjects' shoulders. A rod was placed under the box so subjects did not hold the weight of the box. A cloth was draped around the subjects to block out ambient light. The computer monitor was connected to a laptop computer, from which the experiment was run and which was hidden from subjects' view. A PowerPoint display using gray circles of 284, 192, 150, 77, and 41 lumens on a black background was used as light magnitudes. Lumens were converted to percent grey scale (83.922, 69.804, 41.176, 24.706, and 2.745, resp.) which was the magnitude scale used for analysis. The investigator was seated in the room with the subjects during experimentation. After subjects had been presented a circle of light, they were asked to tell the researcher a modified Borg scale number that corresponded to the perceived lightness of the circle. A practice trial was first given with cues of "light" and "dark" to familiarize the subject with the grayscale levels. Then, the grayscale circles were presented to the subject in two trials in randomized block order. Each magnitude of grayscale was presented five times in each trial. Thus, each subject was presented each visual grayscale a total of 10 times. Subjects were given a 2–5-minute break in between each trial.

2.8. Statistical Analysis. The outcome measure for the five perception modalities was Borg scale ME as a function of modality magnitude. For all modalities, the Borg scale ME results were averaged for each modality magnitude. For resistive respiratory loading, the slope was determined by plotting Borg scale (ME) against resistive (R) load on a log ME/log R scale. The slope for pressure threshold (PT) respiratory loading was determined on a log ME/log PT load scale. Weight ME slope was determined by plotting Borg scale against weight on a log ME/log ounces scale. For auditory ME slope, the mean Borg scale for each sound intensity was plotted versus the corresponding decibel (dB) on a log ME-dB scale. Visual ME slope was found by plotting the estimated grayscale on a log ME/log gray scale plot.

If a stimulus was given a Borg scale rating of zero on more than 5 presentations, then that stimulus was considered undetected and not included in the regression analysis. The slope was determined by linear regression analysis, and the average slope was determined for each group. The age distribution was the same for all 3 groups. All groups had age averages and ranges that are not significantly different. Overall range is 11–25 years. This raised the issue of combining the "children" (11–18 yrs) with "adults" (19–25 yrs). A Pearson correlation analysis was performed to determine if there was a significant correlation between age and modality slope. An ANOVA was used to test for group-by-modality differences followed by a Tukey's post hoc analysis. Significance was set at $P < 0.05$.

3. Results

There were no significant differences in age, gender, or race between the three groups and no significant difference in severity of asthma between the asthma control group, A, (subjects without a history of life-threatening asthma) and LTA group. All subjects inspired to their target line for each test breath for magnitude estimation of resistive and pressure threshold inspiratory loads. This indicates that each subject was adequately presented each load and was able to perform the task. There was no significant difference between age and perceptual measure thus, the results for children (age 11–18) and adults (age 19–25) were pooled.

The log ME/log R slopes for inspiratory resistive loading were 0.926, 0.921, and 0.726 for NA, A, and LTA groups, respectively. There was no significant difference between the NA and A groups for the group mean slope magnitude estimation of inspiratory resistive loads (Figure 1). The LTA subjects' resistive load magnitude estimation was significantly

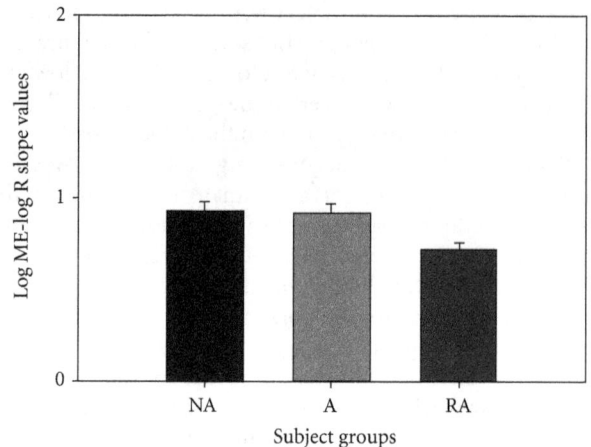

FIGURE 1: Resistive load magnitude estimation was significantly lower ($P < 0.05$) for LTA subjects than for both NA and A groups. There was no significant difference between the NA and A groups.

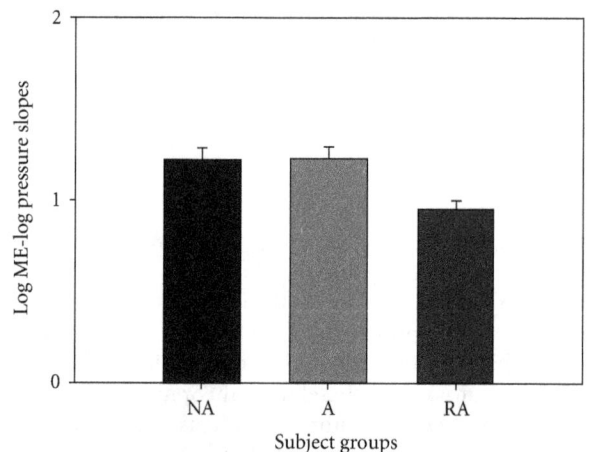

FIGURE 2: There was no significant difference between the slopes for the 3 groups, NA, A, and LTA, for inspiratory PT load ME.

lower ($P < 0.05$) than the group mean slope magnitude estimation for both NA and A groups (Figure 1). There was a significant ($P = 0.05$) group effect for log ME/log Pmax for R load slopes. The log ME/log Pmax R slope for LTA subjects was significantly less than the NA and A groups.

There was no significant difference between the slopes for the 3 groups, NA, A, and LTA, for inspiratory PT load ME (Figure 2). The log ME/log PT slopes for this modality were 1.224, 1.213, and 0.954 for the NA, A, and LTA groups, respectively. There was also no significant difference between the 3 groups for the PT log ME/log Pmax slopes.

Weight magnitude estimation slopes on a log ME/log ounces scale resulted in values of 1.414, 1.285, and 1.214 for NA, A and LTA groups, respectively, (Figure 3). None of these values reached statistical significance.

There was no significant difference between any of the group in auditory magnitude estimation testing (Figure 4). Slope values were 0.373, 0.379, and 0.452 for NA, A, and LTA groups, respectively.

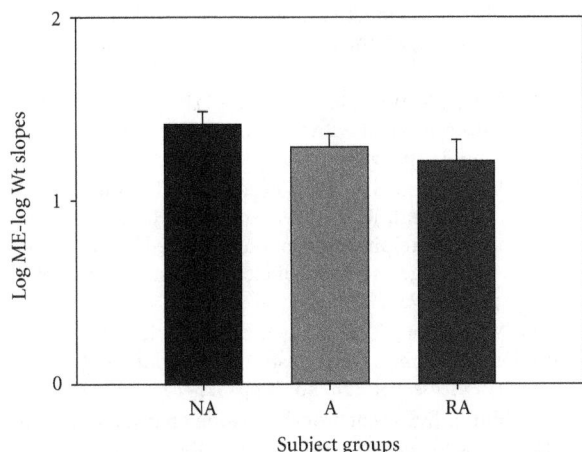

FIGURE 3: There was no significant difference between the slopes for the 3 groups, NA, A, and LTA, for weight ME on log ME/log ounces scale.

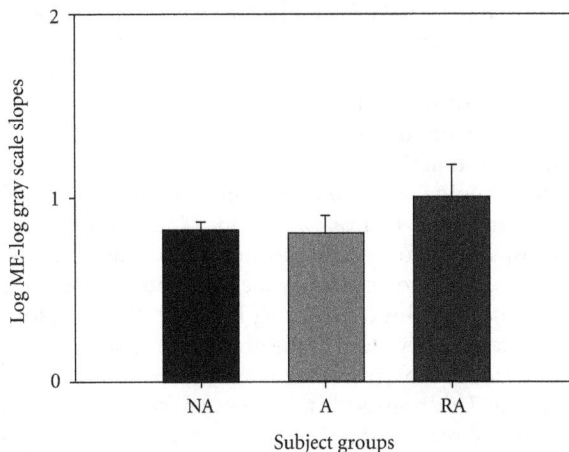

FIGURE 5: There was no significant difference between the slopes for the 3 groups, NA, A, and LTA for visual grayscale magnitude estimation testing.

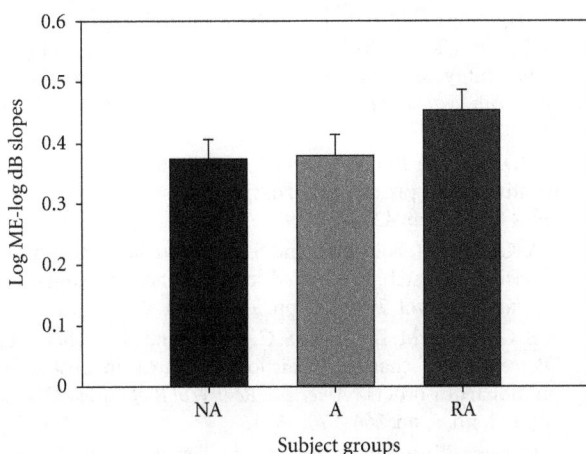

FIGURE 4: There was no significant difference between the slopes for the 3 groups, NA, A, and LTA, for auditory magnitude estimation testing.

Visual gray scale magnitude estimation was plotted on a log Borg/log gray scale plot. The average slope values for this plot were 0.787, 0.810, and 1.009 for NA, A, and LTA groups, respectively, (Figure 5) and were not significantly different.

4. Discussion

The perceptual sensitivity to resistive and pressure threshold respiratory loads, weight heaviness, sound intensity, and light grayscale contrast were determined for LTA, A, and NA subjects. Similar to previous reports [2, 4], LTA subjects were poor perceivers of inspiratory resistive loads, which was evidence by the significantly decreased log ME/log R slope in LTA subjects compared to A and NA subjects. LTA patients had a reduced perceptual sensitivity to inspiratory resistive loads but normal perceptual sensitivity to all other sensory modalities. LTA patients did not exhibit a general respiratory perception deficit, a general somatosensory deficit nor an

overall sensory deficit. While the LTA subjects are poor perceivers of inspiratory resistive loads, this deficit in respiratory perception is specific to inspiratory resistive loads and is not due to perceptual deficits in other sensory modalities.

Asthmatics with LTA are a high-risk asthmatic group due to their poor perception of respiratory resistive loads. If a patient does not feel respiratory loads during an acute asthma attack, they will be less likely to treat their condition with rescue medication. The present study demonstrated that LTA asthmatics' perception deficit is specific to only resistive respiratory loading. We did not find a significant decrease in the LTA group's magnitude estimation of pressure threshold (Figure 2), weight (Figure 3), auditory (Figure 4), or visual loads (Figure 5). Mean slope magnitude estimations for NA, A, and LTA groups for weight were comparable to previously reported values [31, 32]. Group mean auditory magnitude estimation slopes were comparable to previous studies, where slope of sound magnitude estimation versus tone level (in dB) was an average of 0.36 [26] and 0.292 [34]. We observed that our mean slope magnitude estimation of 0.373–0.452 was comparable to previously reported values. Visual gray scale measurements were slightly lower than previously reported studies [25], but this may be due to the previous study measuring reflectance rather than relative gray scale.

If LTA asthmatics had an overall sensory deficit, we would have observed a reduced mean magnitude estimation slope of all modalities we studied. Since we did not observe a reduced mean slope, it is suggested that LTA asthmatics do not have an overall sensory deficit. Alternatively, if this unique group of patients had a somatosensory deficit, we would have observed a reduced perception of both respiratory load protocols and weight sensation. Again, we did not observe such a phenomenon, so, it is suggested that these patients do not have an overall somatosensory deficit. If the LTA group had a general respiratory perception deficit, we would have observed a reduced perception of magnitude estimation of both resistive and pressure threshold loads. Since we only observed a significant decrease in perception in resistive respiratory loads, we suggest that this group of subjects does not have an overall respiratory deficit. This study shows that LTA asthmatics have a specific deficit only in perception of resistive respiratory loads. This finding is consistent with our previous findings of reduced perception in resistive respiratory load magnitude estimation [2, 4].

These findings are also consistent with the nature of the dangers presented to LTA asthmatics. These subjects have been hospitalized for an acute asthma attack. The perception of extrinsic resistive respiratory loads has been shown to be comparable to intrinsic respiratory loads [4]. We chose to use extrinsic respiratory loads in the present study since they are an easier and less obtrusive manner of determining resistive perception. This resistive loading mechanism is comparable to one of the many asthma symptoms that occur during an acute attack. Extrinsic resistive respiratory loading provides us a tool to observe and measure respiratory perception that correlates to some acute asthma symptoms. Pressure threshold loading produces a different sensation that is not directly related to asthma symptoms. Naturally, weight, auditory, and visual load perception have little relevance in an acute asthma attack. Thus, the only LTA subject perception deficit found in this study was that directly related to asthma symptoms.

This study shows that LTA asthmatics have a perception deficit that is specific for some of the symptoms of an acute asthma attack. This is an important observation because LTA asthma places these patients at an increased risk for hospitalization or death due to asthma. Not perceiving their respiratory distress during an acute asthma attack and therefore decreasing likelihood of timely treatment with rescue medication often cause this increased risk. Identifying the extent of LTA asthmatics' perception deficit is an important step in developing methods and approaches to treating this unique group of patients to better manage their disease.

Acknowledgment

This paper was supported by the National Institutes of Health (NIH) Grant no. HL48792.

References

[1] P. W. Davenport, M. Cruz, A. A. Stecenko, and Y. Kifle, "Respiratory-related evoked potentials in children with life-threatening asthma," *American Journal of Respiratory and Critical Care Medicine*, vol. 161, no. 6, pp. 1830–1835, 2000.

[2] Y. Kifle, V. Seng, and P. W. Davenport, "Magnitude estimation of inspiratory resistive loads in children with life-threatening asthma," *American Journal of Respiratory and Critical Care Medicine*, vol. 156, no. 5, pp. 1530–1535, 1997.

[3] Y. Kikuchi, W. Hida, T. Chonan, C. Shindoh, H. Sasaki, and T. Takishima, "Decrease in functional residual capacity during inspiratory loading and the sensation of dyspnea," *Journal of Applied Physiology*, vol. 71, no. 5, pp. 1787–1794, 1991.

[4] S. M. Julius, K. L. Davenport, and P. W. Davenport, "Perception of intrinsic and extrinsic respiratory loads in children with life-threatening asthma," *Pediatric Pulmonology*, vol. 34, no. 6, pp. 425–433, 2002.

[5] J. M. Sherman and C. L. Capen, "The red alert program for life-threatening asthma," *Pediatrics*, vol. 100, no. 2, pp. 187–191, 1997.

[6] J. H. C. M. Bakers and S. M. Tenney, "The perception of some sensations associated with breathing," *Respiration Physiology*, vol. 10, no. 1, pp. 85–92, 1970.

[7] I. D. Bijl-Hofland, S. G. M. Cloosterman, C. P. van Schayck, F. J. J. V. D. Elshout, R. P. Akkermans, and H. T. M. Folgering, "Perception of respiratory sensation assessed by means of histamine challenge and threshold loading tests," *Chest*, vol. 117, no. 4, pp. 954–959, 2000.

[8] J. G. W. Burdon, E. F. Juniper, and K. J. Killian, "The perception of breathlessness in asthma," *American Review of Respiratory Disease*, vol. 126, no. 5, pp. 825–828, 1982.

[9] N. K. Burki, "Effects of bronchodilation on magnitude estimation of added resistive loads in asthmatic subjects," *American Review of Respiratory Disease*, vol. 129, no. 2, pp. 225–229, 1984.

[10] N. K. Burki, P. W. Davenport, F. Safdar, and F. W. Zechman, "The effects of airway anesthesia on magnitude estimation of added inspiratory resistive and elastic loads," *American Review of Respiratory Disease*, vol. 127, no. 1, pp. 2–4, 1983.

[11] N. K. Burki, K. Mitchell, B. A. Chaudhary, and F. W. Zechman, "The ability of asthmatics to detect added resistive loads," *American Review of Respiratory Disease*, vol. 117, no. 1, pp. 71–75, 1978.

[12] K. R. Chapman and A. S. Rebuck, "Inspiratory and expiratory resistive loading as a model of dyspnea in asthma," *Respiration*, vol. 44, no. 6, pp. 425–432, 1983.

[13] J. A. Gliner, L. J. Folinsbee, and S. M. Horvath, "Accuracy and precision of matching inspired lung volume," *Perception and Psychophysics*, vol. 29, no. 5, pp. 511–515, 1981.

[14] S. B. Gottfried, M. D. Altose, S. G. Kelsen, and N. S. Cherniack, "Perception of changes in airflow resistance in obstructive pulmonary disorders," *American Review of Respiratory Disease*, vol. 124, no. 5, pp. 566–570, 1981.

[15] I. Homma, "Inspiratory inhibitory reflex caused by the chest wall vibration in man," *Respiration Physiology*, vol. 39, no. 3, pp. 345–353, 1980.

[16] C. H. Huang, A. D. Martin, and P. W. Davenport, "Effects of inspiratory strength training on the detection of inspiratory loads," *Applied Psychophysiology Biofeedback*, vol. 34, no. 1, pp. 17–26, 2009.

[17] S. G. Kelsen, T. F. Prestel, and N. S. Cherniack, "Comparison of the respiratory responses to external resistive loading and bronchoconstriction," *Journal of Clinical Investigation*, vol. 67, no. 6, pp. 1761–1768, 1981.

[18] K. J. Killian, C. K. Mahutte, and E. J. M. Campbell, "Magnitude scaling of externally added loads to breathing," *American Review of Respiratory Disease*, vol. 123, no. 1, pp. 12–15, 1981.

[19] R. W. Lansing and R. B. Banzett, "Psychophysical methods in the study of respiratory sensation," in *Respiratory Sensation*, L. Adams and A. Guz, Eds., vol. 90 of *Lung Biology in Health and Disease*, pp. 69–100, Marcel Dekker, New York, NY, USA, 1996.

[20] M. L. Moy, J. W. Weiss, D. Sparrow, E. Israel, and R. M. Schwartzstein, "Quality of dyspnea in bronchoconstriction differs from external resistive loads," *American Journal of Respiratory and Critical Care Medicine*, vol. 162, no. 2, pp. 451–455, 2000.

[21] W. R. Revelette and R. L. Wiley, "Plasticity of the mechanism subserving inspiratory load perception," *Journal of Applied Physiology*, vol. 62, no. 5, pp. 1901–1906, 1987.

[22] O. Taguchi, Y. Kikuchi, W. Hida et al., "Effects of bronchoconstriction and external resistive loading on the sensation of dyspnea," *Journal of Applied Physiology*, vol. 71, no. 6, pp. 2183–
2190, 1991.

[23] F. W. Zechman and R. Wiley, "Afferent inputs to breath-
ing: respiratory sensation," in *Handbook of Physiology*, N. S.
Cherniack and J. G. Widdicombe, Eds., vol. 2 of *Control of
Breathing, I*, Section 3: The Respiratory System, pp. 449–474,
American Physiological Society, Bethesda, Md, USA, 1986.

[24] N. Wolcove, M. D. Altose, S. G. Kelson, P. G. Kondapalli, and
N. S. Cherniack, "Perception of changes in breathing in normal human subjects," *Journal of Applied Physiology*, vol. 50, no.
1, pp. 78–83, 1981.

[25] A. L. Gilchrist and A. Radonjić, "Anchoring of lightness values
by relative luminance and relative area," *Journal of Vision*, vol.
9, no. 9, article 13, 10 pages, 2009.

[26] G. Canévet and B. Scharf, "The loudness of sounds that increase and decrease continuously in level," *Journal of the Acoustical Society of America*, vol. 88, no. 5, pp. 2136–2142, 1990.

[27] M. Epstein and M. Florentine, "Loudness of brief tones measured by magnitude estimation and loudness matching," *Journal of the Acoustical Society of America*, vol. 119, no. 4, pp.
1943–1945, 2006.

[28] R. P. Hellman and J. J. Zwislocki, "Loudness function of a
1000-cps tone in the presence of a masking noise," *Journal of
the Acoustical Society of America*, vol. 36, pp. 1618–1627, 1964.

[29] G. A. Gescheider and B. A. Hughson, "Stimulus context and
absolute magnitude estimation: a study of individual differences," *Perception and Psychophysics*, vol. 50, no. 1, pp. 45–57,
1991.

[30] L. L. Andersen, C. H. Andersen, O. S. Mortensen, O. M.
Poulsen, I. B. T. Bjørnlund, and M. K. Zebis, "Muscle activation and perceived loading during rehabilitation exercises:
comparison of dumbbells and elastic resistance," *Physical
Therapy*, vol. 90, no. 4, pp. 538–549, 2010.

[31] D. F. Cooper, G. Grimby, D. A. Jones, and R. H. T. Edwards,
"Perception of effort in isometric and dynamic muscular con-
traction," *European Journal of Applied Physiology and Occupational Physiology*, vol. 41, no. 3, pp. 173–180, 1979.

[32] D. M. Pincivero, A. J. Coelho, and R. M. Campy, "Perceived
exertion and maximal quadriceps femoris muscle strength
during dynamic knee extension exercise in young adult males
and females," *European Journal of Applied Physiology*, vol. 89,
no. 2, pp. 150–156, 2003.

[33] American Thoracic Society, "Standards for the diagnosis and
care of patients with chronic obstructive pulmonary disease
(COPD) and asthma," *American Review of Respiratory Disease*,
vol. 136, no. 1, pp. 225–244, 1987.

[34] A. A. Collins and G. A. Gescheider, "The measurement of
loudness in individual children and adults by absolute magnitude estimation and cross-modality matching," *Journal of
the Acoustical Society of America*, vol. 85, no. 5, pp. 2012–2021,
1989.

18

Patient's Knowledge and Attitude towards Tuberculosis in an Urban Setting

Saria Tasnim,[1] Aminur Rahman,[2] and F. M. Anamul Hoque[1]

[1] *Department of Obstetrics & Gynaecology, Institute of Child and Mother Health, Matuail, Dhaka 1362, Bangladesh*
[2] *Centre for Injury Prevention Bangladesh, Bangladesh*

Correspondence should be addressed to Saria Tasnim, saif031@gmail.com

Academic Editor: Andrew Sandford

Tuberculosis is a public health problem in Bangladesh. This cross-sectional study was conducted to assess knowledge of TB patients about symptoms, ways of transmission and treatment of tuberculosis, and their perception of the illness. Between March and August 2008, 762 adult TB patients were interviewed at selected DOTS centre of Dhaka city. Male and female distribution was 55.6% and 44.4%, respectively. One quarter of them were illiterate, and more than half had extended family and live in a congested situation. Night fever was the most common symptom known (89.9%), and 56% were aware that it could spread through sneezing/coughing. Television was mentioned as a source of information about TB. The majority expressed a helping attitude towards other TB patients. Although most of them were positive about getting family support, 46.6% mentioned discrimination of separate utensils for food or drink. About 50.5% expressed increased sadness, 39.8% had fear of loss of job/wedges, and 21.4% felt socially neglected. Along with drug treatment the psychosocial reactions of TB patients should be addressed at DOTS centers for better control of the disease.

1. Introduction

Tuberculosis (TB) is a public health problem in many developing countries including Bangladesh. Globally there were 8.8 million incident cases of TB in 2010 [1]. With the rising number of HIV infection and AIDS cases there is a threat of resurgence of TB as this is the most common opportunistic infection in them [2]. TB is the leading cause of death among all infectious diseases and WHO reported that in 2010 there were 1.1 million deaths among HIV-negative people and an additional 0.35 million deaths from HIV associated tuberculosis [1].

The global burden of TB mainly lies in the 22 high burden countries and about 50% of prevalence occurs in 5 countries of South East Asia, namely, India, Indonesia, Bangladesh, and Thailand, Myanmar. Bangladesh rank sixth among the high burden countries with an incident rate of 225 per 100,000 thousand population per year and a mortality rate (exclusive of HIV) of 43 per 100,000 thousand population per year [1].

Millennium development goal 6 implies to halt and begin to reverse the incidence of TB by 2015 and fixed the target (MDG 6 Target 6.C) to reduce prevalence of and death due to TB by 50% compared with a baseline of 1990 by 2015 [3]. The direct observed treatment short course (DOTS) was launched in 1995 as the main strategy in the control of tuberculosis [4]. The strategy includes diagnosis through bacteriology and standardized short-course chemotherapy with full patient support [4].

Bangladesh adopted DOTS strategy in national TB control program (NTP) during fourth population & health plan (1992–1998) and integrated into essential service package under the health and populations sector program (HPSP) in 1998 [5]. Although initially TB services were based in TB clinics and TB hospitals, under the DOTS strategy the services were expanded gradually to primary level of health facility incorporating GO-NGO partnership. Government and NGO community health workers are involved in village level for case detection and awareness building activities. In 2002, DOTS was expanded to Dhaka metropolitan city. By 2006 entire country has been covered by DOTS service [5].

The DOTS strategy relies greatly on passive case finding for TB treatment and its success depends on the patient's health awareness, ability to recognize early sign symptoms,

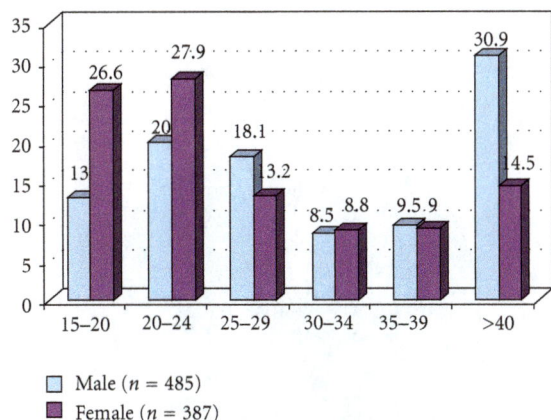

Figure 1: Age distribution ($N = 872$).

Table 1: Sociodemographic characteristics and living condition.

	Male ($n = 485$)	Female ($n = 387$)
Level of education		
Illiterate	25.8	24.5
Institutional	69.6	70.5
Informal	4.5	4.9
Family size	4.89 ± 1.8	5.03 ± 1.9
(Mean ± SD)	(1–13)	(1–12)
No. of living rooms in the house	1.72 ± 0.9	1.56 ± 0.8
(Mean ± SD)	(1–7)	(1–5)
Person living per room	3.27 ± 1.4	3.68 ± 1.6
(Mean ± SD)	(1–8)	(1–10)

Table 2: Distribution according to sex and sources of information about TB.

Sources of information	Male% ($n = 485$)	Female% ($n = 387$)	Total% ($n = 872$)
TV	46.4	47.3	46.8
Doctor's chamber	20.0	16.0	18.2
Family members/friends	14.2	15.0	14.6
Radio	13.4	13.7	13.5
Government Hospital	12.2	8.8	10.7
Billboard	10.1	7.0	8.7
NGO worker	8.5	7.2	7.9
Liflet, poster, and other printed materials	3.9	2.6	3.3
Pharmacy	.8	1.8	1.3

and accessibility to health services for immediate self-reporting [6]. It is important that basic knowledge about the disease and the availability of treatment is clear among community to prevent any undue delay in availing the service. The perceptions of TB prevailing in the community influence the health seeking behavior of people for their symptoms. While care seeking behavior of chest symptomatic has been explored in different studies, there is dearth of information on community perceptions of TB [7]. The current study was done to determine knowledge of TB patients about tuberculosis and their perception of the illness.

2. Method

This was a cross-sectional descriptive study conducted during March to August 2008 in selected DOTS centres of Dhaka metropolitan city. From the list of 73 centres providing DOTS service 27 were selected according to convenience and accessibility. Face to face interview of adult TB patients attending the selected centre for treatment was taken using structured questionnaire. Written informed consent was obtained from all respondents. Data was analysed using SPSS software version 12.

3. Results

Total number of respondents were 872 constituting 55.6% male and 44.4% female, respectively, and more than half of them ($58 > 4\%$) were within 15–29 years (Figure 1). One fourth of them were illiterate, about 70% studied in any institution, mean family size was 4.89 ± 1.8 and 5.03 ± 1.9 among male and female, respectively (Table 1). About 46.8% stated that they get information about TB from television, next was doctors chamber (18.2%), and 87% mentioned about bill boards (Table 2). Regarding symptoms of TB (89.9%) mentioned night fever, tiredness (86.5%), productive cough (80.6%), and (61.6%) mentioned cough more than 3 weeks (Table 3). About mode of transmission of disease 22.9% were ignorant, 56% thought sneezing and cough, smoking 5.4%, and 2.2% mentioned TB is a familial disease (Table 4). Most of them knew that TB can be cured

completely, they opined that the remedial measure is taking specific drugs given in DOTS centre (Table 5). Ninety percent of them can mention the duration of treatment should be 6–8 months (Figure 2). Regarding attitude towards other TB patients 65.7% felt compassionate and desire to help, 28.6% indifferent, and 4.9% would prefer to stay away (Table 6). About self-perception of being TB patient 95.4% got family support, 59.3% are anxious for reduction of family income, 21.9% felt socially neglected, 46.6% expressed that utensils for food/drink are separated for them, and 11.2% felt isolated within family (Table 7).

4. Discussion

Tuberculosis (TB) especially affects the economically most productive age group. The Bangladesh national tuberculosis program has reported that among TB cases three fourth belonged to age group 15–45 years [5]. In the current study, the mean age of the patients was 30.65 ± 13.1 years ranging from 15 to 86 years and female patients were younger than the male patients ($P < 0.05$). Other study from Bangladesh reported 70% cases were within age group 15–44 years and mean age was 36 years [8]. Karim et al. reported mean age for men and women was 41.8 and 33.6 years and among women more teen-agers were diagnosed [6]. Study from

TABLE 3: Symptoms experienced during TB diagnosis.

Symptoms during TB Diagnosis	Male% ($n = 485$)	Female% ($n = 387$)	Total% ($n = 872$)
Night fever	91.5	87.9	89.9
Fatigue/tiredness	89.1	83.2	86.5
Productive cough	87.8	72.1	80.8
Loss of weight	70.5	68.2	69.5
Cough more than 3 weeks	66.6	55.3	61.6
Nausea	56.9	58.7	57.7
Severe headache	53.2	59.2	55.8
Chest pain	51.3	46.8	49.3
Shortness of breath	38.8	35.4	37.3
Fever without cause that lasts >7 days	34.2	30.0	32.3
Haemoptysis	27.8	22.5	25.5

TABLE 4: knowledge on ways of transmission of disease (TB).

Knowledge on transmission of disease	Male% ($n = 485$)	Female% ($n = 387$)	Total% ($n = 872$)
Do not know	18.4	28.2	22.9
Through sneezing/cough	57.1	54.5	56.0
Smoking	8.9	1.0	5.4
Dust	4.9	3.4	4.2
Unhygienic condition	2.9	3.4	3.1
Familial	1.9	2.6	2.2
Through cold	1.9	2.6	2.2
Handshake with TB patients	2.1	1.6	1.8
Irregular diet	.6	1.0	.9
Eating from the same plate	.2	1.0	.6

TABLE 5: Perception about how TB would be cured.

	Male% ($n = 485$)	Female% ($n = 387$)	Total% ($n = 872$)
TB could be cured completely	98.6	97.2	97.9
Remedial measure of TB			
Specific drugs given by health centre/DOTS	96.9	98.2	97.5
Do not know	2.1	1.0	1.6
Herbal remedies	.2	.3	.2
Praying	.8	.5	1.3

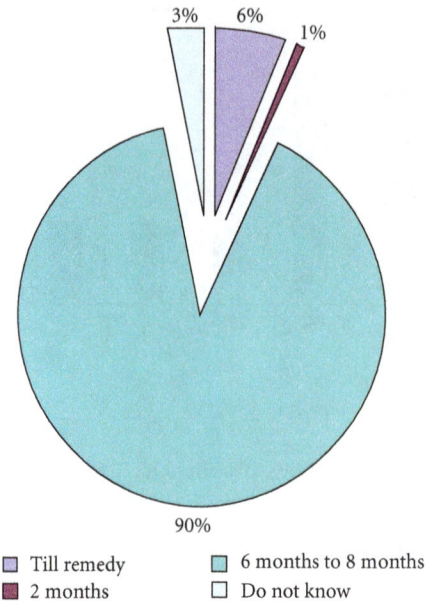

FIGURE 2: Knowledge about duration of TB treatment ($N = 872$).

Legend: Till remedy; 6 months to 8 months; 2 months; Do not know.

TABLE 6: Feeling about other TB patients.

Perception about the TB	Male% ($n = 485$)	Female% ($n = 387$)	Total% ($n = 872$)
I feel compassion and desire to help	66.6	64.6	65.7
I have no particular feeling	28.0	29.2	28.6
I tend to stay away from these people	4.1	5.9	4.9
I fear them because they may infect me	.8	.3	.6

TABLE 7: Perception on being a TB patient.

Perception as TB patients	Male% ($n = 485$)	Female% ($n = 387$)	Total% ($n = 872$)
Family members are cooperative towards me	96.9	93.5	95.4
Fear chance of reduction of family income	66.6	50.1	59.3
Increase sadness	57.9	41.1	50.5
Utensils are separated for me	47.6	45.2	46.6
Threat of loss of job/wages	48.0	29.5	39.8
Feels socially neglected/ low esteem	17.9	25.8	21.4
Most people behave differently	11.8	13.4	12.5
Feel isolated within the family	6.6	17.1	11.2
Family member avoid me	1.2	5.2	3.0

India showed a mean age of 43.02 years (range: 20–90 years) [9]. A study from Nigeria reported mean age of male and female 33.5 and 22.2 years, respectively [2].

Studies show prolonged cough, at times chest pain, loss of weight, fever, difficulty in breathing, and coughing up blood are perceived to be associated with TB by the people [7, 10, 11]. In the present study the symptoms of TB reported by the patients indicated a fairly good level of knowledge. This may be associated with urban setting of the study with better opportunity to access to information and education level of respondents. Croft reported 44% individuals to be aware of cough as TB symptom in a rural area of Bangladesh [12]. Study from India reported that 73.7% cough with sputum, weakness and breathlessness 40.4%, fever 34.3%, and haemoptysis 30% were mentioned as symptoms of TB [9]. In Pakistan most commonly recognized symptom was cough 83.5%, fever 54.7%, chest pain 24.7%, and bloody sputum 24.7% [11].

However, misconceptions about the cause and mode of transmission are also prevalent. In some places TB is believed to be hereditary [10, 13, 14]. Some studies found cause of TB was attributed to smoking and drinking alcohol [7, 15] stamping on sputum [7], sharing eating and drinking utensil, and sleeping with TB patient [11, 16]. Study from Vietnam brought out that men have wider social contacts as compared to women and were more likely to get TB than women [17]. Poor knowledge about TB and traditional misbelieves are associated with delays in case detection [10, 18].

Mass media could play a vital role in success for passive case finding and treatment [3]. In our study television was cited as the main sources of information (46.8) and a small proportion mentioned about radio and bill boards. This reflects positive impact of governments' initiatives of mass awareness utilizing the media. This may also be the reason that 98% could mention that TB can be cured completely through taking specific drugs from DOT centers. In India doctors and health care workers were stated to be the source of the information regarding tuberculosis by 50.2% followed by mass media (33.8%), and (34.7%) mentioned interaction with others in the community [9].

Tuberculosis-related pervasive stigma may worsen the quality of life of its victims [15]. A higher degree of psychiatric morbidity like denial, hopelessness about life, tension/anxiety, and feeling neglected by family and society is common in TB patients [19]. Eram et al. reported the initial reaction to the diagnosis was negative in majority of patients, 98% were hopeful of care, 30% had anxiety/tension, 26% had lost interest from life, and 20% could not explain how they felt [20].

Being diagnosed with TB can create the fear of isolation and discrimination [2]. In HIV prevalent countries TB patients are stigmatized due to assumed coinfection with HIV [10]. Study from Uganda shows the main reason for delayed diagnosis of TB was a lack of recognition of symptoms and the stigma of association with HIV [21]. We do not look for the psychological status of the patients, however, although half of the respondents were optimistic about the support from their family and community but about one fourth felt socially neglected and 17.1% feels isolation within the family.

5. Conclusion

Knowledge about cause and treatment of tuberculosis among TB patients was quite good, however, misconceptions also exist. Misconceptions about transmission of disease lead to discrimination like separate utensils for food or drink. Diagnosis of TB is associated with increase anxiety/tension, fear of loss of wage/earning, and stigma threatening self-esteem and quality of life. Mass media can be better utilized to remove misconceptions. Psychosocial reactions towards TB as revealed in this study should be addressed through counseling and communication during treatment in the DOTS centre. This may contribute to success of the national TB control program.

References

[1] "Global tuberculosis control: epidemiology, strategy, financing," WHO Report, World Health Organization, Geneva, Switzerland, 2011.

[2] O. Christopher and I. Bosede, "Health seeking behaviour of tuberculosis patients in Ekiti State, Nigeria," *Studies on Ethno-Medicine*, vol. 4, no. 3, pp. 191–197, 2010.

[3] Stop TB Partnership and World Health Organization: The Stop TB Strategy: building on and enhancing DOTS to meet the TB-related Millennium Development Goals, Geneva, Switzerland, (WHO/HTM/TB/2006. 368), 2006.

[4] "Resolution WHA44. 8: Tuberculosis control programme," in *Handbook of Resolutions and Decisions of the World Health Assembly and the Executive Board*, vol. 3, World Health Organization, Geneva, Switzerland, 3rd edition, 1993, (1985–1992) (WHA44/1991/REC/1).

[5] Tuberculosis control in Bangladesh, "National tuberculosis control program," Annual Report 2008, Director General of Health Services. Government of Bangladesh, Dhaka, Bangladesh, 2009.

[6] F. Karim, E. Johansson, V. K. Diwan, and A. Kulane, "Community perceptions of tuberculosis: a qualitative exploration from a gender perspective," *Public Health*, vol. 125, no. 2, pp. 84–89, 2011.

[7] S. Ganapathy, B. E. Thomas, M. S. Jawahar, K. J. Selvi, Sivasubramaniam, and M. Weiss, "Perceptions of gender and tuberculosis in a south Indian urban community," *The Indian Journal of Tuberculosis*, vol. 55, no. 1, pp. 9–14, 2008.

[8] G. Ahsan, J. Ahmed, P. Singhasivanon et al., "Gender difference in treatment seeking behaviours of tuberculosis cases in rural communities of Bangladesh," *Southeast Asian Journal of Tropical Medicine and Public Health*, vol. 35, pp. 126–135, 2004.

[9] R. Malhotra, D. K. Taneja, V. D. Dhingra, S. Rajpal, and M. Mehra, "Awareness regarding tuberculosis in a rural population in Delhi," *Indian Journal of Community Medicine*, vol. 27, no. 2, p. 62, 2002.

[10] E. Buregyeya, A. Kulane, R. Colebunders et al., "Tuberculosis knowledge, attitudes and health-seeking behaviour in rural Uganda," *International Journal of Tuberculosis and Lung Disease*, vol. 15, no. 7, pp. 938–942, 2011.

[11] M. U. Mushtaq, U. Shahid, H. M. Abdullah et al., "Urban-rural inequities in knowledge, attitudes and practices regarding tuberculosis in two districts of Pakistan's Punjab province," *International Journal for Equity in Health*, vol. 10, article 8, 2011.

[12] R. P. Croft and R. A. Croft, "Knowledge, attitude and practice regarding leprosy and tuberculosis in Bangladesh," *Leprosy Review*, vol. 70, no. 1, pp. 34–42, 1999.

[13] M. M. Mesfin, T. W. Tasew, I. G. Tareke, G. W. M. Mulugeta, and J. M. Richard, "Community knowledge, attitudes and practices on pulmonary tuberculosis and their choice of treatment supervisor in Tigray, Nothern Ethiopia," *The Ethiopian Journal of Health Development*, vol. 19, pp. 21–27, 2005.

[14] M. E. Edginton, C. S. Sekatane, and S. J. Goldstein, "Patients' beliefs: do they affect tuberculosis control? A study in a rural district of South Africa," *International Journal of Tuberculosis and Lung Disease*, vol. 6, no. 12, pp. 1075–1082, 2002.

[15] M. G. Weiss, C. Auer, D. B. Somma, and A. Abouhia, *Gender and Tuberculosis: Cross-Site Analysis and Implications of a Multi-Country. Study in Bangladesh, India, Malawi and Colombia*, vol. 3 of *TDR Monograph*, WHO, Geneva, Switzerland, 2006.

[16] A. M. Kilale, A. K. Mushi, L. A. Lema et al., "Perceptions of tuberculosis and treatment seeking behaviour in Ilala and Kinondoni Municipalities in Tanzania," *Tanzania Journal of Health Research*, vol. 10, no. 2, pp. 89–94, 2008.

[17] N. H. Long, E. Johansson, V. K. Diwan, and A. Winkvist, "Different tuberculosis in men and women: beliefs from focus groups in Vietnam," *Social Science and Medicine*, vol. 49, no. 6, pp. 815–822, 1999.

[18] N. Shetty, M. Shemko, and A. Abbas, "Knowledge, attitudes and practices regarding tuberculosis among immigrants of Somalian ethnic origin in London: a cross-sectional study," *Communicable Disease and Public Health*, vol. 7, no. 1, pp. 77–82, 2004.

[19] E. Manoharan, K. R. John, A. Joseph, and K. S. Jacob, "Psychiatric morbidity, Patients perspectives of illness and factors associated with poor medication compliance among the tuberculosis in Vellore, South India," *The Indian Journal of Tuberculosis*, vol. 48, pp. 77–80, 2001.

[20] U. Eram, I. A. Khan, Z. Md Tamanna, Z. Khan, N. Khaliq, and A. J. Abidi, "Patient perception of illness and initial reaction to the diagnosis of tuberculosisIndian," *Journal of Community Medicine*, vol. 31, no. 3, 2006.

[21] L. Macfarlane and N. J. Newell, "A qualitative study exploring delayed diagnosis and stigmatization of tuberculosis amongst women in Uganda," *Intenational Health*, vol. 4, no. 2, pp. 143–147, 2012.

19

Low Vital Capacity and Electrocardiographic ST-T Abnormalities in Asymptomatic Adults

Kei Nakajima,[1, 2] Yulan Li,[1] Hiroshi Fuchigami,[3] and Hiromi Munakata[2]

[1] Division of Clinical Nutrition, Department of Medical Dietetics, Faculty of Pharmaceutical Sciences, Josai University,
  1-1 Keyakidai, Sakado, Saitama 350-0295, Japan
[2] Department of Internal Medicine, Social Insurance Omiya General Hospital, 453 Bonsai, Kita, Saitama 331-0805, Japan
[3] Department of Health Care Center, Social Insurance Omiya General Hospital, 453 Bonsai, Kita, Saitama 331-0805, Japan

Correspondence should be addressed to Kei Nakajima, keinaka@josai.ac.jp

Academic Editor: Hisako Matsumoto

Studies have shown that low forced vital capacity (LFVC) is associated with atherosclerosis. However, it is unclear whether LFVC is associated with resting electrocardiographic ST-T abnormalities, a common finding that is prognostic for cardiovascular events. Therefore, pulmonary functions, ST-T abnormalities defined with Minnesota Code, and cardiometabolic risk factors were examined in a cross-sectional study of 1,653 asymptomatic adults without past history of coronary heart diseases. The prevalence of diabetes, metabolic syndrome, and ST-T abnormalities significantly increased with decreasing percent of predicted forced vital capacity (%PFVC). ST-T abnormalities were observed in 73 subjects (4.4% in total). Multiple logistic regression analysis showed that, compared with the highest quartile of %PFVC ($\geq$99.7%), the lowest quartile of %PFVC ($\leq$84.2%) was persistently associated with ST-T abnormalities even after further adjustment for diabetes or metabolic syndrome (odds ratio (95%CI): 2.44 (1.16–5.14) and 2.42 (1.15–5.10), resp.). Similar trends were observed when subjects were divided into quartiles according to percent of predicted forced expiratory volume in 1 second (FEV_1), but not the ratio of FEV_1/FVC. In conclusion, LFVC may be associated with ST-T abnormalities independent of metabolic abnormalities in asymptomatic adults, suggesting a plausible link between impaired pulmonary defects and cardiovascular diseases.

1. Introduction

Accumulating evidence has shown that not only impaired obstructive pulmonary function but also low forced vital capacity (LFVC) and impaired restrictive pulmonary function are associated with increased risk of mortality, partially owing to cardiovascular disease [1, 2]. Some studies have shown that LFVC is associated with arterial stiffness assessed by pulse-wave velocity [3, 4] and coronary artery calcification [5], which may reflect systemic atherosclerosis. In addition, LFVC and a restrictive pattern have been associated with critical metabolic abnormalities such as type 2 diabetes and metabolic syndrome (MetS) [2, 5–8], which are often followed by the development of cardiovascular disease [9, 10]. To date, however, the association between and the underlying mechanism of such pulmonary function defects and subclinical cardiovascular disease have been poorly understood.

Meanwhile, ST depression, T-wave abnormalities, or both (ST-T abnormalities), particularly minor ST-T abnormalities, on the resting electrocardiogram are commonly observed in the general population without coronary heart disease [11–15]. Major ST-T abnormalities are an independent predictor for stroke [13], cardiovascular events, and increased mortality risk in people without heart disease at baseline [11, 12]. Likewise, many studies have provided evidence that even minor ST-T abnormalities are associated with increased risk for future cardiovascular disease independent of traditional risk factors [14, 16, 17], although the prognostic significance of minor ST-T abnormalities has not been well established [14].

In the light of this evidence, we hypothesized that impaired pulmonary functions, especially LFVC, may be associated with ST-T abnormalities irrespective of cardiometabolic risk factors, diabetes, and MetS. So far, no large epidemiological studies have examined the associations between impaired lung functions and ST-T abnormalities in asymptomatic individuals without overt heart disease.

Therefore, we examined lung functions, ST-T abnormalities that comprised major and minor ST-T abnormalities, cardiometabolic risk factors, diabetes, and MetS in a cross-sectional study of asymptomatic adults who underwent an annual checkup. Abnormal pulmonary function was evaluated by continuous pulmonary function variables including the percentage of predicted forced vital capacity (%PFVC).

2. Methods

The current study represents a series of studies performed in collaboration with Josai University, Sakado, Japan, and Social Insurance Omiya General Hospital, Saitama, Japan, that were conducted to explore the causalities and mechanism in lifestyle-related diseases. The study design and protocol have been described elsewhere [8]. The protocol was approved by the Ethical Committee of Josai University and the Council of the Hospital, and informed consent was obtained from all participants.

3. Subjects

Asymptomatic healthy subjects (n = 2,488) were randomly recruited from those who underwent complete medical checkups at their own will at the Health Care Center attached to Omiya General Hospital between April 2009 and March 2010. Most lived or worked close to the hospital (a small portion was treated in the hospital). Individuals who required immediate treatment for suspected cancers, pneumothorax, or infectious pneumonia, including tuberculosis, were not included from the beginning. All recruited subjects, who were free from overt disability and hemiplegia, completed a questionnaire about their lifestyle characteristics. Exclusion criteria of subjects and a flow chart are shown in Figure 1. Since people less than 45 years old are less likely to have ST-T abnormalities, first, subjects outside the age limitation of 45 to 80 years were excluded. Second, subjects with a high C-reactive protein (CRP) level (>10 mg/L) were excluded because of latent critical diseases or inflammation. Third, subjects with abnormal electrocardiograms, with the exception of ST-T abnormalities, were excluded. Subjects with a self-reported medical history of overt coronary heart disease were also excluded. Finally, after additional exclusion of subjects with suspected interstitial pneumonia based on chest X-ray findings and those without available spirometry data, 1,653 subjects (1,014 men and 639 women) were eligible for this analysis.

4. Laboratory Measurements and Determination of MetS and Diabetes

Anthropometric measurements and laboratory tests were carried out after an overnight fast. Waist circumference was measured at the height of the navel. Clinical and biochemical variables were measured automatically with standard methods using an autoanalyzer (Hitachi, Tokyo, Japan). The

diagnosis of MetS was based on the modified Third Report of the National Cholesterol Education Program Expert Panel/Adult Treatment Panel criteria [9] with the following cutoff values: (1) systolic blood pressure of ≥130 mmHg and diastolic blood pressure of ≥85 mmHg; (2) triglycerides of ≥150 mg/dL; (3) low high-density lipoprotein of <40 mg/dL for men and <50 mg/dL for women; (4) fasting plasma glucose of ≥100 mg/dL; (5) waist circumference of ≥90 cm for men and ≥80 cm for women. We took ethnic-specific values for waist circumference into consideration. MetS was diagnosed in subjects fulfilling three or more of the above five criteria. Subjects receiving medication for any of these components were defined as having the component. Diabetes was defined as a fasting plasma glucose of ≥126 mg/dL or HbA1c of ≥6.5% according to the American Diabetes Association criteria [18], or treatment with oral hypoglycemic drugs or insulin. HbA1c was converted to National Glycohemoglobin Standardization Program (NGSP) levels by the formula HbA1c (%) (NGSP) = HbA1c (JDS) (%) + 0.4% [19].

5. Spirometry

Pulmonary function tests were performed with a spirometry analyzer (Autospiro-507, Minato Medical Science Co., Ltd., Osaka, Japan). The test was performed by trained technicians with the subject in a standing position. The %PFVC, percentage of predicted forced expiratory volume in 1 second (%PFEV$_1$), and ratio of forced expiratory volume in 1 second to observed forced vital capacity (FEV$_1$/FVC) were calculated as in our previous report [8]. We quoted the standard predicted values for FVC, FEV$_1$, and FEV$_1$/FVC from data published by the Japanese Respiratory Society in 2001 [20].

6. Electrocardiogram

Standard 12-lead electrocardiograms were recorded with an electrocardiogram recorder (Cardio Base FDX-4521, Fukuda Denshi Co., Ltd., Tokyo, Japan). ST-T abnormalities were defined with the Minnesota Code [21]. Minor ST-T abnormalities included the following: ST junction depression of <0.5 mm (MC 4-3); ST junction depression of >1 mm and ST segment ascent, that is, upslope (MC 4-4); T wave flat, diphasic, or inverted by <1 mm (MC 5-3). Major ST-T abnormalities included (MC 4-1), (MC 4-2), (MC 5-1), and (MC 5-2). The findings were first determined by experienced physicians and subsequently confirmed by trained medical laboratory technicians, all of whom exclusively belong to the Social Insurance Omiya General Hospital and were blinded to individuals' data. The minor and major ST-T abnormalities were combined and analyzed together in this study because, on the checkup sheets, minor and major ST abnormalities were recorded together indistinguishably.

7. Statistical Analysis

Data are expressed as means ± SD or median/geometric mean (interquartile range). Subjects were divided into quartiles according to continuous pulmonary function variables:

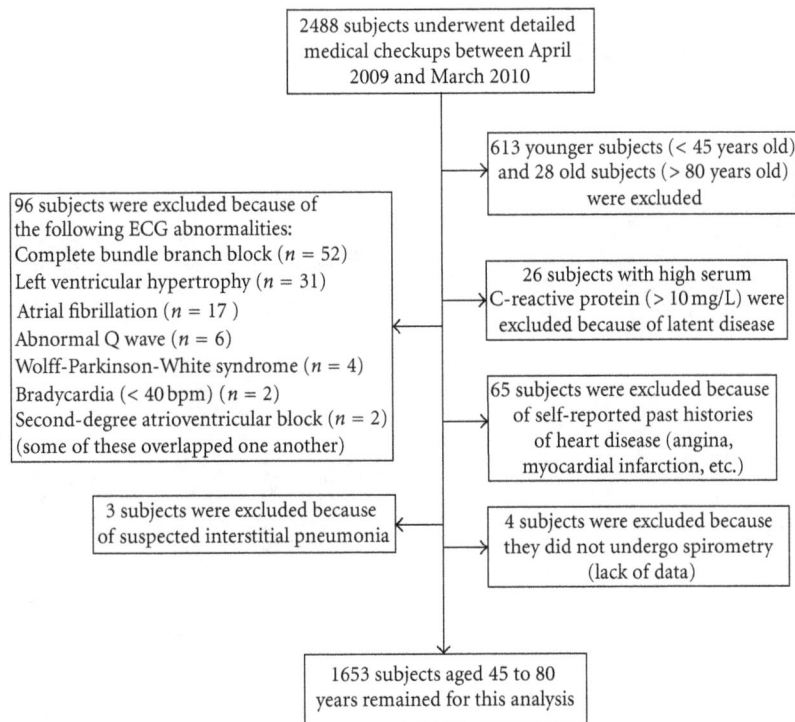

FIGURE 1: Exclusion criteria of subjects and flow chart.

%PFVC, %PFEV$_1$, and FEV$_1$/FVC. P values for continuous variables and categorical variables were determined with ANOVA and the χ^2-test, respectively.

Multivariate logistic regression models were used to examine the associations between the lowest quartiles (Q1) of lung functions and ST-T abnormalities compared with the corresponding highest quartiles (Q4), controlling for clinical confounding factors including diabetes and MetS. This analysis yielded odds ratios (OR) and 95% confidential intervals (95% CI). Tests for linear trends (P for trend) were calculated by treating quartile categories (Q1–Q4) as a continuous variable (i.e., 1–4), and the same model analysis was conducted. In this study, hypertension ($\geq 130/85$ mmHg) was considered as a special confounder that substantially interferes with the associations because hypertension is likely to affect ST-T abnormalities and the decline of FVC [13, 22]. Statistical analyses were performed using SPSS software version 18.0 (SPSS-IBM, Chicago, IL) and Statview version 5.0 (SAS Institute, Cary, NC). Values of $P < 0.05$ were considered to be statistically significant.

8. Results

Overall, most subjects in this study had relatively good profiles in terms of anthropometric and biochemical parameters, including pulmonary functions tests (Table 1). The prevalence of cardiometabolic risk factors, diabetes, MetS, and ST-T abnormalities significantly increased with decreasing %PFVC (toward Q4).

Multiple logistic analysis showed that compared with the highest quartile of %PFVC ($\geq 99.7\%$) (Q1), the lowest

quartile ($\leq 84.2\%$) (Q4) was significantly associated with ST-T abnormalities (Table 2). This association remained significant even after adjustment for age, sex, smoking, alcohol consumption, frequency of exercise, self-reported past history of stroke, waist circumference, and CRP (both as a continuous variable), with significant P for trends. Moreover, extended adjustment for diabetes (Model 4) or MetS (Model 5) attenuated but did not remarkably alter the associations. In these conditions, diabetes and MetS were significantly associated with ST-T abnormalities (OR (95% CI), 2.18 (1.18–4.03), $P = 0.01$ and 2.20 (1.23–3.93), $P = 0.008$, resp.; data not shown).

Likewise, similar trends were observed when subjects were divided into quartiles according to %PFEV$_1$. However, observed associations between lowest quartile of %PFEV$_1$ and ST-T abnormalities were not significant after adjustment for diabetes or MetS. In contrast, no significant associations between lowest quartile of FEV$_1$/FVC and ST-T abnormalities were observed in comparison with the highest quartile of FEV$_1$/FVC, irrespective of adjustments for confounders.

Meanwhile, the lowest quartile of %PFVC was significantly associated with hypertension ($\geq 130/85$ mmHg) (OR (95%CI), 1.76 (1.30–2.38), $P = 0.0003$, data not shown) compared with the highest quartile, even after full adjustments for confounders in Model 3 of Table 2. However, the significant association between LFVC and ST-T abnormalities persisted after further adjustments for confounders in Model 3 of Table 2, plus hypertension or medication for hypertension (OR (95%CI), 2.43 (1.15–5.11), $P = 0.02$ and 2.58 (1.23–5.40), $P = 0.01$, resp., data not shown).

TABLE 1: Clinical characteristics of subjects according to %PFVC quartiles.

	Total	Q1 (highest)	Q2	Q3	Q4 (lowest)	P values
n	1,653	412	413	414	414	
Men, n (%)	1,014 (61.3)	205 (49.8)	248 (60.0)	273 (65.9)	288 (69.6)	<0.0001
Age, y	58.2 ± 8.6	58.6 ± 8.6	57.3 ± 8.3	58.3 ± 8.5	58.6 ± 8.9	0.12
BMI, kg/m^2	23.3 ± 3.1	22.8 ± 2.6	23.1 ± 3.0	23.3 ± 3.0	23.9 ± 3.1	<0.0001
Waist circumference, cm	82.3 ± 8.5	80.5 ± 7.5	81.8 ± 8.56	82.6 ± 8.3	84.3 ± 9.2	<0.0001
Systolic blood pressure, mmHg	123 ± 19.0	120 ± 17.9	123 ± 18.1	124 ± 19.6	127 ± 19.9	<0.0001
Diastolic blood pressure, mmHg	76.9 ± 12.6	74.3 ± 12.2	77.4 ± 12.1	77.5 ± 12.7	78.6 ± 12.8	<0.0001
Triglyceride, mg/dL	96 (69–138)	84 (63–120)	90 (66–133)	103 (74–142)	107 (74–155)	<0.0001
HDL-C, mg/dL	62.0 ± 15.3	64.8 ± 15.1	62.2 ± 15.3	61.5 ± 15.5	59.4 ± 15.1	<0.0001
Fasting plasma glucose, mg/dL	102 ± 18.5	99.8 ± 16.2	101 ± 16.2	103 ± 18.6	106 ± 22.1	<0.0001
HbA1c, % (NGSP)	5.4 ± 0.6	5.3 ± 0.6	5.3 ± 0.5	5.4 ± 0.6	5.5 ± 0.7	<0.0001
CRP, mg/L	0.51 (0.30–0.80)	0.44 (0.30–0.60)	0.49 (0.30–0.70)	0.54 (0.30–0.90)	0.60 (0.30–1.00)	<0.0001
FVC, mL	3,133 ± 763	3,500 ± 834	3,274 ± 729	3,046 ± 661	2713 ± 574	<0.0001
FEV$_1$, mL	2,496 ± 618	2,761 ± 645	2,605 ± 593	2,442 ± 559	2,176 ± 513	<0.0001
%PFVC (range)	92.3 (55.6–138)	108 (99.7–138)	95.5 (91.9–99.6)	88.0 (84.3–91.8)	78.4 (55.6–84.2)	—
%PFEV$_1$	89.1 ± 13.4	103 ± 10.3	91.9 ± 7.7	85.3 ± 7.3	76.0 ± 9.9	<0.0001
FEV$_1$/FVC ratio, %	79.9 ± 6.8	79.2 ± 5.7	79.8 ± 6.4	80.3 ± 6.6	80.2 ± 8.1	0.11
ST-T abnormalities, n (%)	73 (4.4)	11 (2.7)	13 (3.1)	18 (4.3)	31 (7.5)	0.003
Metabolic syndrome, n (%)	298 (18.0)	51 (12.4)	58 (14.0)	80 (19.3)	109 (26.3)	<0.0001
Components of metabolic syndrome						
Elevated waist circumference, n (%)	515 (31.2)	111 (26.9)	119 (28.8)	129 (31.2)	156 (37.7)	0.006
Elevated blood pressures, n (%)	690 (41.7)	134 (32.5)	163 (39.5)	186 (44.9)	207 (50.5)	<0.0001
Elevated triglyceride, n (%)	342 (20.7)	61 (14.8)	78 (18.9)	94 (22.7)	109 (26.3)	0.0003
Low HDL-C, n (%)	99 (6.0)	22 (5.3)	22 (5.3)	19 (4.6)	36 (8.7)	0.06
Elevated fasting plasma glucose, n (%)	749 (45.3)	152 (36.9)	182 (44.0)	189 (45.7)	226 (54.6)	<0.0001
Diabetes, n (%)	158 (9.6)	27 (6.5)	35 (8.5)	37 (8.9)	59 (14.3)	0.001
Medical history of						
Stroke, n (%)	29 (1.8)	9 (2.2)	2 (0.5)	7 (1.7)	11 (2.7)	0.10
Medications for						
Hypertension, n (%)	322 (19.5)	60 (14.6)	78 (18.9)	93 (22.5)	91 (22.0)	0.02
Hypercholesterolemia, n (%)	202 (12.2)	48 (11.7)	43 (10.4)	58 (14.0)	53 (12.8)	0.43
Diabetes, n (%)	63 (3.6)	10 (2.4)	13 (3.1)	12 (2.9)	24 (5.8)	0.04
Current smoker, n (%)	382 (23.1)	94 (22.8)	86 (20.8)	92 (22.2)	110 (26.6)	0.24
Daily alcohol consumption, n (%)	547 (33.1)	143 (34.7)	133 (32.2)	144 (34.9)	127 (30.7)	0.51
Regular exercise, n (%)	599 (36.3)	155 (37.6)	144 (34.9)	161 (38.9)	139 (33.6)	0.37

Data are means ± SD. Triglyceride and CRP are expressed as medians and geometric means with interquartile range, respectively. %PFVC is expressed as means (range).

Regular exercise: ≥30 min exercise per session ≥2 days/week. Elevated waist circumference: ≥90 cm for men and ≥80 cm for women. Elevated blood pressures: ≥130/85 mmHg. Elevated triglyceride: ≥150 mg/dL. Low HDL-C: <40 mg/dL for men and <50 mg/dL for women. Elevated fasting plasma glucose: ≥100 mg/dL.

[a]Proportion of T-wave abnormalities of all ST-T abnormalities in each quartile.

P values for continuous variables and categorical variables were determined with ANOVA and the χ^2-test, respectively.

BMI: body mass index; HDL-C: high-density lipoprotein cholesterol; CRP: C-reactive protein; FVC: forced vital capacity; FEV$_1$: forced expiratory volume in 1 second; %PFVC: percentage of predicted forced vital capacity; %PFEV$_1$: percentage of predicted forced expiratory volume in 1 second; FEV$_1$/FVC: ratio of forced expiratory volume in 1 second to observed forced vital capacity; NGSP: National Glycohemoglobin Standardization Program.

TABLE 2: Odds ratio (95% CI) of lung function quartiles for ST-T abnormalities.

	Q1 (highest)	Q2	Q3	Q4 (lowest)	P for trend*
%PFVC, n	412	413	414	414	
Model 1	1	1.19 (0.52–2.68)	1.66 (0.77–3.55)	2.95 (1.46–5.95)[†]	0.0007
Model 2	1	1.33 (0.59–3.03)	1.83 (0.85–3.95)	3.27 (1.60–6.69)[†]	0.0004
Model 3	1	1.30 (0.56–3.00)	1.74 (0.79–3.81)	2.59 (1.23–5.42)[§]	0.006
Model 4	1	1.29 (0.56–2.97)	1.74 (0.79–3.83)	2.44 (1.16–5.14)[§]	0.009
Model 5	1	1.29 (0.56–3.00)	1.69 (0.77–3.73)	2.42 (1.15–5.10)[§]	0.01
%PFEV$_1$, n	412	415	414	412	
Model 1	1	0.67 (0.31–1.47)	1.06 (0.53–2.13)	1.87 (1.002–3.51)[§]	0.02
Model 2	1	0.78 (0.36–1.72)	1.35 (0.66–2.77)	2.42 (1.23–4.75)[§]	0.003
Model 3	1	0.76 (0.34–1.69)	1.16 (0.56–2.42)	2.09 (1.04–4.21)[§]	0.02
Model 4	1	0.75 (0.34–1.69)	1.10 (0.53–2.31)	2.00 (0.99–4.0.4)	0.02
Model 5	1	0.76 (0.34–1.70)	1.13 (0.54–2.35)	2.00 (0.99–4.06)	0.02
FEV$_1$/FVC, n	412	413	416	412	
Model 1	1	1.41 (0.76–2.63)	0.71 (0.34–1.46)	0.94 (0.48–1.86)	0.42
Model 2	1	1.38 (0.74–2.59)	0.60 (0.28–1.26)	0.74 (0.36–1.56)	0.15
Model 3	1	1.56 (0.82–2.98)	0.69 (0.32–1.48)	0.94 (0.44–1.98)	0.41
Model 4	1	1.52 (0.80–2.91)	0.69 (0.32–1.49)	0.94 (0.44–1.98)	0.42
Model 5	1	1.55 (0.81–2.97)	0.69 (0.32–1.50)	0.93 (0.44–1.97)	0.41

Data are expressed as odds ratio (95% confidence interval) with references of highest quartiles (Q1).
Model 1: unadjusted; Model 2: adjusted for age, sex, height, and current smoking (versus nonsmokers); Model 3: Model 2 plus adjustment for daily alcohol consumption (versus infrequent/no alcohol consumption), regular exercise (versus no regular exercise), waist circumference, log-transformed CRP, and self-reported past history of stroke; Model 4: Model 3 plus adjustment for diabetes; Model 5: Model 3 plus adjustment for MetS.
* P values correspond to tests for linear trends across quartile treated as a continuous value.
[†] $P < 0.005$, [§] $P < 0.05$ for each association.

9. Discussion

This study was conducted to investigate the relationship of impaired lung functions with resting electrocardiographic ST-T abnormalities in a cross-sectional analysis of asymptomatic adults without past history of heart disease. We found that LFVC and probably low FEV$_1$, but not low FEV$_1$/FVC, were significantly associated with ST-T abnormalities, which was attenuated by further adjustment for cardiometabolic risk factors, diabetes (presumably mostly type 2 diabetes in this study), or MetS, but remained significant. Notably, cardiometabolic risk factors included circulating CRP and waist circumference, surrogate markers of systemic inflammation, and amount of abdominal fat, respectively. Collectively, the current findings suggest that LFVC, which often reflects restrictive pulmonary function pattern, may be independently associated with ST-T abnormalities irrespective of clinical confounders, diabetes, and MetS, whereas obstructive pulmonary function defects are not.

So far, no clinical study has examined the relationship of LFVC with electrocardiographic abnormalities with the exception of a study by Sideris and Katsadoros [23]. This study reported a negative correlation between vital capacity and number of abnormalities, such as a rightward shift of the P-wave and clockwise rotation of QRS, but it did not address ST or T-wave abnormalities. Thus, to our knowledge, this study is the first to demonstrate the association

between LFVC and ST-T abnormalities, which is conceivably prognostic for cardiovascular events in asymptomatic people [14, 16, 17].

According to previous studies, LFVC and restrictive pulmonary defects have been associated with coronary artery calcification [5] and arterial stiffness [3, 4]. Because artery calcification and arterial stiffness generally reflect atherosclerosis and ischemic cardiovascular diseases, the current results are consistent with these previous studies. Generally, ST-T abnormalities are observed in various conditions, such as ischemia, hypokalemia, cardiomyopathy, and pulmonary embolism [15]. Ohira et al. [13] mentioned that minor ST-T abnormalities may reflect an end-organ effect of long-term hypertension because hypertensive men with minor ST-T abnormalities tended to have longer durations of hypertension in their study. Indeed, arterial stiffness assessed with pulse-wave velocity is substantially affected by hypertension [24]. Furthermore, a recent study showed that decline in FVC predicted incident hypertension in young apparently healthy individuals [22]. Actually, in our study, LFVC was robustly associated with hypertension, even after full adjustments for critical confounders. Nevertheless, the significant association between LFVC and ST-T abnormalities persisted after further adjustments for confounders plus hypertension or medication for hypertension. Therefore, although hypertension likely contributes in part to the observed associations through the close interrelationship of lung with cardiovascular system, other unknown factors may principally interfere with the associations between LFVC and ST-T abnormalities.

Considering that LFVC was associated with ST-T abnormalities independently of cardiometabolic factors, circulating CRP, diabetes, and MetS, which are proatherosclerotic and proinflammatory [9, 10], several factors not examined in this study, such as insulin resistance, oxidative stress, or subclinical hypoxia, might interfere with the relationship between LFVC and ST-T abnormalities. In accordance with this, previous studies have hypothesized that insulin resistance is a fundamental element for the pathophysiology of LFVC and restrictive lung function [2, 6, 7].

Meanwhile, many studies in the past decade have shown that a predisposition for cardiovascular disease and impaired pulmonary functions (low vital capacity and low FEV_1) are associated with low birth weight [25, 26], possibly via physiological alterations such as increased adrenocortical and sympathoadrenal responses to an adverse fetal environment [27]. LFVC and ST-T abnormalities might then relate to such potential factors as epiphenomena.

Alternatively, physicochemical factors might interfere with the associations. Of note, the American Heart Association recently updated its scientific statement to describe that exposure to particulate-matter air pollution contributes to cardiovascular morbidity and mortality [28]. It highlighted several possible biological mechanisms secondary to pulmonary oxidative stress, inflammation, and an impaired lung autonomic nervous system that might result in vascular dysfunction and ST-segment depression irrespective of metabolic abnormalities.

Several limitations should be mentioned. First, because of the nature of cross-sectional studies, causality remains unknown and must be elucidated in large prospective studies. Second, it was not possible to distinguish between major and minor ST-T abnormalities in this study because the electrocardiogram findings on individual checkup sheets in combinations of major and minor ST-T abnormalities were recorded together indistinguishably. However, most ST-T abnormalities were likely to be minor ST-T abnormalities because the prevalence of minor ST-T abnormalities is approximately 2-fold greater than that of major ST-T abnormalities in the Japanese population [13].

Third, all subjects in this study were instructed by staff members trained in spirometry, and the subjects performed a few rehearsals. Nevertheless, it was not clear whether all subjects had acceptable results in the actual test, especially the elderly, regardless of cognitive status, physical performance, or education level. This is likely to result in potential bias of the outcomes.

Finally, most subjects were healthy with good profiles in terms of various parameters, although a small portion of them had several critical conditions such as diabetes or history of stroke. Therefore, the current findings may not be applicable to other populations that have more cardiometabolic risk factors and ST-T abnormalities, where the observed associations, if any, might be dependent on hypertension, diabetes, or metabolic syndrome.

10. Conclusion

LFVC may be associated with ST-T abnormalities independently of cardiometabolic risk factors, diabetes, and MetS in asymptomatic adults without overt heart disease. Our results suggest that there is a mechanism linking low vital capacity with common electrocardiographic abnormalities and that this mechanism is prognostic for increased risk for cardiovascular diseases, which needs to be confirmed in further larger studies.

Disclosure

The present research was not supported by specific grants from any funding agency in the public, commercial, or not-for-profit sectors.

Conflict of Interests

The authors declare no conflict of interests.

References

[1] S. Guerra, D. L. Sherrill, C. Venker, C. M. Ceccato, M. Halonen, and F. D. Martinez, "Morbidity and mortality associated with the restrictive spirometric pattern: a longitudinal study," *Thorax*, vol. 65, no. 6, pp. 499–504, 2010.

[2] F. L. Fimognari, S. Scarlata, and R. Antonelli-Incalzi, "Why are people with "poor lung function" at increased atherothrombotic risk? A critical review with potential therapeutic indications," *Current Vascular Pharmacology*, vol. 8, no. 4, pp. 573–586, 2010.

[3] M. Zureik, A. Benetos, C. Neukirch et al., "Reduced pulmonary function is associated with central arterial stiffness in men," *American Journal of Respiratory and Critical Care Medicine*, vol. 164, no. 12, pp. 2181–2185, 2002.

[4] C. E. Bolton, J. R. Cockcroft, R. Sabit et al., "Lung function in mid-life compared with later life is a stronger predictor of arterial stiffness in men: the Caerphilly Prospective Study," *International Journal of Epidemiology*, vol. 38, no. 3, pp. 867–876, 2009.

[5] H. Y. Park, S. Y. Lim, J. H. Hwang et al., "Lung function, coronary artery calcification, and metabolic syndrome in 4905 Korean males," *Respiratory Medicine*, vol. 104, no. 9, pp. 1326–1335, 2010.

[6] D. A. Lawlor, S. Ebrahim, and G. D. Smith, "Associations of measures of lung function with insulin resistance and Type 2 diabetes: findings from the British Women's Heart and Health Study," *Diabetologia*, vol. 47, no. 2, pp. 195–203, 2004.

[7] F. L. Fimognari, P. Pasqualetti, L. Moro et al., "The association between metabolic syndrome and restrictive ventilatory dysfunction in older persons," *Journals of Gerontology A*, vol. 62, no. 7, pp. 760–765, 2007.

[8] K. Nakajima, Y. Kubouchi, T. Muneyuki, M. Ebata, S. Eguchi, and H. Munakata, "A possible association between suspected restrictive pattern as assessed by ordinary pulmonary function test and the metabolic syndrome," *Chest*, vol. 134, no. 4, pp. 712–718, 2008.

[9] S. M. Grundy, J. I. Cleeman, S. R. Daniels et al., "Diagnosis and management of the metabolic syndrome: an American Heart Association/National Heart, Lung, and Blood Institute

scientific statement," *Circulation*, vol. 112, no. 17, pp. 2735–2752, 2005.

[10] S. Mottillo, K. B. Filion, J. Genest et al., "The metabolic syndrome and cardiovascular risk: a systematic review and meta-analysis," *Journal of the American College of Cardiology*, vol. 56, no. 14, pp. 1113–1132, 2010.

[11] K. Cullen, N. S. Stenhouse, K. L. Wearne, and G. N. Cumpston, "Electrocardiograms and 13 year cardiovascular mortality in Busselton study," *British Heart Journal*, vol. 47, no. 3, pp. 209–212, 1982.

[12] Y. Liao, K. Liu, A. Dyer et al., "Sex differential in the relationship of electrocardiographic ST-T abnormalities to risk of coronary death: 11.5 year follow-up findings of the Chicago Heart Association Detection Project in Industry," *Circulation*, vol. 75, pp. 347–352, 1987.

[13] T. Ohira, H. Iso, H. Imano et al., "Prospective study of major and minor ST-T abnormalities and risk of stroke among Japanese," *Stroke*, vol. 34, no. 12, pp. e250–e253, 2003.

[14] A. Kumar and D. M. Lloyd-Jones, "Clinical significance of minor nonspecific ST-segment and T-wave abnormalities in asymptomatic subjects: a systematic review," *Cardiology in Review*, vol. 15, no. 3, pp. 133–142, 2007.

[15] E. B. Hanna and D. L. Glancy, "ST-segment depression and T-wave inversion: classification, differential diagnosis, and caveats," *Cleveland Clinic Journal of Medicine*, vol. 78, no. 6, pp. 404–414, 2011.

[16] M. L. Daviglus, Y. Liao, P. Greenland et al., "Association of nonspecific minor ST-T abnormalities with cardiovascular mortality: the Chicago western electric study," *Journal of the American Medical Association*, vol. 281, no. 6, pp. 530–536, 1999.

[17] P. Greenland, X. Xie, K. Liu et al., "Impact of minor electrocardiographic ST-segment and/or T-wave abnormalities on cardiovascular mortality during long-term follow-up," *American Journal of Cardiology*, vol. 91, no. 9, pp. 1068–1074, 2003.

[18] American Diabetes Association, "Diagnosis and classification of diabetes mellitus," *Diabetes Care*, vol. 33, supplement 1, pp. S62–S69, 2010.

[19] Y. Seino, K. Nanjo, N. Tajima et al., "Report of the committee on the classification and diagnostic criteria of diabetes mellitus," *Journal of Diabetes Investigation*, vol. 1, no. 5, pp. 212–228, 2010.

[20] Japanese Respiratory Society, *Reference values of spirogram and arterial blood gas levels in Japanese*, Japanese Respiratory Society, Tokyo, Japan, 2001.

[21] R. J. Prineas, R. S. Crow, and H. Blackburn, *The Minnesota Code Manual of Electrocardiographic Findings: Standards and Procedures for Measurement and Classification*, John Wright-PSG, Littleton, Mass, USA, 1982.

[22] D. R. Jacobs Jr., H. Yatsuya, M. O. Hearst et al., "Rate of decline of forced vital capacity predicts future arterial hypertension: the coronary artery risk development in young adults study," *Hypertension*, vol. 59, pp. 219–225, 2012.

[23] D. A. Sideris and D. P. Katsadoros, "Some correlations between electrocardiographic findings and lung volumes in pulmonary diseases," *Journal of Electrocardiology*, vol. 7, no. 4, pp. 295–300, 1974.

[24] A. Milan, F. Tosello, A. Fabbri et al., "Arterial stiffness: from physiology to clinical implications," *High Blood Pressure and Cardiovascular Prevention*, vol. 18, no. 1, pp. 1–12, 2011.

[25] R. J. Hancox, R. Poulton, J. M. Greene, C. R. McLachlan, M. S. Pearce, and M. R. Sears, "Associations between birth weight, early childhood weight gain and adult lung function," *Thorax*, vol. 64, no. 3, pp. 228–232, 2009.

[26] L. Pei, G. Chen, J. Mi et al., "Low birth weight and lung function in adulthood: retrospective cohort study in China, 1948–1996," *Pediatrics*, vol. 125, no. 4, pp. e899–e905, 2010.

[27] D. I. W. Phillips, A. Jones, and P. A. Goulden, "Birth weight, stress, and the metabolic syndrome in adult life," *Annals of the New York Academy of Sciences*, vol. 1083, pp. 28–36, 2006.

[28] R. D. Brook, S. Rajagopalan, C. A. Pope III et al., "Particulate matter air pollution and cardiovascular disease: an update to the scientific statement from the American Heart Association," *Circulation*, vol. 121, pp. 2331–2378, 2010.

20

Outcomes after Bronchoscopic Procedures for Primary Tracheobronchial Amyloidosis: Retrospective Study of 6 Cases

Ihsan Alloubi,[1] Matthieu Thumerel,[1] Hugues Bégueret,[2] Jean-Marc Baste,[1] Jean-François Velly,[1] and Jacques Jougon[1]

[1] *Thoracic Surgery Department, Victor Segalen Bordeaux 2 University and Haut Lévêque Hospital, CHU de Bordeaux, 33604 Pessac Cedex, France*
[2] *Pathology Department, Victor Segalen Bordeaux 2 University and Haut Lévêque Hospital, CHU de Bordeaux, 33604 Pessac Cedex, France*

Correspondence should be addressed to Ihsan Alloubi, ialloubi@yahoo.fr

Academic Editor: Leif Bjermer

Respiratory amyloidosis is a rare disease which refers to localized aberrant extracellular protein deposits within the airways. Tracheobronchial amyloidosis (TBA) refers to the deposition of localized amyloid deposits within the upper airways. Treatments have historically focused on bronchoscopic techniques including debridement, laser ablation, balloon dilation, and stent placement. We present the outcomes after rigid bronchoscopy to remove the amyloid protein causing the airway obstruction in 6 cases of tracheobronchial amyloidosis. This is the first report of primary diffuse tracheobronchial amyloidosis in our department; clinical features, in addition to therapy in the treatment of TBA, are reviewed. This paper shows that, in patients with TBA causing airway obstruction, excellent results can be obtained with rigid bronchoscopy and stenting of the obstructing lesion.

1. Introduction

Primary isolated tracheobronchial amyloidosis (PTBA) is a very uncommon disease caused by aberrant extracellular deposition of amyloid fibrils, which is an inert, eosinophilic, and proteinaceous material [1]. The precise mechanism that causes amyloidosis is unknown. The natural history of this disorder and the efficacy of potential therapies have not been clearly defined. Hence we sought to investigate the long-term outcome of patients with PTBA who underwent invasive bronchoscopic treatment and stenting of the obstructing lesion.

2. Material and Methods

Our institute serves as a regional referral center for interventional bronchoscopy procedures. We retrospectively analyzed the medical records of all patients who were refereed to our institute for evaluation and management of symptomatic PTBA between January 2000 and October 2011. Patient data were retrieved from our local database (Epithor logiciel French cardiothoracic database society). Institutional review board approval was obtained. Informed consent for each bronchoscopy was obtained prior to the procedure.

Each patient underwent a standard preoperative assessment, including physical examination, routine laboratory tests, spirometry, the six-minute walk test, chest radiography, and computed tomography of the chest. This paper included immunoelectrophoretic analysis of plasma and urine, salivary gland and rectal biopsies and X-rays of flat bones to look for myeloma.

An initial diagnostic flexible bronchoscopy was performed for each patient to identify the type, location, and severity of the disease. The diagnostic gold standard of amyloid is by histological confirmation through Congo red staining, which produces red-green birefringence under crossed polarised light [2]. Most tissue specimens, ranging from needle biopsies to open surgical resections, can be studied.

Rigid bronchoscopy was performed in all patients. Anesthetic induction permitted continued spontaneous ventilation by the patient until rigid bronchoscopy secured a stable

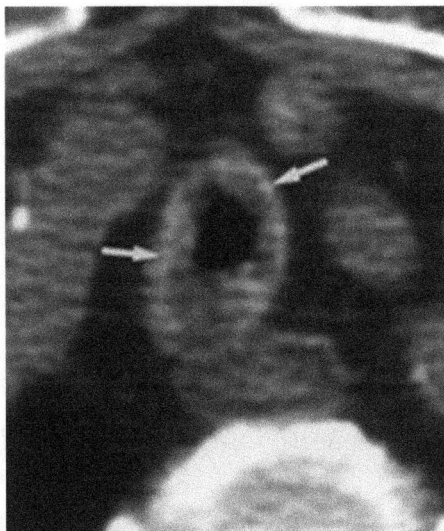

FIGURE 1: CT scan with amyloid deposits narrowing the tracheal diameter.

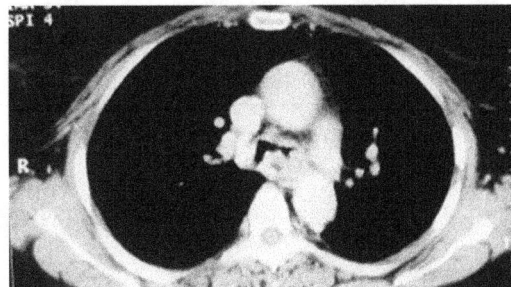

FIGURE 2: Wall thickening of the main bronchi with bilaterally luminal narrowing.

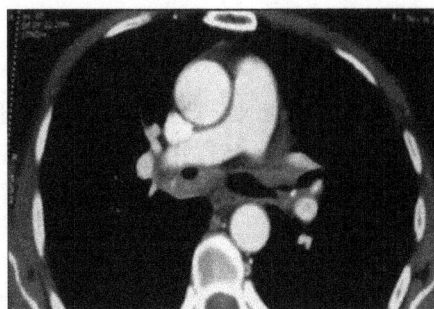

FIGURE 3: Computed tomography of the chest showing significant tracheobronchial wall thickening with narrowing of intermediate trunk.

airway. Rigid-bronchoscopic debulking, with adjunctive laser therapy or electrocautery, was performed for airway recanalization. If endobronchial obstruction is accompanied by marked extrinsic compression or severe stenosis, the placement of a stent may be indispensable.

Early outcomes were assessed by patient symptoms and signs, and late outcomes were assessed by patient follow-up visits, follow-up bronchoscopy, or discussion with referring physician. Patients were considered cured when free of symptoms for at least one year after the last interventional procedure. Statistical analysis descriptive data are presented as mean (±SD) or median (range).

3. Results

Between 2000 and November 2011, 2758 patients were seen in our department for trachea-bronchial endoscopy. In this cohort we identified six patients with histological evidence of amyloidosis. Sex ratio was 1/1, mean age 72 years, ranging from 56 years to 83 years. All patients presented with signs and symptoms of upper airway obstruction including shortness of breath, stridor, cough, dyspnea, and wheezing and presented with typical flow volume curve that demonstrates fixed airway obstruction.

In all patients, serum protein electrophoresis result was normal. A rectal biopsy specimen did not show any evidence of rectal amyloidosis. The diagnosis of bronchial amyloidosis was made and several investigations were undertaken. The results of urine analysis (for 24 h proteinuria and creatinuria) and protein profiles were within normal limits. An electrocardiogram, echocardiography, and abdominal ultrasound showed no abnormalities.

The plasma cell clones that underlie systemic amyloidosis are often subtle and may not be detected by bone marrow examination or immunofixation of serum and urine.

Flexible fibroscopy was performed in all cases; localized tracheobronchial amyloidosis was manifested by completely

irregular surface of the tracheal and bronchial mucosa with prominent reddish and white-yellowish plaques, extending along the entire wall of the trachea and bronchus reducing its diameter by more than 50% with luminal narrowing and stenosis (Figure 1).

All patients underwent rigid bronchoscopy to remove the amyloid protein causing the airway obstruction. One patient presented both tracheobronchial lesions manifesting as bilateral bronchial thickening and narrowing the proximal bronchi diameter (Figure 2).

In another patient, the main bronchi and their major divisions were the only ones affected, but in these the deposits were massive and caused extreme narrowing (Figure 3). Thus the stem bronchi to upper lobes were affected.

We practiced laser therapy by neodymium:yttrium aluminium-garnet (Nd:YAG) prior to mechanical debulking, and we think that this procedure decreases intrabronchial bleeding secondary to interventional bronchoscopy (Figure 4). The median duration of the procedure was 45 minutes (range 35–60 minutes). A satisfactory tracheal size and resolution of symptoms were obtained after multiple sessions of rigid endoscopy (three to five) under general anesthesia in four patients (Figure 5). In two others patients, the examination showed an extreme stenosis of the height trachea by tumor-like, vulnerable tissue without improvement after repeating bronchoscopy (resection and dilatation) and restenosis. A Dumon silicone stent was then inserted to alleviate the obstruction; the patients recovered well and were discharged without dyspnea. After this therapy

TABLE 1: Characteristics of six patients with tracheobronchial amyloidosis.

Age (y)/sex	Common symptoms	Localization/bronchoscopic description	Treatment	Followup/outcomes
70/M	Dyspnea	Tracheal/tumor	Forceps debulking Laser resection	6 months/no followup
72/F	Hemoptysis	Tracheal/nodular	Laser resection Forceps debulking	One year/died of respiratory failure
56/F	Cough, hoarseness	Laryngeal and tracheal Tumor, nodular	Laser resection Forceps debulking with stent	Two years/stable
83/F	Dyspnea, pneumonia	Tracheal and main stem bronchus submucosal	Forceps debulking Laser resection	3 years/stable
82/M	Thoracic pain, cough	Trachea, main stem bronchus Bilateral superior lobar bronchus submucosal	Laser resection Forceps debulking	Few days/died of cardiac attack (atherosclerosis)
72/M	Hemoptysis, cough, dyspnea	Bronchus/nodular, tumor	Laser resection	Five years/stable

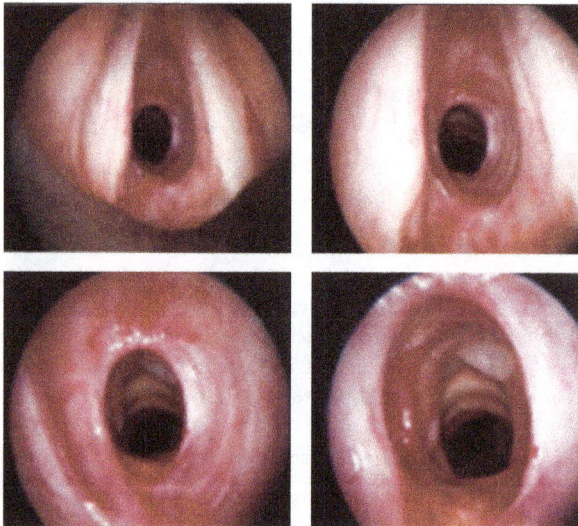

FIGURE 4: Tracheobronchial amyloidosis in a 55-year-old man. Bronchoscopic image shows subglottic stenosis and irregular mucosal thickening with diffuse nodular deposits that involve all portions of the trachea.

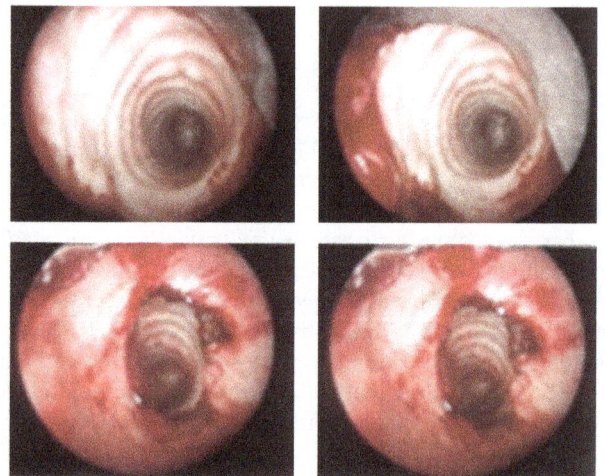

FIGURE 5: On bronchoscopy, this is the appearance of debulking with laser therapy; the left tracheal wall is edematous and narrowed.

there was an excellent clinical response; there was no stridor or rhonchi with symptomatic improvement. Followup bronchoscopy after six months revealed almost permeable caliber of tracheobronchial tree.

There were no intraoperative and perioperative deaths. Procedure complications were relatively manageable and included severe bleeding in three cases; laser treatment stopped the bleeding and resulted in a successful recanalization of the airways after forceps debulking. Granulation tissue formation with stenosis required recurrent laser treatments in two cases. Over a median followup of 15 months (range 6–24 months), 02 patients (33%) died. Timing from the first intervention to death ranged from 15 days to 12 months. The causes of death were respiratory failure after recurrent obstruction in one patient, and cardiac attack in other patients; death cases were due to exacerbation of the

underlying condition and not directly related to the interventional procedure. Three patients were currently being followed up without any progression of symptoms. We have unfortunately no information about the last patient. The characteristics of our patients are summarized in Table 1.

4. Discussion

TBA is characterized by amyloid deposits primarily in the trachea and large bronchi, with extension at times into segmental bronchi. Submucosal vessels are frequently involved [1].

Patients with severe central airway obstruction from TBA involvement have disabling symptoms of dyspnea, respiratory distress, and obstructive pneumonia. For many of these patients, in the absence of intervention, their airway pathology may be the direct cause of death from suffocation [2].

Bronchoscopy is the cornerstone in the diagnosis of TBA that allows better visualization of the lesions and has the advantage of allowing excision of amyloid deposits for histopathological analysis. Diagnosis requires histological confirmation through biopsy, in which sections stained with Congo red reveal greenish birefringence under polarized-light microscopy [1, 2].

This paper shows that in patients with TBA causing airway obstruction, excellent results can be obtained with rigid bronchoscopy, using subjective patient symptoms to assess success in this series; 100% of patients had an immediate and significant improvement in their respiratory symptoms after bronchoscopic debridement with forceps debulking.

All patients were treated by endoscopic debulking with two stent placements during rigid bronchoscopy, each of them with excellent clinical and functional results. In one of these patients regular endoscopic and clinical control exams were performed in the 5 years following the initial treatment, showing stable disease, requiring no further therapeutic intervention until today.

The advantages of rigid bronchoscopy in treating TBA are well known and include airway safety, the ability to perform mechanical debulking, and the ease of blood and airway secretion cleaning [3]. Laser ablation therapy was initially described as efficient in the control of local tracheobronchial amyloidosis [4, 5]. We have used Nd:YAG (neodymium:yttrium aluminum-garnet) laser therapy in all patients prior to forceps debulking with rigid bronchoscopy. We think that repeated bronchoscopic intervention with debridement of luminal obstruction with Nd:YAG laser therapy remains the standard therapeutic approach to upper and mid-airway TBA. It is thought to be preferable and safer and to reduce the major bleeding. The bleeding during bronchoscopy was described and prevalence is most likely due to fragility of submucosal vessels infiltrate with amyloid protein [6].

Overall there have been very few reports of long-term observation of TBA; unfortunately, there is no known effective treatment. Treatment options range from observation and clinical-radiological followup to forceps debulking, local aggressive radiotherapy, and laser ablation therapy. A Dumon silicone stent can be an alternative to alleviate the obstruction; many patients were treated successfully with rigid bronchoscopy and stenting and have a prompt improvement in their symptoms, and relief of impending suffocation [5, 7]. The lack of an untreated control group, or systematic followup, prevents firm conclusions about the intermediate and long-term efficacy of airway debulking. The immediately dramatic improvement in patient symptoms, seen in 100% of patients in this series, creates enthusiasm and optimism in the interventional bronchoscopists. Although, it is seems that repeated rigid bronchoscopic debridement and laser treatments did not prevent progressive airways narrowing in patients dying from TBA, in the study by Hui and colleagues [8], follow-up data were available for 7 of 14 patients with tracheobronchial amyloidosis, and 3 of these patients died of respiratory failure or recurrent pneumonia secondary to bronchial obstruction. In our series, follow-up data were available for three patients in which the disease may remain stable for five years.

5. Conclusion

TBA is a rare disease resulting from abnormal protein deposition within the airway submucosa. There is no cure, although forceps debulking with rigid bronchoscopy with laser therapy can improve the outlook for these patients. Despite the size of this series, in our knowledge, Bronchoscopic treatment modalities can provide durable successful results in patients with TBA with a relatively low rate of complications that can rescue the patient from imminent death and assure an improved quality of life.

Acknowledgments

The authors thank members of the Pathology Department and the Department of Thoracic Surgery (Haut Levêque Medical Center) for assistance in management of these challenging patients.

References

[1] S. A. Capizzi, E. Betancourt, and U. B. S. Prakash, "Tracheobronchial amyloidosis," *Mayo Clinic Proceedings*, vol. 75, no. 11, pp. 1148–1152, 2000.

[2] M. E. Howard, J. Ireton, F. Daniels, D. Langton, N. D. Manolitsas, and P. Fogarty, "Pulmonary presentations of amyloidosis," *Respirology*, vol. 6, pp. 61–64, 2001.

[3] J. D. Gillmore and P. N. Hawkins, "Amyloidosis and the respiratory tract," *Thorax*, vol. 54, no. 5, pp. 444–451, 1999.

[4] M. Paccalin, E. Hachulla, C. Cazalet et al., "Localized amyloidosis: a survey of 35 French cases," *Amyloid*, vol. 12, no. 4, pp. 239–245, 2005.

[5] H. Gibbaoui, S. Abouchacra, and M. Yaman, "A case of primary diffuse tracheobronchial amyloidosis," *Annals of Thoracic Surgery*, vol. 77, no. 5, pp. 1832–1834, 2004.

[6] R. H. Falk and M. Skinner, "The systemic amyloidoses: an overview," *Advances in Internal Medicine*, vol. 45, pp. 107–137, 2000.

[7] S. Hanon, T. de Keukeleire, B. Dieriks et al., "Primary tracheobronchial amyloidosis: a series of 3 cases," *Acta Clinica Belgica*, vol. 62, no. 1, pp. 56–60, 2007.

[8] A. N. Hui, M. N. Koss, L. Hochholzer, and W. D. Wehunt, "Amyloidosis presenting in the lower respiratory tract. Clinicopathologic, radiologic, immunohistochemical, and histochemical studies on 48 cases," *Archives of Pathology and Laboratory Medicine*, vol. 110, no. 3, pp. 212–218, 1986.

21

The Effect of Ventilation, Age, and Asthmatic Condition on Ultrafine Particle Deposition in Children

Hector A. Olvera,[1,2] **Daniel Perez,**[2] **Juan W. Clague,**[3] **Yung-Sung Cheng,**[4] **Wen-Whai Li,**[2] **Maria A. Amaya,**[5] **Scott W. Burchiel,**[6] **Marianne Berwick,**[6] **and Nicholas E. Pingitore**[3,5]

[1] *Center for Environmental Resource Management, University of Texas at El Paso, 500 W. University Avenue, El Paso, TX 79968, USA*
[2] *Civil Engineering Department, University of Texas at El Paso, 500 W. University Avenue, El Paso, TX 79968, USA*
[3] *Geological Sciences Department, University of Texas at El Paso, 500 W. University Avenue, El Paso, TX 79968, USA*
[4] *Aerosol and Dosimetry Program, Lovelace Respiratory Research Institute, 2425 Ridgecrest Dr. SE, Albuquerque, NM 87108-5127, USA*
[5] *School of Nursing, University of Texas at El Paso, 500 W. University Avenue, El Paso, TX 79968, USA*
[6] *Center for Environmental Health Sciences, University of New Mexico, Los Lunas, NM 87131, USA*

Correspondence should be addressed to Hector A. Olvera, holvera@utep.edu

Academic Editor: Cecilie Svanes

Ultrafine particles (UFPs) contribute to health risks associated with air pollution, especially respiratory disease in children. Nonetheless, experimental data on UFP deposition in asthmatic children has been minimal. In this study, the effect of ventilation, developing respiratory physiology, and asthmatic condition on the deposition efficiency of ultrafine particles in children was explored. Deposited fractions of UFP (10–200 nm) were determined in 9 asthmatic children, 8 nonasthmatic children, and 5 nonasthmatic adults. Deposition efficiencies in adults served as reference of fully developed respiratory physiologies. A validated deposition model was employed as an auxiliary tool to assess the independent effect of varying ventilation on deposition. Asthmatic conditions were confirmed via pre-and post-bronchodilator spirometry. Subjects were exposed to a hygroscopic aerosol with number geometric mean diameter of 27–31 nm, geometric standard deviation of 1.8–2.0, and concentration of 1.2×10^6 particles cm^{-3}. Exposure was through a silicone mouthpiece. Total deposited fraction (TDF) and normalized deposition rate were 50% and 32% higher in children than in adults. Accounting for tidal volume and age variation, TDF was 21% higher in asthmatic than in non-asthmatic children. The higher health risks of air pollution exposure observed in children and asthmatics might be augmented by their susceptibility to higher dosages of UFP.

1. Introduction

Particles smaller than 100 nm, due to their size, can elude human defense mechanisms, penetrate deep into the body, reach the bloodstream, and accumulate in sensitive target sites such as bone marrow, lymph nodes, spleen, heart, brain, and the central nervous system [1–9]. The distinctive translocation properties of nanoparticles have prompted their application as drug carrying vectors and in early detection, diagnosis, and treatment of diseases [7, 10–19]. Unfortunately, such translocation properties might also explain why ultrafine particles (UFP) significantly contribute to the elevated health risks associated with urban air pollution

[3, 20–22]. In particular, UFPs have been shown to impact the cardiovascular, pulmonary, and central nervous systems, especially in children, the elderly, and those with respiratory diseases [5, 20–26]. Exposure to UFPs has also been linked to pulmonary inflammation and increased susceptibility to respiratory infections as well as increased risk of cancer, chronic obstructive pulmonary diseases, and exacerbation of asthma [27–38].

Despite extensive research on the health effects of air pollution, the fundamental mechanisms by which UFP could induce disease remain elusive. Further research (e.g., absorption, biopersistence, carcinogenicity, translocation to other tissues or organs, etc.) is necessary to support a comprehensive assessment of the risks associated with human inhalation exposure to UFP. Advances in the epidemiology, toxicology, and pharmacology of nanoparticles hinge on the ability to accurately determine dose-based susceptibility associated with inhalation exposure. As prevalence of asthma and other respiratory illnesses remains high among children, understanding their underlying susceptibility to air pollution is urgent [39–43]. In asthmatics, greater UFP deposition might be induced by enhanced diffusional mechanisms caused by airway obstruction and increased alveolar volumes. In children, however, developing respiratory physiology and changes in breathing patterns could further induce deposition variability [44–46]. In adults, asthmatic conditions have been observed to significantly increase UFP deposition [47]. In children, the effect of asthmatic conditions on deposited fraction of ultrafine particles remains undetermined. The objective of this study was to explore the effect of ventilation, developing respiratory physiology, and asthmatic condition on the deposition efficiency of poly-dispersed hygroscopic ultrafine particles in children. Deposition efficiencies of healthy adults were determined to serve as reference of fully developed respiratory physiologies. The International Commission on Radiological Protection deposition model [48] was employed as an auxiliary tool to assess the independent effect of ventilation on deposition efficiency.

2. Methods

2.1. Subjects. The Institutional Review Board for the protection of human subjects participating in research at the University of Texas at El Paso approved the research protocol (no. 93915). Informed written consent forms were obtained from subjects or their legal guardians in the case of children. Assent forms were obtained directly from children. The experiment was conducted on a group of 22 male subjects, 5 nonasthmatic adults, 8 nonasthmatic children, and 9 clinically diagnosed asthmatic children. Non-smoking adults between 25 and 35 years of age with no history of asthmatic symptoms were recruited at the University of Texas at El Paso. Children between the ages of 9 and 16, from nonsmoking households, were randomly selected from an existent cohort of 500 children. The cohort was built for purposes of a larger epidemiological study for which children asthmatic status was confirmed as described next. Suspected asthmatics were identified based on the standardized asthmatic symptom prevalence questionnaire from the International Study of Asthma and Allergies in Childhood (ISAAC) [49]. Subsequently, lung function tests (spirometry and bronchodilator response) were performed following the American Thoracic Guidelines (ATS) [50]. A forced expiratory volume in 1 s (FEV_1) $\geq$ 90% of predicted was used as a healthy threshold. A forced expiratory volume in 1 s (FEV_1) $\leq$ 80% of predicted, a ratio of FEV_1 to forced vital capacity (FVC) $\leq$ 75%, and a positive bronchodilator response were used as asthmatic thresholds. A positive bronchodilator response was defined as an increase in FEV_1 $\geq$ 15% and/or $\geq$200 mL from baseline after inhalation of 400 μg of albuterol.

2.2. Experimental Design. The experiment was conducted between February and May, 2010. Deposition measurements were conducted during uncontrolled breathing. Breathing frequency (breaths per minute, bpm), tidal volume (liters, L), and minute ventilation (liters per minute, lpm) were recorded with a pneumotachograph (PNT) during exposure. Height, weight, and body mass index (BMI) were also documented. The variables were categorized into groups representing varying ventilation and physiological conditions. The ventilation group included breathing frequency, minute ventilation, and tidal volume, whereas the physiological group included BMI, height, weight, and age. The objective was to evaluate the combined influence of varying ventilation and physiology on UFP deposition, by paring and controlling for variables from these two groups. Pulmonary function immediately before exposure was assessed by means of forced expiratory volume and forced vital capacity measured with an EasyOne spirometer (NDD Medical Technologies, Andover, MA) following previously documented protocols [51]. Pearson correlation was employed to assess associations between variables. Deposition means between groups were compared by two-tailed Student's *t*-tests with $P < 0.05$ denoting significance [52]. The effect of asthmatic condition adjusted for ventilation and physiological variability was explored via one-way analyses of covariance (ANCOVA) [53]. The International Commission on Radiological Protection (ICRP 66) deposition model [48] was employed to assess the effect of varying ventilation independently.

2.3. Exposure. Subjects were exposed to polydisperse sodium chloride (NaCl) produced via atomization (TSI. Inc., Model 3076) of a salt-deionized water solution of 1% by mass. The NaCl aerosol had a geometric mean mobility diameter (GMD) of 27–31 nm, a geometric standard deviation (GSD) of 1.8–2.0, and a total concentration of 1.2×10^6 particles cm^{-3}. The particle number concentration is comparable to the levels of ultrafine particle typically observed near dense traffic highways [54–56]. Sodium chloride particles were used because they do not exacerbate asthmatic symptoms. The system was extensively characterized with NaCl particles and particle shift and loss were known to be minimal [57]. Two size-resolved deposited fraction (DF) curves for particles with mobility diameters in the range 10–200 nm were determined per subject per measurement. Each measurement was duplicated on a nonconsecutive day. Each DF curve measurement was obtained during a 12-minute exposure period. A short period was desired to facilitate children's participation. The exposure period was defined as the shortest time span for which consistent measurements were achieved. Exposure was through a silicone mouthpiece assisted by a nose-clip. The use of a mouthpiece has been observed to affect breathing patterns by increasing minute ventilations during respiratory measurements [58]. The instrumentation employed to measure the ultrafine particle concentrations requires the capture and retention of uncontaminated exhaled breath samples; thus the use of a mouthpiece was necessary. By controlling for ventilation in the ANCOVA mouthpiece-induced breathing variability was also accounted for.

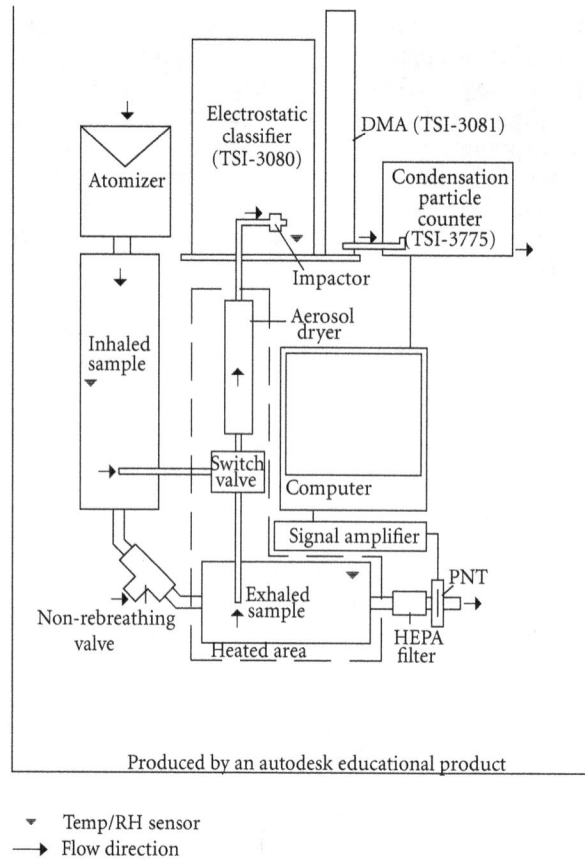

Produced by an autodesk educational product

▼ Temp/RH sensor
→ Flow direction

FIGURE 1: Layout of flow-through breath sampling system.

2.4. *Deposition Measurements.* A scanning mobility particle sizer (SMPS 3936-L75, TSI Inc. USA) was employed to determine particle size distributions and number concentrations in breath samples. Breath samples were delivered to the SMPS via a well-characterized flow-through system [57]. To accommodate children's breathing conditions and further reduce particle loss, a custom-made aluminum non-rebreathing valve and a smaller exhaled sample tank (2.5 L) were introduced to the system originally presented by Löndahl et al. [57]. The non-rebreathing valve had a dead space of 19.5 cm^3. The temperature of the exhaled sample was maintained at 37°C until dried to prevent condensation and minimize size shift due to coagulation. To avoid the effects of temperature on concentration due to air volume changes, inhale and exhale samples were dried and cooled to identical conditions before reaching the SMPS. The system operated at ambient pressure. A diagram of the flow-through system is shown in Figure 1.

The inherent particle loss in the modified system was measured as in Löndahl et al. [57] and was reduced to 5% as compared to the 10% previously reported. The highest size-dependent particle loss was below 5 ± 0.8% and occurred at the smallest measured particle size (5.9 nm) and it decreased with particle size. Measurements for particles smaller than

10 nm were discarded. Deposition fractions were estimated as follows:

$$\mathrm{DF}_{\mathrm{human}}\left(d_{p,i}\right) = 1 - \frac{C_{\mathrm{ex}}\left(d_{p,i}\right)}{C_{\mathrm{in}}\left(d_{p,i}\right) \cdot \left(1 - \mathrm{DF}_{\mathrm{equip}}\left(d_{p,i}\right)\right)}, \quad (1)$$

where $d_{p,i}$ is the particle diameter in size channel i, C_{in} and C_{ex} are the particle concentrations in the inhaled and exhaled samples, respectively, and $\mathrm{DF}_{\mathrm{equip}}$ is the particle loss incurred in the system. The equation is valid for depositional losses occurring in any part of the system between the two sampling ports providing that the particles do not change size during measurements. The SMPS produced DF curves consisting of 99 logarithmically spaced size bins within a mobility diameter size range of 10–200 nm. To further minimize the effect of particle size shift on the DF measurements, the number of size-bins was reduced to 33 by increasing the size range of the bins. Total deposited fraction (TDF) of the NaCl aerosol in the particle size range of 10 nm–225 nm was calculated as in the equation by using the total number concentration for the inhaled and exhaled breath samples.

2.5. *Model.* Deposition in the respiratory tract of healthy subjects was estimated with the empirical ICRP 66 model

TABLE 1: Measurements by participating subject.

Subject	Condition	Sex	Age	Weight (kg)	Height (cm)	Chest width (cm)	BMI	BMI %ile	f (bpm)	V_t (L)	V_E (L/min)	TDF
A	Asthmatic	M	9	33.8	137	76	18.1	80	24.0 ± 1.41	.14 ± .01	3.24 ± .02	.49 ± .00
B	Asthmatic	M	9	36.6	142	77	18.2	81	16.0 ± .00	.26 ± .01	4.08 ± .11	.46 ± .03
C	Asthmatic	M	10	36.3	145	71	17.4	63	22.0 ± 5.66	.16 ± .05	3.27 ± .21	.61 ± .05
D	Asthmatic	M	10	42.0	147	76	19.4	85	18.5 ± .71	.23 ± .02	4.17 ± .55	.60 ± .01
E	Asthmatic	M	12	56.8	162	82	23.5	89	16.8 ± .32	.54 ± .04	9.07 ± .27	.51 ± .03
F	Asthmatic	M	12	56.4	150	81	25.1	96	13.7 ± .00	.66 ± .01	9.04 ± .19	.43 ± .01
G	Asthmatic	M	15	56.6	167	77	20.3	58	9.5 ± 2.12	.37 ± .13	3.38 ± .42	.64 ± .01
H	Asthmatic	M	16	63.5	174	80	21.0	56	7.4 ± .92	.48 ± .01	3.52 ± .34	.65 ± .01
I	Asthmatic	M	12	54.3	158	80	20.5	78	15.2 ± .32	.61 ± .04	9.70 ± .50	.43 ± .01
J	Nonasthmatic	M	11	53.1	160	77	20.8	88	31.5 ± 2.12	.20 ± .05	6.20 ± 1.97	.42 ± .06
K	Nonasthmatic	M	11	45.3	152	70	19.5	80	39.5 ± .71	.17 ± .01	6.72 ± .68	.61 ± .06
L	Nonasthmatic	M	11	40.8	142	74	20.2	85	16.5 ± .46	.61 ± .01	9.98 ± .39	.37 ± .00
M	Nonasthmatic	M	12	61.2	170	84	21.2	86	19.0 ± .00	.24 ± .02	4.47 ± .40	.53 ± .02
N	Nonasthmatic	M	12	57.1	168	76	20.4	81	23.5 ± 2.12	.15 ± .01	3.51 ± .01	.36 ± .04
O	Nonasthmatic	M	12	52.2	155	84	21.8	88	15.2 ± .28	.52 ± .02	7.81 ± .46	.42 ± .01
P	Nonasthmatic	M	15	54.2	170	76	18.9	34	12.5 ± 2.12	.47 ± .15	5.66 ± .87	.55 ± .07
Q	Nonasthmatic	M	16	80.3	176	90	26.2	92	12.5 ± 2.12	.51 ± .12	6.19 ± .43	.55 ± .07
R	Adult	M	21	74.5	174	85	24.6	—	12.9 ± .92	.64 ± .11	8.26 ± .55	.36 ± .06
S	Adult	M	36	86.6	180	91	26.6	—	12.1 ± 1.10	.68 ± .06	8.23 ± .24	.38 ± .00
T	Adult	M	22	78.3	175	84	25.6	—	13.4 ± .67	.62 ± .11	8.31 ± .46	.34 ± .05
U	Adult	M	20	69.4	171	71	23.7	—	16.7 ± .85	.54 ± .09	9.02 ± .76	.30 ± .04
V	Adult	M	29	88.7	181	88	25.8	—	10.00 ± .89	.82 ± .07	9.12 ± .39	.42 ± .02

[*]Mean values ± standard deviation for four experimental repetitions.

[48]. The ICRP 66 was selected for this study as it has been shown to produce comparable results to most deposition models and has been widely referenced in similar studies [47, 57]. The anatomical and physiological reference values for 15- and 10-year-olds provided by the ICRP 66 model were employed in this study. Hygroscopic growth was estimated under the assumption of RH = 99.5% throughout the respiratory tract and immediate particle growth to the equilibrium size [48]. Deposition estimates produced with ICRP 66 model were made for an aerosol with the same characteristics as the one used during the experiments, that is, with a GMD of 30 nm, GSD of 2.0, and a total concentration of 1.2×10^6 particles cm^{-3}.

3. Results

3.1. Child versus Adult.
The dataset is presented in Table 1 and mean and standard deviations of age, sex, BMI, respiratory parameters, and TDF by subject group are summarized in Table 2. The average BMI percentiles by age for all three subject-groups were below the 85 percentile overweight criteria [59]. However, individually six children had a BMI in the overweight percentile range and two in the obese percentile range [59]. As expected, children had higher breathing frequencies and lower tidal volume and minute ventilation than adults [60, 61]. During the uncontrolled breathing measurements TDF for both asthmatic and non-asthmatic children was higher as compared to healthy adults. Specifically, non-asthmatic children had 50% higher TDF than non-asthmatic adults ($P = 0.002$) for ultrafine hygroscopic particles with dry mobility diameters of 10 to 200 nm (see Table 2). The curves in Figure 2 show that the significant differences in size resolved DF between adults and children, occurred for diameters greater than 50 nm.

3.2. Asthmatic versus Non-Asthmatic.
The asthmatic group experienced a decrease of minute volume (V_E) and breathing rate (f) as compared to non-asthmatic subjects. The mean TDF was 14% higher for asthmatic children as compared to non-asthmatics (see Table 3). However, the TDF difference among asthmatic and non-asthmatic children was not significant ($P = 0.212$). The effect of the wide variation of breathing patterns and age within and among the two subjects groups on TDF is further explored in the following sections. As with TDF, the size-dependent DF curves did not suggest a significant difference between the asthmatic and nonasthmatics as shown in Figure 2. The modeled DF curves for healthy 10 and 15 year-olds slightly underestimated the deposition in healthy children, but still performed acceptably well (see Figure 3). Mean V_t and f values shown in Table 1 for asthmatic and non-asthmatic children were employed in the ICRP model to estimate TDF for the two groups. Based solely

TABLE 2: Subject demographics and summarized results*.

Characteristic	Asthmatic (FEV1% < 80)	Nonasthmatic** (FEV1% > 90)	Total children	Adult (control) (FEV1% > 90)
Age (years)	11.67 ± 2.50	12.50 ± 1.93	12.06 ± 2.22	25.60 ± 7.16
Weight (kg)	48.52 ± 11.20	51.79 ± 11.88	51.79 ± 11.74	79.5 ± 8.12
Height (cm)	153.6 ± 12.38	157.35 ± 11.41	157.35 ± 12.28	176.11 ± 4.08
BMI	20.39 ± 2.55	20.74 ± 2.25	20.74 ± 2.37	25.26 ± 1.12
BMI-Percentile	76.22 ± 14.09	77.65 ± 18.69	77.65 ± 15.95	$- \pm -$
f (bpm)	15.98 ± 5.34	18.47 ± 9.71	18.47 ± 7.93	13.01 ± 2.45
V_t (L)	$.38 \pm .20$	$.37 \pm .18$	$.37 \pm .19$	$.66 \pm .34$
V_E (L/min)	5.50 ± 2.85	6.31 ± 1.99	5.88 ± 2.44	$8.59 \pm .44$
TDF***	$.54 \pm .09$	$.48 \pm .10$	$.51 \pm .09$	$.36 \pm .05$

*Mean values ± standard deviation.
**Including a passive smoker.
***Total deposition fraction for an aerosol with GMD of 40 nm, σ_g of 1.9, and mobility diameter range from 10 to 200 nm.

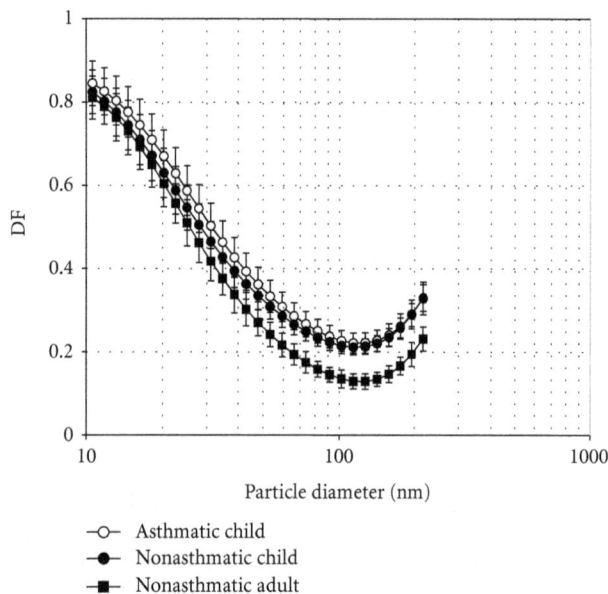

FIGURE 2: Measured deposition fraction curves for all subjects. Error bars represent 95% confidence intervals. The DF curves show a significant difference between children and adults and a nonsignificant difference between asthmatic and non-asthmatic children.

on varying breathing conditions, the ICRP model predicted a positive effect on TDF of 16% and 5% for an "asthmatic" 15-year-old and 10-year-old child, respectively (see Table 3). An age-related effect was also evident from the size-resolved DF curves shown in Figure 3.

3.3. Correlation Analysis. Pearson correlation coefficients for observations from the entire group and for children only are shown in Table 4. For the entire group, significant correlations were observed between TDF and BMI, V_T, and V_E. Age significantly correlated with weight, height, BMI, and f. Whereas BMI was inversely correlated with TDF and f and directly correlated to V_T and V_E. Among children, TDF was

only significantly correlated to V_E. Correlations between age and V_T, and BMI and f were not significant among children. These two pairs of variables, each representing ventilation and a physiological characteristic, were used as covariates to evaluate the effect of asthmatic conditions among children.

3.4. Adjusted Effects. A series of evaluations of the effect of asthmatic condition on TDF while controlling for age, BMI, height, weight, f, V_T and V_E independently did not reveal significant results. However, after controlling for age and V_T or BMI and f, significant effects on TDF due to asthmatic conditions were observed (see Tables 5 and 6). The age-V_T ANCOVA produced the most significant results; $F(1, 13) = 7.419$, $P < .05$ and $20.4\% (w^2 = 0.204)$ of the total variance in TDF was accounted for by the two levels of asthmatic condition controlling for the effect of subject age and tidal volume during the experiment. The adjusted TDF mean for asthmatics (0.552) was 21% higher than for non-asthmatics (0.458) for an age value of 12.06 years and V_t of 0.37 L (see Table 3). The homogeneity-of-regression (slopes) assumption was confirmed as the relationship between the covariates, and the dependent variable did not differ significantly as a function of the independent variable: $F(1, 10) = 1.195$, $P = .300$ for tidal volume and $F(1, 10) = .176$, $P = .684$ for age.

4. Discussion

Bennett and Zeman [58] established that for identical DF values, and independent of particle size, the deposition rate is higher in children than in adults due to higher minute ventilation and smaller lung surface area. Bennett and Zeman [58] also observed that the normalized deposition rate for monodisperse $2 \mu m$ particles was actually 35% higher in children as compared to adults. In this study, it was observed that for UFPs, specifically for hygroscopic particles with mobility diameters between 10 and 200 nm, the total deposited fraction was 50% higher in children as compared to adults (see Table 2). Following the approach presented by Bennett and Zeman [58] and using the same functional

TABLE 3: Summary of total deposited fraction values.

Characteristic	Asthmatic	Nonasthmatic	Effect	Notes
Mean	.544	.476	14%	All subjects
Adjusted Means	.552	.458	21%	ANCOVA
ICRP for 15 year olds*	.507	.438	16%	Based on distinct f and V_t values as shown in Table 2
ICRP for 10 year olds*	.501	.475	5%	Based on distinct f and V_t values as shown in Table 5

*Estimated for an aerosol of GMD = 30 nm, σ_g 2.0, and total concentration 1.2×10^6 particles cm^{-3}.

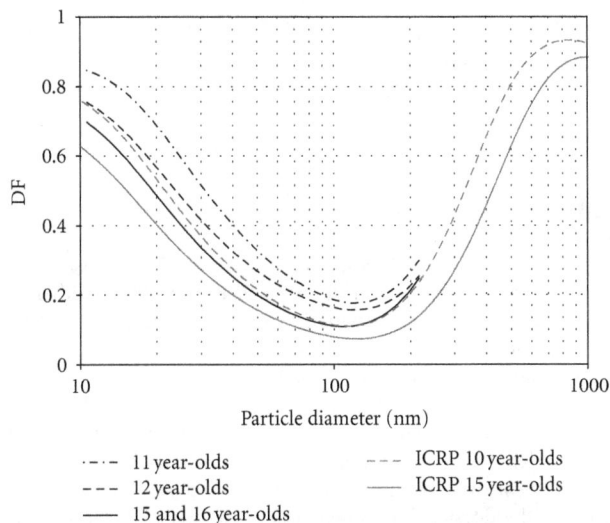

FIGURE 3: Measured and modeled deposition fraction curves by age for non-asthmatics. The curves suggest a strong effect of age on deposition. Age was used as a covariate in the ANCOVA analysis for total deposited fraction. Note reasonable agreement between our measurements and the ICRP model estimates.

residual capacity values for adults (2.87 L) and 12 year olds (1.77 L), the 50% increase in TDF for UFP observed in this study results in a normalized deposition rate 32% higher in healthy children as compared to adults. These results suggest that children are prone to considerably higher dosages of airborne ultrafine particles as compared to adults and that such disposition increases with smaller particle size.

The mean differences in TDF between asthmatic and non-asthmatic children were nonsignificant and strongly affected by age and breathing patterns. For ultrafine hydrophobic particles, Chalupa et al. [47] and Diagle et al. [62] observed significantly higher (42.6%) deposition fractions in asthmatic adults as compared to non-asthmatic adults. However, the effect on total particle deposition variation induced by distinctive breathing patterns among subject groups observed in those studies was undetermined. In this study, after controlling for extraneous variance associated with age and V_T or BMI and f a significant effect due to asthmatic conditions was also observed for children. For children, the estimated adjusted effect of asthmatic condition on TDF was 21%. The ICRP model, based solely on varying breathing conditions between the asthmatic and non-asthmatic groups, predicted an effect between 5% and 16%. The model results suggest that a considerable fraction of the increase

in DF in asthmatics is directly associated with the variation of f, and V_T induced by asthmatic conditions. Enhance diffusional deposition of UFPs might also be associated with airway obstruction and increased lung residual volume, characteristic of asthmatic conditions. In this regard, the disposition to higher dose in asthmatic children might be linked to inflammatory airway conditions, higher minute ventilation, and a smaller lung surface area. The results of this study, which build upon and complement a series of previous studies, suggest that children, and evermore so asthmatic children, receive significantly higher dosages of ultrafine particles than adults with similar exposure.

This study, as well as other deposition studies [47, 63, 64], worked with a small sample size due to constrains of the experimental procedure. The results are preliminary, not only because the subject group is small but also because the breathing conditions were through a mouthpiece and therefore might be unrepresentative of "real" breathing conditions. Still the results clearly substantiate the need for more comprehensive studies on the mechanisms and sources of variability in nanosize particle deposition within the human respiratory tract. Specifically, studies with controlled breathing conditions on asthmatic children, with hydrophobic particles, and on larger groups are necessary. Additional exercises to determine if the accuracy of the ICRP in determining the effect of DF in asthmatic children could be improved by employing subject-specific biometric values would also be valuable. Given the high prevalence of childhood asthma and the potentially higher susceptibility of asthmatic children to air quality impacts, the results of this study were deemed important.

5. Conclusion

The results of this study suggest that for the same exposure, children receive a higher lung dose of UFP as compared to adults and that asthmatic condition further increases deposited fraction. The total deposited fraction and normalized deposition rate were 50% and 32% higher in children than in adults, respectively. After controlling for age and tidal volume variation, TDF was 21% higher in asthmatic than in non-asthmatic children. The effect on TDF of distinctive tidal volume and breathing frequency induced by asthmatic conditions was estimated by the ICRP to be between 16% and 5%, for a 10 to 15 year old age range. The results suggest that the observed higher deposited fraction of UFP in asthmatics is due to causes beyond distinctive breathing patterns and possibly due to diffusional deposition enhanced by inflamed airways. The higher health risk of air pollution exposure

TABLE 4: Pearson correlation coefficients for variables.

		Age	Weight	Height	BMI	f	V_T	V_E	TDF
					Only children				
Age		**1.000**	.836**	.867**	.507*	−.571*	0.478	0.004	0.353
Weight		.865**	**1.000**	.895**	.794**	−0.389	0.427	0.143	0.091
Height		.757**	.922**	**1.000**	0.473	−0.337	0.208	−0.102	0.247
BMI	All Subjects	.743**	.896**	.692**	**1.000**	−0.313	.617**	.494*	−0.166
f		−.459*	−.493*	−.455*	−.441*	**1.000**	−.649**	−0.031	−0.123
V_T		.668**	.692**	.509*	.768**	−.688**	**1.000**	.753**	−0.219
V_E		0.402	.432*	0.215	.627**	−0.174	.798**	**1.000**	−.503*
TDF		−0.385	−0.365	−0.187	−.477*	0.075	−.454*	−.629**	**1.000**

**Correlation is significant at the 0.01 level (2-tailed).
*Correlation is significant at the 0.05 level (2-tailed).

TABLE 5: Analysis of covariance for total deposited fraction by asthmatic condition.

Source	SS	df	MS	F	P
Age	0.057	1	0.057	12.199	0.004
Tidal volume	0.04	1	0.04	8.578	0.012
Asthmatic condition	0.035	1	0.035	7.419	0.017
Error	0.061	13	0.005		
Total	0.142	16			

TABLE 6: Analysis of covariance for total deposited fraction by asthmatic condition.

Source	SS	df	MS	F	P
BMI	0.047	1	0.047	7.778	0.015
f	0.022	1	0.022	3.608	0.080
Asthmatic condition	0.043	1	0.043	7.154	0.019
Error	0.081	13	0.006		
Total	0.140	16			

commonly observed in children, and asthmatics might be linked to higher dosages of UFP, as compared to adults and healthy individuals.

The subject group studied was small, composed of only males, and the breathing conditions were through a mouthpiece, and therefore might be unrepresentative of "real" breathing conditions. Given the high prevalence of asthma among children the suggested susceptibility to UFP levels is of importance and warrants further research.

Acknowledgments

This work was supported by grant number S11 ES013339 from the National Institute of Environmental Health Sciences (NIEHS) and the National Institutes of Health (NIH). Its contents are solely the responsibility of the authors and do not necessarily represent the official views of the NIEHS, NIH, or HEI. The authors would like to thank Dr. Jakob Löndahl for his technical assistance and valuable comments.

References

[1] W. G. Kreyling, M. Semmler, F. Erbe et al., "Translocation of ultrafine insoluble iridium particles from lung epithelium to extrapulmonary organs is size dependent but very low," *Journal of Toxicology and Environmental Health—Part A*, vol. 65, no. 20, pp. 1513–1530, 2002.

[2] A. Nemmar, M. F. Hoylaerts, P. H. M. Hoet et al., "Ultrafine particles affect experimental thrombosis in an *in vivo* hamster model," *American Journal of Respiratory and Critical Care Medicine*, vol. 166, no. 7, pp. 998–1004, 2002.

[3] G. Oberdörster, "Pulmonary effects of inhaled ultrafine particles," *International Archives of Occupational and Environmental Health*, vol. 74, no. 1, pp. 1–8, 2001.

[4] G. Oberdörster, Z. Sharp, V. Atudorei et al., "Extrapulmonary translocation of ultrafine carbon particles following whole-body inhalation exposure of rats," *Journal of Toxicology and Environmental Health—Part A*, vol. 65, no. 20, pp. 1531–1543, 2002.

[5] S. K. Park, M. S. O'Neill, P. S. Vokonas, D. Sparrow, and J. Schwartz, "Effects of air pollution on heart rate variability: the VA normative aging study," *Environmental Health Perspectives*, vol. 113, no. 3, pp. 304–309, 2005.

[6] P. H. M. Hoet, I. Brüske-Hohlfeld, and O. V. Salata, "Nanoparticles—known and unknown health risks," *Journal of Nanobiotechnology*, vol. 2, no. 1, article 12, 2004.

[7] G. Oberdörster, E. Oberdörster, and J. Oberdörster, "Nanotoxicology: an emerging discipline evolving from studies of ultrafine particles," *Environmental Health Perspectives*, vol. 113, no. 7, pp. 823–839, 2005.

[8] G. Oberdörster, Z. Sharp, V. Atudorei et al., "Translocation of inhaled ultrafine particles to the brain," *Inhalation Toxicology*, vol. 16, no. 6-7, pp. 437–445, 2004.

[9] G. Oberdörster and M. J. Utell, "Ultrafine particles in the urban air: to the respiratory tract—ang beyond?" *Environmental Health Perspectives*, vol. 110, no. 8, pp. A440–A441, 2002.

[10] S. Fiorito, A. Serafino, F. Andreola, A. Togna, and G. Togna, "Toxicity and biocompatibility of carbon nanoparticles," *Journal of Nanoscience and Nanotechnology*, vol. 6, no. 3, pp. 591–599, 2006.

[11] B. Gopalan, I. Ito, C. D. Branch, C. Stephens, J. A. Roth, and R. Ramesh, "Nanoparticle based systemic gene therapy for lung cancer: molecular mechanisms and strategies to suppress nanoparticle-mediated inflammatory response," *Technology in Cancer Research and Treatment*, vol. 3, no. 6, pp. 647–657, 2004.

[12] J. M. Koziara, P. R. Lockman, D. D. Allen, and R. J. Mumper, "The blood-brain barrier and brain drug delivery," *Journal of Nanoscience and Nanotechnology*, vol. 6, no. 9-10, pp. 2712–2735, 2006.

[13] J. Kreuter, "Nanoparticulate systems for brain delivery of drugs," *Advanced Drug Delivery Reviews*, vol. 47, no. 1, pp. 65–81, 2001.

[14] P. R. Lockman, J. Koziara, K. E. Roder et al., "In vivo and in vitro assessment of baseline blood-brain barrier parameters in the presence of novel nanoparticles," *Pharmaceutical Research*, vol. 20, no. 5, pp. 705–713, 2003.

[15] P. R. Lockman, R. J. Mumper, M. A. Khan, and D. D. Allen, "Nanoparticle technology for drug delivery across the blood-brain barrier," *Drug Development and Industrial Pharmacy*, vol. 28, no. 1, pp. 1–13, 2002.

[16] P. R. Lockman, M. O. Oyewumi, J. M. Koziara, K. E. Roder, R. J. Mumper, and D. D. Allen, "Brain uptake of thiamine-coated nanoparticles," *Journal of Controlled Release*, vol. 93, no. 3, pp. 271–282, 2003.

[17] S. Mansouri, Y. Cuie, F. Winnik et al., "Characterization of folate-chitosan-DNA nanoparticles for gene therapy," *Biomaterials*, vol. 27, no. 9, pp. 2060–2065, 2006.

[18] C. Medina, M. J. Santos-Martinez, A. Radomski, O. I. Corrigan, and M. W. Radomski, "Nanoparticles: pharmacological and toxicological significance," *British Journal of Pharmacology*, vol. 150, no. 5, pp. 552–558, 2007.

[19] S. B. Tiwari and M. M. Amiji, "A review of nanocarrier-based CNS delivery systems," *Current Drug Delivery*, vol. 3, no. 2, pp. 219–232, 2006.

[20] G. Oberdorster, R. M. Gelein, J. Ferin, and B. Weiss, "Association of particulate air pollution and acute mortality: involvement of ultrafine particles?" *Inhalation Toxicology*, vol. 7, no. 1, pp. 111–124, 1995.

[21] G. Oberdörster, A. Maynard, K. Donaldson et al., "Principles for characterizing the potential human health effects from exposure to nanomaterials: elements of a screening strategy," *Particle and Fibre Toxicology*, vol. 2, article 8, 2005.

[22] P. Pedata, E. M. Garzillo, and N. Sannolo, "Ultrafine particles and effects on the organism: literature review," *Giornale Italiano di Medicina del Lavoro ed Ergonomia*, vol. 32, no. 1, pp. 23–31, 2010.

[23] D. W. Dockery, H. Luttman-Gibson, D. Q. Rich et al., "Association of air pollution with increased incidence of ventricular tachyarrhythmias recorded by implanted cardioverter defibrillators," *Environmental Health Perspectives*, vol. 113, no. 6, pp. 670–674, 2005.

[24] M. W. Frampton, M. J. Utell, W. Zareba et al., "Effects of exposure to ultrafine carbon particles in healthy subjects and subjects with asthma," *Research Report*, no. 126, pp. 1–47, 2004.

[25] M. W. Frampton, "Does inhalation of ultrafine particles cause pulmonary vasular effects in humans?" *Inhalation Toxicology*, vol. 19, no. 1, pp. 75–79, 2007.

[26] J. Braz Nogueira, "Air pollution and cardiovascular disease," *Revista Portuguesa de Cardiologia*, vol. 28, no. 6, pp. 715–733, 2009.

[27] Y. Bai, A. K. Suzuki, and M. Sagai, "The cytotoxic effects of diesel exhaust particles on human pulmonary artery endothelial cells in vitro: role of active oxygen species," *Free Radical Biology and Medicine*, vol. 30, no. 5, pp. 555–562, 2001.

[28] A. Baulig, M. Garlatti, V. Bonvallot et al., "Involvement of reactive oxygen species in the metabolic pathways triggered by diesel exhaust particles in human airway epithelial cells,"

American Journal of Physiology, vol. 285, no. 3, pp. L671–L679, 2003.

[29] D. Diaz-Sanchez, "The role of diesel exhaust particles and their associated polyaromatic hydrocarbons in the induction of allergic airway disease," *Allergy*, vol. 52, no. 38, supplement, pp. 52–56, 1997.

[30] D. Diaz-Sanchez, M. P. Garcia, M. Wang, M. Jyrala, and A. Saxon, "Nasal challenge with diesel exhaust particles can induce sensitization to a neoallergen in the human mucosa," *Journal of Allergy and Clinical Immunology*, vol. 104, no. 6, pp. 1183–1188, 1999.

[31] D. Diaz-Sanchez, M. Jyrala, D. Ng, A. Nel, and A. Saxon, "In vivo nasal challenge with diesel exhaust particles enhances expression of the CC chemokines rantes, MIP-1α, and MCP-3 in humans," *Clinical Immunology*, vol. 97, no. 2, pp. 140–145, 2000.

[32] D. Diaz-Sanchez, M. Penichet-Garcia, and A. Saxon, "Diesel exhaust particles directly induce activated mast cells to degranulate and increase histamine levels and symptom severity," *Journal of Allergy and Clinical Immunology*, vol. 106, no. 6, pp. 1140–1146, 2000.

[33] E. Garshick, F. Laden, J. E. Hart et al., "Lung cancer and vehicle exhaust in trucking industry workers," *Environmental Health Perspectives*, vol. 116, no. 10, pp. 1327–1332, 2008.

[34] A. L. Holder, D. Lucas, R. Goth-goldstein, and C. P. Koshland, "Cellular response to diesel exhaust particles strongly depends on the exposure method," *Toxicological Sciences*, vol. 103, no. 1, pp. 108–115, 2008.

[35] J. Kagawa, "Health effects of diesel exhaust emissions—a mixture of air pollutants of worldwide concern," *Toxicology*, vol. 181-182, pp. 349–353, 2002.

[36] J. Lewtas, "Air pollution combustion emissions: characterization of causative agents and mechanisms associated with cancer, reproductive, and cardiovascular effects," *Mutation Research*, vol. 636, no. 1–3, pp. 95–133, 2007.

[37] R. O. McClellan, "Health effects of exposure to diesel exhaust particles," *Annual Review of Pharmacology and Toxicology*, vol. 27, pp. 279–300, 1987.

[38] P. Møller, J. K. Folkmann, L. Forchhammer et al., "Air pollution, oxidative damage to DNA, and carcinogenesis," *Cancer Letters*, vol. 266, no. 1, pp. 84–97, 2008.

[39] T. F. Bateson and J. Schwartz, "Children's response to air pollutants," *Journal of Toxicology and Environmental Health—Part A*, vol. 71, no. 3, pp. 238–243, 2008.

[40] H. Moshammer, A. Bartonova, W. Hanke et al., "Air pollution: a threat to the health of our children," *Acta Paediatrica, International Journal of Paediatrics*, vol. 95, no. 453, pp. 93–105, 2006.

[41] M. M. Patel and R. L. Miller, "Air pollution and childhood asthma: recent advances and future directions," *Current Opinion in Pediatrics*, vol. 21, no. 2, pp. 235–242, 2009.

[42] L. J. Akinbami, J. E. Moorman, and X. Liu, "Asthma prevalence, health care use, and mortality: United States, 2005–2009," *National Health Statistics Reports*, 2011, http://www.cdc.gov/nchs/products/hestats.htm.

[43] N. Pearce, N. Aït-Khaled, R. Beasley et al., "Worldwide trends in the prevalence of asthma symptoms: phase III of the International Study of Asthma and Allergies in Childhood (ISAAC)," *Thorax*, vol. 62, no. 9, pp. 757–765, 2007.

[44] W. D. Bennett and G. C. Smaldone, "Human variation in the peripheral air-space deposition of inhaled particles," *Journal of Applied Physiology*, vol. 62, no. 4, pp. 1603–1610, 1987.

[45] J. Heyder, J. Gebhart, and G. Scheuch, "Influence of human lung morphology on particle deposition," *Journal of Aerosol Medicine*, vol. 1, no. 2, pp. 81–88, 1988.

[46] W. D. Bennet, "Human variation in spontaneous breathing deposition fraction: a review," *Journal of Aerosol Medicine*, vol. 1, no. 2, pp. 67–80, 1988.

[47] D. C. Chalupa, P. E. Morrow, G. Oberdörster, M. J. Utell, and M. W. Frampton, "Ultrafine particle deposition in subjects with asthma," *Environmental Health Perspectives*, vol. 112, no. 8, pp. 879–882, 2004.

[48] International Comission on Radiological Protection, *Human Respiratory Tract Model for Radiological Protection*, ICRP, Elsevire Science, Tarrytown, NY, USA, 1994.

[49] M. I. Asher, U. Keil, H. R. Anderson et al., "International study of asthma and allergies in childhood (ISAAC): rationale and methods," *European Respiratory Journal*, vol. 8, no. 3, pp. 483–491, 1995.

[50] M. R. Miller, J. Hankinson, V. Brusasco et al., "Standardisation of spirometry," *European Respiratory Journal*, vol. 26, no. 2, pp. 319–338, 2005.

[51] S. E. Sarnat, A. U. Raysoni, W.-W. Li et al., "Air pollution and acute respiratory response in a panel of asthmatic children along the U.S.-Mexico Border," *Environmental Health Perspectives*, vol. 120, no. 3, pp. 437–444, 2012.

[52] B. W. Brown, "The crossover experiment for clinical trials," *Biometrics*, vol. 36, no. 1, pp. 69–79, 1980.

[53] E. Huitema, *The Analysis of Covariance and Alternatives: Statistical Methods for Experiments, Quasi-Experiments, and Single-Case Studies*, John Wiley & Sons, Hoboken, NJ, USA, 2nd edition, 2011.

[54] Y. Zhu and W. C. Hinds, "Predicting particle number concentrations near a highway based on vertical concentration profile," *Atmospheric Environment*, vol. 39, no. 8, pp. 1557–1566, 2005.

[55] Y. Zhu, W. C. Hinds, S. Kim, S. Shen, and C. Sioutas, "Study of ultrafine particles near a major highway with heavy-duty diesel traffic," *Atmospheric Environment*, vol. 36, no. 27, pp. 4323–4335, 2002.

[56] Y. Zhu, J. Pudota, D. Collins et al., "Air pollutant concentrations near three Texas roadways, Part I: ultrafine particles," *Atmospheric Environment*, vol. 43, no. 30, pp. 4513–4522, 2009.

[57] J. Löndahl, J. Pagels, E. Swietlicki et al., "A set-up for field studies of respiratory tract deposition of fine and ultrafine particles in humans," *Journal of Aerosol Science*, vol. 37, no. 9, pp. 1152–1163, 2006.

[58] W. D. Bennett and K. L. Zeman, "Deposition of fine particles in children spontaneously breathing at rest," *Inhalation Toxicology*, vol. 10, no. 9, pp. 831–842, 1998.

[59] W. H. Dietz and T. N. Robinson, "Use of the body mass index (BMI) as a measure of overweight in children and adolescents," *Journal of Pediatrics*, vol. 132, no. 2, pp. 191–193, 1998.

[60] E. Tabachnik, N. Muller, B. Toye, and H. Levison, "Measurement of ventilation in children using the respiratory inductive plethysmograph," *Journal of Pediatrics*, vol. 99, no. 6, pp. 895–899, 1981.

[61] M. J. Tobin, T. S. Chadha, and G. Jenouri, "Breathing patterns. 1. Normal subjects," *Chest*, vol. 84, no. 2, pp. 202–205, 1983.

[62] C. C. Daigle, D. C. Chalupa, F. R. Gibb et al., "Ultrafine particle deposition in humans during rest and exercise," *Inhalation Toxicology*, vol. 15, no. 6, pp. 539–552, 2003.

[63] J. Löndahl, A. Massling, J. Pagels, E. Swietlicki, E. Vaclavik, and S. Loft, "Size-resolved respiratory-tract deposition of fine and ultrafine hydrophobic and hygroscopic aerosol particles during rest and exercise," *Inhalation Toxicology*, vol. 19, no. 2, pp. 109–116, 2007.

[64] J. Löndahl, A. Massling, E. Swietlicki et al., "Experimentally determined human respiratory tract deposition of airborne particles at a busy street," *Environmental Science and Technology*, vol. 43, no. 13, pp. 4659–4664, 2009.

22

Pulmonary Function Tests in Emergency Department Pediatric Patients with Acute Wheezing/Asthma Exacerbation

Kathryn Giordano,[1] **Elena Rodriguez,**[2] **Nicole Green,**[1] **Milena Armani,**[2] **Joan Richards,**[3] **Thomas H. Shaffer,**[2, 4, 5] **and Magdy W. Attia**[1]

[1] *Department of Emergency Medicine, Nemours/Alfred I. duPont Hospital for Children, Wilmington, DE 19803, USA*
[2] *Nemours Research Lung Center, Nemours/Alfred I. duPont Hospital for Children, Wilmington, DE 19803, USA*
[3] *Department of Respiratory Care, Nemours/Alfred I. duPont Hospital for Children, Wilmington, DE 19803, USA*
[4] *Department of Pediatrics, Jefferson Medical College, Philadelphia, PA 19107, USA*
[5] *Departments of Physiology and Pediatrics, Temple University School of Medicine, Philadelphia, PA 19140, USA*

Correspondence should be addressed to Kathryn Giordano, kfgiorda@nemours.org

Academic Editor: N. Ambrosino

Background. Pulmonary function tests (PFT) have been developed to analyze tidal breathing in patients who are minimally cooperative due to age and respiratory status. This study used tidal breathing tests in the ED to measure asthma severity. *Design/Method.* A prospective pilot study in pediatric patients (3 to 18 yrs) with asthma/wheezing was conducted in an ED setting using respiratory inductance plethysmography and pneumotachography. The main outcome measures were testing feasibility, compliance, and predictive value for admission versus discharge. *Results.* Forty patients were studied, of which, 14 (35%) were admitted. Fifty-five percent of the patients were classified as a mild-intermittent asthmatic, 30% were mild-persistent asthmatics, 12.5% were moderate-persistent asthmatics, and 2.5% were severe-persistent. Heart rate was higher in admitted patients as was labored breathing index, phase angle, and asthma score. *Conclusions.* Tidal breathing tests provide feasible, objective assessment of patient status in the enrolled age group and may assist in the evaluation of acute asthma exacerbation in the ED. Our results demonstrate that PFT measurements, in addition to asthma scores, may be useful in indicating the severity of wheezing/asthma and the need for admission.

1. Introduction

Asthma and other childhood wheezing disorders represent a significant percentage of pediatric emergency department (ED) visits [1]. Management decisions are largely based on exam findings, vital signs, and pulse oximetry [2]. The child and parents' perception of the clinical symptoms are important tools in the guidelines for assessing asthma severity. Dyspnea, cough, wheezing, and exercise intolerance are helpful in making clinical decisions, but it is well known that neither the child nor the parent accurately report these symptoms. Their perceptions often underestimate the severity of the disease [3].

Preschool children (<5 years of age) make up a large percentage of the asthmatics presenting to the pediatric ED; however, because of their inability to cooperate with spirometry or peak flow, they are frequently excluded from research studies. An estimated 40% of children aged 6 to 9 years and 25% of children under 10 years would likely be excluded from participation in trials if spirometry was the objective measure of asthma severity [3, 4]. Pulmonary function tests (PFT) have been developed to analyze tidal breathing in patients who are minimally cooperative due to age or clinical condition (urgency associated with the ED). These include respiratory inductance plethysmography (RIP) and pneumotachography (PT), which have been used extensively in the minimally cooperative neonate and pediatric populations [5–12].

In the present pilot study, we hypothesized that PFT in the ED would provide a predictive value associated with disposition (admission versus discharge) to aid in resource utilization. Since these measurements have not been utilized in this setting, we set out to determine the feasibility of performing these measurements in this setting, the compliance of patients with the evaluation techniques, and the post-hoc predictive value of the results (clinicians were initially blinded to the PFT results at the time of admission). Finally, we were interested in an assessment tool employing tidal breathing analysis that suggests the severity of the wheezing exacerbation. Thus, we are speculating that this objective diagnostic approach may be used in the future to determine from the moment of triage the likelihood that a given patient would require a prolonged ED visit. A decision regarding disposition could then be made early, decreasing the patient's ED length of stay (LOS).

2. Methods and Materials

2.1. Patients and Protocol. We conducted a prospective observational study of 40 patients (aged 3 to 18 years) who presented to the ED with the chief complaint of wheezing or with an asthma exacerbation. The study was reviewed and approved by our Institutional Review Board, and we obtained written, informed parental consent in all cases. Only those patients who were determined to be in mild-to-moderate respiratory distress based on the Emergency Severity Index (ESI v.4) criteria were eligible for enrollment. The ESI v.4 is a five-level triage system based on resource utilization. It is widely used among both adult and pediatric EDs [13]. Exclusion criteria were severe respiratory distress warranting immediate intervention (ESI levels 1 and 2), underlying lung disease (including but not limited to cystic fibrosis or spinal muscular atrophy), and age less than 3 years or greater than 18 years. Once identified by the coinvestigators, the parent/guardian provided consent for enrollment and assent was obtained for patients 7 years and older. The patient then completed an asthma severity questionnaire to give insight to their disease.

Pulmonary function tests were obtained at baseline, prior to implementing standard of care treatment (i.e., protocol-driven care for asthmatic patients). Tests included RIP and inductance bands. We also evaluated the objective monitoring of real tidal volume, respiratory rate, flow patterns, and end-tidal CO_2 by tidal breathing analysis with PT. Below is a detailed explanation of these two noninvasive tidal breathing techniques.

The prescribed clinical treatment was at the discretion of the treating physician. For moderate asthma exacerbation, the treatment regimen includes one nebulized albuterol (dose of 0.15 mg/kg/dose, max 5 mg) and ipratropium bromide (dose of 250 mcg for patients less than 20 kg or 500 mcg for patients greater than 20 kg) followed by either one hour of continuous albuterol nebulization or two additional nebulized albuterol and ipratropium bromide treatments 15 minutes apart with oral corticosteroids (dose of 2 mg/kg, max 60 mg). Mild asthma exacerbations occasionally were treated more conservatively. At times, only one nebulized albuterol treatment was needed with or without

oral corticosteroids. The PFT were therefore performed before the initial treatment was prescribed.

The treating physician was blinded to the results of the PFT measurements. The clinical decisions were based on the standards of care that are currently used in the ED, including vital signs (respiratory rate, heart rate, transcutaneous oxygen saturation [Masimo, Irvine, CA]) and clinical appearance. An asthma score was assigned to each patient. This score was calculated as follows: respiratory rate based on age (less than 7 years: 0: 0–30, 1: 31–45, 2: 46–60, 3: >60; greater than 7 years: 0: 0–20, 1: 21–35, 2: 36–50, 3: >50), wheezing (0: absent, 1: expiratory only, 2: expiratory, and inspiratory, 3: audible without stethoscope), and degree of retractions (0: none, 1: mild, 2: moderate, 3: severe) [4, 14].

2.2. PFT Methods. PFT methods included RIP using the SomnoStarPT Unit (Sensormedics, Yorba Linda, CA) and inductance bands (RespiBands Plus; VIASYS Respiratory Care, Yorba Linda, CA). We also evaluated the objective monitoring of real tidal volume, respiratory rate, flow patterns, and end-tidal CO_2 by tidal breathing analysis with PT. For PT, we used a pediatric respiratory profile monitor (CO2SMO Plus; Novametrix, Wallingford, CT). Initially, patients underwent RIP, in which the relationship between thoracic and abdominal contributions to the respiratory effort was assessed (7–9). Bands containing inductive coils were carefully placed around the rib cage at the level of the axillae and around the abdomen mid-way between the xiphisternal junction and the umbilicus. *We used a noncalibrated RIP method for phase and synchrony evaluations and used an abbreviated two-point RIP-tidal breathing calibration for evaluation of labored breathing index (LBI).* The Respitrace device was used to construct Lissajous loops and for calculation of phase angle between the rib cage and abdominal movement associated with respiration (10, 15, 16). Reported phase angle measurements and other indices of asynchrony were based on the average of at least 10 uniform Lissajous loops. The signals from the RIP bands around the rib cage and the abdomen were treated mathematically as sine waves. The phase angle was then calculated with RespiEvents software 5.2 (NIMS, Miami, FL). This parameter and other thoracoabdominal markers express the degree to which chest and abdominal excursion are out of phase. Normally, the rib cage moves outward during inspiration completely in phase with the outward movement of the abdomen (in phase). With progressive increase in the work of breathing, like in airflow obstruction, the rib cage lags behind abdominal movement (out of phase) becoming asynchronous [10].

Recordings were made with the patient in the sitting position. During the test, raw signals and Konno-Mead (Lissajous) loops were monitored to ensure adequate signal quality and to select suitable breathing sequences for analysis with RespiEvents. In this study, we analyzed phase angle (the phase delay between the thoracic and abdominal excursions, or the degree of thoracoabdominal asynchrony [TAA]), phase relation during total breath (PhRTB%), and LBI.

Pulmonary breathing patterns were assessed using a commercially available neonatal/pediatric pulmonary monitoring system. Airway flow and volume were simultaneously measured over time at the airway opening using a pneumotachometer via face mask; mask integrity was monitored for leaks (less than 10% tidal volume change throughout each breath) and a constant tidal volume breathing frequency history was observed for at least 10 breaths (7–9). Airflow was measured with a low dead space volume pneumotachometer and integrated pressure transducer. Respiratory volumes were determined by integrating time and flow signals. Minute ventilation, respiratory rate, peak expiratory flow, and end-tidal CO_2 were calculated by the algorithms incorporated into the monitoring system unit. Flow and volume data, as well as the calculated parameters, were recorded using a software package that interfaces with the pulmonary monitoring unit (Analysis Plus, Novametrix) [11]. Flow and CO_2 graphs were analyzed in real time and after each measurement. Parameters related to timing of peak tidal expiratory flow were extracted from the tidal-flow-volume loops. Flow, volume, and pressure-volume loops as well as CO_2 graphs are excellent tools for assessing airway obstruction and response to bronchodilator therapy. As an additional safety measurement, the transcutaneous saturation of oxygen (SpO_2) was monitored simultaneously, as per ED asthma care protocol, with a small sensor on the finger of the patient.

Tidal breathing measurements required the child to breathe through a mask for 15–30 seconds; the recordings started when we detected a steady and natural respiratory pattern. Based on previous experience, this technique allows repeatability of the study and the mean of the data can then be analyzed with confidence (9). For example, in a patient with a moderate asthma exacerbation and a respiratory rate of approximately 42 breaths per minute, this reading can be obtained in less than 15 seconds. The data of interest included time to peak tidal expiratory flow (t_{PTEF}), volume at peak tidal expiratory flow (V_{PTEF}), total expiratory time (t_E), expired tidal volume (V_E), and the ratios t_{PTEF}/t_E and V_{PTEF}/V_E [5].

2.3. Statistics. Although this was a feasibility pilot study, we calculated a sample size. We did so with the assumption that the proportion of positive in the population is 0.25 (25% asthma admission rate; internal ED quality assurance data). The effect size was selected as the smallest effect that would be important to detect and was clinically reasonable: 0.2 (based on sensitivity of 80% for the PFT). Alpha was set at 0.05. Data analysis was performed with SPSS 17.0 (Chicago, IL) and graphs were created with GraphPad Prism 5 (GraphPad Software, La Jolla, CA). Quantitative variables were summarized using mean and standard deviation, and categorical variables were summarized using frequencies and percentages. A two-sample *t*-test was used to compare the mean the of quantitative variables, and a chi-square test was used to compare the distribution of categorical variables. A one-tailed *t*-test was chosen to analyze PFT data since normative values are known for the data collected. It is understood that with increased work of breathing indices, the values from the PFT levels trend in a specific direction,

as was seen in our patients. The distributional assumptions were checked before analyses.

3. Results

Over a four-month period during 2010-2011, we screened 44 patients and enrolled 40 patients (91% capture rate). Sixty-five percent of the patients were male, and the mean age was 8.7 years (SD 4.8). Fifty percent self-identified as African American, 25% were Caucasian, and 23% were Hispanic. We categorized the remaining 2% as "other," due to the small number of participants. It is also noteworthy that approximately 30% of the patients were preschoolers (age < 5 years).

Fifty-five percent of the patients were classified as a mild-intermittent asthmatic, 30% were mild-persistent asthmatics, 12.5% were moderate-persistent asthmatics, and 2.5% were severe-persistent. This was a convenience sample in that coinvestigators were present in the ED based on scheduled research hours (4–8 hours a day Monday through Friday). The other four patients were not enrolled because nursing initiated treatment prior to performing PFTs. As stated above, PFTs were performed at baseline, prior to treatment with bronchodilators with or without oral corticosteroids. Patients who were unable to cooperate with the PFTs were not excluded unless no data were collected. Complete RIP data are available for 38 patients (95% compliance), and complete breathing pattern data are available for 37 patients (93% compliance).

Our 93% patient acceptance of the study and high compliance rate give insight to the feasibility of performing such a test in the ED. The majority of patients performed the assessment without difficulty. Patients as young as 3 years were able to perform the task with minimal coaching. The cases where RIP data were not obtained involved two patients, aged 3 and 14 years. The cases where data for the tidal breathing analysis were not obtained involved three patients, aged 17, 10, and 3 years. Age, therefore, was not a confounding factor in compliance. Once consent data were obtained, the initial assessment was performed in 15 minutes or less. The investigators did not have to discontinue any of the tests for patient safety reasons. The older and/or more cooperative patients had easier/shorter assessments.

The main outcome measure of the study was the association of PFT and patient disposition (admitted patients versus discharged patients). Demographic information, pertinent clinical information, and vital signs in the two groups are shown in Table 1. Means, standard deviations, and reference values for data obtained in PFTs are available in Table 2. PFT data are presented in box plot graphs (Figures 1 and 2(a)). Asthma score is also presented as a box plot graph (Figure 2(b)).

The RIP results provided the following data: LBI (Figure 1(a)) was higher in the admitted versus discharged patients ($P = 0.04$). Phase angle (Figure 1(b)) showed a significant difference between the admitted and discharged patients ($P = 0.04$). Together, LBI and phase angle indicate that the TAA was increased in admitted patients. Phase

TABLE 1: Summarized demographic data for 40 patients.

Demographics	Admitted	Discharged	P value*
Sex			
Female	4 (29%)	10 (71%)	0.5
Male	10 (39%)	16 (61%)	0.5
Race			
Caucasian	4 (40%)	6 (60%)	
African American	7 (35%)	13 (65%)	
Hispanic	2 (22%)	7 (78%)	
Other/unknown	1 (100%)	0 (0 %)	
Age (years)	7.4 (4.3)	9.4 (5.0)	0.2
Weight (kg)	32.5 (22.1)	47.3 (38.1)	0.2
Height (cm)	130 (29.9)	136.2 (27.2)	0.2
Length of stay (min)	326.85 (77.4)	221.96 (57.8)	0.07
Vital signs			
Heart rate	121.4 (18.8)	105.4 (20.9)	0.02
Respiratory rate	31.9 (9.2)	26.5 (8.1)	0.06
Pulse oximetry	97.2 (1.8)	97.8 (1.9)	0.3
Asthma score	4.3 (0.91)	3.1 (1.5)	0.01
Pertinent history			
Asthma/wheezing	14 (35%)	26 (65%)	0.7
Allergic rhinitis	10 (33%)	20 (67%)	0.7
Eczema	5 (42%)	7 (58%)	0.6
Exposure to smoke	4 (36%)	7 (64%)	0.9

Values represent number of patients (% of total) or mean (SD). *P value for two-tailed t-test or chi-square.

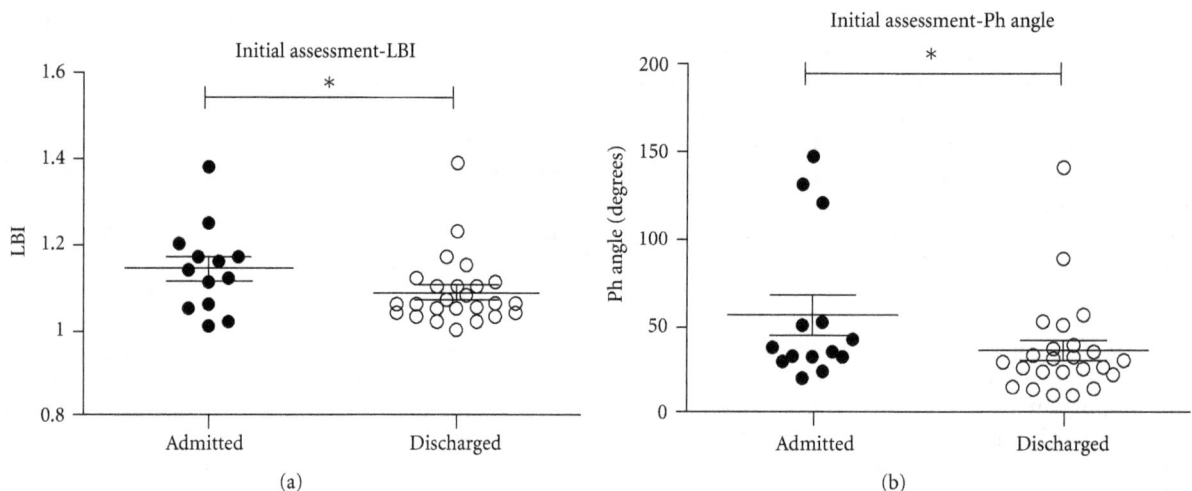

FIGURE 1: Summarized scatter plot results of (a) labored breathing index (LBI) and (b) phase angle (Ph angle) initial assessments as a function of admitted and discharged patients. Data are presented as mean ± SD. *P = 0.04 for 40 patients.

relation (Figure 2(a)) results were not significantly different for the admitted versus discharged patients but did trend up in the admitted group. Compared to the predictive values for healthy children (Table 2), it can be demonstrated that our patients showed significant increases in TAA and thus represent patients presenting with obstructive respiratory disease [6, 12, 15].

Tidal breathing analysis data (Table 2) show that our patient population had a significantly lower tidal volumes ($P < 0.001$) compared with the predicted normal value. The t_{PTEF}/t_E was similar between those patients admitted and discharged, but the value was significantly lower ($P < 0.001$) than the referenced control data [5]. This finding is indicative of the degree of obstruction in our population on presentation to the ED.

Finally, our study supports the strength of the asthma score (Figure 2(b)). Those admitted had a significantly higher ($P < 0.01$) asthma score (two-tailed test).

TABLE 2: Summarized and statistical data for pulmonary function tests (PFT).

	Predicted mean (SEM)	Admitted ($n = 14$) mean (SD)	Discharged ($n = 24$) mean (SD)	*P value
LBI	1.01 (0.01)	1.27 (0.10)	1.08 (0.05)	0.04
Phase angle (°)	15.7 (4.0)	55.5 (43.1)	35.2 (28.3)	0.04
PhRTB (%)	10.1 (1.8)	32.4 (12.1)	28.5 (12.1)	0.17
Asthma score**	n/a	4.3 (0.9)	3.1 (1.5)	0.005
	Predicted average (Range)	Admitted ($n = 14$) mean (SD)	Discharged ($n = 23$) mean (SD)	*P value
$ETCO_2$ (mmHG)	40 (35–45)	34.1 (4.5)	35.2 (3.7)	0.2
Tidal volume (mL/kg)	9 (7–10)	4.7 (1.8)$^\xi$	4.6 (2.0)$^\xi$	0.43
Minute ventilation (L)	7 (5–8)	3.9 (1.2)	4.1 (1.5)	0.3
t_{PTEF}/t_E	0.41 (0.05)	0.21 (0.09)	0.20 (0.08)	0.36
V_{PTEF}/V_E	n/a	1.01 (0.25)	1.0 (0.10)	0.44

LBI: labored breathing index; PhRTB: phase relation during total breath; $ETCO_2$: end-tidal CO_2; t_{PTEF}: time to peak tidal expiratory flow; t_E: total expiratory time; V_{PTEF}: volume at peak tidal expiratory flow; V_E: expired tidal volume. *P value comparing the admitted versus discharged patients; one-tailed t-test. **P value comparing the admitted versus discharged patients; two-tailed t-test ($P < 0.01$). $^\xi$P value comparing admitted and discharged patients to predicted controls; two-tailed t-test, ($P < 0.001$). Predicted values based on known healthy controls (12, 15).

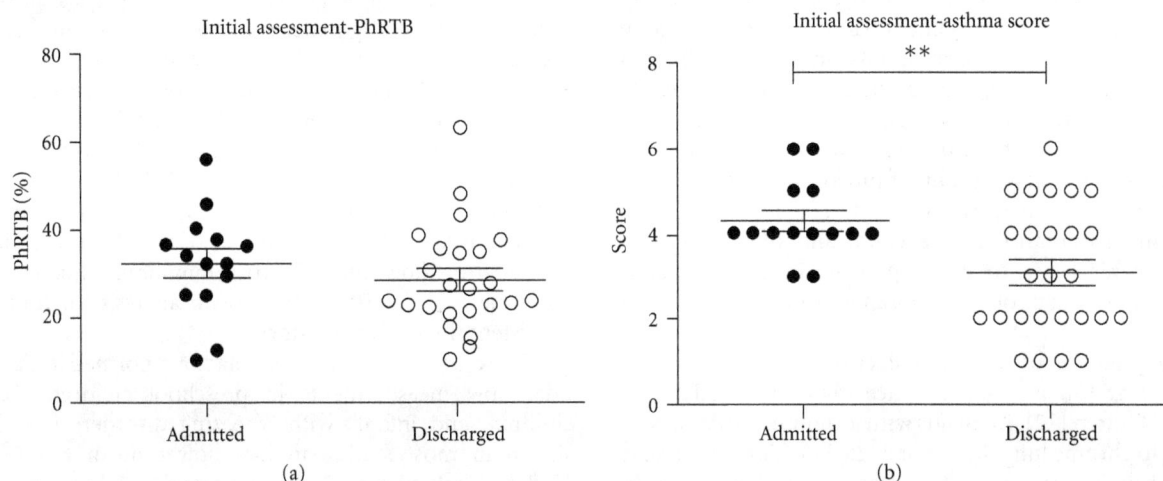

FIGURE 2: Summarized scatter plot results of (a) phase relation during total breath (PhRTB) and (b) asthma score initial assessments as a function of admitted and discharged patients. Data are presented as mean ± SD. **$P < 0.01$ for 40 patients.

4. Discussion

In the United States, asthma accounts for nearly two million ED visits each year [1]. Management decisions are largely subjective and based on exam findings, vital signs, and pulse oximetry [2]. Symptoms are often underestimated by the child and parent. Children with longstanding symptoms are less likely to report symptoms and are more likely to present with hypoxia and a severe, life-threatening asthma exacerbation [3].

In the present pilot study, we demonstrated the feasibility and compliance of noninvasive PFT results in the ED, as well as the predictive value associated with disposition (admission versus discharge) to aid in resource utilization. Since these measurements have not been utilized in this setting, we set out to determine the feasibility of performing these measurements in this setting with the assistance of respiratory therapy, the compliance of patients with the evaluation techniques, and the post-hoc predictive value

of the results (clinicians were initially blinded to the PFT results at the time of admission). Finally, we were interested in a convenient, noninvasive, assessment tool employing tidal breathing analysis that indicates the severity of the wheezing exacerbation. Thus, we are speculating that this objective diagnostic approach may be used in the future to determine from the moment of triage the likelihood that a given patient would require a prolonged ED visit. A decision regarding disposition could then be made early, decreasing the patient's ED length of stay (LOS). Our results supported our hypothesis in that we had a 93% patient acceptance of the study and high compliance rate, which supports the feasibility of performing such a test in the ED. Patients as young as 3 years were able to perform the task with minimal coaching, and age was not a confounding factor in compliance. Once consent data were obtained, the initial assessment was performed in 15 minutes or less.

Pulmonary function tests, including RIP and PT via a mask using a pediatric respiratory profile monitor, have

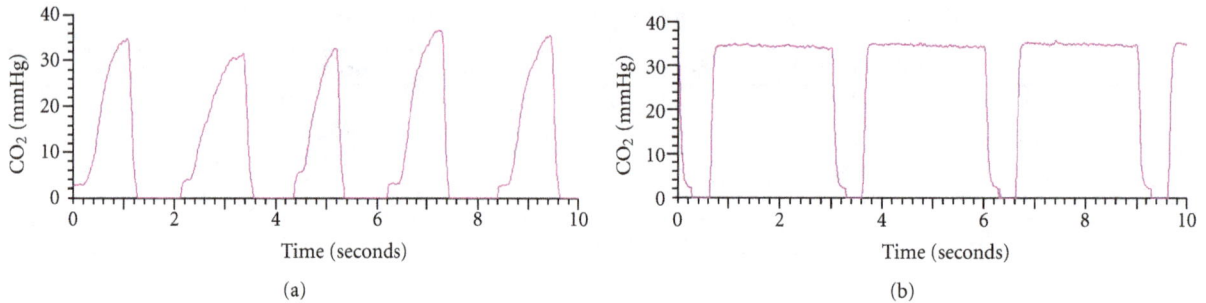

FIGURE 3: Pneumotachography measurements. (a) End-tidal CO_2 pattern in an admitted 12-year-old patient enrolled in our study. Note the rise in end-tidal CO_2 during the last portion of expiration (no clear plateau was observed). (b) End-tidal CO_2 pattern of a control subject (from our pulmonary function test laboratory archives) demonstrating the plateau of normal CO_2 waveform.

been developed to evaluate patients who are minimally cooperative due to age (neonatal/pediatric population) or clinical condition as presented in the ED [5–10, 15, 16]. In earlier studies, these same PFT methods have been utilized in preterm and term infants, infants and children with skeletal dysplasias, and in children with asthma [9, 16–21]. In addition, the American Thoracic Society states that TAA and tidal expiratory flow analyses are promising techniques for assessing lung function in children [5]. Measurements are performed rapidly and repeatedly with minimum disturbance to the child, and there is potential for clinical use to assess patients in acute respiratory distress when other techniques cannot be applied [3].

The presence of TAA is reflective of increased work of breathing [5]. Normal reference values are available in healthy children [12]. In infants with airflow obstruction secondary to chronic lung disease or acute infection, the change in phase angle correlated with changes in lung resistance. In studies involving adolescents with cystic fibrosis and infants with bronchopulmonary dysplasia or bronchiolitis, the phase angle shift calculated from the motion indices of the rib cage versus the abdominal wall was significantly higher when compared to healthy controls [5]. Previous studies have also determined that changes measured by the RIP in infants with airflow obstruction after bronchodilators correlate well with changes in lung resistance and compliance [15]. These data validate the use of RIP in the evaluation and re-evaluation of asthmatics as an objective measure of the severity of asthma/wheezing exacerbation.

As shown in the RIP data, we found that LBI, phase angle, and asthma scores were all significantly higher in those patients admitted versus discharged from the ED. It can be inferred that they had a more severe exacerbation that led to their required admission. Thus, prospective utilization of these parameters in the ED may provide an additional predictive value associated with disposition (admission versus discharge) to aid in resource utilization and to guide therapy. With a larger sample size, it may be possible to predetermine RIP values that further assist in predicting which patients require admission and the type of therapy required. Thus, increased predictability on the decision to admit greatly decreases LOS in the ED.

Furthermore, patient satisfaction would likely increase if LOS in the ED were lessened.

In addition to RIP data, the PT analysis provided pulmonary breathing patterns of tidal flow by simultaneous measurement of flow and volume and by CO_2 analysis of expired gas. As noted in Figure 3, our patients typically demonstrated an uneven rise in end-tidal CO_2 during expiration (compared to normal children). This rise in CO_2 correlates with unequal emptying of CO_2 from lung compartments, indicating lower-airway obstruction. Finally, the PFT equipment allows calculation of the above mentioned indices from flow and CO_2 determinations, thus enabling real-time data collection and breath analysis for leaks and consistent tidal volume history.

There are currently no satisfactory normative data for tidal flow measurements in preschool children. Adults, children, and infants with wheezing disorders have been shown in most studies to have lower mean t_{VEF}/t_E and V_{PTEF}/V_E when compared to controls [5, 22]. In older children, t_{VEF}/t_E has correlated well with FEV_1. Treatment with bronchodilators in wheezing infants and young children has been shown to increase t_{VEF}/t_E. It has been reported that tidal breathing analysis is an objective measurement in asthmatics [3]. In this regard, tidal breathing analysis demonstrated that the patients enrolled in this study had a lower tidal volume compared to the predictive values. Furthermore, a larger sample size may have demonstrated that t_{VEF}/t_E and V_{PTEF}/V_E values correlate better with the current subjective measures for deciding patient admission versus discharge.

Our study had a few inherent limitations. Since the study was a pilot study, the initial results are based on a limited sample size. It is anticipated, however, that these positive outcomes, with regard to feasibility, test compliance, and potential predictability of admission, will enable us to perform a much larger prospective study in which PFT will be utilized in patient disposition and therapy guidance. Post-hoc analysis of the enrolled patients, again due to sample size, did not allow a uniform distribution of patients with regard to gender, age, race, or severity of disease. Furthermore, based on the observational study design, the PFT results could not be utilized to guide therapy or triage patients. With regard to PFT methodology, the RIP techniques have the advantage of being noninvasive, require no calibration or cooperation for phase and synchrony evaluations; however, accurate calibration of the RIP technology is difficult and requires detailed regression analysis using RIP and tidal breathing correlations [15]. In the present study, we used a noncalibrated RIP method for phase and synchrony evaluations and used an abbreviated two point RIP-tidal breathing calibration for evaluation of labored breathing index. Finally, it should be noted that the RIP Lissajous approach was developed for sinusoidal breathing patterns, and not complex patterns associated with some distressed breathing patterns. However, it has been shown that even in distorted loops, the calculated phase angle is still a good estimate of synchrony, and the error has been estimated at <10% [15].

5. Conclusions

Our data support the use of PFTs in the evaluation of asthmatics as an objective measure of the severity of the asthma/wheezing exacerbation in an ED setting. Noneffort-dependent PFTs can provide an objective value that can be used in the evaluation of an acute asthma exacerbation in the ED setting. These tests can be performed safely and efficiently in children with mild-to-moderate asthma on presentation to an ED. PFT results, like the clinical asthma score, are associated with patient disposition (admission versus discharge). As an objective measure of the acuity of an asthmatic patient, PFT results may better guide care, allowing an early decision on whether to admit a patient. This could decrease their LOS. Resource utilization and decreasing LOS in the ED are important in combating the national problem of ED overcrowding and can improve patient satisfaction. Finally, a more accurate sample size and power analysis can be calculated from our preliminary data for future prospective ED studies.

Acknowledgments

This study was funded through Nemours, NIH COBRE Grant 8 P20 GM103464 (the Center for Pediatric Research), and NIGMS T32 GM08562 (ER) pediatric clinical pharmacology fellow funded by NICHD under the Best Pharmaceuticals for Children Act. This work was performed at the Nemours/Alfred I. duPont Hospital for Children. This paper was presented in part at the 2011 Pediatric Academic Societies and Asian Society for Pediatric Research Joint Meeting, Denver, Colorado, and ESPR 2011 52nd Annual Meeting, New Castle, United Kingdom, Pediatric Research.

References

[1] M. Schatz, G. Rachelefsky, and J. A. Krishnan, "Follow-up after acute asthma episodes: what improves future outcomes?" *Proceedings of the American Thoracic Society*, vol. 6, no. 4, pp. 386–393, 2009.

[2] C. A. Camargo Jr., G. Rachelefsky, and M. Schatz, "Managing asthma exacerbations in the emergency department: summary of the national asthma education and prevention program expert panel report 3 guidelines for the management of asthma exacerbations," *Proceedings of the American Thoracic Society*, vol. 6, no. 4, pp. 357–366, 2009.

[3] P. Basek, D. Straub, and J. H. Wildhaber, "Childhood asthma and wheezing disorders," in *Paediatric Pulmonary Function Testing*, J. Hammer and E. Eber, Eds., vol. 33 of *Progress in Respiratory Research Series*, pp. 204–214, Karger, Basle, Switzerland, 2005.

[4] F. M. Ducharme and G. M. Davis, "Respiratory resistance in the emergency department: a reproducible and responsive measure of asthma severity," *Chest*, vol. 113, no. 6, pp. 1566–1572, 1998.

[5] N. Beydon, S. D. Davis, E. Lombardi et al., "An official American thoracic society/european respiratory society statement: pulmonary function testing in preschool children," *American Journal of Respiratory and Critical Care Medicine*, vol. 175, no. 12, pp. 1304–1345, 2007.

[6] C. K. van der Ent, H. J. L. Brackel, J. D. van Laag, and J. M. Bogaard, "Tidal breathing analysis as a measure of airway obstruction in children three years of age and older," *American Journal of Respiratory and Critical Care Medicine*, vol. 153, no. 4, pp. 1253–1258, 1996.

[7] T. H. Shaffer, M. Delivoria-Papadopoulos, E. Arcinue, P. Paez, and A. B. Dubois, "Pulmonary function in premature lambs during the first few hours of life," *Respiration Physiology*, vol. 28, no. 2, pp. 179–188, 1976.

[8] M. J. Wagaman, J. G. Shutack, A. S. Moomjian, J. G. Schwartz, T. H. Shaffer, and W. W. Fox, "Improved oxygenation and lung compliance with prone positioning of neonates," *Journal of Pediatrics*, vol. 94, no. 5, pp. 787–791, 1979.

[9] M. R. Wolfson, J. S. Greenspan, K. S. Deoras, J. L. Allen, and T. H. Shaffer, "Effect of position on the mechanical interaction between the rib cage and abdomen in preterm infants," *Journal of Applied Physiology*, vol. 72, no. 3, pp. 1032–1038, 1992.

[10] J. L. Allen, J. S. Greenspan, K. S. Deoras, E. Keklikian, M. R. Wolfson, and T. H. Shaffer, "Interaction between chest wall motion and lung mechanics in normal infants and infants with bronchopulmonary dysplasia," *Pediatric Pulmonology*, vol. 11, no. 1, pp. 37–43, 1991.

[11] T. L. Miller, T. J. Blackson, T. H. Shaffer, and S. M. Touch, "Tracheal gas insufflation-augmented continuous positive airway pressure in a spontaneously breathing model of neonatal respiratory distress," *Pediatric Pulmonology*, vol. 38, no. 5, pp. 386–395, 2004.

[12] O. H. Mayer, R. G. Clayton Sr., A. F. Jawad, J. M. McDonough, and J. L. Allen, "Respiratory inductance plethysmography in healthy 3- to 5-year-old children," *Chest*, vol. 124, no. 5, pp. 1812–1819, 2003.

[13] Y. Durani, D. Brecher, D. Walmsley, M. W. Attia, and J. M. Loiselle, "The emergency severity index version 4: reliability in pediatric patients," *Pediatric Emergency Care*, vol. 25, no. 8, pp. 504–507, 2009.

[14] F. M. Ducharme and G. M. Davis, "Measurement of respiratory resistance in the emergency department: feasibility in young children with acute asthma," *Chest*, vol. 111, no. 6, pp. 1519–1525, 1997.

[15] J. L. Allen, M. R. Wolfson, K. McDowell, and T. H. Shaffer, "Thoracoabdominal asynchrony in infants with airflow obstruction," *American Review of Respiratory Disease*, vol. 141, no. 2 I, pp. 337–342, 1990.

[16] R. Locke, J. S. Greenspan, T. H. Shaffer, S. D. Rubenstein, and M. R. Wolfson, "Effect of nasal CPAP on thoracoabdominal motion in neonates with respiratory insufficiency," *Pediatric Pulmonology*, vol. 11, no. 3, pp. 259–264, 1991.

[17] K. S. Deoras, J. S. Greenspan, M. R. Wolfson, E. N. Keklikian, T. H. Shaffer, and J. L. Allen, "Effects of inspiratory resistive loading on chest wall motion and ventilation: differences between preterm and full-term infants," *Pediatric Research*, vol. 32, no. 5, pp. 589–594, 1992.

[18] T. L. Miller, C. Palmer, T. H. Shaffer, and M. R. Wolfson, "Neonatal chest wall suspension splint: a novel and noninvasive method for support of lung volume," *Pediatric Pulmonology*, vol. 39, no. 6, pp. 512–520, 2005.

[19] T. L. Miller, T. Cox, T. Blackson, D. Paul, K. Weiss, and T. H. Shaffer, "Pulmonary function assessment in an infant with Barnes syndrome: proactive evaluation for surgical intervention," *Pediatrics*, vol. 118, no. 4, pp. e1264–e1267, 2006.

[20] A. G. Didario, M. A. Whelan, W. H. Hwan et al., "Efficacy of chest physiotherapy in pediatric patients with acute asthma exacerbations," *Pediatric Asthma, Allergy and Immunology*, vol. 22, no. 2, pp. 69–74, 2009.

[21] M. E. Rodriguez, W. G. Mackenzie, C. Ditro, T. L. Miller, A. Chidekel, and T. H. Shaffer, "Skeletal dysplasias: evaluation with impulse oscillometry and thoracoabdominal motion analysis," *Pediatric Pulmonology*, vol. 45, no. 7, pp. 679–686, 2010.

[22] K. H. Carlsen and K. C. L. Carlsen, "Tidal breathing techniques," *European Respiratory Monograph*, vol. 47, pp. 35–45, 2010.

23

Radiotherapy for Oligometastases and Oligo-Recurrence of Bone in Prostate Cancer

Ken-ichi Tabata,[1] Yuzuru Niibe,[2] Takefumi Satoh,[1]
Hideyasu Tsumura,[1] Masaomi Ikeda,[1] Satoru Minamida,[1] Tetsuo Fujita,[1] Daisuke Ishii,[1]
Masatsugu Iwamura,[1] Kazushige Hayakawa,[2] and Shiro Baba[1]

[1] Department of Urology, Kitasato University School of Medicine, 1-15-1 Kitasato, Minami-ku, Sagamihara,
Kanagawa 252-0375, Japan
[2] Department of Radiology and Radiation Oncology, Kitasato University School of Medicine, 1-15-1 Kitasato, Minami-ku, Sagamihara,
Kanagawa 252-0375, Japan

Correspondence should be addressed to Ken-ichi Tabata, ktabata@med.kitasato-u.ac.jp

Academic Editor: Hideomi Yamashita

Purpose. To retrospectively evaluate the clinical significance of radiotherapy for oligometastases of bone in prostate cancer (PCa). *Methods and Materials.* Between 2003 and 2008, 35 PCa patients with oligometastases of bone were treated with radiotherapy. *Results.* The median radiotherapy dose was 40 Gy. The 3-year overall survival rates for all patients, for patients that received a radiotherapy dose of $\geq$40 Gy ($n = 21$) and for those that received <40 Gy ($n = 14$), were 77.2%, 90.5%, and 50.0%, respectively. Fourteen out of 16 patients (87.5%) who had pain were improved 1 month after radiotherapy. The median duration of pain relief was 12 months. Pathological fracture and spinal cord compression (SCC) were not seen at the treated sites but developed at nonirradiated sites in three patients (8.6%) and in one patient (2.8%), respectively. Although the high-dose group ($\geq$40 Gy) achieved better survival than the low-dose group (<40 Gy), it was not independent prognostic factor in multivariable analysis. *Conclusions.* Radiotherapy of bone oligometastases in PCa was effective for long-term pain relief. Pathological fracture and SCC were not seen at the treated sites. A larger clinical trial is warranted to study the actual benefit following radiotherapy for oligometastases of bone in PCa.

1. Introduction

Patients with bone metastases from prostate cancer frequently experience skeletal morbidities as a result of their disease. Skeletal-related events (SREs), such as pathological fractures and spinal cord compression, are major causes of morbidity in patients with prostate cancer and may lead to other comorbidities including pain [1, 2].

Soloway et al. [3] reported an analysis of survival in prostate cancer patients with bone metastases using a semi-quantitative grading system based upon the extent of disease (EOD) on the bone scintigram. They concluded that the EOD on the scintigram correlated with survival. This study also demonstrated that the 2-year survival rate in prostate cancer patients with EOD I, defined as having fewer than six

bone metastases on bone scan, was 94%. Thus the clinical course of prostate cancer patients with a small number of bone metastases is relatively long. Successful management of bone metastases during these periods is essential for reducing the skeletal complications and for maximizing patients' quality of life. Therefore, we must carefully manage metastatic bone disease from an early stage in prostate cancer.

The aim of radiotherapy for metastatic bone disease is not only relief of bone pain but also healing and prevention of pathological fractures, with anticipated effects including improved mobility, function, and quality of life [4, 5]. In addition to these effects, the notion of oligometastases and oligo-recurrence has recently been proposed [6–9], with the suggestion that local therapy to a small number of gross metastatic sites and recurrences may result in prolonged survival or even cure [6–10]. The most favorable prognostic factor of oligometastases is the state of primary lesion, which means that oligometastatic patients with controlled primary lesions achieve significant better survival than those with active primary lesions [11, 12]. The notion of oligo-recurrence overcomes this problem. Oligo-recurrence is the state that cancer patients with one to several metastases or recurrences have controlled primary lesions. Niibe and Hayakawa proposed this notion as oligo-recurrence [9].

The objective of this retrospective study was to evaluate the effect of radiotherapy on bone oligometastases and oligo-recurrence in patients with prostate cancer. We were also interested in the disease behavior in patients with bone oligometastases and oligo-recurrence.

2. Methods and Materials

Between January 2003 and December 2008, 136 Japanese men diagnosed with prostate cancer with bone metastases received radiotherapy directed at the metastatic bone lesions at Kitasato University Hospital, Japan. Their medical records were evaluated retrospectively. Thirty-five of the patients had bone metastases of EOD I, referred to as oligometastases or oligo-recurrence of bone in this study. EOD I has been defined by Soloway et al. [3] as the presence of fewer than six bone metastases on bone scan, with each site being less than 50% the size of a vertebral body. Indications for radiation to metastatic bone sites in patients with EOD I prostate cancer were bone pain or spinal cord compression, pathological fracture, or prevention of SREs.

We analyzed the overall survival and the effect of radiotherapy on pain relief and the incidence of SREs, including pathological fracture and spinal cord compression. Short-term pain relief was determined by comparing symptoms prior to radiotherapy to that 1 month after its completion. Pain relief response was classified as follows by taking the best point from the start of treatment: "response," when pain decreased or the daily dosage of the analgesic was decreased; "no change," when pain was unchanged and the dosage of the analgesic did not change; and "progressive disease," when pain increased or the dosage of the analgesic was increased.

For long-term pain relief, the time to progression was defined as the interval between the initial date of radiotherapy and the date when increased pain or increased dosage of the analgesic was first documented after the best pain relief response at treated sites.

Local treatment for prostate cancer might affect overall survival we divide patients into oligo-recurrence group which has treated enough locally such as prostatectomy and oligometastases group which has not been treated with local therapy for the prostate.

Overall survival was calculated as the time interval from the last day of radiotherapy for bone metastases to the time of death. Progression-free survival for bone pain was defined as the proportion of patients surviving with decreased pain from the onset of pain relief to pain relapse at a treated site. Patients were followed for a median of 36 months (range, 1–70 months) after radiotherapy.

Radiotherapy was performed using one port postero-anterior field for the middle thoracic spine/upper lumbar spine and two ports anteroposterior parallel opposed fields for the other spine, legs, and pelvic bone. The energy of radiotherapy was 6 or 10 MV X-rays.

The survival rate was calculated using the Kaplan-Meier method. Differences in patient characteristics between the two groups were compared by chi-square test or Fisher exact test, as appropriate. Multivariable analysis was performed by employing the Cox proportional hazards regression model to examine the interaction between total radiotherapy dose (≥ 40 Gy versus <40 Gy) and other clinical variables and to estimate the independent prognostic effect of radiotherapy on survival by adjusting for confounding factors. Within the present study population, there were 11 deaths, which allow a maximum of two variables to be included in a multivariable regression model. Therefore all potential confounding factors of radiotherapy dose were reduced to one single composite characteristic by applying a propensity score [13]. The conventional P value < 0.05 was used to determine the level of statistical significance. Analyses were performed with Stata version 11 for Windows (Stata, Chicago, IL, USA).

3. Results

Table 1 shows the baseline characteristics of the study population according to the total radiotherapy dose. In prior treatment to the primary site, radical prostatectomy was performed in 10 patients, and radiotherapy including conformal external beam radiotherapy (3DCRT) alone and high dose rate brachytherapy (HDR) in combination with 3DCRT (HDR/3DCRT) was performed in eight patients. These eighteen patients were to be in the state of oligo-recurrence. Other seventeen patients are called as oligometastases group in this study. All 35 patients received hormonal therapy. Nine patients received Zoledronic acid. There were significant differences in baseline serum prostate-specific antigen, Eastern Cooperative Oncology Group performance status (ECOG PS) and oligostatus between total radiotherapy doses of ≥ 40 Gy and <40 Gy (Table 1).

Treatment characteristics are given in Table 2. The median local radiotherapy dose was 40 Gy (range, 30–50 Gy) in 10–25 fractions. The median biologically effective dose (BED) was 67 Gy$_3$ (range, 50–92 Gy$_3$) if α/β of 3 was applied. The reasons for radiotherapy were pain relief in 16 patients (45.7%), prevention of SREs in 17 patients (48.6%), and spinal cord compression in 2 patients (5.7%).

Figure 1 shows the overall survival curves after radiotherapy for metastatic bone disease. The 3-year overall survival rate for all patients was 77.2%. The overall survival rate of radiotherapy doses of >40 Gy and of <40 Gy was 90.5% and 50.0%, respectively ($P = 0.0116$). There is no significant difference between Oligo-recurrence group and Oligometastases group (Figure 2). A Cox proportional hazards model was applied to estimate the effect of radiotherapy dose on overall survival. The crude hazard ratio (HR) of high-dose group (≥ 40 Gy) compared with low-dose group (<40 Gy) was 0.231 (95% CI, 0.067–0.798; $P = 0.021$), which indicated that high-dose group decreased the hazard of

Table 1: Patient characteristics (35 patients).

Variables	<40 Gy ($n = 14$)	≥40 Gy ($n = 21$)	Total ($n = 35$)	P value*
Age	72 (66–85)	70 (55–93)	71.5 (55–93)[†]	0.206
Baseline PSA (ng/mL)	72.0 (0.3–964)[†]	11.0 (0.1–142)[†]	34.0 (0.1–964)[†]	0.047
ECOG PS				
0–1	8	21	29 (82.9%)	0.002
≥2	6	0	6 (17.1%)	
No. of bone metastases	3 (1–5)[†]	2 (1–5)[†]	2 (1–5)[†]	0.218
CRPC	5 (35.7%)	2 (9.5%)	7 (20%)	0.090
Pain				
Yes	9 (64.3%)	7 (33.3%)	16 (45.7%)	0.094
Spinal cord compression				
Yes	2 (14.3%)	0	2 (5.7%)	0.153
Pathologic fracture				
Yes	4 (28.6%)	1 (4.8%)	4 (14.3%)	0.134
Oligostatus				
oligo-recurrence group	2 (14.3%)	16 (76.2%)	18 (51.4%)	0.000

Abbreviations. PSA: prostate-specific antigen; ECOG PS: Eastern Cooperative Oncology Group performance status; CRPC: castration-resistant prostate cancer.
[†]Median (range).
*Significance of difference between groups determined by chi-square test or Fisher exact test, as appropriate. $P < 0.05$ considered significant.

Table 2: Treatment characteristics.

Variables	Total $n = 35$
Total radiation dose (Gy)	40 (30–50)[†]
Biological effective dose (Gy$_3$)	67 (50–92)[†]
Reasons for radiotherapy	
Pain	16 (45.7%)
Spinal cord compression	2 (5.7%)
Prevention for SREs	17 (48.6%)
Treatment site	
Spine	15 (42.9%)
Femur	17 (48.6%)
Pelvis/hip	3 (8.6%)
Sternum	1 (2.8%)
Ribs	2 (5.7%)
Overall treatment time (days)	28 (12–43)[†]

Abbreviations. SREs: skeletal-related events.
[†]Median (range).

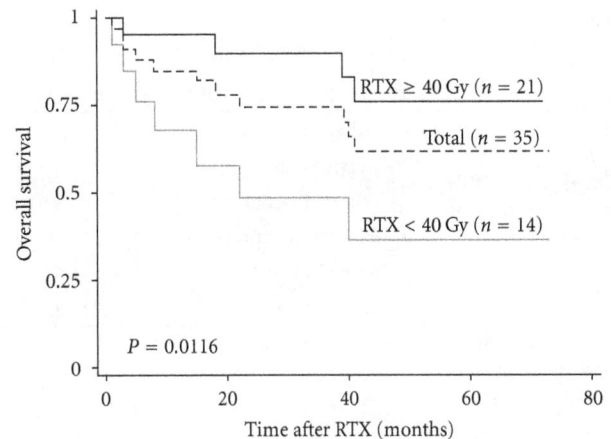

Figure 1: The overall survival curves for all patients ($n = 35$) and those that received a total radiotherapy dose of ≥40 Gy ($n = 21$) or <40 Gy ($n = 14$). RTX, radiotherapy.

death by four times that of low-dose group (Table 4). Then we performed multivariable analysis using propensity score to adjust the effect of receiving high-dose radiotherapy (≥40 Gy) given by other confounding variables including age, baseline PSA, ECOG PS, castration-resistant prostate cancer (CRPC), oligostatus into a single estimator. The results revealed that the HR of radiotherapy dose (≥40 Gy versus <40 Gy) changed to 0.630 (95% CI, 0.098–4.285; $P = 0.637$), which suggests that high-dose radiotherapy was not an independent risk factor for overall survival (Table 4).

The treatment outcomes are shown in Table 3. At 1 month after radiotherapy, 14 out of 16 patients (87.5%) with pain gained relief. Five of these patients (31.3%), however, experienced pain relapse in the treated sites. Figure 3 shows the progression-free survival for bone pain. One-year progression-free survival was 64.8%, and the median duration of pain relief was 12 months (range, 5–68 months). Two patients had a relapse of bone pain within 1 year after radiotherapy in ≥40 Gy and <40 Gy, respectively. With regard to SREs, spinal cord compression and pathological fracture were not seen at treated sites after radiotherapy. On the other hand, there were three patients (8.6%) with pathological fracture and one patient (2.8%) with spinal cord compression in nontreated sites after radiotherapy.

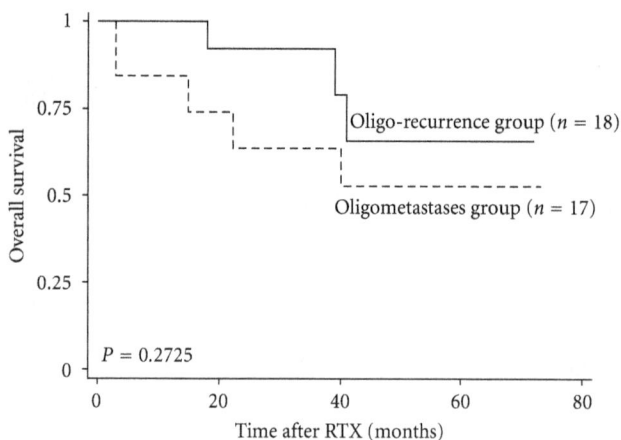

FIGURE 2: The overall survival curves for oligo-recurrence group ($n = 18$) and oligometastases group ($n = 17$). RTX, radiotherapy.

TABLE 3: Treatment outcomes.

Variables		No. of patients (%)
Pain relief ($n = 16$)	Short-term response	14 (87.5)
	No change	2 (12.5)
	Progressive disease	0
	Long-term progression	5 (31.3)
	Time to progression (months)	9 (5–15)[†]
Incidence of SREs after radiotherapy ($n = 35$)	Pathologic fracture	
	Treatment site	0
	Nontreatment site	3 (8.6)
	Spinal cord compression	
	Treatment site	0
	Nontreatment site	1 (2.8)

Abbreviations. SREs: skeletal-related events.
[†]Median (range).

4. Discussion

Prostate cancer is the most frequently diagnosed cancer and is second only to lung cancer as the leading cause of cancer-related deaths among in the USA. In Japan, it is estimated that the incidence and mortality cases for prostate cancer will increase 3-fold by 2020 compared with 2000. Previous studies showed that independent prognostic variables for survival among patients with prostate cancer were patient age, time to androgen-independent disease, the extent of metastatic disease, and number of metastases on bone scan [14]. Several studies have focused on quantifying or stratifying risk according to the extent of bone involvement and the number of metastatic sites of prostate cancer [3, 15–17]. They have shown that the number of metastatic lesions is a powerful prognostic indicator of the outcome in metastatic disease. Among these studies, Soloway et al. [3] reported that a scale based on a count of the number of metastatic bone lesions on bone scan was predictive when ≤5 (EOD I) or >20 (EOD IV)

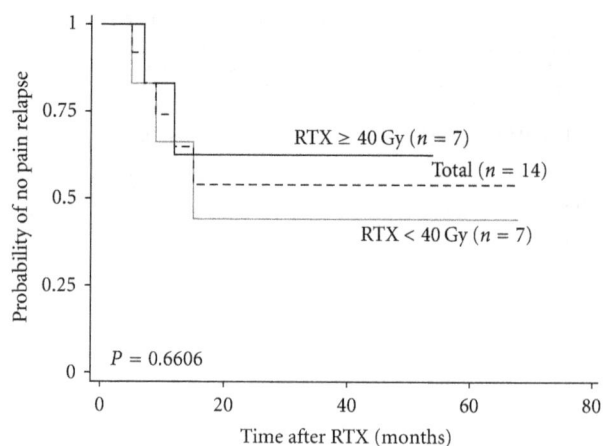

FIGURE 3: The progression-free survival curves for patients with bone pain who had pain relief response at 1 month after radiotherapy ($n = 14$) and with received total radiotherapy dose of ≥40 Gy ($n = 7$) and <40 Gy ($n = 7$). RTX, radiotherapy.

lesions were present. On the basis of this result, we grouped our prostate cancer patients with bone metastases likewise and applied radiotherapy to metastatic bone disease in EOD I cases (i.e., oligometastases and oligo-recurrence of bone in prostate cancer) regardless of the presence of the bone pain. Results of this study revealed that the 3-year overall survival rate after radiotherapy to oligometastases or oligo-recurrence of bone was 77.2% in prostate cancer. To our knowledge, no previous study has examined overall survival in this patient population. Although the widely accepted treatment for patients with metastatic prostate cancer is hormonal therapy, we should manage oligometastases, oligo-recurrence, and polymetastases separately because of their difference in prognosis. Hellman and Weichselbaum [7] reported that local therapy such as radiotherapy and surgery for one or several distant metastatic sites could be efficacious for survival in patients with oligometastases. Niibe et al. [8] and Niibe and Hayakawa [9] also proposed oligo-recurrence, a more strictly defined type of oligometastases, in which one or several metastatic or recurrent lesions occur with the controlled primary lesions. They suggest that the local treatment of the metastatic or recurrent lesions could improve prognosis. Many studies have been performed along these lines [6–10]. Niibe et al. [8] also indicated that high-dose radiotherapy for bone metastases could contribute to patient survival in breast cancer. In the current study, because patient baseline characteristics were different between groups receiving a total radiation dose of ≥40 Gy or <40 Gy and there is few events on survival in each group, usual multivariable analysis could not be performed without propensity score. Therefore, radiotherapy for oligometastases and oligo-recurrence of bone in patients with prostate cancer is worth prospective testing as an approach to improving survival.

The Radiation Therapy Oncology Group (RTOG) has previously studied various treatment fraction regimens for palliation of bone metastases. The RTOG 9714 study, a recent phase III trial centered on prostate cancer and breast cancer

TABLE 4: Univariable and multivariable analysis for the effect of radiotherapy on survival.

Factors	Univariable analysis			Multivariable analysis		
	HR	95% CI	P value*	HR	95% CI	P value*
RTX (≥40 Gy versus <40 Gy)	0.231	0.067–0.798	0.021	0.630	0.098–4.285	0.637
Propensity score†	n/d	n/d	n/d	0.300	0.024–3.763	0.351

Abbreviations. HR: hazard ratio; n/d: not done.
*Analyses were performed using Cox proportional hazard regression.
†Multivariable model indicates adjusted effect of RTX by applying propensity score which is a conditional probability of receiving RTX (≥40 Gy) given by other factors including age, baseline PSA, performance status, castration-resistant prostate cancer, and oligostatus.

with osseous metastases, revealed 8 Gy per single fraction was equal to 30 Gy in 10 fractions for the pain relief of osseous metastases at 3 months after irradiation [18]. However, this study evaluation point for pain relief is very early, at 3 months after radiotherapy. This is not appropriate appreciation for oligometastases and oligo-recurrence because of long-term survival. Niibe et al. reported high-dose radiation contributed to long-term pain relief in breast cancer [8]. Milano et al. also reported high-dose stereotactic body radiotherapy for bone oligometastases, oligo-recurrence was efficacious [19]. Moreover, other investigation in the same population demonstrated that the retreatment rate was significantly higher in the 8 Gy arm (18%) than in the 30 Gy arm (9%) [20].

In Japan, longer courses of radiotherapy with higher total doses of radiation remain the most commonly used, typically with a regimen of 30–40 Gy given in 10–20 treatment sessions. While conventional radiotherapy was used in this study, the results reveal a median duration of pain relief of 12 months, with approximately half of the patients experiencing relapsed bone pain. The bone pain trial which include 34% of prostate cancer patients in patient population showed 40% of pain relapse at 12 months [18]. Although those patient characteristics are different from our study, we considered our result in duration of pain relief is comparable with that study. However, these results indicate that conventional radiotherapy alone for pain relief may be inadequate for oligometastases and oligo-recurrence of bone in prostate cancer. Consequently, for the management of bone pain in patients with prostate cancer, we should consider altering the radiation dose or fraction using high-dose SBRT combining it with treatments such as systemic chemotherapy, zoledronic acid, and painkiller. Punglia et al. [21] reported that as improving systemic therapy, local therapy got survival benefit dramatically. Niibe and Hayakawa [9] also reported the significance of systemic therapy for oligometastases and oligo-recurrence treated by local therapy.

For patients without bone pain in this study, the main purpose of radiotherapy was prevention of SREs, including pathological fracture and spinal cord compression. The current study demonstrated that the complications were not seen in treated sites; however, three patients experienced pathological fracture and one patient had spinal cord compression in a nontreated site after radiotherapy. These results indicate that radiotherapy for metastatic bone disease may potentially decrease the incidence of SREs in treated sites. Both pathological fractures and spinal cord compression

with neurologic deficit negatively affect quality of life [22]. Moreover neurologic recovery is unlikely if spinal compression is not relieved within 24–48 hours [23]. Therefore, efforts have recently been made to predict sites of fracture and to prevent the occurrence of a fracture by prophylactic therapy, which includes radiotherapy [24–26].

Our study has several limitations. Because it is retrospective, patient populations differ between total radiation dose received (≥40 Gy and <40 Gy). There was also no control group, that is, one that did not receive radiotherapy. Therefore, in the future, a large prospective study is required to investigate the actual benefits, including overall survival associated with radiotherapy for oligometastases and oligo-recurrence of bone in prostate cancer.

Conflict of Interests

The authors declare that they have no conflict of Interests.

References

[1] A. Berruti, L. Dogliotti, R. Bitossi et al., "Incidence of skeletal complications in patients with bone metastatic prostate cancer and hormone refractory disease: predictive role of bone resorption and formation markers evaluated at baseline," Journal of Urology, vol. 164, no. 4, pp. 1248–1253, 2000.

[2] R. C. M. Pelger, V. Soerdjbalie-Maikoe, and N. A. T. Hamdy, "Strategies for management of prostate cancer-related bone pain," Drugs and Aging, vol. 18, no. 12, pp. 899–911, 2001.

[3] M. S. Soloway, S. W. Hardeman, D. Hickey et al., "Stratification of patients with metastatic prostate cancer based on extent of disease on initial bone scan," Cancer, vol. 61, no. 1, pp. 195–202, 1988.

[4] S. Koswig and V. Budach, "Recalcification and pain relief following radiotherapy for bone metastases. A randomized trial of 2 different fractionation schedules (10 × 3 Gy vs 1 × 8 Gy)," Strahlentherapie und Onkologie, vol. 175, no. 10, pp. 500–508, 1999.

[5] E. Steenland, J. Leer, H. Van Houwelingen et al., "The effect of a single fraction compared to multiple fractions on painful bone metastases: a global analysis of the Dutch Bone Metastasis Study," Radiotherapy and Oncology, vol. 52, no. 2, pp. 101–109, 1999.

[6] Y. Niibe, M. Kenjo, T. Kazumoto et al., "Multi-institutional study of radiation therapy for isolated para-aortic lymph node recurrence in uterine cervical carcinoma: 84 subjects of a population of more than 5,000," International Journal of Radiation Oncology Biology Physics, vol. 66, no. 5, pp. 1366–1369, 2006.

[7] S. Hellman and R. R. Weichselbaum, "Oligometastases," Journal of Clinical Oncology, vol. 13, no. 1, pp. 8–10, 1995.

[8] Y. Niibe, M. Kuranami, K. Matsunaga et al., "Value of high-dose radiation therapy for isolated osseous metastasis in breast cancer in terms of oligo-recurrence," *Anticancer Research*, vol. 28, no. 6, pp. 3929–3931, 2008.

[9] Y. Niibe and K. Hayakawa, "Oligometastases and oligo-recurrence: the new era of cancer therapy," *Japanese Journal of Clinical Oncology*, vol. 40, no. 2, Article ID hyp167, pp. 107–111, 2010.

[10] T. Inoue, N. Katoh, H. Aoyama et al., "Clinical outcomes of stereotactic brain and/or body radiotherapy for patients with oligometastatic lesions," *Japanese Journal of Clinical Oncology*, vol. 40, no. 8, Article ID hyq044, pp. 788–794, 2010.

[11] Y. Niibe, T. Nishimura, T. Inoue et al., "Oligometastases of brain only in patients with non-small cell lung cancer (NSCLC) treated with stereotactic irradiation (STI): a multi-institutional study," *International Journal of Radiation Oncology*, vol. 78, p. S497, 2010.

[12] J. L. Lopez Guerra, D. Gomez, Y. Zhuang et al., "Prognostic impact of radiation therapy to the primary tumor in patients with non-small cell lung cancer and oligometastasis at diagnosis," *International Journal of Radiation Oncology*, vol. 84, no. 1, pp. 61–67, 2012.

[13] M. S. Cepeda, R. Boston, J. T. Farrar, and B. L. Strom, "Comparison of logistic regression versus propensity score when the number of events is low and there are multiple confounders," *American Journal of Epidemiology*, vol. 158, no. 3, pp. 280–287, 2003.

[14] R. B. Wyatt, R. F. Sánchez-Ortiz, C. G. Wood, E. Ramirez, C. Logothetis, and C. A. Pettaway, "Prognostic factors for survival among Caucasian, African-American and Hispanic men with androgen-independent prostate cancer," *Journal of the National Medical Association*, vol. 96, no. 12, pp. 1587–1593, 2004.

[15] P. Sabbatini, S. M. Larson, A. Kremer et al., "Prognostic significance of extent of disease in bone in patients with androgen-independent prostate cancer," *Journal of Clinical Oncology*, vol. 17, no. 3, pp. 948–957, 1999.

[16] A. Rana, G. D. Chisholm, M. Khan, S. S. Sekharjit, M. V. Merrick, and R. A. Elton, "Patterns of bone metastasis and their prognostic significance in patients with carcinoma of the prostate," *British Journal of Urology*, vol. 72, no. 6, pp. 933–936, 1993.

[17] K. Yamashita, K. Denno, T. Ueda et al., "Prognostic significance of bone metastases in patients with metastatic prostate cancer," *Cancer*, vol. 71, no. 4, pp. 1297–1302, 1993.

[18] J. R. Yarnold, "8 Gy single fraction radiotherapy for the treatment of metastatic skeletal pain: randomised comparison with a multifraction schedule over 12 months of patient follow-up," *Radiotherapy and Oncology*, vol. 52, no. 2, pp. 111–121, 1999.

[19] M. T. Milano, A. W. Katz, M. C. Schell, A. Philip, and P. Okunieff, "Descriptive analysis of oligometastatic lesions treated with curative-intent stereotactic body radiotherapy," *International Journal of Radiation Oncology Biology Physics*, vol. 72, no. 5, pp. 1516–1522, 2008.

[20] W. F. Harstell, C. B. Scott, D. W. Bruner et al., "Randomized trial of short- versus long-course radiotherapy for palliation of painful bone metastases," *Journal of the National Cancer Institute*, vol. 97, no. 11, pp. 798–804, 2005.

[21] R. S. Punglia, M. Morrow, E. P. Winer, and J. R. Harris, "Local therapy and survival in breast cancer," *The New England Journal of Medicine*, vol. 356, no. 23, pp. 2399–2348, 2007.

[22] K. P. Weinfurt, Y. Li, L. D. Castel et al., "The significance of skeletal-related events for the health-related quality of life of patients with metastatic prostate cancer," *Annals of Oncology*, vol. 16, no. 4, pp. 579–584, 2005.

[23] T. Siegal and T. Siegal, "Vertebral body resection for epidural compression by malignant tumors. Results of forty-seven consecutive operative procedures," *Journal of Bone and Joint Surgery—Series A*, vol. 67, no. 3, pp. 375–382, 1985.

[24] D. Rades, F. Fehlauer, R. Schulte et al., "Prognostic factors for local control and survival after radiotherapy of metastatic spinal cord compression," *Journal of Clinical Oncology*, vol. 24, no. 21, pp. 3388–3393, 2006.

[25] A. Bayley, M. Milosevic, R. Blend et al., "A prospective study of factors predicting clinically occult spinal cord compression in patients with metastatic prostate carcinoma," *Cancer*, vol. 92, no. 2, pp. 303–310, 2001.

[26] R. Venkitaraman, Y. Barbachano, D. P. Dearnaley et al., "Outcome of early detection and radiotherapy for occult spinal cord compression," *Radiotherapy and Oncology*, vol. 85, no. 3, pp. 469–472, 2007.

24

Mannose-Binding Lectin Promoter Polymorphisms and Gene Variants in Pulmonary Tuberculosis Patients from Cantabria (Northern Spain)

J.-Gonzalo Ocejo-Vinyals,[1] Lucía Lavín-Alconero,[1]
Pablo Sánchez-Velasco,[1] M.-Ángeles Guerrero-Alonso,[1] Fernando Ausín,[1]
M.-Carmen Fariñas,[2] and Francisco Leyva-Cobián[1]

[1] *Servicio de Inmunología, Hospital Universitario Marqués de Valdecilla, Avenida de Valdecilla s/n, 39008 Santander, Spain*
[2] *Unidad de Enfermedades Infecciosas, Departamento de Medicina Interna, Hospital Universitario Marqués de Valdecilla,*
 Universidad de Cantabria, 39011 Santander, Spain

Correspondence should be addressed to J.-Gonzalo Ocejo-Vinyals, jgocejo@humv.es

Academic Editor: José R. Lapa e Silva

Mannose-binding lectin is a central molecule of the innate immune system. Mannose-binding lectin 2 promoter polymorphisms and structural variants have been associated with susceptibility to tuberculosis. However, contradictory results among different populations have been reported, resulting in no convincing evidence of association between mannose-binding lectin 2 and susceptibility to tuberculosis. For this reason, we conducted a study in a well genetically conserved Spanish population in order to shed light on this controversial association. We analysed the six promoter and structural mannose-binding lectin 2 gene variants in 107 patients with pulmonary tuberculosis and 441 healthy controls. Only D variant and HYPD haplotype were significantly more frequents in controls which would indicate that this allele could confer protection against pulmonary tuberculosis, but this difference disappeared after statistical correction. Neither the rest of alleles nor the haplotypes were significantly associated with the disease. These results would indicate that mannose-binding lectin promoter polymorphisms and gene variants would not be associated with an increased risk to pulmonary tuberculosis. Despite the slight trend of the D allele and HYPD haplotype in conferring protection against pulmonary tuberculosis, susceptibility to this disease would probably be due to other genetic factors, at least in our population.

1. Introduction

Tuberculosis (TB) is one of the world's most important infectious causes of death worldwide. More than 90 million TB patients were reported to WHO between 1980 and 2005, most of them in Asia and sub-Saharan Africa [1]. Spain is one of the European countries with the highest rates of incidence and prevalence of TB [2].

Approximately 90%–95% of individuals infected with *Mycobacterium tuberculosis* (MTB) are able to mount an immune response that halts the progression from latent TB infection to active TB disease. This is one of the main reasons that would indicate the need to identify and treat all those with risk factors for TB disease [3, 4].

Susceptibility to TB seems to be multifactorial, and the development of active disease would probably be the result of a complex interaction between the host and pathogen influenced by environmental and genetic factors. Numerous host genes are likely to be involved in this process [5–7].

Mannose-binding lectin (MBL) is an acute phase protein primarily produced by the liver. One of its main roles is to activate the complement system suggesting that it is one of the most important constituents of the innate immune system [8–12]. The gene encoding MBL has been associated with susceptibility to TB and other infectious diseases [8, 13]. The first mutation in *MBL2*, the gene encoding MBL was found in 1991 [14]. Three structural mutations, affecting codons 52, 54, and 57, in the first exon of the *MBL2* gene (MBL1 is a pseudogene) have been found, and the corresponding alleles were designated D, B, and C, respectively (A is the wild-type allele for all three positions). Moreover, three polymorphisms have also been identified in the *MBL2* promoter and 5'-untranslated regions: H/L at position −550, X/Y at position −221, and P/Q at position +4 [15].

The effect of the three structural mutations in the *MBL2* first exon involves the impairment of MBL multimerization. This caused decreasing ligand binding and, consequently, a lack of complement activation [16]. In general, all these genetic variants result in a phenotype of low serum MBL levels, which influences the susceptibility to TB and the course of different diseases [13, 17, 18].

To date, controversial results have been reported regarding the relationship between structural genetic variants or polymorphisms of the *MBL2* gene and an increased risk of TB in different populations [19–30]. Several studies have found a significant association between the frequency of structural alleles or promoter polymorphisms and serum MBL levels with susceptibility to TB [20, 23, 24, 26–30] while others did not find any significant association [19, 21, 25]. Recently a meta-analysis of 17 human trials considering the effect of *MBL2* genotype and/or MBL levels and TB infection did not found significant association between *MBL2* genotype and pulmonary TB infection [22]. The majority of studies analysed did not report neither the *MBL2* haplotype nor the promoter polymorphisms. The aim of our study was to analyse if gene variants, promoter polymorphisms, haplotypes, or diplotypes could contribute to increase the risk of active pulmonary TB (PTB) in a human immunodeficiency virus negative genetically homogeneous population (Cantabria, Northern Spain), containing newly diagnosed patients with active disease.

2. Material and Methods

2.1. Study Population. To investigate the possible association between *MBL2* polymorphisms and PTB infection in our population, we recruited a total of 107 active PTB patients and 441 randomly selected healthy blood donors from Cantabria (northern Spain). All of them were HIV negative.

The study was conducted at a 1,200-bed community and teaching hospital. Both, blood donors (mean age, 48 years; range, 18–65 years; male/female ratio, 1.3) and PTB patients (mean age, 56 years; range, 23–76 years; male/female ratio, 1.5) were of Caucasian background. The PTB patients group was selected from patients admitted to the Infectious Unit and the Department of Respiratory Medicine (Hospital Universitario Marqués de Valdecilla) from 2008 to 2011 and who fulfilled clinical, radiological, and bacteriological criteria of active PTB according the standards for the diagnosis and classification of TB developed by the American Thoracic Society and the Centers for Disease Control and Prevention (http://www.cdc.gov/mmwr/). Diagnosis of PTB was made clinically and by X-rays and confirmed by bacteriological (microscopy and culture) procedures. We excluded patients with extrapulmonary TB due to dissemination and subsequent involvement of single or multiple nonpulmonary

sites. In the same way, we excluded patients with autoimmune or neoplastic diseases, chronic renal failure, transplant individuals, and patients suffering from alcoholism or drug abuse. Controls had neither previous history of TB nor contact with infected patients. Furthermore, we ruled out the presence of active or latent TB in the control group by performing an interferon-gamma release assay (Quantiferon TB Gold, Cellestis Ltd., Carnegie, Victoria, Australia). All the procedures used in the study conformed to the principles outlined in the Declaration of Helsinki. Informed consent was obtained and data anonymously recorded. The study protocol was accepted and approved by the Research Ethics Board of the Hospital.

2.2. DNA Extraction and Amplification of Genomic DNA for MBL2 Genotyping. Blood was collected in EDTA-stabilized tubes in compliance with approved protocols from our institution. Genomic DNA from patients and controls was extracted from peripheral blood by using the Maxwell 16 Genomic DNA Purification system. For *MBL2* gene amplification and genotyping, we used the INNO-LiPA *MBL2* (Innogenetics Diagnóstica Iberia S.L.U, Barcelona, Spain), following the manufacturer's instructions. The INNO-LIPA *MBL2* is a line probe assay, designed for genotyping the 6 variations in the human *MBL2* gene (−550G > C, −221G > C, +4C > T, R52C, G54D, and G57E) which leads to analyse the seven common haplotypes and the 28 possible resulting diplotypes.

3. Statistical Analysis

Frequencies of alleles and diplotypes of patients and healthy controls were estimated by direct counting. Alleles and genotypic (dyplotypes) frequencies were compared by χ^2 test or the Fisher's exact test when necessary. P values with Yates correction and odds ratio (OR) with 95% confidence intervals (CI) were calculated using SPSS version 12.0 (SPSS Inc, Chicago, IL, USA). $P < 0.05$ was considered statistically significant. Hardy-Weinberg equilibrium (HWE) was tested in patients and controls for all the analysed parameters. Bonferroni correction for multiple comparisons was applied in order to avoid false positive results.

For haplotype analysis, frequencies and linkage disequilibrium were calculated trough the expectation maximization algorithm using the SNPStats web-based tool (http://bioinfo.iconcologia.net/SNPstats/). To determine the linkage disequilibrium between pairs of alleles, we calculated the D' statistic. Comparisons between patients and controls were performed by χ^2 test or the Fisher's exact test considering each haplotype like an allele.

Statistical power was calculated by using the PS power and sample size calculation software version 3.0, (http://biostat.mc.vanderbilt.edu/PowerSampleSize).

4. Results and Discussion

4.1. MBL2 Structural Variants, Promoter Polymorphisms, and Genotypes. Frequencies of *MBL2* alleles are shown in Table 1. All the structural genetic variants and the promoter

TABLE 1: Allelic frequencies of *MBL2* structural variants and promoter polymorphisms in healthy controls and patients with pulmonary tuberculosis.

	Structural variants				Promoter polymorphisms					
	A	B	C	D	L	H	Y	X	P	Q
Controls										
($n = 441$)	0.782	0.143	0.008	**0.067**	0.655	0.345	0.760	0.240	0.815	0.195
PTB Patients										
($n = 107$)	0.836	0.131	0.009	**0.023**	0.678	0.322	0.776	0.224	0.757	0.243
P value[a,b]				**0.014**						
OR				**0.33**						
(95% CI)				**(0.13–0.84)**						

[a] Only D variant showed significant differences between the two groups. The rest of structural and promoter alleles did not show significant differences.
[b] The study had 74% power for detecting an odds ratio (OR) ≥ 2.

TABLE 2: Frequency of *MBL2* haplotypes in controls and PTB patients from Cantabria compared with other previously reported populations.

						Population					
Haplotype	Controls	PTB	CAN	ESK	DAN	JAP	KEN	MOZ	CHIR	MAP	WAR
	($n = 441$)	($n = 107$)	($n = 344$)	($n = 72$)	($n = 250$)	($n = 218$)	($n = 61$)	($n = 154$)	($n = 43$)	($n = 25$)	($n = 190$)
HYPA	0.28	0.30	0.24	0.81	0.31	0.44	0.08	0.06	0.54	0.38	0.75
LYQA	0.23	0.23	0.22	0	0.19	0.16	0.25	0.27	0.01	0	0.01
LYPA	0.07	0.08	0.08	0.04	0.04	0.07	0.13	0.30	0.02	0.08	0.23
LXPA	0.21	0.23	0.19	0.03	0.26	0.11	0.24	0.13	0.01	0.04	0.01
LYPB	0.14	0.13	0.17	0.12	0.11	0.22	0.02	0	0.42	0.46	0
LYQC	0.01	0.01	0.03	0	0.03	0	0.24	0.24	0	0.04	0
HYPD	0.07	0.02[a]	0.07	0	0.06	0	0.04	0	0	0	0.003
H[b]	0.81	0.82	0.82	0.33	0.79	0.72	0.81	0.76	0.54	0.66	0.39

Controls, healthy population from Cantabria, PTB, patients with pulmonary tuberculosis from Cantabria, CAN, and Gran Canaria p; ESK, Eskimo; DAN, Danish; JAP, Japanese; KEN, Kenya; MOZ, Mozambique; CHIR, Chiriguano (South America); MAP, Mapuche (South America); WAR, Warlpiri (Australia) populations.
[a] P value 0.014 (OR 0.33 and 95% CI 0.13–0.84): frequency of HYPD haplotype in PTB patients versus control subjects from Cantabria.
[b] Average heterozygosity of the seven alleles when they were considered together.

polymorphisms were within the range of HWE. The average heterozygosity in the control group was 0.88 when the seven alleles of the *MBL2* gene were analysed, being this frequency higher than others previously reported in different populations [30].

There was no significant difference in the frequencies of the different promoter polymorphisms. Regarding the structural variants, only D allele was significantly more frequent in controls ($P = 0.014$, OR 0.33, and CI 95% 0.13–0.84), but this significance disappeared after Bonferroni correction.

Table 2 shows the frequency of the *MBL2* haplotypes in controls and PTB patients from Cantabria compared with other previously reported populations. As with D structural variant, HYPD showed the same significant difference between PTB patients and controls which disappeared after Bonferroni correction. All the promoter polymorphisms and structural variants conforming the different haplotypes were in linkage disequilibrium ($P < 2e - 16$).

4.2. MBL2 Complete Genotypes (Diplotypes) in PTB Patients and Healthy Controls. The frequencies of all the possible combinations of the seven haplotypes that appeared in both groups are shown in Table 3. No significant differences were

found in any of the complete diplotypes between PTB patients and healthy controls.

All seven haplotypes were present in both groups following the same order of frequency in them, giving rise to 22 different *MBL2* diplotypes in our subjects. Eighteen of these diplotypes were present in both groups, 5 in either the PTB patients or the control group, and six diplotypes were not observed in any of the groups.

HYPA was the most frequent haplotype, followed by LYQA, LXPA, LYPB, LYPA, HYPD, and LYQC, respectively. When we regrouped the 22 observed diplotypes in all the possible genotypic combinations (structural-structural, structural-polymorphism, and polymorphism-polymorphism), we did not find any significant difference (data not shown).

5. Discussion

Innate immunity is one of the most important barriers against invading pathogens. The complement system gets activated when these microorganisms are detected, resulting in biochemical pathways that lead to the destruction of the infectious agent. One of these pathways that make up

TABLE 3: Frequencies of complete diplotypes in Spanish PTB patients and controls.

MBL2 diplotypes*	PTB patients n (%)	Controls n (%)	P value	OR	(95% CI)
LYQA/HYPA	17 (15.9)	54 (12.24)	0.40	1.35	(0.75–2.45)
LYQA/LYPB	10 (9.3)	29 (6.58)	0.43	1.46	(0.69–3.11)
LYQA/LYPA	6 (5.6)	19 (4.31)	0.60	1.32	(0.51–3.39)
LYQA/LYQA	3 (2.8)	19 (4.31)	0.59	0.64	(0.19–2.20)
LYQA/HYPD	1 (0.9)	10 (2.27)	0.70	0.41	(0.05–3.21)
LYQA/LYQC	0 (0)	2 (0.45)	1.0	NA	NA
LYQC/HYPD	0 (0)	1 (0.23)	1.0	NA	NA
LXPA/HYPA	15 (14.0)	45 (10.20)	0.34	1.43	(0.77–2.69)
LXPA/LYQA	10 (9.3)	53 (12.02)	0.54	0.75	(0.37–1.54)
LXPA/LXPA	7 (6.5)	14 (3.17)	0.15	2.14	(0.84–5.43)
LXPA/LYPB	4 (3.7)	31 (7.03)	0.30	0.51	(0.18–1.49)
LXPA/HYPD	3 (2.8)	13 (2.95)	1.0	0.95	(0.27–3.39)
LXPA/LYPA	1 (0.9)	10 (2.27)	0.70	0.41	(0.05–3.21)
LXPA/LYQC	1 (0.9)	2 (0.45)	0.48	2.07	(0.19–23.05)
HYPA/HYPA	10 (9.3)	38 (8.62)	0.96	1.09	(0.53–2.27)
LYPB/HYPA	8 (7.5)	38 (8.62)	0.88	0.86	(0.39–1.89)
LYPB/LYPB	1 (0.9)	7 (1.59)	1.0	0.58	(0.07–4.81)
LYPB/LYQC	1 (0.9)	1 (0.23)	0.35	4.15	(0.26–66.90)
LYPB/HYPD	0 (0)	9 (2.04)	0.22	NA	NA
LYPA/HYPA	4 (3.7)	18 (4.08)	1.0	0.91	(1.30–2.75)
LYPA/LYPB	3 (2.8)	4 (0.91)	0.14	3.15	(0.69–14.30)
LYPA/LYPA	1 (0.9)	2 (0.45)	0.48	2.07	(0.19–23.05)
LYPA/LYQC	0 (0)	1 (0.23)	1.0	NA	NA
LYPA/HYPD	1 (0.9)	2 (0.45)	0.48	2.07	(0.19–23.05)
HYPD/HYPA	0 (0)	14 (3.17)	0.08	NA	NA
HYPD/HYPD	0 (0)	5 (1.13)	0.59	NA	NA

*Frequencies of the rest of combined diplotypes (LYQC/HYPA, LYQC/ LYQC) were 0 in both groups.

the complement system is the lectin pathway in which MBL plays the main role. MBL protein is therefore important, especially in first-line defense against invading pathogens. It has been reported that low levels of circulating MBL may predispose against infectious diseases [8, 31, 32].

Structural variants are found at the coding regions of the MBL2 gene that lead to low or near absent serum MBL levels in heterozygosis and homozygosis, respectively. Low-serum levels of MBL are associated with defects in opsonization, resulting in recurrent infections mainly during infancy [31]. Due to a strong linkage disequilibrium between the polymorphisms present in the promotor and the structural variants in exon 1 of the human MBL2 gene, only seven common haplotypes have been described (HYPA, LYPA, LXPA, LYQA, HYPD, LYPB, and LYQC) which give rise to 28 possible haplotype combinations. The frequencies of the seven haplotypes vary considerably between populations [17, 18]. Among haplotypes carrying the wild-type A allele, HYPA results in the production of higher amounts of MBL, whereas LXPA is associated with lower serum MBL levels.

Several groups have studied MBL2 genetic variants and PTB, suggesting a partial protective effect of heterozygosity for MBL2 variant alleles against PTB [33–35], whereas others have pointed toward a susceptibility to PTB for homozygous carriers of MBL2 variant alleles [36].

Previous studies have found controversial results, at least at a genetic level. Some authors have reported a lower frequency of allele B in Afro-Americans, but not in Caucasian or in the so-called "Hispanic" TB patients [28]. However, other reports have not found any significant differences in the frequency of structural MBL2 alleles between PTB Caucasian patients and control subjects. Nevertheless, when they included the promoter polymorphisms according to high serum MBL levels (YA/YA, YA/XA, XA/XA, and YA/O), low MBL levels (XA/O), and deficient MBL individuals (O/O),a significant difference in diplotype frequency was revealed [25, 27, 29]. Finally, another study has found a significantly increased frequency of O/O diplotype of structural polymorphism and of Y/Y diplotype of promoter polymorphisms in HIV-TB+ patients compared with controls [24].

In the present study, we have investigated whether structural variations or promoter polymorphisms in the MBL2 gene considering them individually of regrouped might be associated with PTB in Northern Spain. Our results after statistical correction show that there is no differences neither in the frequencies of polymorphisms in the promoter and 5′-untranslated region nor in the structural variants of the exon 1 of the MBL2 gene between PTB patients and control subjects when we considered them individually.

Lack of concordance of our results and those from other studies, specifically another Spanish report that studied MBL2 gene variants in the population from Canary Islands, [27] could be explained, at least, by the genetic characteristics of both pathogens and hosts. There are, consequently, two possibilities to understand these differences among insular and peninsular Spaniards.

First of all, it should be considered the different ethnic background of geographically apart populations [37–40]. Genetic studies have demonstrated that an aboriginal African background still persists in inhabitants from Canary Islands. Estimates of genetic contribution to the Canary Islanders from their putative parental populations based on mtDNA and other genetic markers are 43% Berbers, 35% Peninsular Spaniards, and 21% Guineans (being the Spanish nuclear contribution due to males and practically all the Berber and Guinean due to females). On the other hand, Cantabrians, at the North of the Iberian Peninsula, appear as a semi-isolated result of an ancient indigenous substrate more or less mixed with more recent immigrants. This population seems to be a genetically well-differentiated community, as deduced from uniparental and autosomal markers, perhaps to a higher level than their neighbours, the Basques, the most reputed European isolate on linguistic grounds [41–43].

Secondly, another explanation could be due to the genetic background within M. tuberculosis because variability among different strains of M. tuberculosis in their surface, oligosaccharides, might have led to differences in the MBL levels associated with resistance or susceptibility against PTB [27, 44, 45]. Consequently, when geographic variation in pathogen polymorphism is superimposed on host genetic heterogeneity, considerable variation may occur in detectable allelic association [5]. These factors could explain our findings in the analysed Northern Spanish population.

6. Conclusion

The results obtained in our study show a significant higher prevalence of MBL2 D allele and HYPD haplotype in controls than in PTB patients (6.7% versus 2.3%, $P = 0.014$, OR 0.33, and CI 95% 0.13–0.84).

Although after statistical correction, the significance disappeared; this trend of the P values to significance could indicate a role of D allele and HYPD haplotype in conferring protection against PTB. For this reason, we cannot argue that MBL2 D allele or HYPD haplotype would act as a factor of resistance to PTB, and susceptibility to this disease would probably be determined by other environmental and genetic factors, at least in our population [20, 46–50].

Conflict of Interests

The authors declare that they have no conflict of interests.

Acknowledgments

This work was partly supported by Grants PI05-0503 and G03-104 to F. Leyva-Cobián. and Grant PI04-1086 to M.-Carmen Fariñas. from the Fondo de Investigaciones Sanitarias (Ministry of Health, Spain). All authors read and approved the final version of the paper for publication.

References

[1] World Health Organization, "Global tuberculosis control: surveillance, planning, financing," WHO Report 2007, World Health Organization, Geneva, Switzerland, (WHO/HTM/TB/2007. 376).

[2] M. Díez, C. Huerta, T. Moreno et al., "Tuberculosis in Spain: epidemiological pattern and clinical practice," International Journal of Tuberculosis and Lung Disease, vol. 6, no. 4, pp. 295–300, 2002.

[3] M. Pai, S. Kalantri, and K. Dheda, "New tools and emerging technologies for the diagnosis of tuberculosis: part I. Latent tuberculosis," Expert Review of Molecular Diagnostics, vol. 6, no. 3, pp. 413–422, 2006.

[4] M. Pai, S. Kalantri, and K. Dheda, "New tools and emerging technologies for the diagnosis of tuberculosis: part II. Active tuberculosis and drug resistance," Expert Review of Molecular Diagnostics, vol. 6, no. 3, pp. 423–432, 2006.

[5] P. Selvaraj, "Host genetics and tuberculosis susceptibility," Current Science, vol. 86, no. 1, pp. 115–121, 2004.

[6] E. Schurr, "Is susceptibility to tuberculosis acquired or inherited?" Journal of Internal Medicine, vol. 261, no. 2, pp. 106–111, 2007.

[7] R. Bellamy, "Genome-wide approaches to identifying genetic factors in host susceptibility to tuberculosis," Microbes and Infection, vol. 8, no. 4, pp. 1119–1123, 2006.

[8] D. L. Worthley, P. G. Bardy, and C. G. Mullighan, "Mannose-binding lectin: biology and clinical implications," Internal Medicine Journal, vol. 35, no. 9, pp. 548–555, 2005.

[9] W. I. Weis, K. Drickamer, and W. A. Hendrickson, "Structure of a C-type mannose-binding protein complexed with an oligosaccharide," Nature, vol. 360, no. 6400, pp. 127–134, 1992.

[10] I. P. Fraser, H. Koziel, and R. A. B. Ezekowitz, "The serum mannose-binding protein and the macrophage mannose receptor are pattern recognition molecules that link innate and adaptive immunity," Seminars in Immunology, vol. 10, no. 5, pp. 363–372, 1998.

[11] S. Thiel, T. Vorup-Jensen, C. M. Stover et al., "A second serine protease associated with mannan-binding lectin that activates complement," Nature, vol. 386, no. 6624, pp. 506–510, 1997.

[12] O. Neth, D. L. Jack, A. W. Dodds, H. Holzel, N. J. Klein, and M. W. Turner, "Mannose-binding lectin binds to a range of clinically relevant microorganisms and promotes complement deposition," Infection and Immunity, vol. 68, no. 2, pp. 688–693, 2000.

[13] D. P. Eisen, "Mannose-binding lectin deficiency and respiratory tract infection," Journal of Innate Immunity, vol. 2, no. 2, pp. 114–122, 2010.

[14] M. Sumiya, M. Super, P. Tabona et al., "Molecular basis of opsonic defect in immunodeficient children," The Lancet, vol. 337, no. 8757, pp. 1569–1570, 1991.

[15] H. O. Madsen, P. Garred, S. Thiel et al., "Interplay between promoter and structural gene variants control basal serum level of mannan-binding protein," Journal of Immunology, vol. 155, no. 6, pp. 3013–3020, 1995.

[16] F. Larsen, H. O. Madsen, R. B. Sim, C. Koch, and P. Garred, "Disease-associated mutations in human mannose-binding lectin compromise oligomerization and activity of the final protein," The Journal of Biological Chemistry, vol. 279, no. 20, pp. 21302–21311, 2004.

[17] P. Garred, F. Larsen, J. Seyfarth, R. Fujita, and H. O. Madsen, "Mannose-binding lectin and its genetic variants," Genes and Immunity, vol. 7, no. 2, pp. 85–94, 2006.

[18] J. L. Casanova and L. Abel, "Human mannose-binding lectin in immunity: friend, foe, or both?" Journal of Experimental Medicine, vol. 199, no. 10, pp. 1295–1299, 2004.

[19] N. Singla, D. Gupta, A. Joshi, N. Batra, J. Singh, and N. Birbian, "Association of mannose-binding lectin gene polymorphism with tuberculosis susceptibility and sputum conversion time," International Journal of Immunogenetics, vol. 39, no. 1, pp. 10–14, 2012.

[20] Z. B. Liu, R. J. Zheng, H. P. Xiao et al., "The correlation between polymorphisms of genes with susceptibility to tuberculosis and the clinical characteristics of tuberculosis in 459 Han patients," Zhonghua Jie He He Hu Xi Za Zhi, vol. 34, no. 12, pp. 923–928, 2011.

[21] H. A. Solğun, D. Taştemir, N. Aksaray, I. Inan, and O. Demirhan, "Polymorphisms in NRAMP1 and MBL2 genes and their relations with tuberculosis in Turkish children," Tuberkuloz ve Toraks, vol. 59, no. 1, pp. 48–53, 2011.

[22] J. T. Denholm, E. S. McBryde, and D. P. Eisen, "Mannose-binding lectin and susceptibility to tuberculosis: a meta-analysis," Clinical and Experimental Immunology, vol. 162, no. 1, pp. 84–90, 2010.

[23] O. P. Dossou-Yovo, C. Lapoumeroulie, M. Hauchecorne et al., "Variants of the mannose-binding lectin gene in the benin population: heterozygosity for the p.G57E allele may confer a selective advantage," Human Biology, vol. 81, no. 5-6, pp. 899–909, 2009.

[24] K. Alagarasu, P. Selvaraj, S. Swaminathan, S. Raghavan, G. Narendran, and P. R. Narayanan, "Mannose binding lectin gene variants and susceptibility to tuberculosis in HIV-1 infected patients of South India," *Tuberculosis*, vol. 87, no. 6, pp. 535–543, 2007.

[25] W. Liu, F. Zhang, Z. T. Xin et al., "Sequence variations in the MBL gene and their relationship to pulmonary tuberculosis in the Chinese Han population," *International Journal of Tuberculosis and Lung Disease*, vol. 10, no. 10, pp. 1098–1103, 2006.

[26] P. Selvaraj, M. S. Jawahar, D. N. Rajeswari, K. Alagarasu, M. Vidyarani, and P. R. Narayanan, "Role of mannose binding lectin gene variants on its protein levels and macrophage phagocytosis with live *Mycobacterium tuberculosis* in pulmonary tuberculosis," *FEMS Immunology and Medical Microbiology*, vol. 46, no. 3, pp. 433–437, 2006.

[27] M. I. García-Laorden, M. J. Pena, J. A. Caminero et al., "Influence of mannose-binding lectin on HIV infection and tuberculosis in a Western-European population," *Molecular Immunology*, vol. 43, no. 14, pp. 2143–2150, 2006.

[28] H. M. El Sahly, R. A. Reich, S. J. Dou, J. M. Musser, and E. A. Graviss, "The effect of mannose binding lectin gene polymorphisms on susceptibility to tuberculosis in different ethnic groups," *Scandinavian Journal of Infectious Diseases*, vol. 36, no. 2, pp. 106–108, 2004.

[29] C. Søborg, H. O. Madsen, A. B. Andersen, T. Lillebaek, A. Kok-Jensen, and P. Garred, "Mannose-binding lectin polymorphisms in clinical tuberculosis," *Journal of Infectious Diseases*, vol. 188, no. 5, pp. 777–782, 2003.

[30] M. I. García-Laorden, A. Manzanedo, A. Figuerola, F. Sánchez-García, and C. Rodríguez-Gallego, "Mannose-binding lectin polymorphisms in a Canary Islands (Spain) population," *Genes and Immunity*, vol. 2, no. 5, pp. 292–294, 2001.

[31] F. Özbaş-Gerçeker, I. Tezcan, A. I. Berkel et al., "The effect of mannose-binding protein gene polymorphisms in recurrent respiratory system infections in children and lung tuberculosis," *Turkish Journal of Pediatrics*, vol. 45, no. 2, pp. 95–98, 2003.

[32] L. E. Mombo, C. Y. Lu, S. Ossari et al., "Mannose-binding lectin alleles in sub-Saharan Africans and relation with susceptibility to infections," *Genes and Immunity*, vol. 4, no. 5, pp. 362–367, 2003.

[33] A. V. S. Hill, "The immunogenetics of human infectious diseases," *Annual Review of Immunology*, vol. 16, pp. 593–617, 1998.

[34] P. Garred, C. Richter, A. B. Andersen et al., "Mannan-binding lectin in the sub-saharan HIV and tuberculosis epidemics," *Scandinavian Journal of Immunology*, vol. 46, no. 2, pp. 204–208, 1997.

[35] E. G. Hoal-van Helden, J. Epstein, T. C. Victor et al., "Mannose-binding protein B allele confers protection against tuberculous meningitis," *Pediatric Research*, vol. 45, no. 4 I, pp. 459–464, 1999.

[36] P. Selvaraj, P. R. Narayanan, and A. M. Reetha, "Association of functional mutant homozygotes of the mannose binding protein gene with susceptibility to pulmonary tuberculosis in India," *Tubercle and Lung Disease*, vol. 79, no. 4, pp. 221–227, 1999.

[37] J. C. Delgado, A. Baena, S. Thim, and A. E. Goldfeld, "Ethnic-specific genetic associations with pulmonary tuberculosis," *Journal of Infectious Diseases*, vol. 186, no. 10, pp. 1463–1468, 2002.

[38] C. Flores, N. Maca-Meyer, J. A. Pérez, A. M. González, J. M. Larruga, and V. M. Cabrera, "A predominant European ancestry of paternal lineages from Canary Islanders," *Annals of Human Genetics*, vol. 67, no. 2, pp. 138–152, 2003.

[39] F. Pinto, A. M. González, M. Hernández, J. M. Larruga, and V. M. Cabrera, "Genetic relationship between the Canary Islanders and their African and Spanish ancestors inferred from mitochondrial DNA sequences," *Annals of Human Genetics*, vol. 60, no. 4, pp. 321–330, 1996.

[40] F. M. Pinto, A. M. González, M. Hernández, J. M. Larruga, and V. M. Cabrera, "Sub-Saharan influence on the Canary Islands population deduced from G6PD gene sequence analysis," *Human Biology*, vol. 68, no. 4, pp. 517–522, 1996.

[41] E. Esteban, J. M. Dugoujon, E. Guitard et al., "Genetic diversity in Northern Spain (Basque Country and Cantabria): GM and KM variation related to demographic histories," *European Journal of Human Genetics*, vol. 6, no. 4, pp. 315–324, 1998.

[42] P. Sánchez-Velasco, J. Escribano de Diego, J. E. Paz-Miguel, G. Ocejo-Vinyals, and F. Leyva-Cobián, "HLA-DR, DQ nucleotide sequence polymorphisms in the Pasiegos (Pas valleys, Northern Spain) and comparison of the allelic and haplotypic frequencies with those of other European populations," *Tissue Antigens*, vol. 53, no. 1, pp. 65–73, 1999.

[43] P. Sánchez-Velasco, E. Gómez-Casado, J. Martínez-Laso et al., "HLA alleles in isolated populations from north Spain: origin of the basques and the ancient Iberians," *Tissue Antigens*, vol. 61, no. 5, pp. 384–392, 2003.

[44] M. Kato-Maeda, P. J. Bifani, B. N. Kreiswirth, and P. M. Small, "The nature and consequence of genetic variability within *Mycobacterium tuberculosis*," *Journal of Clinical Investigation*, vol. 107, no. 5, pp. 533–537, 2001.

[45] B. López, D. Aguilar, H. Orozco et al., "A marked difference in pathogenesis and immune response induced by different *Mycobacterium tuberculosis* genotypes," *Clinical and Experimental Immunology*, vol. 133, no. 1, pp. 30–37, 2003.

[46] N. Keicho, M. Hijikata, and S. Sakurada, "Human genetic susceptibility to tuberculosis," *Nihon Rinsho*, vol. 69, no. 8, pp. 1363–1367, 2011.

[47] R. J. Wilkinson, "Human genetic susceptibility to tuberculosis: time for a bottom-up approach?" *Journal of Infectious Diseases*, vol. 205, no. 4, pp. 525–527, 2012.

[48] J. L. Rowell, N. F. Dowling, W. Yu, A. Yesupriya, L. Zhang, and M. Gwinn, "Trends in population-based studies of human genetics in infectious diseases," *PloS ONE*, vol. 7, no. 2, Article ID e25431, 2012.

[49] T. Qidwai, F. Jamal, and M. Y. Khan, "DNA sequence variation and regulation of genes involved in pathogenesis of pulmonary tuberculosis," *Scandinavian Journal of Immunology*, vol. 75, no. 6, pp. 568–587, 2012.

[50] A. K. Azad, W. Sadee, and L. S. Schlesinger, "Innate immune gene polymorphisms in tuberculosis," *Infection and Immunity*, vol. 80, no. 10, pp. 3343–3359, 2012.

25

Levels of Interferon-Gamma Increase after Treatment for Latent Tuberculosis Infection in a High-Transmission Setting

Iukary Takenami,[1] Brook Finkmoore,[2] Almério Machado Jr.,[3, 4] Krisztina Emodi,[2] Lee W. Riley,[2] and Sérgio Arruda[1, 3]

[1] *Advanced Laboratory of Public Health, Oswaldo Cruz Foundation, Gonçalo Moniz Research Center, Salvador, Bahia 40296 710, Brazil*
[2] *Division of Infectious Diseases & Vaccinology, School of Public Health, University of California, Berkeley, CA 94720, USA*
[3] *Bahia School of Medicine and Public Health, Salvador, Bahia 40290 000, Brazil*
[4] *Hospital Especializado Octávio Mangabeira, Secretary of Health of Bahia State, Salvador, Bahia 40320 350, Brazil*

Correspondence should be addressed to I. Takenami, iukary@yahoo.com.br

Academic Editor: José R. Lapa e Silva

Objectives. We investigated IFN-γ levels before and after a six month course of isoniazid among individuals with latent tuberculosis infection (LTBI) in a high-transmission setting. *Design.* A total of 26 household contacts of pulmonary tuberculosis patients who were positive for LTBI by tuberculin skin test completed six months of treatment and submitted a blood sample for a follow-up examination. The IFN-γ response to *Mycobacterium tuberculosis*-specific antigens was measured, and the results before and after the completion of LTBI treatment were compared. *Results.* Of the 26 study participants, 25 (96%) showed an IFN-γ level higher than their baseline level before treatment ($P \leq 0.001$). Only one individual had a decreased IFN-γ level after treatment but remained positive for LTBI. *Conclusion.* In a high-transmission setting, the IFN-γ level has increased after LTBI treatment. Further studies must be undertaken to understand if this elevation is transient.

1. Introduction

Commercially available interferon-gamma release assays (IGRAs) diagnose *Mycobacterium tuberculosis (M. tb)* infection by measuring interferon-gamma (IFN-γ) released by cells of whole blood after *in vitro* stimulation with *M. tb*-specific antigens, early secreted antigenic target 6 (ESAT-6), and culture filtrate protein 10 (CFP-10) [1]. These diagnostic tests are more specific than the tuberculin skin test (TST) because they include *M. tb*-specific antigens encoded by the region of difference 1 (RD1) which is absent from *Bacillus* Calmette-Guérin (BCG) and most nontuberculous mycobacteria (NTM) [1–3]. A recent meta-analysis concluded that the commercially available IGRAs have excellent specificity to diagnose latent tuberculosis infection (LTBI) and are unaffected by BCG vaccination [4].

The capacity of IGRAs to monitor the treatment response tuberculosis (TB) and LTBI is under investigation. This study was motivated by studies which have found that the level of IFN-γ released by cells of whole blood after *in vitro* stimulation with *M. tb*-specific antigens in commercial IGRAs declines in patients treated with multidrug regimens for active TB [5–7]. Despite these results, some investigators have concluded that IGRAs may not be helpful in monitoring TB treatment because of high intersubject variability and because test reversion is rare [8, 9].

In contrast to treatment of active TB, previous studies on T-cell response before and after treatment for LTBI have shown conflicting results [10–12]. A study from Japan found that the levels of IFN-γ decreased after LTBI treatment although the commercial IGRA result did not revert to negative [11]. Another study in health care workers in India found that IFN-γ levels remain high after LTBI treatment [10]. In Singapore, a study found that LTBI treatment had a differential effect on T-cell responses depending on which RD1 antigen the T-cells were exposed to [12]. It is unclear if the amount of IFN-γ released by T-cells stimulated with the M.tb-specific antigens in commercial IGRAs follow a specific pattern after completion of LTBI treatment. Moreover, it is unknown if specific T-cell responses after LTBI treatment are different in settings where the transmission of M.tb in the community is low compared to setting where transmission is high [10, 13–16]. This study compares the IFN-γ levels, measured by a commercial IGRA, of household contacts (HHCs) of pulmonary TB patients before and after six months of isoniazid (H) for the treatment of LTBI in a high-transmission setting.

2. Study Population and Methods

2.1. Setting. Participants were recruited from Hospital Especializado Octávio Mangabeira (HEOM) a 217-bed public chest-disease hospital in Salvador, Brazil. In 2007, Salvador had a TB incidence of approximately 79 per 100 000 population [17].

2.2. Study Participants. Study participants were HHCs of patients hospitalized with pulmonary TB at HEOM who tested positive for LBTI by TST and completed a six-month course of H [18]. None of the index cases or HHC were taking medication for the management of HIV. The characteristics of the index cases and all HHC are described elsewhere [19]. The characteristics of the HHC who initiated LTBI treatment and their adherence to the six-month regimen are described elsewhere [20]. It is well documented in the literature that HHC with LTBI are at high risk of developing active disease during the two years after infection [21, 22].

The study was approved by the human subjects committees of the Oswaldo Cruz Foundation in Salvador, Brazil, and the University of California at Berkeley, USA. Informed consent was obtained for all study participants.

2.3. Data Collection. Study participants underwent a baseline examination (TST, blood test, and interview) as part of another study [19]. LTBI could only be diagnosed in those who returned to have their TST read. Those eligible for LTBI treatment were offered the six-month supply of H free of charge [20]. Among the HHC who initiated LTBI treatment, HHCs considered to have completed treatment were those who collected six supplies of 30 H tablets from HEOM. A member of the study team (IT) called all HHC who completed LTBI treatment and invited them to return to HEOM for a follow-up examination and blood draw. HHCs were called and asked to participate in the follow-up examination a maximum of four times.

2.4. Treatment. Study participants were given six months of daily H treatment (5 mg/kg, up to 300 mg daily); this is the standard treatment regimen in Brazil [18].

2.5. Laboratory Tests. The TST was administered according to the Mantoux method, by injecting intradermally 2 tuberculin units (in 0.1 mL) of purified protein derivate (RT23 PPD; Staten Serum Institute, Copenhagen, Denmark). TST reaction was 72 hours after an administration by the chest physician on the study team (AMJ). The cut-off point for a positive reaction was ≥ 10 mm induration because this was the cutoff used in the decision to initiate treatment in Brazil at the time of the study, according to the Brazilian Society of Thoracic and Phthisiology [18].

The blood was examined with a commercially available IGRA, the QuantiFERON-TB Gold In Tube (QFT-IT; Cellestis Limited, Carnegie, VIC, Australia). QFT-IT includes the following M.tb-specific proteins: secreted antigenic protein 6 kDa (ESAT-6), culture filtrate protein 10 kDa (CFP-10), and TB7.7 (Rv 2654). The test was performed according to the manufacturers instructions at the immunology laboratory at Gonçalo Moniz Research Center in Salvador, Bahia, Brazil. The cut-off value for a positive response was 0.35 IU/mL. Samples that gave indeterminate results were reprocessed. Blood was drawn for the baseline IGRA before the TST was administered; both were conducted on the same day.

2.6. Statistical Analysis. Data were analyzed using GraphPad Prism v.5.0 (GraphPad Inc., San Diego, CA, USA). Wilcoxon signed rank test was used to compare the median IFN-γ levels before and after H treatment. The difference between the median values at the two time points was considered statistically significant when the P value ≤ 0.05.

3. Results

Of the 101 HHC of pulmonary TB patients who tested positive for LTBI by TST and initiated on LTBI treatment between January 2007 and February 2008, 55 (54.5%) completed six months of therapy with H. Of the 55 HHC, 26 (47.3%) returned to HEOM for the follow-up examination and submitted a second blood sample for a second test. The second blood sample was submitted for follow-up examination between four and 14 months after the completion of LTBI treatment (Figure 1). None of the 26 HHC who returned for the follow-up examination sought medical attention at HEOM for symptoms consistent with TB between the time they concluded LTBI treatment and the follow-up examination.

The median age of the 26 HHC who returned for the follow-up examination was 27 years (IQR 12.0–37.5). Sixteen (61.5%) were women, and 23 (88.5%) had BCG vaccination scars. At baseline examination, the median value of the TST induration was 13 mm (IQR 12.0–16.7) among the 26 HHC who returned for follow-up examination. Of the 29 HHC who did not return for follow-up examination, the median age was 19 years (IQR 11.5–39.0); 15 (51.7%) were male and 28 (96.5%) had a BCG vaccination scar, and the median value of the TST induration was 16 mm (IQR 11.0–19.5) at baseline examination. The sociodemographic, clinical, and laboratory profile of the HHC who did and did not return

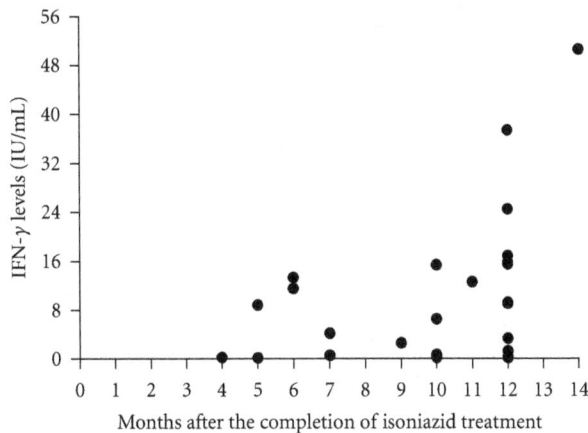

FIGURE 1: The difference between the baseline and follow-up IGRA result according to the number of months elapsed between the completion of H treatment and the follow-up examination. IFN-γ levels were measured by QFT-IT and plotted for each study participant ($n = 26$). H = isoniazid; IFN-γ = interferon-gamma; QFT-IT = QuantiFERON TB Gold in Tube.

for follow-up examinations were not significantly different (data not shown).

Of the 26 HHC who completed H treatment and returned for follow-up examination, 16 (61.5%) were QFT-IT positive, and 10 (38.5%) were QFT-IT negative at baseline examination. All 16 HHC who were QFT-IT positive at baseline tested positive by QFT-IT in the follow-up examination. Of the 10 HHC who were QFT-IT negative at baseline, five (50%) tested negative and five (50%) tested positive by QFT-IT in the follow-up examination. Not one HHC who tested positive by QFT-IT at baseline tested negative after completing H treatment (Figure 2).

Among the 16 HHC who tested positive by QFT-IT before LTBI treatment, the median IFN-γ level to the *M. tb*-specific antigens at baseline evaluation was 5.55 IU/mL; the median IFN-γ level of this group after six-months of H treatment was 12.97 IU/mL (P value = 0.0007) (Figure 3(a)). One individual who tested QFT-IT positive before LTBI treatment had a decreased IFN-γ level after treatment but remained QFT-IT positive (IFN-$\gamma \geq 0.35$ IU/mL) (Figure 3(a)). Among the 10 HHC who tested negative by QFT-IT before LTBI treatment, the median IFN-γ level to the *M. tb*-specific antigens at baseline evaluation was 0.02 IU/mL; the median IFN-γ level of this group after six months of H treatment was 0.32 IU/mL (P value = 0.008) (Figure 3(b)).

The difference in the median value of IFN-γ before and after treatment was 7.42 IU/mL and 0.30 IU/mL in HHC who were QFT-IT positive and those negative at baseline, respectively (P value = 0.0012).

4. Discussion

The treatment of LTBI is a basic strategy for TB control. A six-month course of a single drug, H, is effective in preventing individuals with LTBI from progressing to active disease [23]. It is difficult, however, to monitor LTBI

treatment in individual patients. It is unknown if the results from commercial IGRAs that are approved for the diagnosis of TB and LTBI correlate with clinical outcomes or follow a specific pattern after antibiotic treatment for *M. tb* infection.

The current published data on the effects of LTBI treatment on IFN-γ levels are inconsistent. Studies from low-transmission settings where repeat exposure to *M. tb* is unlikely have found that T-cell IFN-γ levels decline after treatment. One such study in the United Kingdom followed the T-cell responses in students exposed to *M. tb* in a point-source school TB outbreak. Students meeting the UK guideline for the treatment of LTBI by indication from TST results were given both rifampin (R) and H; after the completion of therapy, the levels of IFN-γ response in the students substantially decreased. However, the levels of IFN-γ response also decreased in the students who tested negative by TST and did not undergo treatment [24]. Another study in recent immigrants to the UK showed that T cells produced higher levels of IFN-γ one month after the initiation of treatment for LTBI but towards the end of the LTBI treatment course, the IFN-γ level decreased. This study found that the T-cell response did not change in those with LTBI who were not initiated on treatment. Also, the author showed that peripheral blood mononuclear cells infected with *M. tb* and treated *in vitro* with H, but not R, led to an increase in the number of IFN-γ producing cells. These results suggest that H acts by actively destroying the bacilli through the disruption of the cell wall. Such a process may contribute to the increased release of cell wall-associated antigens, resulting in an increased number of antigens-specific T cells being detected during treatment [15].

Pai et al. (2006) have demonstrated that the baseline of T-cell IFN-γ response among Indian health care workers in a high-transmission setting was high even ten months after the completion of treatment for LTBI [10]. On the other hand, a study by Higuchi et al. (2008) of individuals who had contact with TB patients in Tokyo showed a decline in IFN-γ levels six months after the completion of treatment for LTBI without test reversion [11]. A study conducted in Rome, also an area of low transmission, found a significant decrease in IFN-γ levels in patients after 1-2 months of LTBI treatment and found that response of the majority of the patients became undetectable after six months [16].

Here we found that the IFN-γ levels of individuals with documented LTBI increased after H treatment. Regardless of baseline QFT-IT, 25 of 26 (96%) HHC had a higher IFN-γ level between six and 14 months after the completion of H treatment. Individuals who tested QFT-IT positive at baseline had a greater increase in IFN-γ levels after treatment than did individuals who tested QFT-IT negative at baseline (Figures 3(a) and 3(b)).

Increased production of IFN-γ by T cells may be the result of a massive release of antigens when the *M. tb* bacilli are killed by H treatment [24]. This theory is supported by our finding that HHC who tested positive by QFT-IT at baseline and presumably had a higher bacillary load experienced a greater increase in IFN-γ levels after H therapy than those who tested negative by QFT-IT.

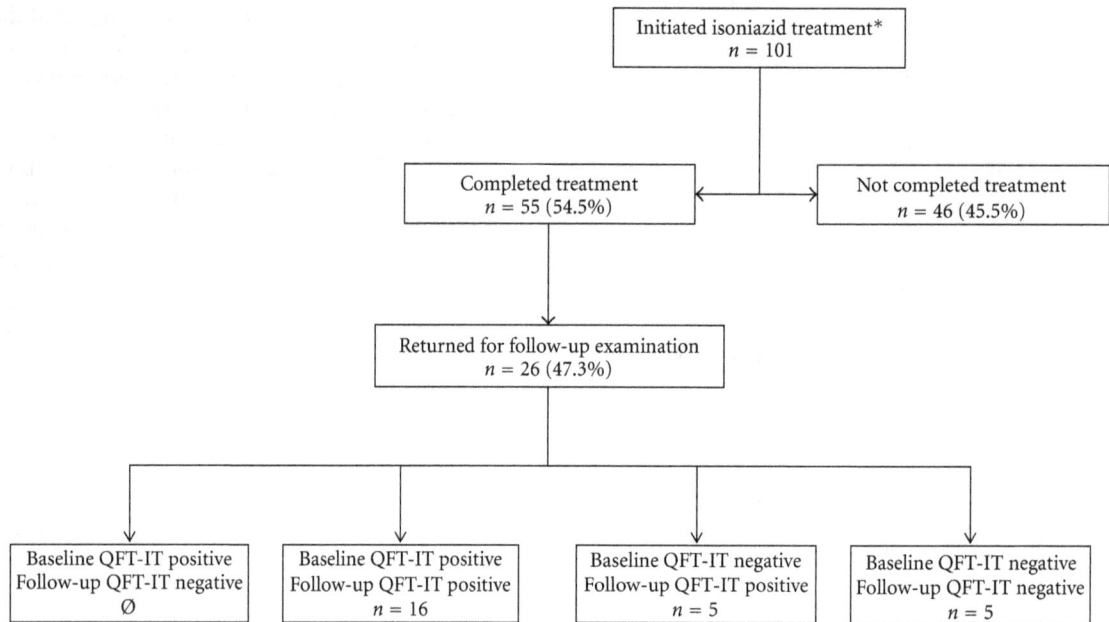

FIGURE 2: Flow chart of the study population and the study participants. *TST ≥ 10 mm. H: isoniazid; QFT-IT: QuantiFERON TB Gold in Tube; TST: tuberculin skin test.

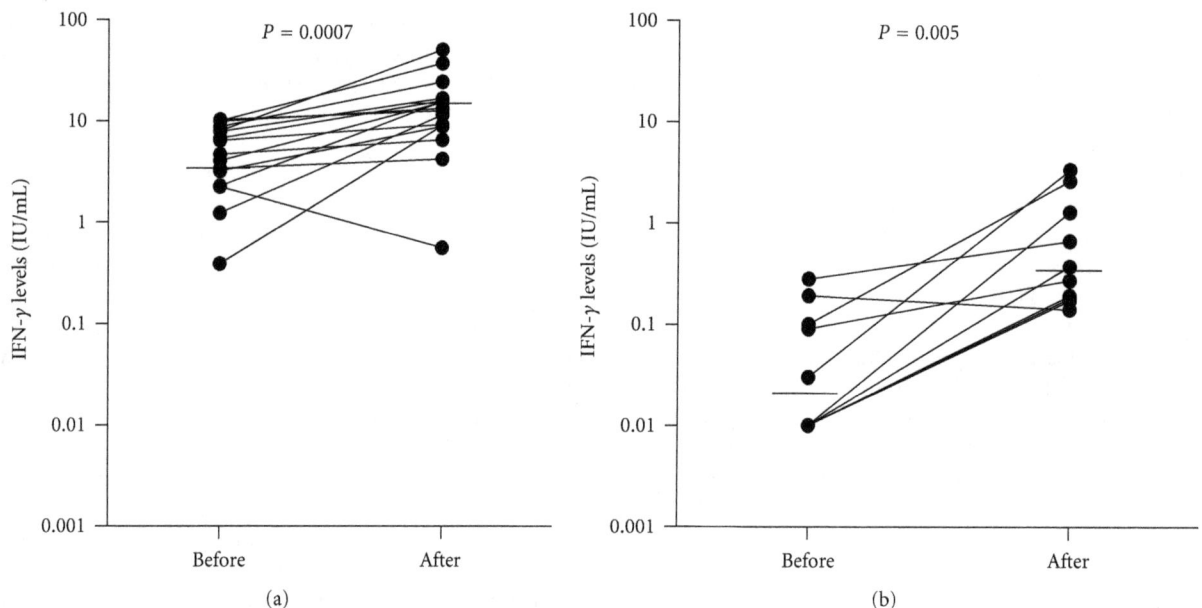

FIGURE 3: IFN-γ levels before and after H treatment for LTBI measured by QFT-IT stratified by baseline QFT-IT result; (a) positive QFT-IT and (b) negative QFT-IT. The solid line represents the median value of IFN-γ levels at the two time points. The differences between the median values in each group before and after H treatment are significant by the Wilconxon's signed rank test ($P = 0.0007$ and $P = 0.005$, resp.). IFN-γ: interferon-gamma; H: isoniazid; QFT-IT: QuantiFERON-TB Gold in Tube.

In combination, effector memory T cells can also upregulate IFN-γ production [25].

TST was unlikely to influence the baseline IGRA, since the HHC submitted the blood sample for baseline testing before the TST was administered. However, the TST given at the baseline evaluation may have interfered with the follow-up IGRA result due to TST-mediated boosting of IGRA responses which has been reported elsewhere [26, 27]. The 26 HHC in this study submitted blood for follow-up IGRA testing between 4 and 14 months after the baseline evaluation that included TST (Figure 1). A recent systematic review suggests that TST affects IGRA responses 3 days after the TST is administered, but its influence may persist for several months [28].

This study was conducted in a high-transmission setting; Salvador has one of the highest incidence rates of TB in Brazil. Therefore, it is possible that some of the HHCs were reinfected with *M. tb* after the completion of treatment and before they submitted blood samples for the follow-up examination. Moreover, follow-up examinations occurred between four and 14 months after the completion of H treatment. This long period of time increases the possibility that elevated IFN-γ levels are due to reinfection. It is also possible that study participants were exposed to environmental mycobacteria which share the ESAT-6 and CFP-10 genes (e.g., *M. kansasii*), and this contributed to elevated production of IFN-γ by T cells. On the other hand, an important aspect that should also be considered is the genetic factors, which has a key role in human phenotypic variability. Several polymorphisms have been described in genes associated with cytokine expression. These polymorphisms could also influence interindividual variability and direct IFN-γ production [29, 30].

IGRAs are not able to accurately estimate IFN-γ production by T cells beyond 10 IU/mL, and two of 26 HHC had IGRA results above this level in the baseline examination, and 10 of 26 HHC had IGRA results above this level in the follow-up examination. These values are likely to overestimate the IFN-γ production and should not be considered to be different than 10 IU/mL.

One of this study's limitations is that the medications were self-administered [20]. We assume that the HHCs who returned to the hospital each month for six months and received H refills were motivated to take the medication. However, we cannot exclude the possibility that some of the 26 HHCs included in this study did not complete the LTBI treatment according the protocol. Another limitation of this study is that less than half of the HHCs who completed H treatment submitted blood for follow-up examination by QFT-IT. There were not substantial epidemiologic differences between those HHCs who returned for the follow-up exam and those who did not. Therefore, it is unlikely that the 26 HHCs who were satisfactorily tested by two IGRAs were a biased group. Another limitation is that the single QFT-IT test for each study participant before and after the completion of H treatment were not taken at the same time. Finally, this study did not have a control group of untreated HHC with LTBI in whom the T-cell responses were monitored at the same time. Limitations in the study design and the lack of active contact-tracing programs through which to monitor individuals at high risk for progressing to active disease precluded data from being collected.

5. Conclusion

The data presented in this study suggest that IGRA results increase in individuals after the completion of LTBI treatment; however, conflicting data from other studies and the limitations of our study do not allow us to exclude the potential role of IGRAs in monitoring LTBI treatment. To further investigate this, larger studies in high-transmission settings must be conducted, which collect data on the T-cell responses of people with LTBI before, during, and after LTBI treatment over a longer time period.

Conflict of Interests

None of the authors of this paper have any conflict of interests.

Acknowledgments

The authors acknowledge the director of the HOEM, the clinical laboratory of the hospital, and the National Institute of Science and Technology in Tuberculosis (INCT-TB) by supporting given to master' student Iukary Takenami. they also thank EBMSP students by their contribution with medical questionnaire interviews. Financial support was provided by NIH Fogarty International Center 5U2RTW 006885.

References

[1] P. Andersen, M. E. Munk, J. M. Pollock, and T. M. Doherty, "Specific immune-based diagnosis of tuberculosis," *The Lancet*, vol. 356, no. 9235, pp. 1099–1104, 2000.

[2] M. Pai, L. W. Riley, and J. M. Colford, "Interferon-γ assays in the immunodiagnosis of tuberculosis: a systematic review," *Lancet Infectious Diseases*, vol. 4, no. 12, pp. 761–766, 2004.

[3] S. Y. Eum, Y. J. Lee, H. K. Kwak et al., "Evaluation of the diagnostic utility of a whole-blood interferon-γ assay for determining the risk of exposure to *Mycobacterium tuberculosis* in Bacille Calmette-Guerin (BCG)-vaccinated individuals," *Diagnostic Microbiology and Infectious Disease*, vol. 61, no. 2, pp. 181–186, 2008.

[4] M. Pai, A. Zwerling, and D. Menzies, "Systematic review: T-cell-based assays for the diagnosis of latent tuberculosis infection: an update," *Annals of Internal Medicine*, vol. 149, no. 3, pp. 177–184, 2008.

[5] A. M. Aiken, P. C. Hill, A. Fox et al., "Reversion of the ELISPOT test after treatment in Gambian tuberculosis cases," *BMC Infectious Diseases*, vol. 6, article 66, 2006.

[6] Y. Kobashi, K. Mouri, S. Yagi, Y. Obase, N. Miyashita, and M. Oka, "Transitional changes in T-cell responses to *Mycobacterium tuberculosis*-specific antigens during treatment," *Journal of Infection*, vol. 58, no. 3, pp. 197–204, 2009.

[7] I. Sauzullo, F. Mengoni, M. Lichtner et al., "In vivo and in vitro effects of antituberculosis treatment on mycobacterial interferon-γ T cell response," *PLoS ONE*, vol. 4, no. 4, Article ID e5187, 2009.

[8] V. Bosshard, P. Roux-Lombard, T. Perneger et al., "Do results of the T-SPOT.TB interferon-γ release assay change after treatment of tuberculosis?" *Respiratory Medicine*, vol. 103, no. 1, pp. 30–34, 2009.

[9] S. Ribeiro, K. Dooley, J. Hackman et al., "T-SPOT.TB responses during treatment of pulmonary tuberculosis," *BMC Infectious Diseases*, vol. 9, article 23, 2009.

[10] M. Pai, R. Joshi, S. Dogra et al., "Persistently elevated T cell interferon-γ responses after treatment for latent tuberculosis infection among health care workers in India: a preliminary report," *Journal of Occupational Medicine and Toxicology*, vol. 1, no. 1, article 7, 2006.

[11] K. Higuchi, N. Harada, and T. Mori, "Interferon-γ responses after isoniazid chemotherapy for latent tuberculosis," *Respirology*, vol. 13, no. 3, pp. 468–472, 2008.

[12] C. B. E. Chee, T. M. S. Barkham, K. W. KhinMar, S. H. Gan, and Y. T. Wang, "Quantitative T-cell interferon-gamma responses to *Mycobacterium tuberculosis*-specific antigens in active and latent tuberculosis," *European Journal of Clinical Microbiology and Infectious Diseases*, vol. 28, no. 6, pp. 667–670, 2009.

[13] S. Carrara, D. Vincenti, N. Petrosillo, M. Amicosante, E. Girardi, and D. Goletti, "Use of a T cell-based assay for monitoring efficacy of antituberculosis therapy," *Clinical Infectious Diseases*, vol. 38, no. 5, pp. 754–756, 2004.

[14] A. Lalvani, "Counting antigen-specific T cells: a new approach for monitoring response to tuberculosis treatment?" *Clinical Infectious Diseases*, vol. 38, no. 5, pp. 757–759, 2004.

[15] K. A. Wilkinson, O. M. Kon, S. M. Newton et al., "Effect of treatment of latent tuberculosis infection on the T cell response to *Mycobacterium tuberculosis* antigens," *Journal of Infectious Diseases*, vol. 193, no. 3, pp. 354–359, 2006.

[16] D. Goletti, M. P. Parracino, O. Butera et al., "Isoniazid prophylaxis differently modulates T-cell responses to RD1-epitopes in contacts recently exposed to *Mycobacterium tuberculosis*: a pilot study," *Respiratory Research*, vol. 8, article 5, 2007, American Thoracic Society, Targeted tuberculin testing and treatment of latent tuberculosis infection, Morbidity and Mortality Weekly Report, vol. 49, pp. 1–51, 2000.

[17] MS—Ministério da Saúde, Brasil, Fundação Nacional de Saúde, Centro Nacional de Epidemiologia, Informe epidemiológico do DATASUS, Brasília, 2009, http://tabnet.datasus.gov.br.

[18] MS—Ministério da Saúde, "II Consenso Brasileiro de Tuberculose—Diretrizes Brasileiras para Tuberculose 2004," *Jornal Brasileiro de Pneumologia*, vol. 30, supplement 1, pp. S2–S56, 2004.

[19] A. Machado, K. Emodi, I. Takenami et al., "Analysis of discordance between the tuberculin skin test and the interferon-gamma release assay," *International Journal of Tuberculosis and Lung Disease*, vol. 13, no. 4, pp. 446–453, 2009.

[20] A. Machado, B. Finkmoore, K. Emodi et al., "Risk factors for failure to complete a course of latent tuberculosis infection treatment in Salvador, Brazil," *International Journal of Tuberculosis and Lung Disease*, vol. 13, no. 6, pp. 719–725, 2009.

[21] N. M. Parrish, J. D. Dick, and W. R. Bishai, "Mechanisms of latency in *Mycobacterium tuberculosis*," *Trends in Microbiology*, vol. 6, no. 3, pp. 107–112, 1998.

[22] S. Radhakrishna, T. R. Frieden, R. Subramani, T. Santha, and P. R. Narayanan, "Additional risk of developing TB for household members with a TB case at home at intake: a 15-year study," *The International Journal of Tuberculosis and Lung Disease*, vol. 11, no. 3, pp. 282–288, 2007.

[23] B. L. Johnston and J. M. Conly, "Re-examining treatment of latent tuberculosis infection," *Canadian Journal of Infectious Diseases*, vol. 12, no. 4, pp. 211–214, 2001.

[24] K. Ewer, K. A. Millington, J. J. Deeks, L. Alvarez, G. Bryant, and A. Lalvani, "Dynamic antigen-specific T-cell responses after point-source exposure to *Mycobacterium tuberculosis*," *American Journal of Respiratory and Critical Care Medicine*, vol. 174, no. 7, pp. 831–839, 2006.

[25] J. Geginat, F. Sallusto, and A. Lanzavecchia, "Cytokine-driven proliferation and differentiation of human naïve, central memory and effector memory CD4$^+$ T cells," *Pathologie Biologie*, vol. 51, no. 2, pp. 64–66, 2003.

[26] E. M. S. Leyten, C. Prins, A. W. J. Bossink et al., "Effect of tuberculin skin testing on a *Mycobacterium tuberculosis*-specific interferon-γ assay," *European Respiratory Journal*, vol. 29, no. 6, pp. 1212–1216, 2007.

[27] R. N. Van Zyl-Smit, M. Pai, K. Peprah et al., "Within-subject variability and boosting of t-cell interferon-γ responses after tuberculin skin testing," *American Journal of Respiratory and Critical Care Medicine*, vol. 180, no. 1, pp. 49–58, 2009.

[28] R. N. Van Zyl-Smit, A. Zwerling, K. Dheda, and M. Pai, "Within-subject variability of interferon-g assay results for tuberculosis and boosting effect of tuberculin skin testing: a systematic review," *PLoS ONE*, vol. 4, no. 12, Article ID e8517, 2009.

[29] P. Selvaraj, K. Alagarasu, M. Harishankar, M. Vidyarani, D. Nisha Rajeswari, and P. R. Narayanan, "Cytokine gene polymorphisms and cytokine levels in pulmonary tuberculosis," *Cytokine*, vol. 43, no. 1, pp. 26–33, 2008.

[30] D. López-Maderuelo, F. Arnalich, R. Serantes et al., "Interferon-γ and interleukin-10 gene polymorphisms in pulmonary tuberculosis," *American Journal of Respiratory and Critical Care Medicine*, vol. 167, no. 7, pp. 970–975, 2003.

26

Successful Smoking Cessation in COPD: Association with Comorbidities and Mortality

H. Kupiainen,[1,2] **V. L. Kinnula,**[2] **A. Lindqvist,**[2] **D. S. Postma,**[3] **H. M. Boezen,**[4] **T. Laitinen,**[1,2] **and M. Kilpeläinen**[1]

[1] *Department of Pulmonary Diseases and Clinical Allergology, Turku University Hospital and University of Turku, Kiinamyllynkatu 13, 20520 Turku, Finland*
[2] *Clinical Research Unit for Pulmonary Diseases and Division of Pulmonology, Helsinki University Central Hospital, Tukholmankatu 8C, 00290 Helsinki, Finland*
[3] *Department of Pulmonology, University Medical Center Groningen, Hanzeplein 1, 9700 RB Groningen, The Netherlands*
[4] *Department of Epidemiology, University Medical Center Groningen, Hanzeplein 1, 9700 RB Groningen, The Netherlands*

Correspondence should be addressed to H. Kupiainen, henna.kupiainen@helsinki.fi

Academic Editor: Andrew Sandford

Smoking cessation is the cornerstone of COPD management, but difficult to achieve in clinical practice. The effect of comorbidities on smoking cessation and risk factors for mortality were studied in a cohort of 739 COPD patients recruited in two Finnish University Hospitals. The diagnosis of COPD was done for the first time on average 5.5 years prior to the enrollment. Data from the medical records and followup questionnaires (years 0, 1, 2, and 4) have been analyzed. The patients' lung function varied greatly; mean FEV_1 58% of predicted. A total of 60.2% of men and 55.6% of women had been able to quit smoking. Alcohol abuse (OR 2.1, 95% CI 1.4–3.3) and psychiatric conditions (OR 1.8, 95% CI 1.2–2.7) were strongly related to low success rates of quitting. Among current smokers high nicotine dependency was again explained by alcohol abuse and psychiatric conditions. Non-quitters were younger than quitters, but their mortality rates remained significantly higher even when the model was adjusted for impairment of lung functions and comorbidities. In conclusion, co-existing addiction and psychiatric diseases significantly decreased the success rates in smoking cessation and increased mortality among the patients.

1. Introduction

Smoking is by far the strongest risk factor of COPD. Smoking cessation has been shown to decelerate the progression of the disease and reduce mortality [1, 2]. In addition, smoking cessation is associated with a significant reduction of COPD exacerbations [3] and hospital admissions [4]. Data on predictors of smoking cessation relies almost entirely on population studies [5, 6]. COPD patients on the other hand comprise a heterogeneous group of patients who, in addition to heavy smoking, often display a variety of addictive characteristics, such as alcohol abuse [7] and certain psychiatric disorders [8]. Except for the shown efficacy of cessation medication, such as nicotine-replacement therapy, bupropion, and varenicline [9, 10], there are sparse studies on the clinical characteristics of COPD patients who either succeed or fail

in quitting smoking. A previous study has shown that a significant number of COPD patients continued smoking despite of their attempts to quit, underlining the importance of smoking cessation programs in clinical practice [11]. Among Polish smokers simple smoking cessation advice was shown to be more efficient among patients who displayed bronchial obstruction than among smokers with normal lung functions, suggesting that the awareness of COPD may improve the patient's motivation for quitting [12]. In these studies cumulative clinical data from medical records was not available.

We have followed a cohort of 739 COPD patients since the year 2006–07 by gathering their medical records into a single database [13]. The source data covers all health care providers, and the participants' medical history extends up to 5–10 years of prior to the enrollment. The patients are followed for 10 years with the questionnaires mailed every other year, currently the patients are on their fourth follow-up year.

Using this longitudinal clinical and questionnaire data, our aim in the present study is to report the clinical predictors that increase the risk of failure in smoking cessation among COPD patients. Our second aim was to find out whether smoking cessation had an effect on mortality in this hospital-based COPD population that represented all severity stages of the disease.

2. Study Subjects and Methods

2.1. Study Subjects. Hospital Discharge Registries were used to identify all in- and out-patients who had visited the Pulmonary Clinics of the Helsinki University Central Hospital (HUCH) and Turku University Hospital during the years 1995–2006. The databases were screened by the ICD10 code J44.8 and contained all patients between 18 to 75 years of age. The recruitment of all the identified patients was done through a two-phase mailing campaign. Altogether 844 patients (27%) contacted the researchers by phone and agreed on a visit to the clinical research center in Helsinki or Turku.

The research visits took place in years 2006–07 [13]. The participants gave their written informed consent for collecting and merging their comprehensive medical history from all healthcare providers who had treated them during the past 5–10 years. The participants also agreed to continue their followup through medical records and questionnaires for the next 10 subsequent years. They also donated a blood sample for DNA extraction. The health professionals examined the medical records to confirm the previously given smoking-related COPD or chronic bronchitis diagnosis. The diagnostic procedure described previously in detail [13] was based on clinical outcome, smoking history ≥ 10 pack years, and spirometry verification of airway obstruction. This evaluation led to the exclusion of a total of 105 patients due to fragmented documentation, insufficient diagnostic testing, and misclassifications.

2.2. Smoking-Related Variables. Data regarding the number of pack years and the smoking status were evaluated at two cross sectional time points: at the time of the diagnosis and the enrollment to the current study. The primary source of information for each study subject was the spirometry form. If that data was not available, other time-labeled documents were used. If these were not available, self-reported questionnaire data was used to acquire information about the patient's smoking status. Based on that data, smoking cessation was graded as follows: (1) quitting smoking before the diagnosis of COPD (early quitters), (2) quitting smoking after the diagnosis, either before or during the current study (late quitters), and (3) continued smoking throughout the study (nonquitters). Only the combined results are reported, in case no significant differences between the early and late quitters could be discovered.

2.3. Clinical Variables. The reference values for FEV_1 and FVC used in Finnish clinical practice are validated in large Finnish population samples consisting of males and females with a wide age range [14]. "Cardiovascular diseases" consist of patients diagnosed with one of the following diseases: coronary, cerebrovascular, or peripheral artery occlusive disease diagnosed by an internist. The category "diabetes" includes patients with type 1 and 2 disease. Chronic alcoholism, alcohol use disorder, and treatment of alcohol-use-related disorders were all categorized as "alcohol abuse". A wide range of psychotic disorders and long-lasting clinical depression and anxiety with a need for regular medication were combined as "psychiatric condition". The category "cancer" included all malignant solid tumors and malignant haematological diseases. The deaths were verified from the National Death Registry.

2.4. Health Related Quality of life and Nicotine Dependence. The summary scores of the participant's general (15D) [15, 16] and airway specific (AQ20) health-related quality of life [16] were obtained at the recruitment visit and from the 1st follow-up questionnaire. Both questionnaires have been validated and standardized internationally [15, 16]. The score of 15D varies from 0 (= dead) to 1 (= full health) and in AQ20 from 0 (= no symptoms or worries over the disease) to 20 (= full range of symptoms and worries over the disease). The patients' nicotine dependence was evaluated with the Fageström nicotine dependency test (FNDT) [17]. Data for this analysis was collected as a part of the fourth year follow-up questionnaire. At that time point 155 patients were still regular smokers. We were able to compute the Fageström's score for 140 of them.

The study approach was approved by the Coordinating Ethics Committee of the Helsinki and Uusimaa Hospital District, and the permission to conduct this research was granted by the Helsinki and Turku University Hospitals.

2.5. Statistical Analysis. The statistical software package SPSS (version 18.0) was used to compute differences in distributions of demographic and clinical variables between study groups. Differences in continuous variables were tested using the nonparametric Mann-Whitney U-test and in categorical variables the Chi-square or Fisher exact tests. Multivariate logistic regression model for smoking cessation was created with clinically relevant continuous traits and all comorbidities as independent variables. The dependent variable was quitting smoking either before or after COPD diagnosis, and the independent variables included were gender, age (per year), FEV_1 (categorized into four classes >80% normal, 65–80% mild, 40–65% moderate, and <40% severe), pack years, alcohol abuse, psychiatric condition, cardiovascular disease, diabetes, and cancer. A similar analysis was done for all-cause mortality: age, gender, smoking cessation, lung functions, and comorbidities were analyzed by univariate analysis and used in a multiple logistic regression model. The Fageström nicotine dependency score was analyzed with linear regression using gender, age, FEV_1, alcohol abuse, psychiatric conditions requiring medication, diabetes,

TABLE 1: Demographics and clinical characteristics of quitters and nonquitters.

Characteristics	All N = 739 (%)	Quitters[1] N = 433 (%)	Nonquitters N = 306 (%)	P value
Men	473 (64)	285 (60.3)	188 (39.7)	NS
Women	266 (36)	148 (55.6)	118 (44.4)	
Age, mean (±SD) in years	64.0 (6.8)	65.3 (6.6)	62.3 (6.8)	<0.001
Duration of COPD mean (±SD) in years	5.5 (4.1)	5.8 (4.4)	5.2 (3.8)	NS
BMI (kg/m^2) (±SD)	26.5 (5.3)	26.5 (5.2)	26.5 (5.5)	NS
Pack years (±SD)	41 (23)	43 (24)	38 (22)	0.01
Baseline mean (±SD)				
FEV$_1$% predicted	58.4 (18.9)	56.3 (18.4)	61.3 (19.3)	<0.001
FVC % predicted	73.6 (18.1)	72.6 (17.9)	74.9 (18.3)	0.04
FEV$_1$/FVC %	64.0 (13.9)	62.7 (14.4)	65.8 (13.0)	0.002
After bronchodilatation mean (±SD)				
FEV$_1$% predicted	62.1 (18.3)	60.3 (18.1)	64.4 (18.4)	0.004
FVC % predicted	77.8 (17.3)	77.4 (17.2)	78.4 (17.3)	NS
FEV$_1$/FVC %	64.4 (13.9)	63.0 (14.4)	66.4 (13.0)	0.002
N (%) of patients with				
FEV$_1$% >80	87 (12.0)	41 (9.6)	46 (15.4)	
FEV$_1$% 65–80	191 (26.4)	100 (23.5)	91 (30.5)	0.005 for trend
FEV$_1$% 40–64	309 (42.7)	196 (46.1)	113 (37.9)	
FEV$_1$% <40	139 (18.8)	88 (20.7)	48 (16.1)	
General-health-related QoL score (range 0-1) (±SD)	0.79 (0.11)	0.80 (0.10)	0.78 (0.12)	0.05
Airway specific QoL score (range 20–0) (±SD)	8.25 (5.03)	7.98 (4.77)	8.63 (5.35)	NS
Comorbidities N (%)				
Cardiovascular diseases	216 (29.2)	141 (32.6)	75 (24.5)	0.02
Diabetes	121 (16.4)	72 (16.7)	49 (16.1)	NS
Alcohol abuse	129 (17.8)	49 (11.5)	80 (26.6)	<0.001
Psychiatric disorder	177 (24.1)	75 (17.5)	102 (33.6)	<0.001
Cancer	78 (10.6)	49 (11.3)	29 (9.5)	NS
Deceased during the followup	114 (15.3)	52 (12.2)	62 (20.7)	0.002

[1] Early and late quitters combined.

and cardiovascular diseases as independent variables in the model.

The study approach was approved by the Coordinating Ethics Committee of the Helsinki and Uusimaa Hospital District, and the permission to conduct this research was granted by the Helsinki and Turku University Hospitals.

3. Results

3.1. Clinical Characteristics of the Cohort.
The cohort ($N = 739$) represented smoking-related chronic bronchitis and COPD of all severity stages (Table 1). FEV$_1$ ranged from 15 to 100%, mean 58% of predicted [13]. The COPD diagnosis was given for the first time when the participants were on average 58 years of age. During the enrollment to the present study, the average age was 64 years. The participants were diagnosed on average 5.5 years prior to the enrollment, which happened during the years 2006–07, and prospectively they have been followed so far for 4 years. One hundred fourteen patients had deceased during the study (annual mortality 3.8%).

3.2. Gender Differences in Smoking Behavior.
In the cohort 36% of the participants were women (Table 1). There were no significant differences in age or duration of COPD between genders. However, the number of pack years among men was significantly higher than among women (45 versus 33 pack years, $P \leq 0.001$). When COPD was first diagnosed, women were more frequently current smokers than men (80% versus 68%, $P < 0.001$). At the time of enrollment to the present study, the difference between genders was diminished (40% of men and 44% of women current smokers).

3.3. Quitting History.
At the time of the enrollment, a total of 58.6% ($n = 433$) patients had quit smoking. 28% ($n = 207$) of the patients quitted before and 30.6% ($n = 226$) after the COPD diagnosis was set. Minor, but statistically significant, differences were observed between the groups. The quitters were on average older (65 versus 62 years of age, $P = 0.001$) and reported more pack years (43 versus 38, $P = 0.011$) than nonquitters (Table 1). Their disease was more

TABLE 2: Independent risk factors for failure in smoking cessation by multivariate logistic regression analysis.

Variables	Adjusted OR	95% CI
Female gender	1.08	0.75–1.55
Aging by one year	**0.96**	**0.93–0.99****
FEV$_1$% of predicted		
>80	1.00	
65–80	0.84	0.48–1.46
40–64	0.60	0.35–1.02
<40	0.59	0.32–1.09
Number of pack years increased by one	0.99	0.99–1.00
Alcohol abuse	**2.12**	**1.35–3.34****
Psychiatric disorder	**1.83**	**1.23–2.71****
Cardiovascular diseases	0.78	0.53–1.15
Diabetes	1.07	0.68–1.68
Cancer	0.85	0.49–1.47

Response (nonquitter = 1, quitter = 0) **$P \leq 0.01$ *$P \leq 0.05$.

advanced (FEV$_1$ 60.3 versus 64.4% predicted, $P = 0.004$ and FEV$_1$/FVC ratio 63.0 versus 66.4, $P = 0.002$).

3.4. Comorbidities and Quitting. With respect to co-morbidities alcohol abuse and psychiatric conditions were the most significant risk factors associated with failure in smoking cessation. The prevalence of alcohol abuse (26.6% versus 11.5%P values ≤ 0.001) and psychiatric conditions (33.6% versus 17.5%, $P \leq 0.001$) were both higher among nonquitters than quitters. Cardiovascular diseases were more prevalent among early quitters compared to late or nonquitters, 44.4% and 31.3%, respectively, $P = 0.005$.

Multivariate logistic regression for smoking cessation was analyzed with clinical traits and comorbidities as independent variables (Table 2). Of the comorbid conditions, alcohol abuse and psychiatric conditions remained independent risk factors for failure in smoking cessation. The two conditions were partially overlapping. The prevalence of both conditions was 14.0% (42/299) among nonquitters and 3.1% (13/421) among quitters ($P < 0.001$). Gender or degree of airway obstruction did not contribute in smoking cessation significantly. The older a person was, the greater the chance of success in quitting.

3.5. Mortality in the Cohort. Altogether 114 (15.3%) patients had died by June 2011. Mortality rates were significantly higher among nonquitters (20.7%) compared to those among quitters (12.2%, $P = 0.002$). Clinical characteristics that had an effect on mortality are shown in Table 3. In the multivariate model, failure in quitting was strongly associated with increased mortality (OR 2.50, 95% CI 1.55–4.03). Of the comorbidities, cancer (OR 3.08, 95% CI 1.70–5.59) and alcohol abuse (OR 2.03, 95% CI 1.14–3.61) had an independent explanatory role in mortality. Similarly, moderate (OR 3.2, 95% CI 1.3–8.4) and severe (OR 5.6, 95% CI 2.5–17.5) impairment of lung function was associated with increased mortality, but cardiovascular

diseases, diabetes, and psychiatric conditions lost the effect in the adjusted model.

3.6. Nicotine Dependence among the Current Smokers. Nicotine dependence was evaluated using the Fagerström nicotine dependency test. The mean score among the patients was 4.3 (SD 2.4). The FNDT score did not correlate with FEV$_1$ of predicted values. Based on linear regression adjusted with age, gender, FEV$_1$, and comorbidities (cardiovascular diseases, diabetes, and cancer), alcohol abuse was the strongest explanatory variable for a high score (beta-value 0.260, $P = 0.003$). Also psychiatric conditions had an independent explanatory value (beta-value 0.183, $P = 0.04$).

4. Discussion

In the Finnish elderly population at large, smoking does not exceed 20% among men or 10% among women [18]. In this hospital-based COPD cohort, 40% of men and 44% of women continued smoking on average 5.5 years after their COPD had been diagnosed for the first time. Current smoking was significantly more prevalent among the patients who had alcohol abuse and/or psychiatric conditions. Compared to current smokers, the quitters of the cohort were older, reported more pack years, and had more advanced COPD frequently accompanied by cardiovascular disease, suggesting that the quitting takes place rather late in life and among patients with a disabling disease.

Our findings support and expand the previous findings made on quitting smoking in COPD [11, 12, 19]. In a large questionnaire study ($n = 58\,482$) made among the US Veterans, former smokers were older and had more cardiac comorbidities, but better mental health than current smokers [19]. Smoking cessation is strongly recommended in patients with cardiovascular disease and diabetes [20]. In the present study cardiovascular disease seemed to be a strong wake-up call to early smoking cessation and partially explained the better quit rates among males compared to those among females. Diabetes showed not as clear a relationship to smoking cessation, although a similar trend was observed.

COPD patients have been reported to display a twofold risk for depression compared to the general population [21, 22]. Even though presently largely ignored, tobacco dependence among individuals with a mental illness, especially schizophrenia, anxiety and depression, is very high [6, 8, 23, 24]. This might be explained by a robust bidirectional connection between nicotine dependence and vulnerability to psychopathology and susceptibility to certain psychiatric disorders [22]. It has also been reported that heavy drinking impairs success of quitting among COPD patients [11]. In the Finnish population over 50 years of age, hazardous drinking has been reported in 8% of men and 2% of women [25]. In the present COPD cohort the prevalence of alcohol abuse was 1.8 times higher among men and 5 times higher among women and was strongly related to nonquitting.

The Fagerström nicotine dependency test was included in the 4th year follow-up questionnaire and thus gave us information only from the most persistent smokers. The FNDT score of the present COPD cohort was in accordance

TABLE 3: Underlining clinical characteristics that predict mortality of the COPD patients during the four-year followup.

Variables	Patient $N = 739$	Deceased %	Crude OR	95% CI	P value	Adjusted OR	95% CI	P value
Aging by one year			1.05	1.02–1.09	0.002	1.07	1.03–1.11	0.001
Gender								
Male	466	18.0	1.00			1.00		
Female	259	11.6	0.60	0.38–0.93	0.022	0.81	0.48–1.435	NS
Smoking cessation								
Yes	426	12.2	1.00			1.00		
No	299	20.7	1.88	1.26–2.82	0.002	2.50	1.55–4.03	<0.001
Cardiovascular diseases								
No	514	13.0	1.00			1.00		
Yes	211	22.3	1.91	1.26–2.89	0.002	1.52	0.94–2.46	NS
Diabetes								
No	606	14.5	1.00			1.00		
Yes	117	22.8	1.68	1.03–2.75	0.036	1.38	0.79–2.43	NS
Alcohol abuse								
No	584	13.7	1.00			1.00		
Yes	128	24.2	2.01	1.26–3.22	0.003	2.03	1.14–3.61	0.016
Psychiatric condition								
No	544	14.9	1.00			1.00		
Yes	175	17.1	1.18	0.75–1.87	NS	1.32	0.77–2.26	NS
Cancer								
No	649	13.7	1.00			1.00		
Yes	74	32.4	3.02	1.77–5.16	<0.001	3.08	1.70–5.59	<0.001
FEV_1% of predicted								
>80%	87	5.7	1.00			1.00		
80–65%	191	9.9	1.81	0.65–5.02	NS	2.12	0.68–6.67	NS
65–40%	306	16.5	3.24	1.25–8.40	0.015	3.76	1.27–11.15	0.017
<40%	136	28.7	6.59	2.48–17.51	<0.001	8.77	2.88–26.68	<0.001

Response (dead = 1, alive = 0).

with previous studies [26]. It has been reported, however, that low FEV_1 and a high number of pack years indicate strong nicotine dependence [23]. Thus it was somewhat surprising that low FEV_1 in the present study did not significantly associate with the nicotine dependence. The variance found in FEV_1 among these long-term persistent smokers is, however, significantly smaller than in general population and thus decreases our power to detect potential association. The association between alcohol abuse and FNDT score in our study further proves the fact that addictive behavior cumulates [27].

Mortality was higher among nonquitters despite of their younger age and better lung functions. The increased mortality was confirmed irrespective of comorbidities, such as cancer or cardiovascular diseases. The fact that quitters are older, have lower lung function, more pack years, and CVD suggests reversed causality; a "healthy smoker" effect in which patients quit smoking only when they are older and have disabling illnesses. However, this does not directly lead to higher mortality rates. It seems that reversed causality is present but is confounded by the addictive profile of nonquitters with physical and mental problems and death at earlier age [2].

In the present study all the COPD patients (with the recruitment rate of 27%) treated in the clinic were invited to the study without further selection. Often in corresponding study designs the patient cohort has been rather small [28] or excluded relevant subgroups, such as patients with certain comorbidities, addictions, or obesity [29]. In randomized clinical trials, combined pharmacotherapy and counseling seem to lead to best long-term abstinence rates [9]. Participants' compliance, however, is of great importance in those types of studies [30, 31]. Therefore, patients with various mental and substance abuse diseases—to begin with—do not often volunteer and secondly, are generally excluded from clinical trials. This may improve the abstinence results of randomized trials and underestimate the significance of addictions in COPD. In clinical practice these patients may benefit from tight collaboration between their pulmonologist and psychiatrist when their cessation program is tailored. Comanagement of depression and smoking cessation has already shown to be feasible and safe. It increased the quit attempts and the success in cessation did not increase the risk of exacerbation of depression [32].

In addition to above-mentioned strengths our observational study design included also weaknesses. The cumulative clinical data was mainly based on retrospective medical records which were not originally produced for research purposes and therefore prevented us from the further dissection of the severity of psychiatric conditions or alcohol abuse. The smoking history reported by the patients in different cross sectional time points showed some inconsistencies. It seemed difficult for patients to remember when they had started and stopped smoking especially when that had happened a long time ago. At COPD diagnosis and during active treatment the data was more current and thus more adequate. That is why the data should be considered more like rough estimates rather than precise knowledge of patients pack years, starting and quitting dates. The Finnish Current Care Guidelines on Tobacco dependence and cessation and on COPD treatment are followed in the Finnish hospitals, but unfortunately no validated stopping program has been used [33]. In the Turku University Central Hospital patients were systematically referred to an individual or group counseling given by a registered nurse that improved the quit rates (66% versus 54%) suggesting that greater counseling efforts pay off among the COPD patients.

The present study emphasizes the heterogeneous clinical background of COPD patients, the role of coexisting diseases on smoking cessation, and the importance of quitting in the prognosis of COPD. New treatment options that comprehensively recognize patients' mental health and addiction profiles, and evaluate the patient's need of psychiatric help and/or medication, may benefit certain patient groups in their smoking cessation and could reduce mortality in these patient groups.

Acknowledgments

The authors would like to thank clinical research nurses Ms. Kerstin Ahlskog, Kirsi Sariola, and Päivi Laakso for their skillful patient recruitment, Ms. Tuula Lahtinen for the monitoring of the project, Siiri and Nelli Carlsson for their data analysis, and the former personnel of Geneos Ltd for the planning and implementing the patient recruitment. This study was supported by the funding of Helsinki University Hospital (HUS EVO), University of Helsinki, the Finnish Anti-Tuberculosis Association Foundation, Yrjö Jahnsson Foundation, the Research Foundation of the Pulmonary Diseases, Ida Montin Foundation, and Väinö and Laina Kivi Foundation.

References

[1] M. Pelkonen, I. L. Notkola, H. Tukiainen, M. Tervahauta, J. Tuomilehto, and A. Nissinen, "Smoking cessation, decline in pulmonary function and total mortality: a 30 year follow up study among the finnish cohorts of the seven countries study," *Thorax*, vol. 56, no. 9, pp. 703–707, 2001.

[2] N. S. Godtfredsen, T. H. Lam, T. T. Hansel et al., "COPD-related morbidity and mortality after smoking cessation: Status of the evidence," *European Respiratory Journal*, vol. 32, no. 4, pp. 844–853, 2008.

[3] D. H. Au, C. L. Bryson, J. W. Chien et al., "The effects of smoking cessation on the risk of chronic obstructive pulmonary

disease exacerbations," *Journal of General Internal Medicine*, vol. 24, no. 4, pp. 457–463, 2009.

[4] N. S. Godtfredsen, J. Vestbo, M. Osler, and E. Prescott, "Risk of hospital admission for COPD following smoking cessation and reduction: a Danish population study," *Thorax*, vol. 57, no. 11, pp. 967–972, 2002.

[5] N. S. Godtfredsen, E. Prescott, M. Osler, and J. Vestbo, "Predictors of smoking reduction and cessation in a cohort of Danish moderate and heavy smokers," *Preventive Medicine*, vol. 33, no. 1, pp. 46–52, 2001.

[6] A. Agrawal, C. Sartor, M. L. Pergadia, A. C. Huizink, and M. T. Lynskey, "Correlates of smoking cessation in a nationally representative sample of U.S. adults," *Addictive Behaviors*, vol. 33, no. 9, pp. 1223–1226, 2008.

[7] R. F. Leeman, S. A. McKee, B. A. Toll et al., "Risk factors for treatment failure in smokers: relationship to alcohol use and to lifetime history of an alcohol use disorder," *Nicotine and Tobacco Research*, vol. 10, no. 12, pp. 1793–1809, 2008.

[8] D. M. Ziedonis, B. Hitsman, J. C. Beckham et al., "Tobacco use and cessation in psychiatric disorders: National Institute of Mental Health report," *Nicotine and Tobacco Research*, vol. 10, no. 12, pp. 1691–1715, 2008.

[9] E. J. Wagena, R. M. van der Meer, R. J. W. G. Ostelo, J. E. Jacobs, and C. P. van Schayck, "The efficacy of smoking cessation strategies in people with chronic obstructive pulmonary disease: results from a systematic review," *Respiratory Medicine*, vol. 98, no. 9, pp. 805–815, 2004.

[10] B. M. Sundblad, K. Larsson, and L. Nathell, "High rate of smoking abstinence in COPD patients: smoking cessation by hospitalization," *Nicotine and Tobacco Research*, vol. 10, no. 5, pp. 883–890, 2008.

[11] J. S. Schiller and H. Ni, "Cigarette smoking and smoking cessation among persons with chronic obstructive pulmonary disease," *American Journal of Health Promotion*, vol. 20, no. 5, pp. 319–323, 2006.

[12] D. Gorecka, M. Bednarek, A. Nowinski, D. Kaminski, P. Bielen, J. Kolakowski et al., "Predictors of success in smoking cessation among participants of spirometric screening for COPD," *Pneumonol Alergol Pol*, vol. 69, no. 11-12, pp. 611–616, 2001.

[13] T. Laitinen, U. Hodgson, H. Kupiainen et al., "Real-world clinical data identifies gender-related profiles in chronic obstructive pulmonary disease," *Journal of Chronic Obstructive Pulmonary Disease*, vol. 6, no. 4, pp. 256–262, 2009.

[14] A. A. Viljanen, P. K. Halttunen, K. E. Kreus, and B. C. Viljanen, "Spirometric studies in non-smoking, healthy adults," *Scandinavian Journal of Clinical and Laboratory Investigation*, vol. 42, no. 159, pp. 5–20, 1982.

[15] H. Sintonen, "The 15D instrument of health-related quality of life: properties and applications," *Annals of Medicine*, vol. 33, no. 5, pp. 328–336, 2001.

[16] E. A. Barley, F. H. Quirk, and P. W. Jones, "Asthma health status measurement in clinical practice: validity of a new short and simple instrument," *Respiratory Medicine*, vol. 92, no. 10, pp. 1207–1214, 1998.

[17] T. F. Heatherton, L. T. Kozlowski, R. C. Frecker, and K. O. Fagerstrom, "The Fagerstrom test for nicotine dependence: a revision of the fagerstrom tolerance questionnaire," *British Journal of Addiction*, vol. 86, no. 9, pp. 1119–1127, 1991.

[18] T. Sulander, S. Helakorpi, O. Rahkonen, A. Nissinen, and A. Uutela, "Smoking and alcohol consumption among the elderly: trends and associations, 1985–2001," *Preventive Medicine*, vol. 39, no. 2, pp. 413–418, 2004.

[19] S. G. Adams, J. A. Pugh, L. E. Kazis, S. Lee, and A. Anzueto, "Characteristics associated with sustained abstinence from smoking among patients with COPD," *American Journal of Medicine*, vol. 119, no. 5, pp. 441–447, 2006.

[20] S. C. Campbell, R. J. Moffatt, and B. A. Stamford, "Smoking and smoking cessation—the relationship between cardiovascular disease and lipoprotein metabolism: a review," *Atherosclerosis*, vol. 201, no. 2, pp. 225–235, 2008.

[21] T. P. Ng, M. Niti, C. Fones, K. B. Yap, and W. C. Tan, "Comorbid association of depression and COPD: a population-based study," *Respiratory Medicine*, vol. 103, no. 6, pp. 895–901, 2009.

[22] N. Breslau, M. M. Kilbey, and P. Andreski, "Vulnerability to psychopathology in nicotine-dependent smokers: an epidemiologic study of young adults," *American Journal of Psychiatry*, vol. 150, no. 6, pp. 941–946, 1993.

[23] J. M. Williams and D. Ziedonis, "Addressing tobacco among individuals with a mental illness or an addiction," *Addictive Behaviors*, vol. 29, no. 6, pp. 1067–1083, 2004.

[24] A. K. McClave, S. R. Dube, T. W. Strine, K. Kroenke, R. S. Caraballo, and A. H. Mokdad, "Associations between smoking cessation and anxiety and depression among U.S. adults," *Addictive Behaviors*, vol. 34, no. 6-7, pp. 491–497, 2009.

[25] J. T. Halme, K. Seppä, H. Alho et al., "Hazardous drinking: prevalence and associations in the Finnish general population," *Alcoholism Clinical and Experimental Research*, vol. 32, no. 9, pp. 1615–1622, 2008.

[26] D. K. Kim, C. P. Hersh, G. R. Washko et al., "Epidemiology, radiology, and genetics of nicotine dependence in COPD," *Respiratory Research*, vol. 12, p. 9, 2011.

[27] J. R. Hughes and D. Kalman, "Do smokers with alcohol problems have more difficulty quitting?" *Drug and Alcohol Dependence*, vol. 82, no. 2, pp. 91–102, 2006.

[28] C. P. Hersh, D. L. DeMeo, E. Al-Ansari et al., "Predictors of survival in severe, early onset COPD," *Chest*, vol. 126, no. 5, pp. 1443–1451, 2004.

[29] N. R. Anthonisen, J. E. Connett, P. L. Enright, and J. Manfreda, "Hospitalizations and mortality in the lung health study," *American Journal of Respiratory and Critical Care Medicine*, vol. 166, no. 3, pp. 333–339, 2002.

[30] R. Strassmann, B. Bausch, A. Spaar, J. Kleijnen, O. Braendli, and M. A. Puhan, "Smoking cessation interventions in COPD: a networkmeta-analysis of randomised trials," *European Respiratory Journal*, vol. 34, no. 3, pp. 634–640, 2009.

[31] D. Tashkin, R. Kanner, W. Bailey et al., "Smoking cessation in patients with chronic obstructive pulmonary disease: a double-blind, placebo-controlled, randomised trial," *The Lancet*, vol. 357, no. 9268, pp. 1571–1575, 2001.

[32] C. J. Segan, R. Borland, K. A. Wilhelm et al., "Helping smokers with depression to quit smoking: collaborative care with quitline," *Medical Journal of Australia*, vol. 195, no. 3, pp. S7–S11, 2011.

[33] "Finnish current care guidelines," 2009, http://www.kaypahoito.fi/web/english/guidelines.

27

Dietary Flaxseed Oil Protects against Bleomycin-Induced Pulmonary Fibrosis in Rats

Joshua Lawrenz,[1] Betty Herndon,[2] Afrin Kamal,[3] Aaron Mehrer,[4] Daniel C. Dim,[3]
Cletus Baidoo,[3] David Gasper,[1] Jonathan Nitz,[1] Agostino Molteni,[3] and Richard C. Baybutt[1]

[1] Department of Applied Health Science, Wheaton College, 501 College Avenue, Wheaton, IL 60187, USA
[2] Department of Basic Medical Sciences, School of Medicine, University of Missouri-Kansas City (UMKC), USA
[3] Department of Pathology and Pharmacology, School of Medicine, University of Missouri-Kansas City (UMKC), 2411 Holmes Street, Kansas City, MO 64108, USA
[4] Department of Anesthesiology, School of Medicine, University of Missouri-Kansas City (UMKC), Kansas City, MO 64108, USA

Correspondence should be addressed to Richard C. Baybutt, richard.baybutt@wheaton.edu

Academic Editor: S. L. Johnston

Bleomycin, a widely used antineoplastic agent, has been associated with severe pulmonary toxicity, primarily fibrosis. Previous work has shown a reduction in bleomycin-induced lung pathology by long-chain omega-3 fatty acids. Treatment by short-chain omega-3 fatty acids, α-linolenic acid, found in dietary flaxseed oil may also reduce lung fibrosis, as previously evidenced in the kidney. To test this hypothesis, 72 rats were divided between diets receiving either 15% (w/w) flaxseed oil or 15% (w/w) corn oil (control). These groups were further divided to receive either bleomycin or vehicle (saline) via an oropharyngeal delivery, rather than the traditional intratracheal instillation. Lungs were harvested at 2, 7, and 21 days after bleomycin or saline treatment. Animals receiving flaxseed oil showed a delay in edema formation ($P = 0.025$) and a decrease in inflammatory cell infiltrate and vasculitis ($P = 0.04$ and 0.007, resp.). At days 7 and 21, bleomycin produced a reduction in pulmonary arterial lumen patency ($P = 0.01$), but not in rats that were treated with flaxseed oil. Bleomycin-treated rats receiving flaxseed oil had reduced pulmonary septal thickness ($P = 0.01$), signifying decreased fibrosis. Dietary flaxseed oil may prove beneficial against the side effects of this highly effective chemotherapeutic agent and its known toxic effects on the lung.

1. Introduction

Bleomycin is a group of glycopeptides that binds iron and oxygen in vivo to produce an active drug, effective in cancer treatment. In the last few decades, many Americans were diagnosed with Hodgkin's lymphoma and testicular cancer, and a majority received bleomycin as part of their chemotherapeutic regimen. A large study from 1986 to 2003 found that out of 141 Hodgkin's lymphoma patients treated with bleomycin, 18% developed pulmonary toxicity, and of those patients 24% died [1]. Currently, no known treatments exist to prevent pulmonary toxicity in these patients. In short, bleomycin's fibrotic side effects are so common that it is widely used to create animal models of pulmonary fibrosis.

Bleomycin's active intermediate is believed to induce both single-and double-strand DNA cleavage in neoplastic cells [2]. The chemotherapeutic mechanism results from the chelation of iron ions with oxygen, which leads to production of DNA-cleaving superoxide, and also hydroxide free radicals [3–5]. It is the increased production of reactive oxygen species (ROS) that may be critical in producing proinflammatory eicosanoids that lead to bleomycin's pulmonary toxicity, and may eventually lead to lung fibrosis [6–9]. In recent literature, the presence of several ROS has been found in clinical cases of idiopathic pulmonary fibrosis [10, 11], and decreased production of ROS has been shown to protect mice against bleomycin-induced pulmonary fibrosis [12]. In addition, a reduction in antioxidants has been reported in

IPF lungs, and the resulting oxidant-antioxidant imbalance has been suggested in the progression of IPF [13, 14].

Though it still remains unclear the role which oxidation plays in the inflammatory and profibrotic response found in pulmonary fibrosis, oxidative stress seems to be associated with the disease as previously described. As a means of attenuating oxidative damage, long chain omega-3 fatty acids, eicosapentaenoic acid (EPA), and docosahexaenoic acid (DHA) have been found effective due to their protective antioxidant properties [15, 16]. In addition, we have previously shown that fish oil containing EPA and DHA protects against lung inflammation and pulmonary fibrosis in a monocrotaline-induced lung fibrosis model [17]. Another research group has shown that fish oil prevents bleomycin-induced lung inflammation and pulmonary fibrosis [18]. Thus, the long chain omega-3 fatty acids, eicosapentaenoic acid (EPA) and docosahexaenoic acid (DHA), are thought to be responsible for these protective effects. In addition, the essential omega-6 fatty acid, γ-linolenic acid (GLA) has also been shown to be a potent antioxidant [19], and has been found to attenuate bleomycin-induced lung fibrosis in hamsters [20]. Whether short chain omega-3 fatty acids have a similar protective effect is not known.

Shorter-chain omega-3 fatty acids such as α-linolenic acid (ALA) in flaxseed oil do not necessarily have similar biological effects as the longer chain omega-3 fatty acids found in fish oil. For example, long chain fatty acids EPA and DHA have been shown to have cardioprotective effects, while the short chain fatty acid ALA did not reduce or benefit cardiovascular disease outcomes in a recent review [21]. Recent studies also found that low doses of fish oil (0.7–7% energy), not flaxseed oil, suppressed inflammation, as evidenced by decreased thromboxane B_2 and serum TNF-α levels, markers for inflammation [22]. On the other hand, a recent study indicates that dietary ALA in rapeseed oil has antioxidant properties, as it inhibits lipid peroxidation in animals after acute brain ischemia [23]. Also, dietary ALA has been shown to elicit an anti-inflammatory effect in cultured peripheral blood mononuclear cells by inhibiting the proinflammatory cytokine production of IL-6 and TNF-α [24]. Furthermore, a research group at the University of Manitoba has found substantial evidence that dietary flaxseed oil protects against fibrosis in the kidney [25–29].

Therefore, there seem to be similarities and differences in the biological function of the shorter chain omega-3 fatty acid, ALA found in flaxseed oil, and its close relatives GLA, EPA, and DHA. All have been shown to have antioxidant properties, and both anti-inflammatory and antifibrotic effects under certain conditions. To our knowledge, no one has investigated whether ALA found in dietary flaxseed oil protects against bleomycin-induced lung fibrosis. This is the purpose of the present study.

2. Materials and Methods

2.1. Animals and Treatment.
Weanling male Harlan Sprague-Dawley rats (Indianapolis, IN, USA) were housed in stainless steel cages at approximately 24°C with a 12-hour light-dark cycle. Animal care and use were approved by the

Institutional Animal Care and Use Committee (IACUC) of Wheaton College. Animals were housed in an animal facility approved by the American Association for the Advancement of Laboratory Care (AALAC). The rats had ad libitum access to food and water.

A total of 72 rats weighing 40–60 g each were randomly assigned to one of four groups (18 rats per group). All rats were fed a standard AIN-93G diet [30] containing either corn oil (15% w/w) or flaxseed oil (15% w/w). The antioxidant activity of tert-Butylhydroquinone (TBHQ), an effective preservative for unsaturated oils, was not significantly different than that of the small amounts of natural tocopherols found in the corn oil and was substantially less than the amount used in studies that evaluated the antioxidant role of TBHQ [31]. To minimize fat oxidation, the powdered diets were stored in Ziploc freezer bags, and stored at −20°C. The diets were purchased from Dyets Inc., (Bethlehem, PA,). Food consumption was measured by calculating the difference between the preweighed and unconsumed diet. Food was provided daily and the leftovers discarded. Body weights were recorded every week.

After four weeks of dietary treatment of the respective diets, bleomycin was administered. About 5 mL of Trifluralin anesthesia was used to saturate a piece gauze placed in a bell jar. Rats were placed in the covered jar became anesthetized after five seconds of gaseous exposure to Trifluralin, and remained anesthetized for about 30 seconds. During this time, bleomycin or its vehicle (saline) was administered oropharyngeally in a 400 μL solution (8 U/kg body weight) to half of the rats in each respective group, according to a previously published method [32]. The tongue was secured by tissue forceps in such a way as to prevent swallowing, and the rats aspirated the bleomycin solution that was administered via pipette into the oral cavity. The four treatment groups consisted of rats were instilled with the vehicle and fed a corn oil diet (VC), the vehicle and fed a flaxseed oil diet (VF), bleomycin and fed a corn oil diet (BC), and bleomycin and fed a flaxseed oil diet (BF). At the termination of the experiment, blood was collected from the rats, followed by organ removal of the lungs, liver, kidneys, and heart at 2, 7, or 21 days after bleomycin administration.

2.2. Assessment of the Lung Histological Damage.
Histological evaluation of lung tissue was performed in a semiquantitative manner as previously described [33–36]. Briefly, the left lung was removed and then prepared with 10% buffered formalin, and fixed for 1 week. The right lung was immediately frozen in liquid nitrogen and stored at −80°C for analysis. Formalin-fixed lungs were then embedded in paraffin blocks and sections were prepared for hematoxylin eosin staining and Masson-Trichrome collagen staining. For evaluation of pulmonary damage, slides were scored by two pathologists who were unaware of the experimental protocol and their scores were averaged to obtain a single score. Observed changes were evaluated in the thickening of the alveolar septa, and interseptal, intra-alveolar, and vascular areas were examined for the presence of hemorrhaging, inflammatory cells, or collagen deposition (fibrosis).

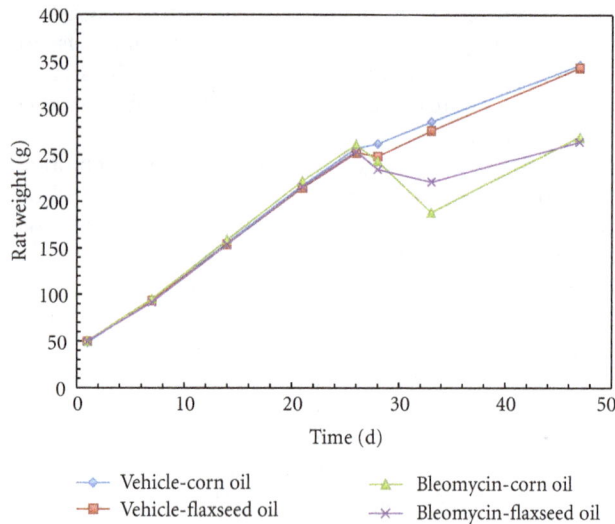

FIGURE 1: Weight gain in rats fed 15% (w/w) corn oil or 15% (w/w) flaxseed oil diet. Bleomycin and vehicle administration occurred at day 26. Data are expressed as means ± SEM, $n = 13–15$. At day 33 (or 7 days after bleomycin administration), there was significantly less weight loss in the BF treated rats than the BC treated rats ($P < 0.03$).

TABLE 1: (a) Body weight gain or loss shown by experimental group after bleomycin treatment. (b) Food intake averages by experimental group after bleomycin treatment.

(a)

	VC	VF	BC	BF
2 days	0.6 ± 2.3^a	0.8 ± 1.9	-17.5 ± 5.3	-20.7 ± 1.6
7 days	23.6 ± 2.2	31.0 ± 1.8	-71.7 ± 2.5	$-37.6 \pm 15.4^*$
21 days	97.3 ± 1.7	88.4 ± 11.9	4.2 ± 62.4	16.9 ± 31.0

Rat weights measured each week, number of rats: $n = 3–5$.
[a]Data are expressed as mean ± SEM. The numerical values are expressed as grams (g).
Significant differences are noted in a row for the respective measurement. The level of significance is $P < 0.05$.
*BC versus BF groups, $P < 0.03$.

(b)

VC	VF	BC	BF
23.0	22.2	3.4	$11.7^{*,a}$

Food intake measured daily, number of rats: $n = 13–18$.
[a]Data are expressed as mean ± SEM. The numerical values are expressed as grams (g).
Significant differences are noted in a row for the respective measurement. The level of significance is $P < 0.05$.
*BC versus BF groups, $P < 0.001$.

Particular evidence was given to the fibrosis (collagen deposition) expressed in the vasculature, the septa, and the peribronchial musculature. Subjective scoring ranging from 5 (presence of borderline damage) to 40 (very severe and extensive damage with destruction of a large portion of the parenchyma) was assigned to the components of the lung previously stated. The total score reported was the mean ± standard error of the mean of the individual scores for each category. Values for each group of treated animals were averaged and reported separately.

The method for determining lumen patency and media/ adventitia ratio has been previously published in different models of lung injury including exposure to radiation, development of pulmonary hypertension and fibrosis, and damage induced by vitamin A deficiency [33–38]. Briefly, the luminal diameter of vessels divided by their external or vascular diameter was the measurement associated with lumen patency. The outer diameter of the media divided by the outer diameter of the adventitia provided the media/adventitia ratio, which was used as a measure of adventitial edema. Both ratios were evaluated in five small caliber pulmonary arteries for each rat in each group. The mean value of the five vessel measurements for each rat was reported for statistical analysis. The thickness of the arteriolar wall and the percentage of small artery lumen occlusion (diameter ranges from 20 to 100 μm) were measured in photographs at 100X and 400X magnifications.

2.3. Statistical Analysis. Data were expressed as means ± SEM. The experiment was analyzed as a 2 × 2 factorial design. Differences among groups for inflammatory cell infiltrate, septal thickness, emphysema, medial vasculitis, and edema were determined using a two-way analysis of variance (ANOVA) followed by least significant difference (LSD) multiple comparison tests (SAS Institute Inc., Cary, NC, USA). For the semiquantitative analysis, group data were compared by a one-way analysis of variance with Tukey posttest. These were calculated using StatView software. The level of significance was $P < 0.05$ for all comparisons.

3. Results

3.1. Morbidity and Mortality. No rats died during the four-week dietary treatment prior to bleomycin treatment. Four rats died during the administration of bleomycin or its vehicle due to too much exposure to anesthesia. These four rats were excluded from statistical analyses. Six rats died after bleomycin treatment and before their sacrifice date. Two BC rats died on day 3 (after bleomycin treatment) and one BC rat died on day 8. Two BF rats died on day 2 and one BF rat died on day 8. Localized darkening areas (hemorrhaging) were observed on the lung surfaces in rats that died on day 8. Otherwise, all rats survived and were sacrificed at 2, 7, or 21 days after bleomycin treatment.

3.2. Body Weight Gain and Food Intake after Bleomycin Treatment. The average daily food intake for the bleomycin-treated rats was significantly less than the vehicle group ($P < 0.03$). The food intake of the BF group was significantly more than the BC group ($P < 0.001$). There was also significantly less weight loss in the BF-treated rats than the BC-treated rats at 7 days ($P < 0.03$). The findings are summarized in Table 1 and Figure 1.

TABLE 2: Relative (normalized to body weight) weights (g) of organs at 7 days after bleomycin treatment and averaged by experimental group.

7 days	VC	VF	BC	BF
Lung	4.3 ± 0.1^a	4.0 ± 0.1	15.5 ± 0.1	$10.3 \pm 1.0^*$
Heart	4.9 ± 0.1	4.2 ± 0.3	5.5 ± 0.1	$4.6 \pm 0.2^*$
Liver	33.0 ± 0.6	32.7 ± 0.2	37.8 ± 1.9	$32.3 \pm 0.8^*$
Left kidney (LK)	4.1 ± 0.1	4.2 ± 0.1	5.3 ± 0.2	$4.6 \pm 0.1^*$
Right kidney (RK)	4.1 ± 0.1	4.2 ± 0.1	5.4 ± 0.1	$4.8 \pm 0.1^*$

Organ tissue weights measured at the time of sacrifice, number of rats: $n =$ 3–5.

No significant differences were found at days 2 and 21.

[a]Data are expressed as mean $\pm$ SEM; all values to 10^{-3}.

Significant differences comparing BC and BF groups are noted in a row for the respective tissue.

*BC versus BF groups, $P < 0.05$.

3.3. Gross Organ Evaluation.

At gross evaluation, the vehicle-treated rat lungs (VC and VF) at 2 days, 7 days and 21 days appeared to be normal. Discoloration, or localized darkening areas (hemorrhaging) and a cobblestone appearance were observed in the lungs of BC rats at 7 days, and to a more severe extent at 21 days. There were no abnormal damages on the rat lung surfaces at 2 days. In contrast, bleomycin-treated rats fed a flaxseed oil diet were seen to have less organ discoloration and surface hemorrhaging. Other organs appeared similar to the controls.

3.4. Organ Tissue Weights.

The relative weights of the respective organs of bleomycin-treated rats were all significantly higher when compared to the organs of the vehicle controls ($P < 0.001$ for all but liver where $P < 0.002$). The average relative weights of all five of the organs (lung, liver, heart, left kidney, and right kidney) in the BF treated rats were significantly less than that of the BC-treated rats at 7 days ($P < 0.05$). The findings are summarized in Table 2.

3.5. Overview.

It is evident that bleomycin-induced damage starts already in the bronchi and septa at 48 hours and progresses throughout the experiment. At day 7, the presence of collagen and vasculitis is already severe, and the damage persists up to 21 days substantially unchanged (Figures 2, 3(a), 3(b), and 3(c)). On the other hand, a strong protective effect is exerted by the flaxseed oil diet.

It has to be noted that some pulmonary damage as septal inflammation and bronchitis is also present in the rats receiving the vehicle and corn oil diet (Figure 4). The flaxseed oil diet protects the bronchi and the lungs also from the vehicle-induced inflammatory effect (Figure 5). Only bleomycin causes severe vasculitis indicating that this compound presents strong similarities with other models of damage of this organ: exposure to radiation [38] or hypoxia [39] and administration of monocrotaline [40].

3.6. Lung Histological Results.

In general, dietary corn oil and flaxseed oil treatment had no significant or severe morphological damages on the lungs of the rats without the bleomycin treatment as shown by H&E staining (Figure 4). It is interesting to note that we found a small inflammatory effect in the vehicle control on day 2 immediately after saline administration. Bleomycin treatment was evaluated by the presence of septal edema and inflammation, medial and adventitial vasculitis, bronchitis, lumen patency changes, and septal thickness. The BF group showed less severe edema formation ($P = 0.025$), a decrease in septal inflammation ($P = 0.04$), and a decrease in vasculitis ($P = 0.007$) compared to the BC group (Figure 4). Differences were more significant at days 7 after bleomycin treatment than at day 2.

Furthermore, five small caliber pulmonary arteries of each rat in each group were evaluated for bleomycin-induced pulmonary vasculitis, by measuring pulmonary lumen patency and the ratio of media diameter/adventitia diameter. At days 7 and 21, bleomycin produced a significant reduction in pulmonary lumen patency ($P = 0.01$) but not of the media/adventitial diameter. However, this significant reduction of the lumen patency was not evident when the rats were on the flaxseed oil diet (Figure 5). Also, the BF group showed a significantly reduced pulmonary septal thickness at day 7 and 21 compared to the BC group ($P = 0.013$) (Figures 3(b), and 3(c)).

The histological changes induced by bleomycin and the two diets observed with H&E staining were reinforced and further supported by the trichrome staining (Figures 3(a), 3(b), and 3(c)) of septal and bronchial inflammatory vasculitis. Increased presence of peribronchial, perivascular, and interseptal collagen was well evident in BC rat lungs, especially at days 7 and 21. The flaxseed oil diet reduced the damaging effect of bleomycin especially in rats sacrificed at 21 days. A small bronchial and septal inflammatory response was also observed in VC rat lungs, but not in VF rat lungs. Figure 2 summarizes the histopathological changes observed with the trichrome staining of the lungs. The trichrome data supports the previously reported H&E information at the histological evaluation.

Histological data in the lungs of rats sacrificed 48 hours after bleomycin instillation already indicate that both bleomycin and the vehicle produce varied degrees of bronchial damage and septal inflammation with the corn oil diet; damage is less evident in the animals fed the flaxseed oil diet. After 7 days, the bleomycin-induced damage is very severe without signs of improvement two weeks later. At both interval times however, the flaxseed oil diet significantly mitigates the bleomycin-induced effects and also the minor damaging effect of the vehicle (Figure 2). The flaxseed oil effect is particularly evident on the hyperproduction of collagen, thus protecting the organ from one of the most severe side effects of bleomycin as an antineoplastic drug: the onset of organ fibrosis.

4. Discussion

The purpose of this study was to determine whether dietary flaxseed oil prevented bleomycin-induced lung fibrosis. These results indicate that flaxseed oil was effective in protecting lung tissue from bleomycin-induced pulmonary toxicity in rats indicated by increased lumen patency and reduced

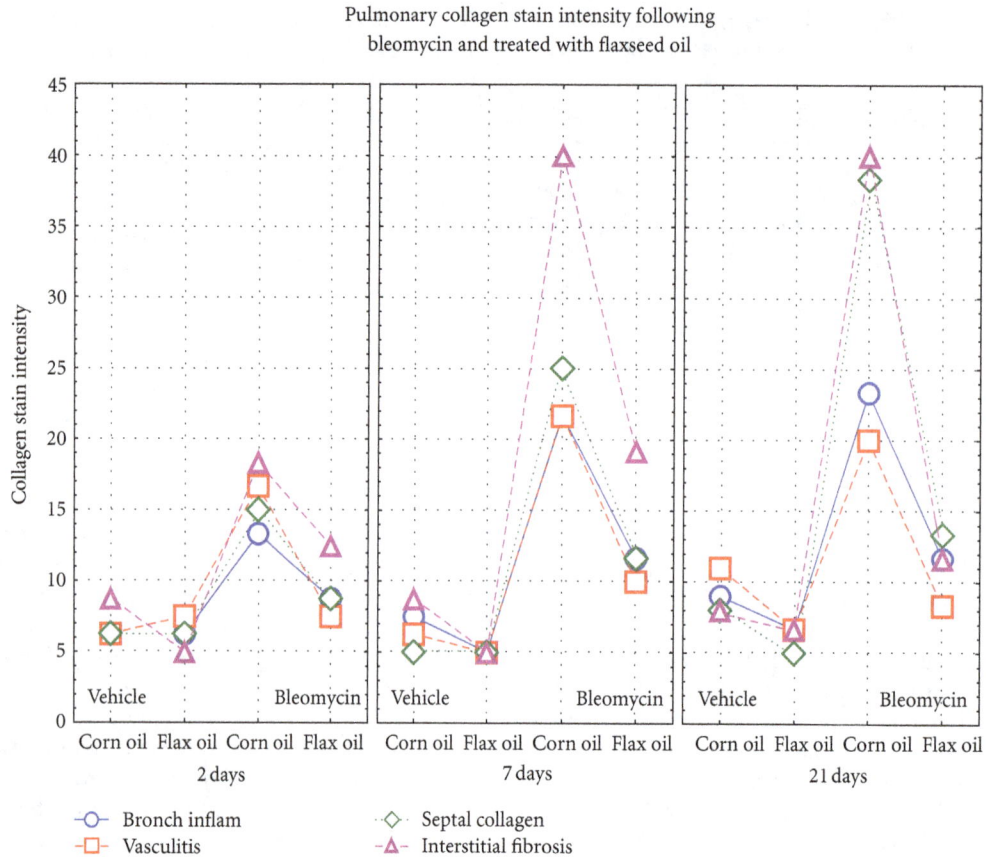

FIGURE 2: Qualitative evaluation of the pathological scores of the various treatment groups at each time interval point. (Staining: Masson's trichrome). The symbols represent the mean of all the rats in each group. Scoring of pathology: Ranges from 5: borderline damage, progressing to a high of 40: very severe and extensive damage. Scoring of stain intensity: estimated area of blue stain on a series of high-power fields with trichrome staining. Abbreviations: Bronch. Inflam.: Bronchial Inflammation with loss of epithelium, loss of cilia, and increased number of inflammatory cells. Vasculitis: Thickening of the media of vessels and reduction of lumen patency. Septal collagen: Presence of blue stained fibers on trichrome stain. Interstitial fibrosis: Presence of fibers in the septa stained by trichrome.

pulmonary septal thickness, decreased inflammatory cell infiltrate, delayed edema formation, reduced vasculitis, and pulmonary and peribronchial fibrosis.

To our knowledge, the present study is the first evidence that flaxseed oil prevents lung fibrosis using a bleomycin rat model. In the present study, we observed the short chain fatty acids in flaxseed oil to be equally effective in protecting against fibrosis as long chain fatty acids in past studies [17, 18]. Others have shown that dietary flaxseed decreases lung fibrosis and inflammation in the lungs of mice at four months after X-ray-radiation-therapy-(XRT-) induced pneumonopathy [41].

A potential mechanism to explain the anti-inflammatory role of flaxseed oil involves lung eicosanoid production. Long chain omega-3 fatty acid (EPA+DHA) eicosanoid derivatives are known to produce less active proinflammatory products than those of the typical omega-6 eicosanoid precursor, arachidonic acid [42], and in a previous work, we have showed that fish oil (EPA+DHA) protects against lung inflammation and pulmonary fibrosis in a monocrotaline-induced lung fibrosis model [17]. In addition, ALA deriva-tives have also been shown to have some anti-inflammatory

action by competitively inhibiting the transformation of arachidonic acid to leukotrienes [43, 44]. Furthermore, ALA decreases production of the profibrotic PGE-2 series precursor, arachidonic acid [45]. Also, a bleomycin-induced lung fibrosis study in hamsters found that the omega-6 fatty acid γ-linolenic acid inhibited fibrosis, via its elongation in vivo to dihomo-γ-linoleic acid with little formation of arachidonic acid, suggesting a potential role for eicosanoid metabolites [20].

Another potential protective mechanism of flaxseed oil against bleomycin-induced pulmonary fibrosis may include specific cytokines. The presence of platelet-derived growth factor (PDGF) has been observed in the bleomycin model of pulmonary fibrosis [46]. The expression of PDGF was elevated in the early stage of disease and reached its peak at day 7 in bleomycin treated groups [46]. In addition, the gene expression of another profibrotic cytokine, transforming growth factor beta-1, has been previously found to be elevated around day 6 in the rat bleomycin model [8]. Similarly, we found pulmonary injury to be most severe at day 7, and also the difference due to flaxseed oil to be great at day 7 and even greater at day 21 (Figures 2, 3(b), and 3(c)).

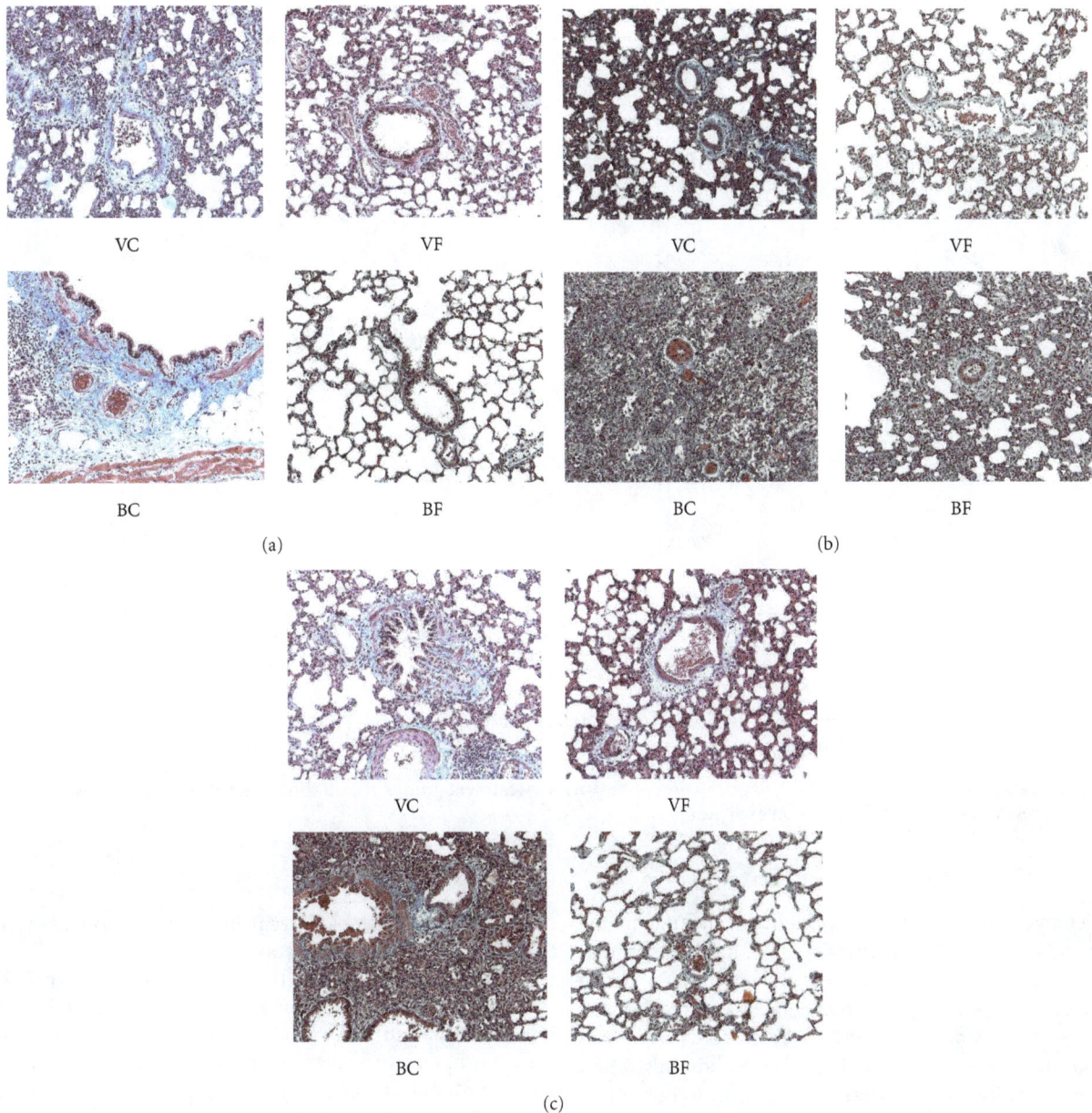

FIGURE 3: (a) Histological sections of rat lungs of the four groups sacrificed at day 2. Mild septal congestion and bronchial inflammatory reaction is found in rats treated with the vehicle and corn oil. Severe septal and bronchial inflammation and the increased presence of collagen (blue) are seen in bleomycin treated rats on the corn oil diet. Inflammation and vascular thickness are less severe when the diet is flaxseed oil. Stain: Masson's Trichrome, 200X. (b) Histological sections of rat lungs of the four groups sacrificed at day 7. The VC-treated rat lungs show modest septal inflammation and a mild increase of adventitial edema and fibrosis. No damage was observed in VF treated rats. Bleomycin treated rats on the corn oil diet present diffuse inflammation and septal thickening, severe vascular thickening with markedly decreased lumen patency and bronchitis with increased presence of collagen (blue). Bleomycin treated rats on the flaxseed oil diet had less severe damage with not so prominent septal thickness, more patent arterial lumina and less fibrosis. Stain: Masson's Trichrome, 200X. (c) Histological sections of rat lungs of the four groups sacrificed at day 21. The vehicle and corn oil caused diffuse septal and bronchial inflammation with increased collagen (blue) around the bronchial pulmonary arteries, and in the septa. No similar damage was observed in VF rats. Septal and bronchial inflammation is very severe in lungs of rats receiving bleomycin and on the corn oil diet, with vasculitis and fibrosis. The peribronchial arterioles were particularly involved with almost total obstruction of their lumen. Flaxseed oil diet markedly attenuated the bleomycin-induced damage both as septal inflammation and vasculitis. While the lungs of bleomycin + corn oil-treated rats were similar at 7 and 21 days, the lungs of bleomycin + flaxseed oil-treated rats were markedly improved at 21 days versus those of rats sacrificed after 7 days. Stain: Masson's Trichrome, 200X. Abbreviations used: VC (vehicle, corn oil), VF (vehicle, flax seed oil), BC (bleomycin, corn oil), and BF (bleomycin, flax seed oil).

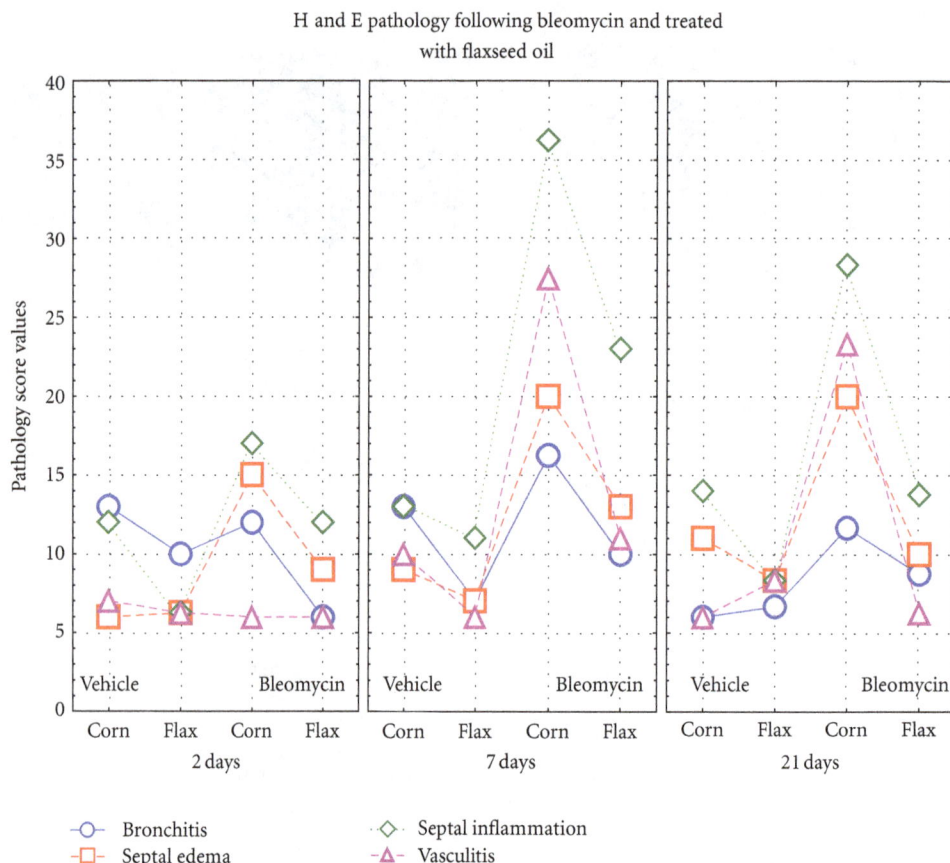

FIGURE 4: Qualitative evaluation of the pathological scores of the various treatment groups at each time interval point. (Staining: H&E). The symbols represent the mean of all the rats in each group.

Bleomycin is not the only compound eliciting in the lungs and other organs, specifically the kidneys, inflammation, and vasculitis and eventually leading to fibrosis. Strong analogies are observed with other models of experimental lung injuries causing similar histopathological damage such as exposure to radiation [38] or hypoxia [39], administration of monocrotaline [40], or lung fat embolism consequent to injection of triolein [37]. In all of these models, the renin-angiotensin system is involved, and treatments with angiotensin converting enzyme inhibitors (Captopril) [47, 48] or angiotensin type 1 receptor blockers (Losartan) [49–53] are effective. Another potential mechanism by which flaxseed oil prevents fibrosis in the bleomycin model may be by the angiotensin pathway. In preliminary and unreported data, we recently found a decreased production of angiotensin peptides in the flaxseed oil treated rats. The role of other components of the respiratory system such as clara cells, osteopontin, angiotensin peptides, smooth muscle actin, mast cells, and different cytokines should also be evaluated in the response to the treatment of flaxseed oil, especially in lieu of the observation that one of the most efficient protectors in the above-mentioned models of damage, Captopril, is also a powerful antioxidant [54]. Defining the precise mechanism for the flaxseed oil-mediated

protection against bleomycin-induced pulmonary fibrosis remains an intriguing question for future studies.

It is important to note because the conversion of ALA to longer chain omega-3 fatty acids is typically less efficient in humans than in rats, the effects of ALA-fibrotic protection via formation of longer chain omega-3 fatty acids cannot be ruled out in the rat model [55]. There does remain considerable uncertainty as to the extent to which short chain ALA is converted into the longer chain EPA and DHA in humans. Some have reported that ALA's conversion into long chain derivatives is limited in humans [55, 56], whereas others have found ALA supplementation to increase the amount of EPA [57, 58]. Future fatty acid tissue analysis should help to define the fatty acid metabolites involved.

The pathological effects of bleomycin did not appear to be due to malnutrition prior to bleomycin treatment, because there was no difference in the average weight gain across groups due to the source of dietary fat. The significant loss of body weight in bleomycin treated groups (BC and BF) after bleomycin administration suggests that the animal is responding to the toxicity (Figure 1). When flaxseed oil was administered along with bleomycin, the average weight loss was significantly reduced and paired with a greater food intake, indicating the protective effects on health maintenance of flaxseed oil over corn oil (Table 1).

(a)

(b)

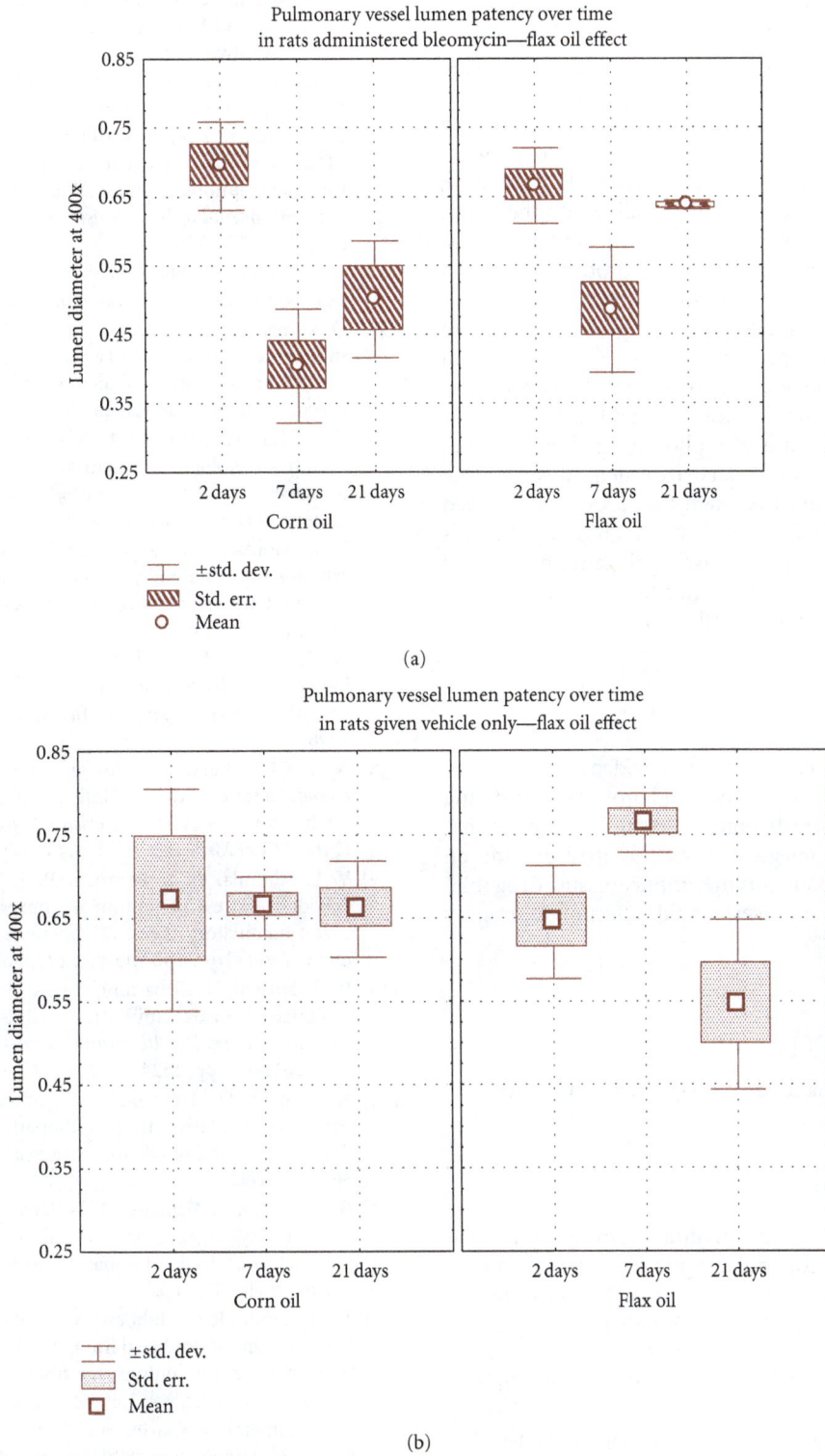

FIGURE 5: Lumen patency of small caliber pulmonary arteries and arterioles of the four groups at each time interval point. BC-treated rats show marked wall thickening and reduced lumen patency at day 7 and 21. No significant differences were observed in the lumen patency of arteries of rats instilled with the vehicle. The symbols represent means, boxes represent standard error, and the whiskers represent standard deviation values.

It is important to note that in this study we adopted an oropharyngeal delivery of bleomycin that has proven to be an effective way to administer bleomycin. A previous study has shown that the oropharyngeal delivery of bleomycin creates a more representative human fibrotic lung disease than traditional intratracheal instillation [32]. There was, however, a slight inflammation in the vehicle control via the oropharyngeal delivery of saline likely due to a "water boarding" effect (Figure 3(a)). As noted in the methods, we administered on average 400 μL of saline into the lungs, which could be the cause of this slight inflammation. Interestingly, the flaxseed oil appeared to protect also against this "water boarding" effect (Figures 3(a), 3(c), and 5).

Lastly, this study was able to show a protective effect of flaxseed oil against the bleomycin-induced fibrosis within only a four-week period of dietary treatment. This apparently provides sufficient time for the omega-3 fatty acids to become incorporated into the phospholipid membranes [17]. The four weeks of dietary treatment was half the length of time of dietary treatment that previously showed a protective effect of fish oil against the fibrosis [18]. This difference in feeding time may have significant implications in considering testing the protective effects of omega-3 fatty acids against fibrosis in the clinical setting.

5. Conclusions

In summary, our results provide first evidence that dietary flaxseed oil decreases inflammation and protects against lung fibrosis in bleomycin-treated rats. These results suggest that ingestion of dietary omega-3 fatty acids may provide an effective protection plan for the antineoplastic drug bleomycin by reducing the deleterious side effect of pulmonary fibrosis.

Conflict of Interests

The authors declare that there is no conflict of interests.

Acknowledgments

The authors thank Provost Stanton L. Jones and Dean Dorothy F. Chappell for their financial support enabling summer student research opportunities at Wheaton College. The authors thank Dr. William M. Struthers for the use of his laboratory, and Lisa K. Hilde and Owen N. Handy for their technical assistance. The authors thank the Chair of the Anesthesiology at the, School of Medicine University of Missouri-Kansas City, Dr. E. E. Fibuch M.D., Jennifer Rawls, and all the personnel of the pathology laboratories of the Truman Medical Center at the University of Missouri at Kansas City for their skillful technical assistance in the preparation of the chemical and histological material. This research was funded by the Aldeen and Alumni Association grants from Wheaton College with its motto "For Christ and His Kingdom."

References

[1] W. G. Martin, K. M. Ristow, T. M. Habermann, J. P. Colgan, T. E. Witzig, and S. M. Ansell, "Bleomycin pulmonary toxicity has a negative impact on the outcome of patients with Hodgkin's lymphoma," *Journal of Clinical Oncology*, vol. 23, no. 30, pp. 7614–7620, 2005.

[2] A. Moeller, K. Ask, D. Warburton, J. Gauldie, and M. Kolb, "The bleomycin animal model: a useful tool to investigate treatment options for idiopathic pulmonary fibrosis?" *International Journal of Biochemistry and Cell Biology*, vol. 40, no. 3, pp. 362–382, 2008.

[3] J. Chen and J. Stubbe, "Bleomycins: towards better therapeutics," *Nature Reviews Cancer*, vol. 5, no. 2, pp. 102–112, 2005.

[4] D. Kumar, H. Hirao, S. Shaik, and P. M. Kozlowski, "Proton-shuffle mechanism of O–O activation for formation of a high-valent oxo-iron species of bleomycin," *Journal of the American Chemical Society*, vol. 128, no. 50, pp. 16148–16158, 2006.

[5] Z. D. Xu, M. Wang, S. L. Xiao, C. L. Liu, and M. Yang, "Synthesis, biological evaluation and DNA binding properties of novel bleomycin analogues," *Bioorganic and Medicinal Chemistry Letters*, vol. 13, no. 15, pp. 2595–2599, 2003.

[6] R. H. Goldstein, K. Miller, J. Glassroth et al., "Influence of asbestos fibers on collagen and prostaglandin production in fibroblast and macrophage co-cultures," *Journal of Laboratory and Clinical Medicine*, vol. 100, no. 5, pp. 778–785, 1982.

[7] N. R. Grande, C. M. de Sá, and A.P. Águas, "Lung fibrosis induced by bleomycin: structural changes and overview of recent advances," *Scanning Microscopy*, vol. 12, pp. 487–494, 1998.

[8] N. I. Chaudhary, A. Schnapp, and J. E. Park, "Pharmacologic differentiation of inflammation and fibrosis in the rat bleomycin model," *American Journal of Respiratory and Critical Care Medicine*, vol. 173, no. 7, pp. 769–776, 2006.

[9] V. L. Kinnula, C. L. Fattman, R. J. Tan, and T. D. Oury, "Oxidative stress in pulmonary fibrosis: a possible role for redox modulatory therapy," *American Journal of Respiratory and Critical Care Medicine*, vol. 172, no. 4, pp. 417–422, 2005.

[10] P. Montuschi, G. Ciabattoni, P. Pared et al., "8-Isoprostane as a biomarker of oxidative stress in interstitial lung diseases," *American Journal of Respiratory and Critical Care Medicine*, vol. 158, no. 5, pp. 1524–1527, 1998.

[11] K. Psathakis, D. Mermigkis, G. Papatheodorou et al., "Exhaled markers of oxidative stress in idiopathic pulmonary fibrosis," *European Journal of Clinical Investigation*, vol. 36, no. 5, pp. 362–367, 2006.

[12] B. Manoury, S. Nennan, O. Leclerc et al., "The absence of reactive oxygen species production protects mice against bleomycin-induced pulmonary fibrosis," *Respiratory Research*, vol. 6, article 11, 2005.

[13] A. M. Cantin, R. C. Hubbard, and R. G. Crystal, "Glutathione deficiency in the epithelial lining fluid of the lower respiratory tract in idiopathic pulmonary fibrosis," *American Review of Respiratory Disease*, vol. 139, no. 2, pp. 370–372, 1989.

[14] M. Peltoniemi, R. Kaarteenaho-Wiik, M. Säily et al., "Expression of glutaredoxin is highly cell specific in human lung and is decreased by transforming growth factor-β in vitro and in interstitial lung diseases in vivo," *Human Pathology*, vol. 35, no. 8, pp. 1000–1007, 2004.

[15] J. M. R. Frenoux, E. D. Prost, J. L. Belleville, and J. L. Prost, "A polyunsaturated fatty acid diet lowers blood pressure and improves antioxidant status in spontaneously hypertensive rats," *Journal of Nutrition*, vol. 131, no. 1, pp. 39–45, 2001.

[16] N. Okabe, T. Nakamura, T. Toyoshima, O. Miyamoto, F. Lu, and T. Itano, "Eicosapentaenoic acid prevents memory impairment after ischemia by inhibiting inflammatory response and oxidative damage," *Journal of Stroke and Cerebrovascular Diseases*, vol. 20, no. 3, pp. 188–195, 2011.

[17] R. C. Baybutt, C. Rosales, H. Brady, and A. Molteni, "Dietary fish oil protects against lung and liver inflammation and fibrosis in monocrotaline treated rats," *Toxicology*, vol. 175, no. 1–3, pp. 1–13, 2002.

[18] J. I. Kennedy Jr., D. B. Chandler, J. D. Fulmer, M. B. Wert, and W. E. Grizzle, "Dietary fish oil inhibits bleomycin-induced pulmonary fibrosis in the rat," *Experimental Lung Research*, vol. 15, no. 2, pp. 315–329, 1989.

[19] W. Peschel, W. Dieckmann, M. Sonnenschein, and A. Plescher, "High antioxidant potential of pressing residues from evening primrose in comparison to other oilseed cakes and plant antioxidants," *Industrial Crops and Products*, vol. 25, no. 1, pp. 44–54, 2007.

[20] V. A. Ziboh, M. Yun, D. M. Hyde, and S. N. Giri, "γ-linolenic acid-containing diet attenuates bleomycin-induced lung fibrosis in hamsters," *Lipids*, vol. 32, no. 7, pp. 759–767, 1997.

[21] C. Wang, W. S. Harris, M. Chung et al., "N-3 Fatty acids from fish or fish-oil supplements, but not α-linolenic acid, benefit cardiovascular disease outcomes in primary- and secondary-prevention studies: a systematic review," *American Journal of Clinical Nutrition*, vol. 84, no. 1, pp. 5–17, 2006.

[22] M. K. Duda, K. M. O'Shea, A. Tintinu et al., "Fish oil, but not flaxseed oil, decreases inflammation and prevents pressure overload-induced cardiac dysfunction," *Cardiovascular Research*, vol. 81, no. 2, pp. 319–327, 2009.

[23] C. Nguemeni, B. Delplanque, C. Rovère et al., "Dietary supplementation of alpha-linolenic acid in an enriched rapeseed oil diet protects from stroke," *Pharmacological Research*, vol. 61, no. 3, pp. 226–233, 2010.

[24] G. Zhao, T. D. Etherton, K. R. Martin, P. J. Gillies, S. G. West, and P. M. Kris-Etherton, "Dietary α-linolenic acid inhibits proinflammatory cytokine production by peripheral blood mononuclear cells in hypercholesterolemic subjects," *American Journal of Clinical Nutrition*, vol. 85, no. 2, pp. 385–391, 2007.

[25] M. R. Ogborn, E. Nitschmann, H. Weiler, D. Leswick, and N. Bankovic-Calic, "Flaxseed ameliorates interstitial nephritis in rat polycystic kidney disease," *Kidney International*, vol. 55, no. 2, pp. 417–423, 1999.

[26] M. R. Ogborn, E. Nitschmann, N. Bankovic-Calic, H. A. Weiler, and H. Aukema, "Dietary flax oil reduces renal injury, oxidized LDL content, and tissue n-6/n-3 FA ratio in experimental polycystic kidney disease," *Lipids*, vol. 37, no. 11, pp. 1059–1065, 2002.

[27] M. R. Ogborn, E. Nitschmann, N. Bankovic-Calic, H. A. Weiler, and H. M. Aukema, "Effects of flaxseed derivatives in experimental polycystic kidney disease vary with animal gender," *Lipids*, vol. 41, no. 12, pp. 1141–1149, 2006.

[28] D. Sankaran, N. Bankovic-Calic, C. Y. C. Peng, M. R. Ogborn, and H. M. Aukema, "Dietary flax oil during pregnancy and lactation retards disease progression in rat offspring with inherited kidney disease," *Pediatric Research*, vol. 60, no. 6, pp. 729–733, 2006.

[29] D. Sankaran, N. Bankovic-Calic, L. Cahill, C. Yu-Chen Peng, M. R. Ogborn, and H. M. Aukema, "Late dietary intervention limits benefits of soy protein or flax oil in experimental polycystic kidney disease," *Nephron*, vol. 106, no. 4, pp. e122–e128, 2007.

[30] P. G. Reeves, F. H. Nielsen, and G. C. Fahey, "AIN-93 purified diets for laboratory rodents: final report of the American Institute of Nutrition ad hoc writing committee on the reformulation of the AIN-76A rodent diet," *Journal of Nutrition*, vol. 123, no. 11, pp. 1939–1951, 1993.

[31] M. J. Gonzalez, R. A. Schemmel, L. Dugan, J. I. Gray, and C. W. Welsch, "Dietary fish oil inhibits human breast carcinoma growth: a function of increased lipid peroxidation," *Lipids*, vol. 28, no. 9, pp. 827–832, 1993.

[32] H. F. Lakatos, H. A. Burgess, T. H. Thatcher et al., "Oropharyngeal aspiration of a silica suspension produces a superior model of silicosis in the mouse when compared to intratracheal instillation," *Experimental Lung Research*, vol. 32, no. 5, pp. 181–199, 2006.

[33] R. C. Baybutt and A. Molteni, "Dietary β-carotene protects lung and liver parenchyma of rats treated with monocrotaline," *Toxicology*, vol. 137, no. 2, pp. 69–80, 1999.

[34] R. C. Baybutt, L. Hu, and A. Molteni, "Vitamin A deficiency injures lung and liver parenchyma and impairs function of rat type II pneumocytes," *Journal of Nutrition*, vol. 130, no. 5, pp. 1159–1165, 2000.

[35] A. Molteni, W. F. Ward, C. H. Ts'ao, and N. H. Solliday, "Monocrotaline-induced cardiopulmonary damage in rats: amelioration by the angiotensin-converting enzyme inhibitor CL242817," *Proceedings of the Society for Experimental Biology and Medicine*, vol. 182, no. 4, pp. 483–493, 1986.

[36] W. F. Ward, A. Molteni, N. H. Solliday, and G. E. Jones, "The relationship between endothelial dysfunction and collagen accumulation in irradiated rat lung," *International Journal of Radiation Oncology Biology Physics*, vol. 11, no. 11, pp. 1985–1990, 1985.

[37] T. E. McIff, A. M. Poisner, B. Herndon et al., "Fat embolism: evolution of histopathological changes in the rat lung," *Journal of Orthopaedic Research*, vol. 28, no. 2, pp. 191–197, 2010.

[38] W. F. Ward, A. Molteni, C. H. Ts'ao, and N. H. Solliday, "Radiation injury in rat lung. IV. Modification by D-penicillamine," *Radiation Research*, vol. 98, no. 2, pp. 397–406, 1984.

[39] A. Molteni, R. M. Zakheim, K. B. Mullis, and L. Mattioli, "The effect of chronic alveolar hypoxia on lung and serum angiotensin I converting enzyme activity," *Proceedings of the Society for Experimental Biology and Medicine*, vol. 147, no. 1, pp. 263–265, 1974.

[40] A. Molteni, W. F. Ward, C. H. Ts'ao, C. D. Port, and N. H. Solliday, "Monocrotaline-induced pulmonary endothelial dysfunction in rats," *Proceedings of the Society for Experimental Biology and Medicine*, vol. 176, no. 1, pp. 88–94, 1984.

[41] J. C. Lee, R. Krochak, A. Blouin et al., "Dietary flaxseed prevents radiation-induced oxidative lung damage, inflammation and fibrosis in a mouse model of thoracic radiation injury," *Cancer Biology and Therapy*, vol. 8, no. 1, pp. 47–53, 2009.

[42] G. Schmitz and J. Ecker, "The opposing effects of n-3 and n-6 fatty acids," *Progress in Lipid Research*, vol. 47, no. 2, pp. 147–155, 2008.

[43] J. Dobryniewski, S. D. Szajda, N. Waszkiewicz, and K. Zwierz, "Biology of essential fatty acids (EFA)," *Przeglad Lekarski*, vol. 64, no. 2, pp. 91–99, 2007.

[44] D. H. Hwang, M. Boudreau, and P. Chanmugam, "Dietary linolenic acid and longer-chain n-3 fatty acids: comparison of effects on arachidonic acid metabolism in rats," *Journal of Nutrition*, vol. 118, no. 4, pp. 427–437, 1988.

[45] L. A. Marshall and P. V. Johnston, "Modulation of tissue prostaglandin synthesizing capacity by increased ratios of dietary alpha-linolenic acid to linoleic acid," *Lipids*, vol. 17, no. 12, pp. 905–913, 1982.

[46] M. Song, B. He, and Z. Qiu, "Expressions of TNF alpha, PDGF in alveolar type II epithelial cells of rats with bleomycin-induced pulmonary fibrosis," *Zhonghua Jie He He Hu Xi Za Zhi*, vol. 21, no. 4, pp. 221–223, 1998.

[47] A. Molteni, W. F. Ward, and C. H. Ts'ao, "Monocrotaline-induced pulmonary fibrosis in rats: amelioration by captopril and penicillamine," *Proceedings of the Society for Experimental Biology and Medicine*, vol. 180, no. 1, pp. 112–120, 1985.

[48] W. F. Ward, Y. T. Kim, A. Molteni, and N. H. Solliday, "Radiation-induced pulmonary endothelial dysfunction in rats: modification by an inhibitor of angiotensin converting enzyme," *International Journal of Radiation Oncology Biology Physics*, vol. 15, no. 1, pp. 135–140, 1988.

[49] A. Molteni, "Applications of angiotensin converting enzyme inhibitors and of angiotensin II receptor blockers in pharmacology and therapy: an update," *Current Pharmaceutical Design*, vol. 13, no. 12, pp. 1187–1190, 2007.

[50] A. Molteni, L. F. Wolfe, W. F. Ward et al., "Effect of an angiotensin II receptor blocker and two angiotensin converting enzyme inhibitors on transforming growth factor-β (TGF-β) and α-Actomyosin (α SMA), important mediators of radiation-induced pneumopathy and lung fibrosis," *Current Pharmaceutical Design*, vol. 13, no. 13, pp. 1307–1316, 2007.

[51] A. Molteni, R.C. Baybutt, T. Li, and B.L. Herndon, "Interactive effects of an antioxidant (retinoic acid) and an angiotensin converting enzyme inhibitor (Captopril) on an experimental model of pulmonary fibrosis," *Current Pharmaceutical Design*, vol. 13, pp. 1327–1333, 2007.

[52] A. Molteni, J. E. Moulder, E. P. Cohen et al., "Prevention of radiation-induced nephropathy and fibrosis in a model of bone marrow transplant by an angiotensin II receptor blocker," *Experimental Biology and Medicine*, vol. 226, no. 11, pp. 1016–1023, 2001.

[53] T. E. McIff, A. M. Poisner, B. Herndon, K. Lankachandra, A. Molteni, and F. Adler, "Mitigating effects of captopril and losartan on lung histopathology in a rat model of fat embolism," *Journal of Trauma*, vol. 70, no. 5, pp. 1186–1191, 2011.

[54] A. Molteni, W. Ward, C. H. Ts'ao, and N. Solliday, "Monocrotaline-induced cardiopulmonary injury in rats: modification by thiol and nonthiol ACE inhibitors," *Clinical and Experimental Hypertension A*, vol. 9, no. 2-3, pp. 381–385, 1987.

[55] L. M. Arterburn, E. B. Hall, and H. Oken, "Distribution, interconversion, and dose response of n-3 fatty acids in humans," *American Journal of Clinical Nutrition*, vol. 83, no. 6, supplement, pp. 1467S–1476S, 2006.

[56] M. R. Fokkema, D. A. J. Brouwer, M. B. Hasperhoven, I. A. Martini, and F. A. J. Muskiet, "Short-term supplementation of low-dose γ-linolenic acid (GLA), α-linolenic acid (ALA), or GLA plus ALA does not augment LCPω3 status of Dutch vegans to an appreciable extent," *Prostaglandins Leukotrienes and Essential Fatty Acids*, vol. 63, no. 5, pp. 287–292, 2000.

[57] J. K. Chan, B. E. McDonald, J. M. Gerrard, V. M. Bruce, B. J. Weaver, and B. J. Holub, "Effect of dietary α-linolenic acid and its ratio to linoleic acid on platelet and plasma fatty acids and thrombogenesis," *Lipids*, vol. 28, no. 9, pp. 811–817, 1993.

[58] C. R. Harper, M. E. Edwards, A. P. DeFilipis, and T. A. Jacobson, "Flaxseed oil increases the plasma concentrations of cardioprotective (n-3) fatty acids in humans," *Journal of Nutrition*, vol. 136, no. 1, pp. 83–87, 2006.

28

Loss of Asthma Control in Pediatric Patients after Discontinuation of Long-Acting Beta-Agonists

Adrian R. O'Hagan, Ronald Morton, and Nemr Eid

Division of Pediatric Pulmonology, University of Louisville, Louisville, KY 40202, USA

Correspondence should be addressed to Adrian R. O'Hagan, adrian.ohagan@louisville.edu

Academic Editor: Leif Bjermer

Recent asthma recommendations advocate the use of long-acting beta-agonists (LABAs) in uncontrolled asthma, but also stress the importance of stepping down this therapy once asthma control has been achieved. The objective of this study was to evaluate downtitration of LABA therapy in pediatric patients who are well-controlled on combination-inhaled corticosteroid (ICS)/LABA therapy. Clinical and physiologic outcomes were studied in children with moderate-to-severe persistent asthma after switching from combination (ICS/LABA) to monotherapy with ICS. Of the 54 patients, 34 (63%) were determined to have stable asthma after the switch, with a mean followup of 10.7 weeks. Twenty (37%) had loss of asthma control leading to addition of leukotriene receptor antagonists, increased ICS, or restarting LABA. There were 2 exacerbations requiring treatment with systemic steroids. In patients with loss of control, there was a statistically significant decline in FEV_1 (-8% versus -1.9%, $P = 0.03$) and asthma control test (-3.2 versus -0.5, $P = 0.03$). This did not approach significance for $FEF_{25-75\%}$, exhaled nitric oxide, lung volumes or airway reactivity. No demographic, asthma control measures, or lung function variables predicted loss of control. Pediatric patients with moderate-to-severe persistent asthma who discontinue LABA therapy have a 37% chance of losing asthma control resulting in augmented maintenance therapies. Recent recommendations of discontinuing LABA therapy as soon as control is achieved should be evaluated in a prospective long-term study.

1. Introduction

Since the introduction of long-acting $\beta2$-agonists (LABAs) in the 1990s and their approval in the United States in 1994, there has been data showing their benefit on lung function and clinical outcomes [1]. These agents are widely used for asthma treatment in combination with inhaled steroids, and may be overused [2, 3]. Reports of increased adverse events in patients receiving this therapy, as noted in the Salmeterol Nationwide Surveillance (SNS) study, led the US Food and Drug Administration (FDA) to request a safety and monitoring trial that started enrollment in 1996 [4]. However, enrollment was stopped in 2003 related to increased asthma-related deaths in patients receiving salmeterol [5]. Despite uncertainty regarding concomitant use of anti-inflammatory therapy in this study, a black box warning for LABAs was introduced. The FDA, after comprehensive reviews and public discussions at multiple

advisory meetings in 2005, 2007, and 2008, released new safety requirements for combination therapy in February, 2010 [4]. The FDA recommended that "LABAs should be used for the shortest duration of time required to achieve control of asthma symptoms and discontinued, if possible, once asthma control is achieved" [6].

While there are data showing that for both pediatric and adult patients whose asthma is not well controlled, the addition of LABA therapy is clinically superior to doubling the inhaled corticosteroid dose or the addition of a leukotriene receptor antagonist [7, 8]; there are little data or clinical practice guidelines on how best to step off LABA therapy. Previous studies have shown that the removal of LABA leads to lower lung function and less well-controlled asthma, but there are no pediatric data available [9, 10]. Current asthma guidelines suggest stepping down the dose of inhaled corticosteroids rather than discontinuation of LABA [11]. This leaves clinicians torn between having to choose between FDA and expert opinion in the management of their patients with persistent asthma. Unfortunately, the safety risks will not be clarified until the multinational, randomized, and double-blinded prospective combined FDA and Pharma initiative is completed in about 6 years [12].

This investigator-initiated study was designed to evaluate short-term clinical outcome after the discontinuation of LABA therapy in a population of well-controlled children with asthma.

2. Methods

This study included patients with moderate-to-severe persistent asthma on the basis of the criteria recommended by the National Asthma Education and Prevention Program [11], and an ability to perform reproducible spirometry. Patients were excluded if they had concomitant primary pulmonary disease (e.g., cystic fibrosis and primary ciliary dyskinesia). All patients were followed at the Childhood Asthma Care and Education Center at Kosair Children's Hospital, Louisville, Ky, USA, every three to four months. Asthma control was based on criteria [11] that included asthma control test score (ACT) $\geq$ 20 [13] and normal or near normal spirometric data. Once these criteria were met, the maintenance therapy was switched from combination therapy to ICS monotherapy. The choice of inhaled steroid was made by the pulmonologist after consideration of insurance coverage, patient factors, and physician preference. Once the LABA was discontinued, the patients remained on bioequivalent doses of inhaled steroids [11, 14]. For example, patients on fluticasone/salmeterol combination were switched 1 to 1 (microgram-microgram) to either fluticasone propionate-HFA (FP-HFA), or beclomethasone-HFA (BDP-HFA), mometasone furoate (MF), or ciclesonide (CIC). Patients on budesonide/formoterol combinations were switched 2 to 1 to BDP-HFA, FP-HFA, MF, or CIC. Standardized education was completed by an asthma educator to review device and spacer technique.

Patients were reevaluated after 8 weeks of therapy. Information recorded included symptom control (cough, wheeze, shortness of breath, and nocturnal symptoms), use of rescue medications including oral steroids, spirometry, lung volumes, exhaled nitric oxide, and ACT scoring. Throughout the study, patients using MDI had to use it with a spacer device with inspiratory flow signal (Aerochamber, Monaghan Medical Corporation, Plattsburgh, NY, USA). All patients received education by a respiratory therapist before the start of the study on device technique. Standard spacer technique included slow inhalation with 10 sec breath hold before exhalation and 4–6 regular tidal breaths/activation. All patients understood and adequately reproduced the technique. None of the patients developed hoarseness or oral candidiasis during the study. Patients were instructed to wash and clean their spacer once a week. Atopy was defined by positive allergy skin test or Immunocap *in vitro* quantitative assay, use of immunotherapy, or physician-diagnosed allergic rhinosinusitis.

Compliance was discussed with each patient on each visit. At each visit, patients were required to give the names

TABLE 1: Baseline patient characteristics.

	All
Patients, n	54
Age, y	10.9 (6–18)
Male sex (%)	33 (61%)
Caucasian race (%)	44 (81%)
Duration of asthma, yr	7.4 (1–15)
LTRA use (%)	25 (46%)
ACT	23.5 ± 1.9
FVC, % predicted	104.8 ± 11.6
FEV$_1$, % predicted	102.3 ± 11.8
FEF$_{25-75}$, % predicted	98.1 ± 24.7

Abbreviations—LTRA: leukotriene receptor antagonists; ACT: asthma control test; FVC: forced vital capacity; FEV$_1$: forced expiratory volume in 1 second; FEF$_{25-75}$: forced expiratory flow at 25–75% of FVC.

and the daily doses of all of their asthma medications, including the inhaled steroids. Patients were also asked about their compliance with each medication, including inhaled steroids, and the information was confirmed with the parents.

Patients were considered to be uncontrolled if they met one of the following: systemic steroid use due to asthma exacerbation, drop in FEV$_1$ of at least 12% or FEF$_{25-75\%}$ of 25%, or a decrease in ACT score to <20. The primary outcome was maintenance of asthma control. Secondary outcomes included the change in FEV$_1$, FEF$_{25-75\%}$ or ACT score, and the value of exhaled nitric oxide (eNO).

Lung function was assessed at each clinic visit by spirometry which was performed according to the American Thoracic Society Standardization of Spirometry Guidelines (1995) [15]. The value recorded for FEV$_1$ was the highest of three American Thoracic Society- acceptable curves from three separate tests. The prediction equation of Polgar and Promadhat was used to determine predicted values [16]. All evaluation was done using the same spirometer (Koko Trek spirometer, Ferraris, Louisville, CO, USA), plethysmograph (MedGraphics Elite Series, Medical Graphics Corporation, St. Paul, MN, USA) and nitric oxide analyzer (Niox Mino, Aerocrine, New Providence, NJ, USA). Pneumotachometer used was Model Number 91-000. Calibration was done daily.

All statistical analysis was performed with SPSS, version 19.0.0 (IBM). The Spearman correlation was utilized due to noncontinuous or not normally distributed data. The test used with continuous outcomes between groups was the t-test if normally distributed or the Mann Whitney if not normally distributed. The institutional review board approved this retrospective review.

3. Results

3.1. Patient Characteristics and Medication Use. A summary of select variables pertinent to our analysis is presented in Table 1. All patients were receiving inhaled corticosteroids and long-acting beta-agonist therapy. Eight patients were receiving the fluticasone-salmeterol combination in one single device, and 43 the budesonide-formoterol combination and the remaining 3 ciclesonide and formoterol by separate devices. All of the budesonide-formoterol combinations were delivered by HFA. Three of the fluticasone-salmeterol combinations were delivered by HFA. Patients were enrolled over a nine-month period, from March through December.

Of those on fluticasone-salmeterol, 4 were started on Mometasone, 3 on Beclomethasone, and 1 on fluticasone. Of those on budesonide-formoterol: 21 were started on Mometasone, 18 on Beclomethasone, and 4 on budesonide. The remaining 3 on Ciclesonide had their formoterol discontinued, remaining on Ciclesonide alone.

3.2. Asthma Control at Followup. Patients were followed at 10.7 weeks (+/− 5.2, range 1–24). Thirty-four (63%) had maintained asthma control based on symptoms and spirometry in accordance with NHLBI guidelines. The remaining 20 (37%) had loss of asthma control. Of these, 8 had a decline in ACT score to <20 with associated spirometric evidence of increased airflow obstruction. Eight patients had a decrease in ACT score alone, including 2 patients that required a 5-day course of oral prednisone due to an asthma exacerbation. The remaining 8 patients had an increase in airflow obstruction without a decrease of ACT to <20. No patients required hospitalization during the followup period. All patients received bronchodilator testing at followup. Only 1 patient in the uncontrolled group had evidence of airway hyperresponsiveness.

Of the patients who had uncontrolled asthma at followup, 14 were initially receiving the budesonide-formoterol combination. Of these, 8 had been switched to beclomethasone, 4 to mometasone, and 2 remained on budesonide. Of the 3 patients on fluticasone-salmeterol that were uncontrolled, they were switched to beclomethasone, mometasone and fluticasone. All three of the patients receiving ciclesonide-formoterol and switched to ciclesonide alone had uncontrolled asthma at followup.

These findings prompted the restarting of LABA therapy in 18 patients. In the other 2 patients, the ICS was doubled in one due to elevated exhaled nitric oxide and LTRA was started in the other due to known underlying atopy.

A summary of the between-group differences of those maintaining and losing control is provided in Table 2. There were no differences at baseline that predicted who could successfully have their LABA therapy stopped. This includes which anti-inflammatory therapy the patients were receiving and what steroid moiety they were subsequently changed to. At followup there were significant group differences in terms of symptomatic and spirometric control. Figures 1, 2, and 3 display scatterplots of individual patient's change in lung function and ACT scores. In the controlled, group those with a decrease in lung function had percent predicted values over 100%, normal FEV_1/FVC, ratio and unchanged ACT. Likewise, those with a decrease in ACT had unchanged spirometric data and were felt to clinically have either a viral upper respiratory illness or allergic rhinosinusitis. Eleven patients in the controlled group and 7 in the uncontrolled

TABLE 2: Patient characteristics comparing those that maintained asthma control off LABA therapy at followup (controlled) and those that experienced loss of asthma control (uncontrolled). *represents $P < 0.05$.

	Controlled	Uncontrolled
Patients, n	34	20
Time to f/u, weeks	10.3	11.5
Age, yr	11.3	10.2
Male sex (%)	22 (65)	11 (55)
Caucasian (%)	27 (79)	16 (80)
Insurance, government (%)	7 (21)	8 (40)
Smoke exposure, negative (%)	19 (56)	14 (70)
Atopy (%)	27 (79)	15 (75)
Duration of asthma, yr	7.6	6.4
LTRA use (%)	15 (44)	10 (50)
ACT, baseline	23.5	23.4
FVC, baseline % pred	105 ± 11.6	104 ± 12.1
FEV_1, baseline % pred	102 ± 11.8	100 ± 10.5
FEF_{25-75}, baseline	101 ± 22.2	93 ± 28.7
Change ACT	−0.5 ± 4.1	−3.2 ± 3.9*
Change FEV_1, % pred	−1.9 ± 11.0	−8.0 ± 8.5*
Change FEF_{25-75}, % pred	−10.8 ± 16.4	−16.9 ± 13.8
TLC, %	105.9 ± 22.0	100.4 ± 11.2
RV/TLC	0.22 ± 0.07	0.31 ± 0.09*
eNO	23.8 ± 25.6	26.7 ± 25.8
Exacerbation	0	2
Hospitalization	0	0

group had lung function and exhaled nitric oxide evaluation at followup. There was no significant difference in exhaled nitric oxide or evidence of hyperinflation. However, the uncontrolled group did have a significantly elevated residual volume over total lung capacity ratio (RV/TLC) (0.31 versus 0.22, $P < 0.05$) indicating more air trapping in the group off LABA therapy. No group differences were present based on date of study enrollment.

4. Discussion

Asthma guidelines have advocated step-down therapy once asthma is well controlled [11]; however, there is little evidence for how this should be accomplished. With the FDA recommending strongly against the use of LABA therapy [6], this study was designed to evaluate whether pediatric patients with well-controlled persistent asthma on combination ICS/LABA therapy were able to maintain short-term asthma control with the discontinuation of their LABA component. Thirty-seven percent of the patients had loss of asthma control necessitating systemic steroids or augmentation of their baseline controller therapy. The loss of spirometric control in a subset of these patients, without a significant increase in symptoms, points to the importance of obtaining objective measures of pulmonary function in the management of pediatric asthma, whenever a therapy change is contemplated.

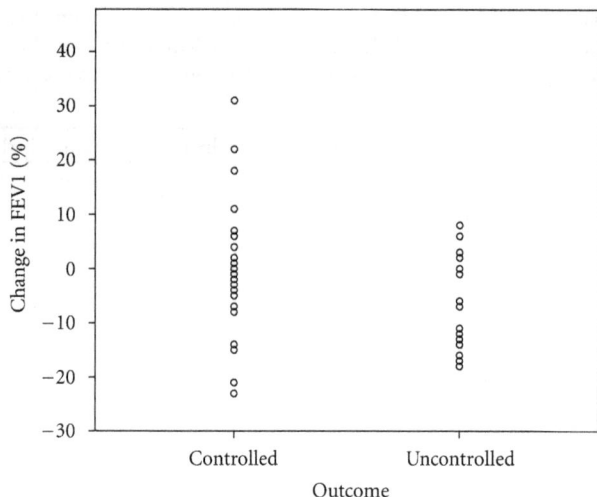

FIGURE 1: Scatterplot showing patient's change in FEV_1 (% predicted) comparing those that maintained asthma control off LABA therapy at followup (controlled) and those that experienced loss of asthma control (uncontrolled).

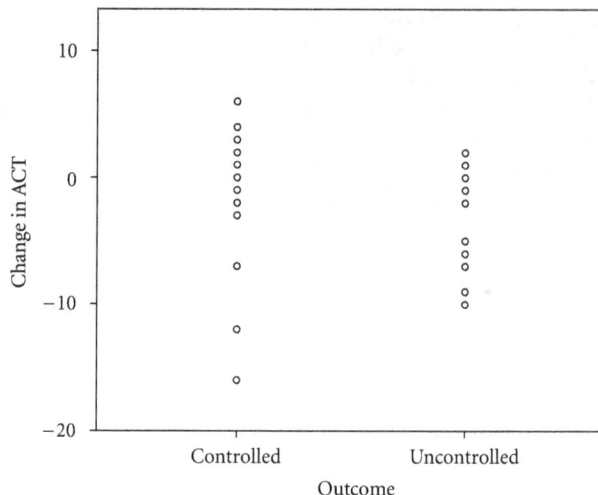

FIGURE 3: Scatterplot showing patient's change in ACT score comparing those that maintained asthma control off LABA therapy at followup (controlled) and those that experienced loss of asthma control (uncontrolled).

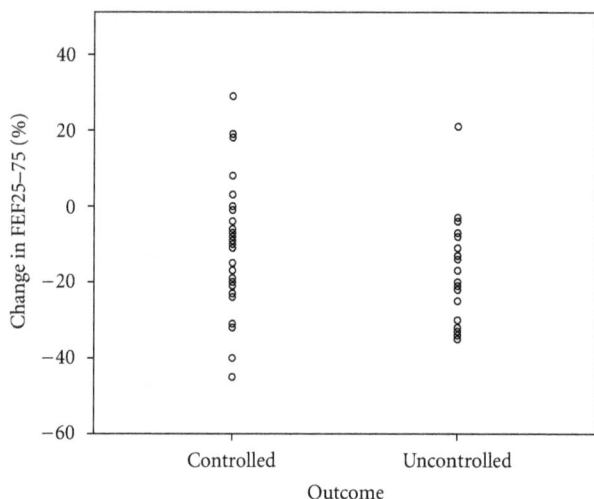

FIGURE 2: Scatterplot showing patient's change in FEF_{25-75} (% predicted) comparing those that maintained asthma control off LABA therapy at followup (controlled) and those that experienced loss of asthma control (uncontrolled).

This study highlights the challenges faced by clinicians on a daily basis. For patients with uncontrolled asthma, there is evidence regarding the utility of adding LABA therapy. Conversely, there are little data, specifically in pediatric patients, on the discontinuation of LABA therapy. Studies from the early 1990s were the first to illustrate the beneficial effects of adding LABA therapy for patients with uncontrolled asthma [17, 18]. The publication of the Formoterol and Corticosteroids Establishing Therapy (FACET) study in 1997 added to the growing body of evidence and led to widespread use of these agents [19].

This double-blind, placebo-controlled study involving 852 adult asthmatics showed a significant reduction in asthma exacerbations over a 1-year period in those treated with formoterol in addition to ICS. Recent meta-analyses have shown the improvement in clinical control, with decreased clinical symptoms and exacerbations, and improved objective measures of pulmonary function with the use of LABA therapy [20, 21]. The recent publication of the Best Add-on Therapy Giving Effective Responses (BADGER) study extended the role of LABA in uncontrolled pediatric asthma [8].This randomized, double-blind, three-period crossover trial for 48 weeks evaluated the response to increased ICS and the addition of LABA or montelukast in pediatric patients with uncontrolled asthma. The response to LABA step-up therapy was the most likely to provide the best response of the three.

The effectiveness of LABA therapy in the management of asthma has been dampened by safety concerns since the time of their FDA approval. The available data and their interpretation regarding safety implications has been ongoing, culminating in 2010 with the release of specific label changes for LABA and planning for a safety megastudy. The label change included "stop use of LABA, if possible, once asthma control is achieved and maintain use of an asthma-controller medication, such as inhaled corticosteroid" [5].

How best to step off LABA therapy is an open question based on available data. Maintaining LABA while reducing the dose of ICS has been shown to maintain control [22]. Extending the SMART (single maintenance and reliever therapy) use of the combination ICS/formoterol product may be another option [23]. Both options, however, advocate the continued use of a LABA. Studies looking at stopping the LABA component have uniformly shown worsening symptoms or quality of life, increased SABA therapy, or worsened pulmonary function [22]. Unfortunately, these studies did not include a pediatric population.

This first report of the loss of asthma control in the pediatric setting is limited by the lack of a control or comparison group, randomization, and blinding. These are inherent biases in an observational study evaluating a universal change in a clinical practice. However, each patient in effect acted as his/her own control, since their degree of control was compared to themselves before the clinical change. During this time our patient care goals were to stop LABA therapy entirely, so a comparison group of lower dose ICS/LABA combination was not considered. With the group's normal spirometry one could postulate that our patients were overtreated for their asthma. However, that strengthens the findings since control should have been maintained by the decrease in therapy. We were unable to get lung volume and exhaled nitric oxide measurements on all of the patients at followup as desired. Reasons for this included patients being seen for a sick visit, insurance coverage, or parent preference. Nor are those measurements part of our routine practice, so baseline measurements are not available. However, there was a statistically significant increase in RV/TLC ratio in the group that lost control despite the small patient number. With the dose of ICS being stable one would not expect the eNO to change significantly with the discontinuation of LABA.

In a secondary analysis, there was no association of lack of control with race or ethnic group. However, this study was not powered to do so, nor did it include genetic polymorphism analysis. Studies have shown a differential response to asthma therapy based on racial demographic [24, 25]. The Badger trial showed that for LABA therapy, this was the add-on therapy most likely to improve control. Whereas in African Americans subjects, this therapy was shown to be no better than increasing ICS at improving control [8]. And recently, the Asthma Clinical Research Network (ACRN) showed an increased rate of treatment failure in African Americans being treated with LABA therapy regardless of concomitant use of other controller therapy, including ICS [25]. This finding would serve to add credence to the SMART study which showed increased risks in African Americans treated with LABA [5]. These differential responses may be related to socioeconomic or other unknown factors. Perhaps the decision for LABA therapy will be personalized in the future, and based on risk-benefit profile and genetic polymorphisms.

Those eight of our patients who had a significant decline in airflow despite no noticeable worsening of symptoms further reminds us of the role of spirometry in asthma management. The Expert Panel Report 3 (EPR-3) recommends the use of spirometry in the diagnosis and periodic monitoring of patients with asthma [11]. The use of symptoms alone has been shown to underrepresent the degree of asthma severity [26]. Symptoms are fairly reliable indexes of asthma control; however, symptoms and lung function do not always correlate. Some patients who are poorly controlled based on objective measures of lung function perceive few, if any, symptoms. These "poor perceivers of airflow obstruction" are at increased risks of asthma morbidity and mortality [27].

5. Conclusion

The goals of most asthma guidelines, as well as the recent FDA concerns, can be met in most patients. However, this study adds to the mounting literature of a group of asthmatics who gain better control on LABA therapy and subsequently lose control when it is discontinued. Clearly, LABA therapy is not acceptable as monotherapy, and the use of combination ICS/LABA therapy in one single device precludes this option. If achieving symptomatic and spirometric control is the goal in pediatric asthma, the availability of LABA therapy as an added option appears necessary. Future prospective trials looking at LABA and stratifying risk by race, gender, and phenotypic response will help further to clarify their role.

Disclosure

Study approval obtained from the University of Louisville Institutional Review Board, Presented in part at American College of Allergy, Asthma & Immunology annual meeting, Nov 6, 2011.

Acknowledgments

The authors appreciate the work of those who contributed to this study including Doctor Jordan Smallwood, Janet Tomazin, and the staff and patients at the University of Louisville Pediatric Pulmonary clinic.

References

[1] Cochrane Review 2010, "Addition of long-acting beta2-agonists to inhaled corticosteroids versus same dose inhaled corticosteroids for chronic asthma in adults and children," http://www.thecochranelibrary.com/userfiles/ccoch/file/CD0-05535.pdf.

[2] H. Bisgaard and S. Szefler, "Long-acting $\beta2$ agonists and paediatric asthma," The Lancet, vol. 367, no. 9507, pp. 286–288, 2006.

[3] H. S. Friedman, N. S. Eid, S. Crespi, T. K. Wilcox, and G. Reardon, "Retrospective claims study of fluticasone propionate/salmeterol fixed-dose combination use as initial asthma controller therapy in children despite guideline recommendations," Clinical Therapeutics, vol. 31, no. 5, pp. 1056–1063, 2009.

[4] B. A. Chowdhury and G. D. Pan, "The FDA and safe use of long-acting beta-agonists in the treatment of asthma," The New England Journal of Medicine, vol. 362, no. 13, pp. 1169–1171, 2010.

[5] H. S. Nelson, S. T. Weiss, E. K. Bleecker, S. W. Yancey, and P. M. Dorinsky, "The salmeterol multicenter asthma research trial: a comparison of usual pharmacotherapy for asthma or usual pharmacotherapy plus salmeterol," Chest, vol. 129, no. 1, pp. 15–26, 2006.

[6] Food and Drug Administration, "FDA drug safety communication: new safety requirements for long-acting inhaled asthma medications called long-acting beta-agonists," 2010, http://www.fda.gov/Drugs/DrugSafety/PostmarketDrugSafetyInformationforPatientsandProviders/ucm200776.htm.

[7] R. A. Pauwels, C. G. Lofdahl, D. S. Postma et al., "Effect of inhaled formoterol and budesonide on exacerbations of asthma. Formoterol and Corticosteroids Establishing Therapy (FACET) International Study Group," *The New England Journal of Medicine*, vol. 337, pp. 1405–1411, 1997.

[8] R. F. Lemanske Jr., D. T. Mauger, C. A. Sorkness et al., "Step-up therapy for children with uncontrolled asthma receiving inhaled corticosteroids," *The New England Journal of Medicine*, vol. 362, no. 11, pp. 975–985, 2010.

[9] E. D. Bateman, L. Jacques, C. Goldfrad, T. Atienza, T. Mihaescu, and M. Duggan, "Asthma control can be maintained when fluticasone propionate/salmeterol in a single inhaler is stepped down," *Journal of Allergy and Clinical Immunology*, vol. 117, no. 3, pp. 563–570, 2006.

[10] P. Godard, P. Greillier, B. Pigearias, G. Nachbaur, J. L. Desfougeres, and V. Attali, "Maintaining asthma control in persistent asthma: comparison of three strategies in a 6-month double-blind randomised study," *Respiratory Medicine*, vol. 102, no. 8, pp. 1124–1131, 2008.

[11] National Asthma Education and Prevention Program, "Expert panel report 3 (EPR-3): guidelines for the diagnosis and management of asthma-summary report 2007," *Journal of Allergy and Clinical Immunology*, vol. 120, no. 5, supplement, pp. S94–S138, 2007.

[12] B. A. Chowdhury, S. M. Seymour, and M. S. Levenson, "Assessing the safety of adding LABAs to inhaled corticosteroids for treating asthma," *The New England Journal of Medicine*, vol. 364, no. 26, pp. 2473–2475, 2011.

[13] R. A. Nathan, C. A. Sorkness, M. Kosinski et al., "Development of the asthma control test: a survey for assessing asthma control," *Journal of Allergy and Clinical Immunology*, vol. 113, no. 1, pp. 59–65, 2004.

[14] H. Derendorf, R. Nave, A. Drollmann, F. Cerasoli, and W. Wurst, "Relevance of pharmacokinetics and pharmacodynamics of inhaled corticosteroids to asthma," *European Respiratory Journal*, vol. 28, no. 5, pp. 1042–1050, 2006.

[15] American Thoracic Society, "Standardization of spirometry. 1994 Update," *American Journal of Respiratory and Critical Care Medicine*, vol. 152, pp. 1107–1136, 1995.

[16] G. Polgar and V. Promadhat, *Pulmonary Function Testing in Children: Techniques and Standards*, WB Saunders, Philadelphia, Pa, USA, 1971.

[17] A. Woolcock, B. Lundback, N. Ringdal, and L. A. Jacques, "Comparison of addition of salmeterol to inhaled steroids with doubling of the dose of inhaled steroids," *American Journal of Respiratory and Critical Care Medicine*, vol. 153, pp. 1481–1488, 1996.

[18] A. P. Greening, P. W. Ind, M. Northfield, and G. Shaw, "Added salmeterol versus higher-dose corticosteroid in asthma patients with symptoms on existing inhaled corticosteroid," *The Lancet*, vol. 344, no. 8917, pp. 219–224, 1994.

[19] R. A. Pauwels, C. G. Lofdahl, D. S. Postma et al., "Effect of inhaled formoterol and budesonide on exacerbations of asthma," *The New England Journal of Medicine*, vol. 337, pp. 1405–1411, 1997.

[20] M. N. Chroinin, T. J. Lasserson, I. Greenstone, and F. M. Ducharme, "Addition of long-acting beta-agonists to inhaled corticosteroids for chronic asthma in children," *Cochrane Database of Systematic Reviews*, no. 3, article CD007949, 2009.

[21] M. N. Chroinin, I. Greenstone, T. J. Lasserson, and F. M. Ducharme, "Addition of inhaled long-acting beta2-agonists to inhaled steroids as first line therapy for persistent asthma in steroid-naive adults and children," *Cochrane Database of Systematic Reviews*, no. 4, article CD005307, 2009.

[22] L. Rogers and J. Reibman, "Stepping down asthma treatment: how and when," *Current Opinion in Pulmonary Medicine*, vol. 18, pp. 70–75, 2012.

[23] K. R. Chapman, N. C. Barnes, A. P. Greening, P. W. Jones, and S. Pedersen, "Single maintenance and reliever therapy (SMART) of asthma: a critical appraisal," *Thorax*, vol. 65, no. 8, pp. 747–752, 2010.

[24] M. Naqvi, H. Tcheurekdjian, J. A. DeBoard et al., "Inhaled corticosteroids and augmented bronchodilator responsiveness in Latino and African American asthmatic patients," *Annals of Allergy, Asthma and Immunology*, vol. 100, no. 6, pp. 551–557, 2008.

[25] M. E. Wechsler, M. Castro, E. Lehman et al., "Impact of race on asthma treatment failures in the asthma clinical research network," *American Journal of Respiratory and Critical Care Medicine*, vol. 184, pp. 1247–1253, 2011.

[26] S. M. Dostaler, J. G. Olajos-Clow, T. W. Sands et al., "Comparison of asthma control criteria: importance of spirometry," *Journal of Asthma*, vol. 48, pp. 1069–1075, 2011.

[27] R. Magadle, N. Berar-Yanay, and P. Weiner, "The risk of hospitalization and near-fatal and fatal asthma in relation to the perception of dyspnea," *Chest*, vol. 121, no. 2, pp. 329–333, 2002.

29

Cigarette and Waterpipe Smoking Decrease Respiratory Quality of Life in Adults: Results from a National Cross-Sectional Study

Salamé Joseph,[1] Salameh Pascale,[2] Khayat Georges,[3] and Waked Mirna[4]

[1] *Faculty of Medical Sciences, Lebanese University, Beirut 961, Lebanon*
[2] *Faculties of Pharmacy and of Public Health, Lebanese University, Beirut 961, Lebanon*
[3] *Hôtel-Dieu de France Hospital and Faculty of Medicine, Saint Joseph University, Beirut 961, Lebanon*
[4] *Saint George Hospital University Medical Center and Faculty of Medicine, Univerity of Balamand, Beirut 961, Lebanon*

Correspondence should be addressed to Salameh Pascale, pascalesalameh1@hotmail.com

Academic Editor: Edgardo D'Angelo

Background. Chronic obstructive pulmonary disease (COPD) is gaining an importance over the world, and its effect on quality of life is better grasped. Our objective was to use the Clinical COPD Questionnaire (CCQ) to describe the respiratory quality of life in the Lebanese population, stressing on differences between smokers and nonsmokers. *Methods*. Using data from a cross-sectional national study, we checked the construct validity and reliability of the CCQ. Factors and items correlation with postbronchodilator FEV1/FVC were reported, in addition to factors and scale association with COPD and its severity. We then conducted a multiple regression to find predictors of quality of life. *Results*. The CCQ demonstrated excellent psychometric properties, with adequacy to the sample and high consistency. Smokers had a decreased respiratory quality of life versus nonsmokers, independently of their respiratory disease status and severity. This finding was confirmed in COPD individuals, where several environmental factors, lower education, and cumulative smoking of cigarette and of waterpipe were found to be independent predictors of a lower quality of life, after adjusting for COPD severity. *Conclusions*. Smoking decreases the respiratory quality of life of Lebanese adults; this issue has to be further emphasized during smoking cessation and patients' education.

1. Introduction

Chronic obstructive pulmonary disease is increasing over the world; it is expected to rank third in 2020 as a cause of mortality [1]. In Lebanon, we had demonstrated that the prevalence of respiratory diseases is quite high (COPD and chronic bronchitis in particular) in the population aged 40 and above, paralleling the high prevalence of smoking cigarettes and waterpipes [2]. Although COPD is known to decrease the patients' quality of life [3], a low percentage (20%) of individuals are diagnosed and treated for COPD in Lebanon. The others are still experiencing chronically respiratory symptoms and consequent limitations without seeking help [2]. However, according to the GOLD (Global initiative for obstructive lung disease) guidelines [4] and their updated version [5], the aim of clinical control in patients with COPD includes health-related quality of life goals (improved exercise tolerance and emotional function)

added to clinical goals (prevention of disease progression and minimization of symptoms).

Several tools have been developed to evaluate quality of life in patients with chronic respiratory diseases [6, 7], but none of them has been validated for use in the Lebanese population. Moreover, the Saint George Respiratory Questionnaire is long [8], while the American Thoracic Society questionnaire evaluates only symptoms [9]. However, the Chronic COPD Questionnaire (CCQ) seems to have excellent psychometric properties, along with simplicity of application [10]; it is also the first questionnaire that incorporates both clinician and patient guideline goals in the clinical control evaluation of patients with COPD in general clinical practice [11]. It was showed to be the best patient-reported outcome tool to assess functional performance [12]. Although the new recommendations issued by the GOLD steering committee [5] adopted the COPD Assessment Test (CAT) questionnaire as the first one to be used without neglecting the value of the CCQ, we had conducted the study before the issuing of these recommendations.

Our objective was to describe the respiratory quality of life in the Lebanese population using data from a cross-sectional national study on the prevalence of COPD [2], stressing on differences between smokers and nonsmokers.

2. Methods

2.1. Study Design. Data for this analysis was taken from a cross-sectional study, using a multistage cluster sample all over Lebanon. This study was carried out between October 2009 and September 2010, using a multistage cluster sample (n = 2201) across Lebanon. From the list of communities in Lebanon (includes a total of 2782 villages, towns, and cities), one hundred communities were randomly selected with randomization performed on a computerized software. Afterwards, through a representative of local authorities, individuals were randomly chosen to be interviewed, from a provided list of dwelling households aged 40 years and above. All individuals of the household were solicited, if they were eligible.

2.2. Procedure. After an oral informed consent, subjects underwent a baseline spirometry (Micro Lab, Micro Medical Limited, UK), conducted by a trained technician, and answered a standardized questionnaire. Thirty minutes after the inhalation of 2 puffs of ipratropium bromide (18 μg/actuation) and albuterol sulfate (103 μg/actuation) (Combivent) in a pressurised metered-dose aerosol unit, a postbronchodilator spirometry was performed. The best result out of 3 trials was taken into account. Spirometric quality was checked, and FEV6/FVC was ≤100% in more than 99.2% of measurements. Additional methodological details are presented in a separate publication [2].

2.3. Questionnaire and Procedure. The standardized questionnaire included sections about sociodemographic characteristics, respiratory diseases and symptoms, and a thorough smoking history evaluation. Moreover, respiratory-related quality of life was measured by the Clinical COPD Questionnaire (CCQ) [10], while the MRC dyspnea scale was used to evaluate dyspnea [13]. The questionnaires were administered in Arabic local language; the translation process was as follows: first, two of the researchers, both bilingual, forward translated the questions into Arabic; instructions were given to them in the approach to translating, emphasizing conceptual rather than literal translations, as well as the need to use natural and acceptable language for the broadest audience. Second, discrepancies were resolved by consensus between them and two other researchers: this panel thus included the original translators, experts in health, as well as experts with experience in instrument development and translation. Third, an independent translator with no knowledge of the questionnaire back translated the questions into English. Translation discrepancies were resolved by consensus between the researchers and the translator. Fourth, the questionnaire was pilot tested on

20 individuals; all questions were deemed clear by these individuals, and no further changes were made to the initial questions.

2.4. Definitions. Chronic Obstructive Pulmonary Disease (COPD) was defined and classified according to GOLD guidelines (FEV1/FVC < 0.70 postbronchodilator) [14], and according to the lower limit of normal (FEV1/FVC postbronchodilator < 5th percentile of the healthy population having the same age and gender of the individual) [15]. Individuals were finally classified as having COPD if they fulfilled one of the definitions described above. Chronic bronchitis was defined by the declaration of morning cough and expectorations for more than 3 months a year over more than two years in individuals with no COPD [14]. On the other hand, an individual was considered "healthy" from the respiratory point of view if he had no respiratory symptoms and no respiratory disease. Moreover, patients with a partially reversible obstruction (postbronchodilator FEV1/FVC that does not go back to normal) are considered with a mixed disorder of asthma and COPD; they are termed "reversible COPD." Further methodology details are presented in another publication [2].

Cumulative dosing of cigarettes was calculated as the mean number of daily packs multiplied by the duration of smoking (pack*years), while that of waterpipe was calculated as the mean number of weekly waterpipes multiplied by the duration of smoking (waterpipe*years). Cigarette and waterpipe dependence were defined according to Fagerström Test for Nicotine Dependence (FTND) [16] and Lebanese Waterpipe Dependence Scale (LWDS-11) [17], respectively.

2.5. Statistical Analysis. SPSS version 17.0 was used to enter and analyze data. Weighting was performed according to the numbers published by the Lebanese Central Administration of Statistics in 2007, taking into account gender, age, and dwelling region [18]. Cluster effect was taken into account, according to Rumeau-Rouquette and collaborators [19].

A P value of 0.05 was considered significant. The Chi^2 test was used for cross tabulation of qualitative variables in bivariate analysis, and odds ratios (OR) were calculated. ANOVA and Kruskal-Wallis tests were used to compare between three groups or more, and Pearson correlation coefficient were used to correlate between quantitative variables. Bonferroni adjustment was used for ANOVA post hoc tests of between groups comparison.

To confirm the CCQ construct validity in the Lebanese population, a factorial analysis was launched for CCQ items, using the principal component analysis technique, with a promax rotation since the extracted factors were found to be significantly correlated. The Kaiser-Meyer-Olkin measure of sampling adequacy and Bartlett's test of sphericity were ensured to be adequate. The retained number of factors corresponded to Eigenvalues higher than one. Factors loading of items were recorded. Moreover, Cronbach's alphas were recorded for reliability analysis for the total score and for subscale factors. The total CCQ score represents the sum of the 10 CCQ items divided by 10 (as recommended in the

CCQ manual) [10], while the factors 1 & 2 are the sums of their respective items. Factors and items correlation with postbronchodilator spirometric FEV1/FVC were reported, in addition to factors and scale association with COPD and its severity.

Afterwards, backward linear multiple regression was performed for multivariate analyses, with CCQ score as the dependent variable, and sociodemographic characteristics and other potentially harmful exposures as the independent variables; after ensuring model adequacy to data, relationship linearity, dependent variable normality, and lack of collinearity between covariates. We used this method to find significant predictors of respiratory quality of life in all individuals, in patients with COPD and in nonsmokers. Moreover, partial correlation with CCQ score was presented, taking other covariates into account.

3. Results

3.1. Sample Description. Among 2201 individuals, 978 were considered healthy (44.5%) from the respiratory point of view. Moreover, 233 (10.6%) had COPD, 204 (9.3%) had asthma, 51 (2.3%) had a reversible COPD, 326 (14.8%) had chronic bronchitis, 72 (3.3%) had a restrictive disease, and 336 individuals (15.3%) had miscellaneous respiratory symptoms (MRS). In the following analysis we will exclude patients with asthma, restrictive disease, and miscellaneous respiratory symptoms.

Thus, patients with COPD ($n = 284$), chronic bronchitis ($n = 326$), and healthy individuals ($n = 978$) will only be included. For them, mean postbronchodilators FEV1/FVC significantly differed: 0.62 (SD = 0.09) for COPD patients, 0.83 (SD = 0.05) for chronic bronchitis, and 0.85 (SD = 0.03) for healthy individuals ($P < 0.001$ for all comparisons). Healthy individuals have never been hospitalized for respiratory problems, while COPD and chronic bronchitis patients have both been hospitalized (mean number of hospitalizations is 0.26 for COPD and 0.36 for chronic bronchitis; $P = 0.090$).

3.2. Sociodemographic and Health Characteristics. In Table 1, we present sociodemographic characteristics of different individuals' categories. We note significant differences in percentages of COPD and chronic bronchitis for all categories. Individuals with obstructive diseases were included older ages, more males, less educated, retired, nonmarried, more obese individuals with more cardiac problems, in the regions of Bekaa and South Lebanon ($P < 0.001$ for all). Moreover, 22.2% of patients with COPD and 17.2% of those with chronic bronchitis are getting inhalation therapy.

Smokers had the higher rates of COPD and of chronic bronchitis, compared with never smokers. While mixed smokers had significantly higher prevalences of both diseases versus exclusive smokers, current waterpipe smokers had rates similar to never smokers, while previous waterpipe smokers included more COPD than previous cigarette smokers, with no chronic bronchitis cases (Table 1).

3.3. Clinical COPD Questionnaire (CCQ) Factor Analyses. Although the CCQ questions were part of the cross-sectional study questionnaire, and they were asked to the whole sample, the factorial analysis that was run over the sample of healthy individuals, COPD and chronic bronchitis patients (Total $n = 1588$). CCQ items converged over a solution of two factors that had an Eigenvalue over 1, explaining a total of 67.91% of the variance. A Kaiser-Meyer-Olkin measure of sampling adequacy of 0.876 was found, with a significant Bartlett's test of sphericity ($P < 0.0001$).

The first one, representing "dyspnea and dysfunction", explained 56.30% of the variance; the second factor, representing "chronic bronchitis" explained 11.61% of the variance. Moreover, high Cronbach's alpha were found for factor 1 (0.909), factor 2 (0.859), and the full scale (0.910) (Table 2).

3.4. Quality of Life in Disease Categories. There were significant differences between the means of respiratory quality of life score (Table 3) ($P < 0.001$). Looking at the means, the lowest CCQ quality of life was found for reversible and irreversible COPD patients and chronic bronchitis, compared with healthy individuals. We also compared respiratory CCQ score in COPD grades: there was a significant increase in CCQ along with COPD severity grades ($P < 0.001$). In individuals declaring being treated by inhalation therapy (including short acting and long acting anticholinergics, beta agonists, and steroids), quality of life was significantly lower versus individuals not declaring so ($P < 0.001$). Moreover, we found a significant correlation between the CCQ and the MRC dyspnea scale ($r = 0.763$; $P < 0.001$); individuals with an MRC dyspnea scale higher than zero had significantly worse quality of life (Table 3).

3.5. Quality of Life and Smoking. For previous smoking, we note significantly a higher CCQ score for all types of smoking, including cigarette, waterpipe, and mixed smoking ($P < 0.001$), compared with never smokers; mixed smokers have significantly higher CCQ versus other categories, while cigarette and waterpipe smoking had nonsignificant differences. As for current smoking, no significant difference was found between waterpipe smoking and never smokers; however, cigarette and mixed smokers had significantly higher sores for CCQ (Table 4).

For patients with chronic bronchitis and COPD, any previous smoker had significantly lower CCQ versus never smokers; mixed smokers had significantly higher values than cigarette and never smokers. In current smokers, cigarette and mixed smokers had significantly higher QOL versus waterpipe and never smokers. No significant difference was found between never smokers and waterpipe smokers, and no significant difference was found between cigarette and mixed smokers (Table 4).

On the other hand, there were clear positive dose-effect relationships between different smoking types cumulative doses and quality of life score (the higher the cumulative dose of smoking, the lower the quality of life): correlation coefficients between CCQ and cumulative doses were all

TABLE 1: Sociodemographic characteristics of the study population.

Characteristic	Healthy (n = 978)	COPD (reversible and irreversible) (n = 284)	Chronic bronchitis without COPD (n = 326)	Total* (n = 1588)
Region				
Beirut	57.4%	21.3%	21.3%	277
Mount Lebanon	67.2%	14.8%	17.9%	687
North Lebanon	67.3%	17.1%	15.6%	263
South Lebanon	55.6%	15.3%	29.1%	196
Bekaa plain	43.0%	29.1%	27.9%	165
Gender				
Male	58.9%	20.9%	20.2%	774
Female	64.2%	14.9%	20.9%	812
Age class				
40–44 years	79.4%	6.2%	14.3%	321
45–49 years	78.6%	9.0%	12.4%	266
50–54 years	70.0%	11.5%	18.5%	227
55–59 years	58.8%	16.1%	25.1%	199
60–64 years	48.2%	29.9%	21.8%	197
65 years and more	37.8%	32.5%	29.6%	378
Education				
Illiterate	50.5%	17.6%	31.9%	91
<8 years of school	46.9%	22.1%	31.0%	290
8–12 years of school	54.2%	24.5%	21.4%	323
12.1–15 years of school	61.3%	21.3%	17.4%	432
University studies	79.1%	7.3%	13.6%	441
Work status				
Currently working	71.5%	13.1%	15.4%	846
Retired	42.0%	31.2%	26.8%	231
Not finding a job	66.7%	20.0%	13.3%	15
Do never work	53.6%	19.8%	26.6%	496
Marital status				
Married	62.2%	17.5%	20.3%	1303
Single	64.1%	12.8%	23.1%	156
Widow or divorced	51.2%	28.1%	20.7%	121
Body Mass Index				
No obesity	62.7%	17.8%	19.5%	1261
Obesity	53.8%	20.2%	25.9%	247
Cardiac problem				
No	66.1%	16.2%	17.7%	1331
Yes	38.4%	26.4%	35.3%	258
Inhalation therapy				
No	66.6%	15.0%	18.4%	1477
Yes	0	52.9%	47.1%	111
Current smoking				
Never smokers	84.1%	4.5%	11.4%	552
Cigarette smokers	45.3%	24.6%	30.1%	479
Waterpipe smokers	83.7%	4.8%	11.5%	104
Mixed smokers	50.6%	27.2%	22.2%	81

TABLE 1: Continued.

Characteristic	Healthy (n = 978)	COPD (reversible and irreversible) (n = 284)	Chronic bronchitis without COPD (n = 326)	Total* (n = 1588)
Previous smokers				
Never smokers	84.1%	4.5%	11.4%	552
Cigarette smokers	46.8%	26.9%	26.3%	308
Waterpipe smokers	65.5%	34.5%	0	55
Mixed smokers	30.0%	42.9%	27.1%	70

*All P values were <0.001.

TABLE 2: Factorial analysis of the Clinical COPD Questionnaire.

Items	Factor loading	Factors correlation*	Correlation with FEV1/FVC*
Factor 1**		Factor 1	−0.436
Had dyspnea at rest	0.480	0.771	−0.356
Had dyspnea on effort	0.607	0.876	−0.422
Was unable to do strenuous effort such as going up stairs	0.701	0.871	−0.451
Was unable to do moderate effort such as walking	0.776	0.896	−0.430
Was anxious about breathing difficulties or getting a cold	0.671	0.786	−0.340
Was depressed because of respiratory problems	0.715	0.733	−0.227
Was unable to socialize (talking, visiting, ...)	0.949	0.767	−0.291
Was unable to do daily activities/dressing ...	0.925	0.819	−0.313
Factor 2**		Factor 2	−0.442
Had sputum production	0.980	0.959	−0.414
Had cough	0.937	0.956	−0.439
Total scale			−0.464

*All correlations were significant (P < 0.001); factor 1 correlation with CCQ was 0.980; factor 2 correlation with CCQ was 0.829; **Cronbach's alpha = 0.910 for the full scale, 0.909 for factor 1 and 0.859 for factor 2; factor 1 correlation coefficient with factor 2 was 0.700.

positive ($P < 0.001$); CCQ means differed for previous and current cigarette smoking, for previous and current waterpipe smoking, and for current cigarette and waterpipe dependence classes ($P < 0.001$). Again, similar results are found for COPD and chronic bronchitis patients (Table 5).

3.6. Predictors of Quality of Life. Predictors of respiratory quality of life, measured by CCQ, are presented in Table 6, by decreasing order of importance: cumulative cigarette dose, older age, having at least one smoker in the family, lower education, female gender, any heart disease, heating house by diesel, cumulative waterpipe dose, heating house by hot air, and having at least one smoker at work were significant predictors of a lower respiratory quality of life (higher CCQ score; $P < 0.05$ for all); ever living close to a local power plant (electricity generator) was important but its effect did not reach statistical significance ($P < 0.10$) (Table 6).

In COPD individuals, by decreasing order of importance, CCQ was significantly affected by cumulative cigarette dose, declared inhalation therapy, female gender, lower education, having at least one smoker in the family, older age, cumulative waterpipe dose, having a cardiac problem, not heating home centrally, and COPD severity grading (Table 6).

Finally, we present in a multivariate analysis the predictors of quality of life in never smokers, by decreasing order of importance. We found that lower education, having a cardiac problem, heating home by hot air, older age, heating its house by diesel, ever living close to a heavy traffic road (<100 m), and occupational exposure to toxic fumes were all significantly associated with a lower quality of life; having at least one smoker in the family was important but their effect did not reach statistical significance ($P \leq 0.10$) (Table 6).

In the study sample (healthy, COPD and chronic bronchitis individuals), cumulative dosing of cigarettes ($r = 0.404$; $P < 0.001$) and cumulative dosing of waterpipe ($r = 0.078$; $P < 0.001$) were both significantly correlated with CCQ score. In the COPD and chronic bronchitis subgroup, these values were, respectively: $r = 0.263$ ($P < 0.001$) and $r = 0.103$ ($P = 0.003$).

4. Discussion

In this study, we were able to describe the quality of life of Lebanese residents aged 40 years and more. The CCQ demonstrated excellent psychometric properties, with an excellent adequacy to a cross-sectional sample and high consistency. As expected, the respiratory related quality of life of COPD patients was decreased relative to healthy individuals; in addition, patients with chronic bronchitis without COPD and reversible COPD disorders also demonstrated a lower quality of life versus healthy individuals. These results have already been found by others: Weatherall and collaborators'

TABLE 3: Respiratory-related quality of life (CCQ[1]) scores.

Categories	Number	Score mean	Score standard deviation
Respiratory diseases			
Healthy	978	0.31	0.60
COPD[2]	233	2.45	1.50
Chronic bronchitis	326	2.12	1.61
Reversible COPD[2]	51	2.06	1.76
Total	1588	1.05	1.44
P value for ANOVA[3]	<0.001		
COPD grades[4]			
Grade 1 (FEV1 $\geq$ 0.8)	37	2.48	1.39
Grade 2 (0.5 $\leq$ FEV1 < 0.8)	124	2.44	1.49
Grade 3 (0.3 $\leq$ FEV1 < 0.5)	43	3.03	1.55
Grade 4 (FEV1 < 0.3)	8	3.63	1.68
P value for ANOVA	<0.001		
Individuals with all COPD[5]			
Taking inhalation therapy	63	3.00	1.48
Not taking inhalation therapy	221	2.21	1.53
P value for ANOVA	<0.001		
Individuals with chronic bronchitis			
Taking inhalation therapy	56	3.42	1.60
Not taking inhalation therapy	270	1.85	1.48
P value for ANOVA	<0.001		
MRC dyspnea scale[6]			
MRC = 0	999	0.33	0.67
MRC > 0	589	2.27	1.57
P value for ANOVA	<0.001		

[1] CCQ: Clinical COPD Questionnaire; [2] COPD: Chronic Obstructive Pulmonary Disease according to GOLD and LLN5% definitions; [3] For CCQ, healthy individuals significantly differed from all disease categories ($P < 0.001$); COPD, chronic bronchitis and reversible COPD disorders did not differ significantly ($P > 0.05$); [4] COPD classification according to GOLD guidelines; [5] Patients with reversible and irreversible COPD; [6] MRC: Medical Research Council scale for dyspnea.

TABLE 4: Quality of life, obstructive diseases, and smoking types.

Score	Total sample		COPD and Chronic bronchitis subgroup	
Smoking type	Number	Mean (Standard deviation)	Number	Mean (Standard deviation)
Previous smoking				
Never	553	0.45 (0.89)	268	1.33 (1.43)
Cigarette	309	1.56 (1.65)	306	2.15 (1.60)
Waterpipe	55	1.24 (1.41)	33	2.22 (1.40)
Mixed smoking	69	2.21 (1.73)	58	2.95 (1.35)
P value ANOVA/Kruskal-Wallis		<0.001*		<0.001[†]
Current smoking				
Never	553	0.45 (0.89)	268	1.33 (1.43)
Cigarette	479	1.37 (1.52)	513	1.82 (1.49)
Waterpipe	104	0.44 (1.00)	45	1.18 (1.47)
Mixed smoking	80	1.27 (1.55)	51	1.99 (1.57)
P value ANOVA/Kruskal-Wallis		<0.001**		<0.001**

* No significant difference between cigarette and waterpipe; significant difference between any smoking type and mixed smoking ($P \leq 0.001$); no significant difference between cigarette and waterpipe smokers; ** No significant difference between never smokers and waterpipe smokers; no significant difference between cigarette and mixed smokers; [†] any previous smoker had significantly lower CCQ versus never smokers; mixed smokers had significantly higher values than cigarette and never smokers.

Table 5: Quality of life and smoking doses relationship.

Score/smoking type	Number	All sample	P value ANOVA	Number	COPD and chronic bronchitis subgroup	P value ANOVA	Correlation coefficient
Previous cigarette smoking							
Never smokers	558	0.45 (0.88)		267	1.33 (1.44)		
1–18 pack-years	94	0.99 (1.39)	<0.001	74	1.65 (1.45)	<0.001[¶]	0.332[‡]
18.1–56 pack-years	139	1.42 (1.58)		135	2.06 (1.57)		
>56 pack-years	120	2.71 (1.59)		144	2.84 (1.48)		
Previous waterpipe smoking							
Never smokers	558	0.45 (0.88)		270	1.32 (1.43)		
0.1–29.9 waterpipe-years	42	1.29 (1.54)	<0.001	26	2.44 (1.36)	<0.001[¶]	0.126[‡]
30+ waterpipe-years	67	2.36 (1.69)		59	3.02 (1.28)		
Current cigarette smoking							
Never smokers	617	0.51 (0.93)		343	1.30 (1.40)		
1–18 pack-years	139	0.61 (0.92)	<0.001[†]	92	1.02 (1.08)	<0.001[*]	0.307[‡]
18.1–45 pack-years	163	1.28 (1.49)		159	1.88 (1.40)		
45+ pack-years	274	2.18 (1.69)		215	2.42 (1.59)		
Current waterpipe smoking							
Never smokers	574	0.45 (0.88)		281	1.30 (1.42)		
0.1–20 waterpipe-years	66	0.32 (0.76)	<0.001[†]	19	0.96 (1.16)	0.001[*]	0.203[‡]
20+ waterpipe-years	86	1.35 (1.65)		58	2.08 (1.69)		
Current cigarette dependence							
Fagerström 0–5 Low dependence	1259	0.89 (1.35)		833	1.74 (1.56)		
Fagerström 6-7 Moderate dependence	116	1.39 (1.48)	<0.001[*]	128	1.93 (1.39)	<0.001[*]	0.256[‡]
Fagerström 8–10 High dependence	108	2.43 (1.65)		149	2.43 (1.56)		
Current waterpipe dependence							
LWDS-11 0–9 Low dependence	74	0.36 (0.66)		33	0.86 (0.87)		
LWDS-11 10–16 Moderate dependence	40	0.63 (1.06)	<0.001[*]	21	1.64 (1.39)	<0.001[*]	0.435[‡]
LWDS-11 17+ High dependence	59	1.52 (1.76)		35	2.46 (1.75)		

[†] No significant difference between never and low-level smokers; [*] no significant difference between low and moderate dependence; [¶] no significant difference between low and moderate smoking level [‡] $P < 0.001$ for correlation coefficients.

work for COPD [20], and Maleki-Yazdi and collaborators' [21] for chronic bronchitis are some examples.

There was also significantly lower quality of life in previous and current smokers in the same disease category versus nonsmokers; one exception is for current smokers of waterpipe. This could be explained with the fact that waterpipe smoking in Lebanon is a relatively new trend, with the majority of waterpipe smokers having a low duration of smoking. However, a dose-effect relationship was clear for the effect of all types of smoking on QOL, with lower quality of life scores in patients with heavier smoking cumulative doses; this result was even found for current waterpipe smokers. Smokers had a decreased respiratory quality of life versus nonsmokers, independently of their respiratory disease. The association of cigarette smoking with lower quality of life has been found by Kotz and collaborators using the CCQ [12], and by Geijer and collaborators, where smoking induced limitations of physical functioning [22]; it was also indirectly shown by Papadopoulos and collaborators, with smoking cessation improving quality of life [23]. For waterpipe, this association seems of lower magnitude; nevertheless, it has

been demonstrated by Tavafian and collaborators using the SF-36 [24].

The relationship between other factors and lower quality of life was also confirmed in COPD individuals: besides cumulative smoking of cigarette and of waterpipe that was previously discussed, several indoor and outdoor environmental factors, age, gender, and lower education were found to be independent predictors of a lower quality of life, after adjusting for COPD severity grades. In fact, it has been shown that persons who have similar reductions in forced expiratory volume in 1st second and exercise capacity and similar levels of dyspnea have a wide range of HRQL, suggesting that other variables contributed to quality of life, such as age and gender [25].

In never smokers, older age, lower education, having a cardiac problem, heating its house by hot air or by diesel, occupational exposure to toxic fumes, ever living close to a heavy traffic road, and having at least one smoker in the family were all associated with a lower respiratory quality of life. We had already showed that these factors were

TABLE 6: Predictors of lower respiratory quality of life (CCQ).

Factor	Beta	P value	Standardized beta	Partial correlation
In all individuals (healthy, COPD and chronic bronchitis)*				
Cumulative cigarette smoking (pack∗years)	0.001	<0.001	0.399	0.404
Older age	0.021	<0.001	0.168	0.155
At least one smoker in the family	0.328	<0.001	0.111	0.129
Lower education	0.126	<0.001	0.108	0.117
Female gender	0.273	<0.001	0.095	0.090
Any heart disease	0.301	<0.001	0.077	0.089
Heating house by diesel	0.205	0.003	0.062	0.083
Cumulative waterpipe smoking (waterpipe∗years)	0.002	<0.001	0.064	0.078
Heating house by hot air	0.281	0.008	0.055	0.066
At least one smoker at work	0.166	0.048	0.044	0.051
Ever lived close to a local power plant	0.11	0.094	0.035	0.048
In all COPD individuals¶				
Cumulative cigarette smoking (pack∗years)	0.001	<0.001	0.260	0.263
Inhalation therapy	0.802	<0.001	0.198	0.219
Female gender	0.371	0.002	0.116	0.123
Lower education level	0.165	0.002	0.125	0.123
At least one smoker in the family	0.380	0.003	0.107	0.117
Older age	0.016	0.008	0.115	0.105
Cumulative waterpipe smoking (waterpipe∗years)	0.002	0.003	0.103	0.103
Having a cardiac problem	0.285	0.031	0.08	0.086
Not heating home by central heating	0.315	0.046	0.071	0.080
COPD severity grading	0.097	0.085	0.065	0.069
In nonsmokers†				
Lower educational level	0.256	<0.001	0.318	0.272
Any cardiac problem	0.622	<0.001	0.202	0.217
Heating house by hot air	0.433	0.001	0.111	0.123
Older age	0.010	0.011	0.106	0.094
Heating house by diesel	0.201	0.018	0.08	0.089
Ever lived close to a heavy traffic road (<100 m)	0.215	0.024	0.097	0.084
Occupational exposure to toxic fumes	0.214	0.032	0.072	0.080
At least one smoker in the family	0.106	0.103	0.047	0.059

*$R = 0.590$ and $R^2 = 0.348$ for the model; factors not retained in the model include heating house by butane gas, wood, and central heating, cooking on gas, being occupationally exposed to toxics and ever living close to a heavy traffic road ($P > 0.05$); ¶$R = 0.500$ and $R^2 = 0.250$ for the model; factors not included in the model include ever living close to a heavy traffic road, heating house by hot air, by wood, diesel, being occupationally exposed to toxics, ever living close to a power plant, and at least one smoker at work ($P > 0.05$). †$R = 0.492$ and $R^2 = 0.242$ for the model; factors not included in the model include gender, ever living close to a power plant, at least one smoker at work, heating its house by butane gas, wood, central heating, and cooking on gas ($P > 0.05$).

independently associated with chronic bronchitis [26] and COPD [2]; this may explain their association with lower respiratory quality of life.

One noticeable result is the lower quality of life in individuals declaring being treated with inhalation therapy; one explanation could be the fact that patients who are more symptomatic in general are the ones who go and seek a physician's help. In fact, in our study, patients with COPD and chronic bronchitis who admitted being treated by inhaled therapy also declared having more chronic cough, expectorations, and wheezing than those without therapy; they also had more severe disease staging (results not shown). This issue may further be explained by the delay in diagnosis and treatment of individuals, the noncompliance to treatment of some individuals, and the irreversible nature

of the disease. Additional studies are necessary to clarify this point.

Despite excellent results in this epidemiological setting, the value of the CCQ scale to evaluate the respiratory quality of life in the Lebanese population should additionally be tested in clinical settings. Moreover, we suggest a comparison of performance with the CAT scale that was shown to be superior to CCQ as a tool for monitoring the impact of symptom variability on the lives of patients with COPD [5]. Other limitations of our work include a possibility of selection bias, and information bias coupled with the used questionnaire. However, the demonstrated dose-effect relationship and the multivariate analyses are considered strong points of this work. Nevertheless, given this data was collected from a Lebanese population, predictive factors native to the Mediterranean region such as smoking a waterpipe may not be generalized to the general worldwide population.

5. Conclusions

In conclusion, we were able to describe the respiratory quality of life of Lebanese residents aged 40 years or more, using a valid tool. We found a lower quality of life in smokers versus nonsmokers, even in the same respiratory disease category and severity grade. A dose-effect relationship was also shown with lower quality of life with higher severity of the disease and higher cumulative smoking. This issue should be further emphasized during patients' education and smoking cessation.

Abbreviations

ANOVA: Analysis of variance
CAT: COPD assessment test
CCQ: Clinical COPD Questionnaire
COPD: Chronic obstructive pulmonary disease
GOLD: Global initiative for obstructive lung disease
MRS: Miscellaneous respiratory symptoms
OR: Odds ratio.

Authors' Contribution

S. Joseph has been involved in drafting the paper and data interpretation. K. Georges contributed to conception and interpretation of data. S. Pascale was involved in the study conception and design, data collection, and data analysis. W. Mirna was involved in study conception, manuscript correction and gave the final approval of the version to be published. All authors read and approved the final paper.

Acknowledgment

This work was funded by an educational grant from Boehringer Ingleheim—Lebanon Company. All authors have no competing interest to declare. The author(s) declare that they have no competing interests.

References

[1] K. F. Rabe, S. Hurd, A. Anzueto et al., "Global strategy for the diagnosis, management, and prevention of chronic obstructive pulmonary disease: GOLD executive summary," *American Journal of Respiratory and Critical Care Medicine*, vol. 176, no. 6, pp. 532–555, 2007.

[2] M. Waked, G. Khayat, and P. Salameh, "COPD Prevalence in Lebanon: a cross-sectional descriptive study," *Clinical Epidemiology*, vol. 3, pp. 315–323, 2011.

[3] E. Ståhl, A. Lindberg, S. A. Jansson et al., "Health-related quality of life is related to COPD disease severity," *Health and Quality of Life Outcomes*, vol. 3, article 56, 2005.

[4] L. M. Fabbri and S. S. Hurd, "for the GOLD Scientific Committee. Global strategy for the diagnosis, management

and prevention of COPD: 2003 update," *European Respiratory Journal*, vol. 22, pp. 1–2, 2003.

[5] Global Initiative for Chronic Obstructive Lung Disease, "Global Strategy for the Diagnosis, Management and Prevention of Chronic Obstructive Pulmonary Disease," 2011, http://www.goldcopd.org/.

[6] M. Weatherall, S. Marsh, P. Shirtcliffe, M. Williams, J. Travers, and R. Beasley, "Quality of life measured by the St George's respiratory questionnaire and spirometry," *European Respiratory Journal*, vol. 33, no. 5, pp. 1025–1030, 2009.

[7] J. W. H. Kocks, G. M. Asijee, I. G. Tsiligianni, H. A. Kerstjens, and T. van der Molen, "Functional status measurement in COPD: a review of available methods and their feasibility in primary care," *Primary Care Respiratory Journal*, vol. 20, no. 3, pp. 269–275, 2011.

[8] P. W. Jones, F. H. Quirk, and C. M. Baveystock, "The St George's respiratory questionnaire," *Respiratory Medicine*, vol. 85, pp. 25–31, 1991.

[9] B. G. Ferris, "Epidemiology standardization project," *The American Review of Respiratory Disease*, vol. 118, no. 6, part 2, pp. 1–88, 1978.

[10] T. van der Molen, B. W. M. Willemse, S. Schokker, N. H. T. ten Hacken, D. S. Postma, and E. F. Juniper, "Development, validity and responsiveness of the clinical COPD questionnaire," *Health and Quality of Life Outcomes*, vol. 1, no. 1, article 13, 2003.

[11] S. Damato, C. Bonatti, V. Frigo et al., "Validation of the Clinical COPD questionnaire in Italian language," *Health and Quality of Life Outcomes*, vol. 3, article 9, 2005.

[12] D. Kotz, G. Wesseling, P. Aveyard, and O. C. P. Van Schayck, "Smoking cessation and development of respiratory health in smokers screened with normal spirometry," *Respiratory Medicine*, vol. 105, no. 2, pp. 243–249, 2011.

[13] C. M. Fletcher, P. C. Elmes, A. S. Fairbairn, and C. H. Wood, "The significance of respiratory symptoms and the diagnosis of chronic bronchitis in a working population," *British Medical Journal*, vol. 2, no. 5147, pp. 257–266, 1959.

[14] P. M. Gold, "The 2007 GOLD guidelines: a comprehensive care framework," *Respiratory Care*, vol. 54, no. 8, pp. 1040–1049, 2009.

[15] T. J. Cole and P. J. Green, "Smoothing reference centile curves: the LMS method and penalized likelihood," *Statistics in Medicine*, vol. 11, no. 10, pp. 1305–1319, 1992.

[16] E. T. Moolchan, A. Radzius, D. H. Epstein et al., "The fagerstrom test for nicotine dependence and the diagnostic interview schedule: do they diagnose the same smokers?" *Addictive Behaviors*, vol. 27, no. 1, pp. 101–113, 2002.

[17] P. Salameh, M. Waked, and Z. Aoun, "Waterpipe smoking: construction and validation of the Lebanon Waterpipe Dependence Scale (LWDS-11)," *Nicotine and Tobacco Research*, vol. 10, no. 1, pp. 149–158, 2008.

[18] Central Administration of Statistics, "Central Administration of Statistics The National Study for Households Living Conditions in 2007," Beirut, 2008, http://www.cas.gov.lb/.

[19] C. Rumeau-Rouquette, G. Breart, and R. Padieu, *Methods in Epidemiology: Sampling, Investigations, Analysis*, Paris, France, 1985.

[20] M. Weatherall, S. Marsh, P. Shirtcliffe, M. Williams, J. Travers, and R. Beasley, "Quality of life measured by the St George's respiratory questionnaire and spirometry," *European Respiratory Journal*, vol. 33, no. 5, pp. 1025–1030, 2009.

[21] M. R. Maleki-Yazdi, C. K. Lewczuk, J. M. Haddon, N. Choudry, and N. Ryan, "Early detection and impaired quality of life in COPD GOLD stage 0: a pilot study," *Journal of*

Chronic Obstructive Pulmonary Disease, vol. 4, no. 4, pp. 313–320, 2007.

[22] R. M. M. Geijer, A. P. E. Sachs, T. J. M. Verheij, H. A. M. Kerstjens, M. M. Kuyvenhoven, and A. W. Hoes, "Quality of life in smokers: focus on functional limitations rather than on lunq function?" *British Journal of General Practice*, vol. 57, no. 539, pp. 477–482, 2007.

[23] G. Papadopoulos, C. I. Vardavas, M. Limperi, A. Linardis, G. Georgoudis, and P. Behrakis, "Smoking cessation can improve quality of life among COPD patients: validation of the clinical COPD questionnaire into Greek," *BMC Pulmonary Medicine*, vol. 11, article 13, 2011.

[24] S. S. Tavafian, T. Aghamolaei, and S. Zare, "Water pipe smoking and health-related quality of life: a population-based study," *Archives of Iranian Medicine*, vol. 12, no. 3, pp. 232–237, 2009.

[25] T. Hajiro, K. Nishimura, M. Tsukino, A. Ikeda, and T. Oga, "Stages of disease severity and factors that affect the health status of patients with chronic obstructive pulmonary disease," *Respiratory Medicine*, vol. 94, no. 9, pp. 841–846, 2000.

[26] P. Salameh, M. Waked, G. Khayat et al., "Waterpipe smoking and dependence are associatedwith chronic bronchitis: a case control study," *Eastern Mediterranean Health Journal*. In press.

30

Predicted Aerobic Capacity of Asthmatic Children: A Research Study from Clinical Origin

Lene Lochte

Centre for Child and Adolescent Health, Section of Aetiological Epidemiology, School of Social and Community Medicine, Faculty of Medicine and Dentistry, University of Bristol, Bristol BS8 2BN, UK

Correspondence should be addressed to Lene Lochte, l.lochte@bristol.ac.uk

Academic Editor: Luke Howard

Objective. To compare longitudinally PAC of asthmatic children against that of healthy controls during ten months. *Methods.* Twenty-eight asthmatic children aged 7–15 years and 27 matched controls each performed six submaximal exercise tests on treadmill, which included a test of EIA (exercise-induced asthma). Predicted aerobic capacity (mLO_2/min/kg) was calculated. Spirometry and development were measured. Physical activity, medication, and "ever asthma/current asthma" were reported by questionnaire. *Results.* Predicted aerobic capacity of asthmatics was lower than that of controls ($P = 0.0015$) across observation times and for both groups an important increase in predicted aerobic capacity according to time was observed ($P < 0.001$). FEV_1 of the asthmatic children was within normal range. The majority (86%) of the asthmatics reported pulmonary symptoms to accompany their physical activity. Physical activity (hours per week) showed important effects for the variation in predicted aerobic capacity at baseline ($F = 2.28$, $P = 0.061$) and at the T4 observation ($F = 3.03$, $P = 0.027$) and the analyses showed important asthma/control group effects at baseline, month four, and month ten. Physical activity of the asthmatics correlated positively with predicted aerobic capacity. *Conclusion.* The asthmatic children had consistently low PAC when observed across time. Physical activity was positively associated with PAC in the asthmatics.

1. Introduction

Children with asthma often experienced breathlessness during physical activity and therefore tended to avoid vigorous physical activity with disadvantageous consequences to their physical conditioning [1, 2].

There are few paediatric pulmonary conditions in which physical activity has had such potentially harmful effect on patients, not only by limiting exercise capability, but also by acting as a direct stimulus to the underlying pathophysiology [3]. Exercise-induced asthma (EIA) has been recognized as one major manifestation of untreated asthma [4] with physical activity acknowledged as a powerful trigger of asthmatic disease [3, 5].

Physical activity in paediatric asthma has been influenced by physical as well as psychosocial variables. The comprehensive psychosocial variables included attitudes towards exercise. Asthmatic children have demonstrated negative attitudes towards physical activity [6] to be influenced by the limitations that they experienced in safely and unrestrictedly to join physical activities [5].

The cardiopulmonary fitness of asthmatic children was often suboptimal. Some studies revealed lower predicted aerobic capacity (PAC) among asthmatic children than with healthy controls [7–9]; yet, most such observations were cross-sectional. Evidence of PAC in healthy children was well established whereas PAC of asthmatic youths was scarcely documented, in particular from longitudinal observation.

The author hypothesized that the asthmatic children would demonstrate a different PAC than that of their healthy peers when observed over time. Therefore, the aim of the present study was to longitudinally compare PAC of asthmatic children against that of healthy controls during ten months.

2. Materials and Methods

2.1. Subjects. Twenty-eight asthmatic children and 27 controls without asthma volunteered. Data were collected at pretest, baseline, EIA-test, and following one, four, and ten months (Table 1). Eligible controls at month four were $n = 24$. Data were collected from October 1998 through April 1999.

The asthmatic group was selected according to the diagnose bronchial asthma as defined by the British Thoracic Society [10] and the control group was matched on age (± 1 year), sex, weight (± 5 kg), and height (± 5 cm). The body weight, mean (SD) of asthmatics and controls was 40.0 (17.9) and 38.4 (13.8), respectively. Standing height, mean (SD) of asthmatics and controls was 143.7 (16.1) and 146.7 (17.8), respectively.

The asthmatic children were outpatients at the Paediatric Asthma and Allergy Clinic of Copenhagen University Hospital, Gentofte, Denmark, and they were included consecutively (informed consent obtained from parents) at their first visit. The control children were recruited from school classes of the Capital Region of Denmark and informed consent obtained from parents of the controls. All subjects were Caucasians.

Both groups were free from pulmonary tract infections, that is, forced expiratory volume in one sec (FEV$_1$) was >60% of the expected normal value estimated from height. Descriptive information on the study population is shown in Table 2.

2.2. Questionnaire. Baseline data on asthma, allergy, and physical activity were obtained by a standardised questionnaire, published elsewhere [7]. The questionnaire was dispatched to all children, was identical for asthma and controls, and was completed by the children assisted by their parents.

2.2.1. Asthma and Allergy. The questions on "ever asthma" and "current asthma" have previously been applied in surveys of asthmatic child populations [11]. The questionnaire included questions on pulmonary and allergy symptoms from skin, eyes, nose, lungs and symptoms frequency (daily, weekly, monthly, and/or every half-year).

2.2.2. Physical Activity. Scores of physical activity as reported by hours per week were adopted from validated standards [12] of the Health Behaviour in School-Aged Children (HBSC) study [13]. For hours (h) per week, six response categories were applied: (i) none, (ii) 0.5 h, (iii) 1 h, (iv) 2-3 hs, (v) 4–6 hs, (vi) ≥7 hs. Physical activity referred to vigorous leisure-time physical activity, exercise, or sports outside school hours equivalent to at least slow jogging that made the children sweat or become out of breath.

Eighty-six per cent ($n = 24$) of the asthmatic children reported pulmonary symptoms such as wheezing, dyspnoea, chest tightness, and cough related to exercise. Of these, 46% ($n = 11$) reported allergic reactions such as eczema, 38% ($n = 9$) rhinoconjunctivitis, and 25% ($n = 6$) both eczema

and rhinoconjunctivitis. Hospital journals confirmed that one-fifth of the asthmatic children were atopic and 7% ($n = 2$) had undergone allergy test; 14% ($n = 4$) had family predisposition.

Classification of asthma severity made reference to modified national guidelines, published elsewhere [7], based on present symptoms, lung function (PEFR), and medical treatment. PEFR, peak expiratory flow rate, (L/min) was self-recorded "same day morning and evening measurements" over the course of two weeks using Wright's peak flow meter (Airmed, Harlow, United Kingdom). The best of three PEFR exhalations was used for calculation. From the PEFR measurements, the percentage predicted values of PEFR (PEFR pred) was estimated using standard normal values according to height [14].

One PEFR registration was not returned and one was excluded due to extreme value. Hence, the study population comprised 13 children with mild asthma (PEFR pred >90–100%) 11 children with moderate (PEFR pred = 80–90%), and 2 children suffered severe asthma (PEFR pred <80%).

2.3. Design. The study population was followed prospectively by treadmill exercise tests during ten months.

2.4. Procedures. The age of the children was calculated from the date of birth to the nearest 0.01 years. Each child performed one pretest of PAC to establish running speed (RS) at an individual level according to sex and age, and to preclude training effect [4]. The pretest served to familiarise the child with the clinical environment and procedures. The baseline PAC-test was performed one week after the pretest.

All tests were performed separately with each child in the Clinic during the afternoon, and the asthmatic children performed the EIA-test prior to the pollen season. All instructions given during tests used comparable standards for asthmatic and control children.

A basic exercise warm-up programme preceded each exercise test. No EIA occurred during warmup. As a safety precaution, blood saturation was monitored during each test in all subjects by finger electrode method using Nellcor Symphony N-3000-120 (Nellcor, Boulder, CO, USA).

Body weight (BW) was measured by a spring balance to the nearest 0.1 kg (indoor clothing worn). Standing height was measured by a stadiometer to the nearest 0.1 cm and no shoes were worn during the measurements. Body mass index (BMI) was calculated as BW (kg)/height^2 (m). The anthropometric apparatus was calibrated according to the standards of the manufacturers.

The endocrinological development of children aged ≥10 years was assessed by three methods: (i) the presence of menarche in girls, (ii) sex characteristics (breast size in girls and pubic hair in girls and boys) evaluated according to standards [15] and (iii) the testicular volume of boys estimated by comparison with an ellipsoid of known volume using Prader Orchidometer, Zachmann, 1974, [15]. The results were presented in Table S1 (see Supplementary Material available online at doi:10.1155/2012/854652).

TABLE 1: Matrix of observations.

	Pretest	T0	T-EIA	T1	T4	T10
Age (year) and sex	X					
BMI	X				X	X
Development characteristics	X					
Ever asthma/current asthma	X					
FEV_1		X	X	X	X	X
ΔFEV_1			X			
HR_{rest}					X	
Medical treatment		X	X	X	X	X
Menarche	X				X	X
PAC		X		X	X	X
PEFR					X	
Physical activity (h/week)		X			X	X
RS	X	X	X	X	X	X
Symptoms (allergic/pulmonary)	X					

T0: time point of baseline test, T-EIA: time point EIA-test, T1: time point 1st month test, T4: time point 4th month test, T10: time point 10th month test, BMI: body mass index (kg/m^2), FEV_1: forced expiratory volume in one second (mL), ΔFEV_1: maximal percentage decrease in FEV_1 from baseline, HR_{rest}: heart rate at rest (beats/min), PAC: predicted aerobic capacity (mLO$_2$/min/kg), PEFR: peak expiratory flow rate (L/min), and RS: running speed (km/h).

Majorities of all children measured were distributed at pubic hair stage 1-2 and breast stage 2 or beyond according to the standards [15]. The boys had testicular volumes developed to stage 1-2 in 67% ($n = 6$) and 71% ($n = 5$) of the evaluated asthmatics and controls, respectively.

The PAC-tests were conducted without influencing ongoing medical treatment (corticosteroids: budesonide; β_2-agonist: terbutaline (short term); salmeterol and formoterol (long term).

Prior to the EIA-test the intake of β_2-agonist was discontinued for short term (12 hours) and long term (24 hours). No controls received medication.

HR at rest (HR_{rest}) was monitored following 30 min of rest in a horizontal position. Heart rate (HR (beats/min)) during the PAC and EIA-tests was continuously monitored in all children by a thoracic Polar Sport Tester band (Polar, Kempele, Finland).

FEV_1 (mL) was measured in a standing position by a Vitalograf (Spiropharma, Vitalograf Gold Standard, Klampenborg, Denmark). FEV_1 was measured immediately before, 3, 5, and 10 minutes posttest. At the EIA-test FEV_1 was further measured at 15, 20, and 30 minutes posttest.

At least three forced expirations were performed and children were instructed to blow from maximal inspiration and exhale quickly, forcefully, and for as long as possible into the instrument. Forced expiratory manoeuvres were repeated until two measurements of FEV_1 within 100 mL of each other were obtained. The largest FEV_1 value was used for analysis and from the FEV_1 measurements the percentage predicted values of FEV_1 (FEV_1 pred) were estimated using standard normal values according to height [14]. The accuracy of the vitalograf was verified weekly by a calibrated syringe (Spiropharma), corrected to body temperature, atmospheric pressure, and saturation with water vapour (BTPS). The vitalograf did not need adjustment during the test period.

TABLE 2: Descriptive information, mean ($\pm$SD), of study population by group.

	Baseline		
	Asthma	P	Control
	♂ / ♀		♂ / ♀
N	17 / 11		16 / 11
Age	10.1 (2.5)	ns	9.9 (2.7)
BMI	18.8 (3.8)	= 0.046	17.1 (2.0)
FEV_1	2.2 (0.8)	ns	2.3 (1.0)
PAC	44.3 (7.3)	= 0.009	52.1 (13.4)
RS	7.5 (1.6)	ns	7.7 (1.3)

N: number
Age (years), BMI: body mass index (kg/m^2), FEV_1: forced expiratory volume in one second (L), PAC: predicted aerobic capacity (mLO$_2$/min/kg), RS: running speed (km/h)
P: probability, ns: nonsignificant.

2.4.1. PAC-Test. The PAC-test constituted a submaximal, 5 min exercise test of continuous running on a treadmill (Spiropharma, Cardiogenics no. 2113, Klampenborg, Denmark). The test constituted continuous increments of RS for the first 2 min, and RS was adjusted to a submaximal HR of 170–180 beats per minute (bpm). When HR attained steadystate ($HR_{steadystate}$), the current speed was maintained for 3 min; $HR_{steadystate}$ (bpm) and RS (km/h) were registered for the estimation of PAC (mLO$_2$/min/kg).

2.4.2. EIA-Test. The EIA-test followed standardised guidelines using continuous increments of RS and inclination of the treadmill (Spiropharma, Cardiogenics no. 2113, Klampenborg, Denmark) during 5 minutes. When a submaximal HR of 180–190 bpm was attained, RS was kept constant for the duration of the test. The range of inclination was 5–15% and each subject wore a nose clip.

The pulmonary response from the EIA-test was expressed as the maximal percentage decrease in FEV_1 ($\Delta FEV_1\%$) from baseline (baseline value—lowest recorded postexercise value/baseline value × 100%) [4]. This value was used to assess the occurrence of EIA with the cutoff value set at 15% [4, 16]. No asthmatic children reached the set cut-off. The mean (95% CI) $\Delta FEV_1\%$ was 3.8 (1.5; 6.2) and 1.3 (−1.1; 3.8) in asthma and controls, respectively.

2.4.3. Equation PAC. PAC was estimated by the following variables: maximal heart rate, HR_{max} (220 bpm—age in years) (estimated), $HR_{steadystate} \approx$ 170–180 bpm (measured), and HR_{rest} (measured). The estimation used a constant for child resting metabolic rate, RMR, (4.2 $mLO_2/min/kg$) [17], and VO_2 ($mLO_2/min/kg$). The estimation used laboratory derived VO_2 corresponding to RS at $HR_{steadystate}$ published earlier [2].

The applied equation (below) was a modification of the original equation proposed by Klausen et al. [18]. The calculation resulted in the estimation of PAC adjusted for BW as follows:

$$PAC = RMR + \frac{HR_{max} - HR_{rest}}{HR_{steadystate} - HR_{rest}} \times (VO_2 - RMR). \quad (1)$$

The ambient room temperature and relative humidity were measured before each exercise test by a portable thermohygrograph (Model SL (Sound Level) 435007). The average room temperature and relative humidity of the PAC tests were 19.6 ± 1.9°C and 62.9 ± 10.6%, respectively; for the EIA-test the average room temperature and relative humidity were 19.0 ± 1.0°C and 58.1 ± 5.0%, respectively.

2.5. Statistics. General linear multiple regression analysis was conducted to determine the adjusted effects on PAC (APL*plus, Scientific Time Sharing Corporation, Rockville, MD, USA).

Two-way analysis of variance "repeated measures" was applied to evaluate the variations in the mean values of PAC over time within and between the groups of asthma and control children (SAS, v.8.2 PROC MIXED, SAS Institute Inc., Cary, NC, USA).

Multiple linear regression models were applied to estimate the groups (asthma and controls) specific regression lines using STATA (v.11.2) (Stata Corp, College Station, TX, USA). Age and sex adjustments were performed.

The sample size was calculated to comply with the power estimation, sensitivity $(1 - \beta)$ = 80% and specificity (α) = 0.95. The significance tests applied were twotailed and the significance level set at 5%.

2.6. Ethics. The study was approved by the local Scientific Ethics Committee of Copenhagen County (no. KA 98029 m), the Danish Data Protection Agency (no. 1998-1200-320), and the Institutional Review Board at the Paediatric Asthma and Allergy Clinic of Copenhagen University Hospital,

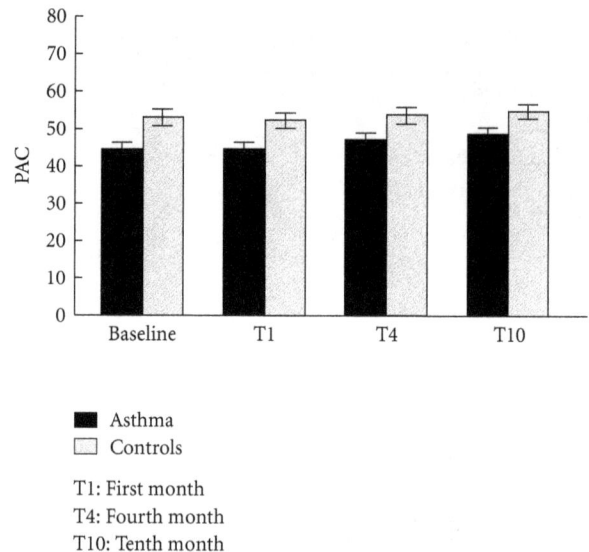

Asthma
Controls

T1: First month
T4: Fourth month
T10: Tenth month

FIGURE 1: Mean PAC ($mLO_2/min/kg$) with SE in the asthmatic and control groups of children according to four observation times.

Gentofte, Denmark. The study followed procedures in accordance with the Declaration of Helsinki (1964).

3. Results

Across the four times of observation, important group differences of PAC (P = 0.0015) between the asthmatic children and controls were seen with asthmatics depicting consistently lower PAC than controls. PAC of both groups of children increased gradually with time (P < 0.001) (Figure 1).

PAC increased with age in the two groups of children. The baseline age effect (F = 14.73, P < 0.001) was illustrated in Figure 2. At baseline the asthmatics showed lower PAC values than controls (group effect: F = 10.35, P = 0.0020).

Figure 3 illustrated the associations between physical activity and PAC at baseline separate for asthmatics and controls. By analysing all children (n = 55) important effects of group (full and reduced models) and marginal effect of physical activity (full model) was found as follows: [(reduced model, effect of group: F = 7.29, P = 0.0093) (R^2 = 0.1209)], [(full model, effect of group: F = 5.52, P = 0.023; effect of physical activity (h/week): F = 2.28, P = 0.061); (R^2 = 0.2898, P = 0.0090)].

Figure 4 illustrated the associations between physical activity and PAC at T4 separate for asthmatics and controls. Analysis of all children (n = 52) at T4 showed important effects of group and physical activity [(reduced model, effect of group: F = 6.86, P = 0.012; effect of physical activity (h/week): F = 3.03, P = 0.027); (R^2 = 0.3040, P = 0.0042)].

Figure 5 illustrated the associations between physical activity and PAC at T10 separate for asthmatics and controls. By analysis of all children (n = 55) at T10 only the effect of group demonstrated importance [(reduced model, effect of group: F = 5.22, P = 0.026) (R^2 = 0.0897)].

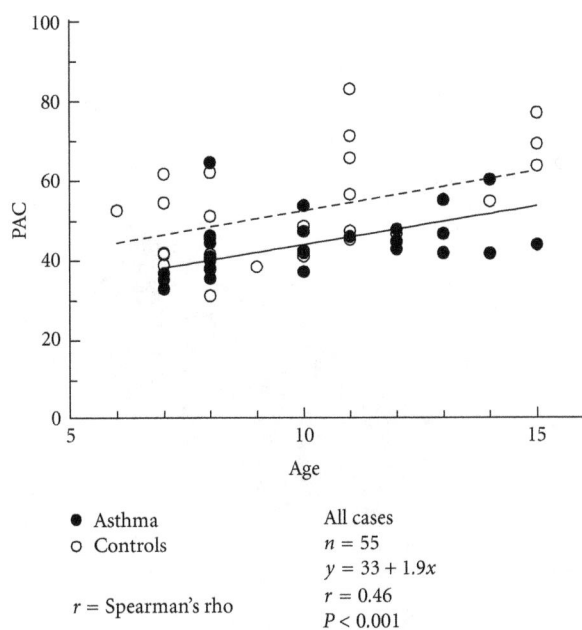

FIGURE 2: Baseline associations of PAC ($mLO_2/min/kg$) by age (years) in asthmatic and control children.

Table S2 showed that in the asthmatic group, approximately 50% of children received medical treatment and the distribution was almost similar at all four time points.

Table S3 illustrated the distributions of "ever asthma" and "current asthma" for asthma and control children. Physical activity (h/week) did not show important effects (ns) for "ever asthma" or "current asthma" in asthmatics or controls (not illustrated).

4. Discussion

The study showed that PAC of the asthmatic children was lower than that of controls and differed between the four times of observation. During the ten months observation time, I found relative consistency in the importance of physical activity effects for PAC, and physical activity explained up to 30% of the variation in PAC. There were consistent and important group differences between asthmatics and controls.

This study was designed to limit well-known bias risks. Laboratory assessment of cardiopulmonary fitness has been documented to require considerable resources whereas the submaximal exercise test overcomes most of these limitations. The PAC-test represented a noninvasive and validated [2] submaximal method and was therefore preferred for the current study.

The requests for study participation followed consecutive order to ensure random selection of the asthmatic children. The procedure for selection of participants was closely monitored to ascertain sufficient time for the individual to contemplate participation. To avoid misclassification from, for example, disproportionate inclusion of highly motivated children (and parents), reflection time prior to giving

consent was extended and further information provided as necessary.

The results showed that physical activity correlated positively with PAC, more consistently so for the asthmatics than controls, but physical activity did not influence "ever asthma" or "current asthma" and therefore these self-reports may not sustain the results. The reports of "ever asthma" and "current asthma," nonetheless, complied with data from other Scandinavian child populations that used the same asthma and physical activity questions [19]. It cannot be excluded, however, that parents of the asthmatics who were well informed of benefits of physical activity for cardiopulmonary fitness in optimal asthma care, could have been overrepresented. Likewise, these parents may have recalled physical activity differently than other parents and could have overreported the physical activity levels of their children.

The study groups originated from slightly varying sociodemographic residential areas of the Capital Region. The variation could have influenced the data collection, for example, self-reports of physical activity in a nonrandom manner. Although unconfirmed, it was also possible that asthmatics and younger children received more support completing the questionnaire than controls.

The results on the endocrinological development of the included children were almost similar in asthmatics and controls. Although asthmatic PAC was consistently lower than that of controls, the stable increase of PAC by age in both groups may illustrate the well-recognized systematic influence of development on VO_2 [20].

The participants with moderate and severe asthma who accounted for almost half of the asthmatic group may in fact have contributed disproportionately to the asthmatic reductions of PAC compared to the mild asthmatic subjects. Earlier findings from studies of severe childhood asthma [8] may lend support to this interpretation.

The asthmatic children demonstrated a similar increase of PAC over time to that seen for the healthy controls. It is plausible that this finding reflected a diminished asthmatic disease activity occurring during the observation time. However, this hypothesis needs to be prespecified and tested separately in future studies.

Indeed poor fitness of asthmatic children has been thoroughly investigated and physical risk factors documented [1, 3, 21, 22]. In healthy children, "previous" physical activity played an important role for the "present" activity level [23]. The reports of physical activity were collected at three different time points during ten months, but the current study was not designed to test for separate effects of physical activity in the asthmatics and controls investigated.

Over the course of the past decade, reviewers of asthmatic children's fitness have demonstrated a shift in their conclusions from previous "asthmatic children being less fit" [3] to current positions that "studies are inconclusive" [24]. This study complied with the former representing the times when data were collected.

The submaximal exercise test has been validated in different populations, and the validity of a submaximal exercise test depended on a predictable relationship between

Baseline PAC by physical activity

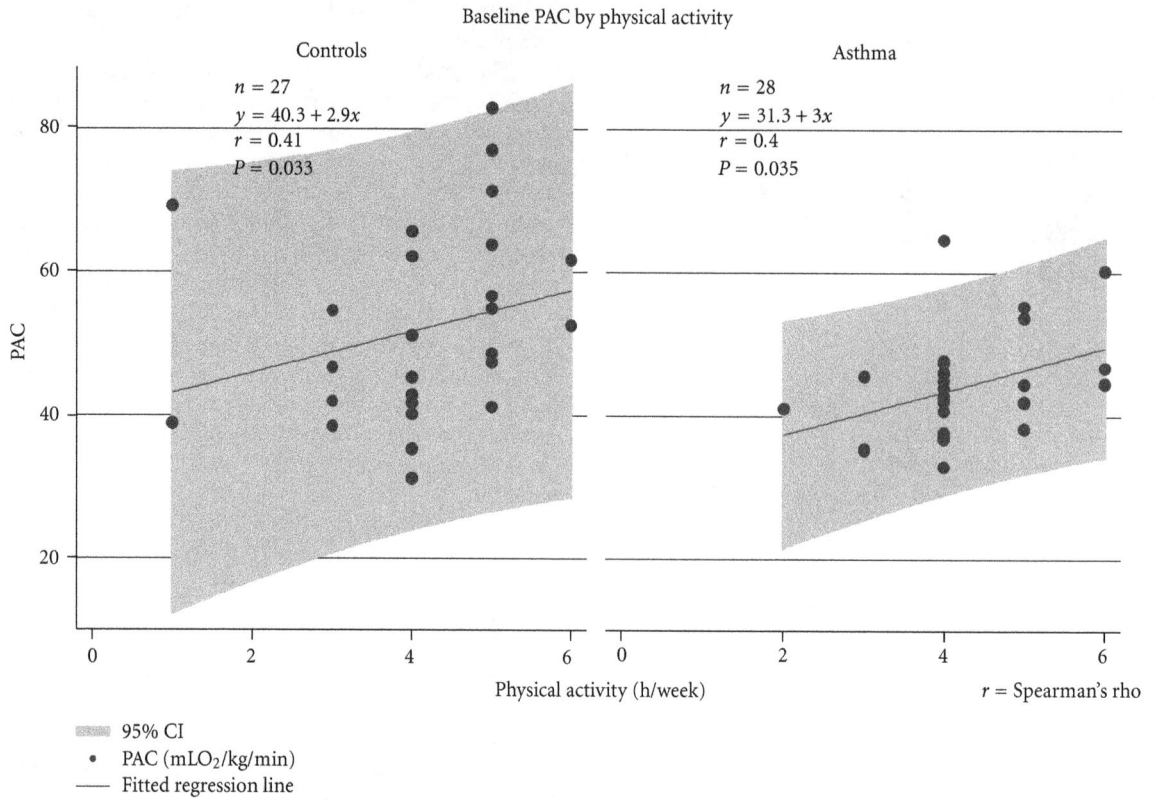

FIGURE 3: Baseline associations between PAC (mLO$_2$/min/kg) and physical activity (h/week) in asthmatics and controls.

T4 PAC by physical activity

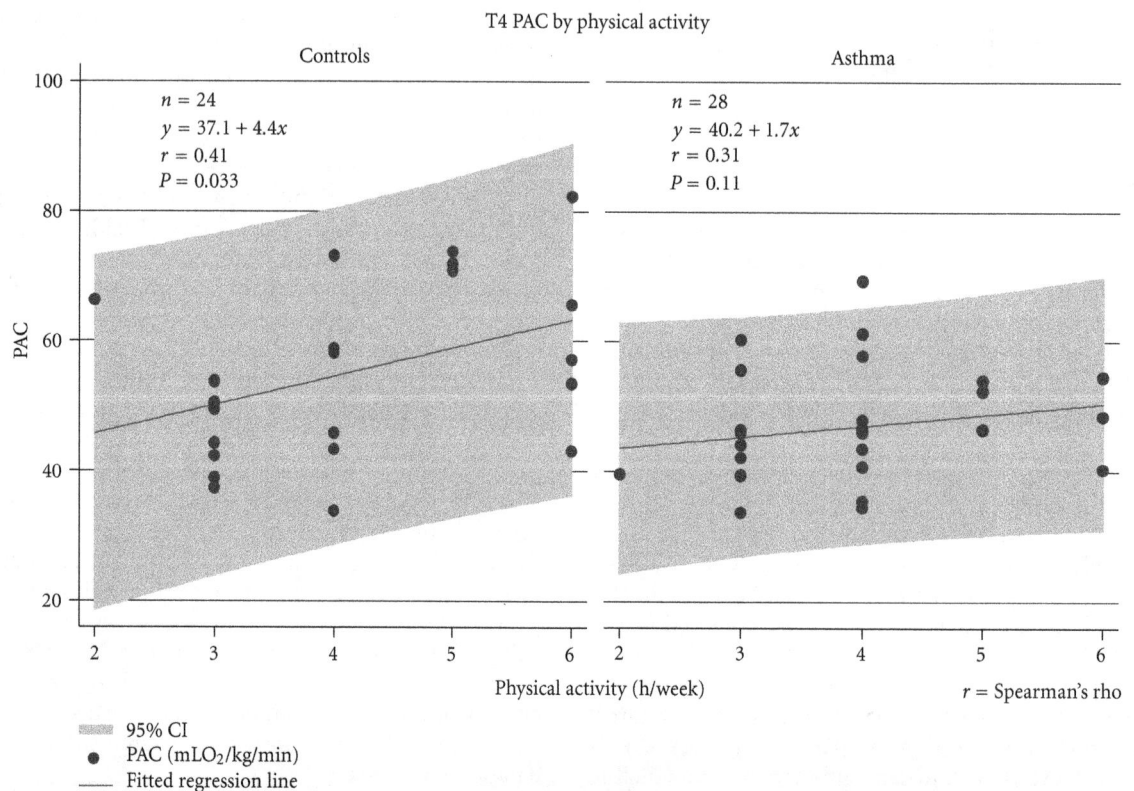

FIGURE 4: T4 associations between PAC (mLO$_2$/min/kg) and physical activity (h/week) in asthmatics and controls.

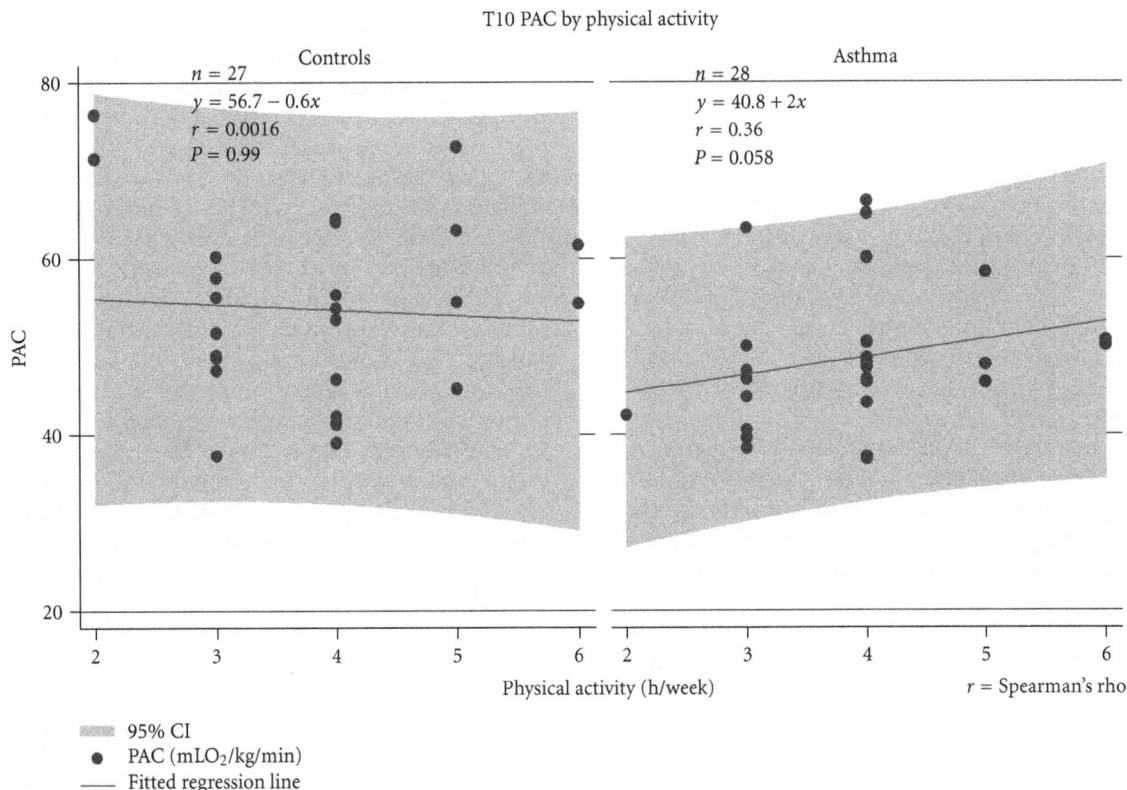

Figure 5: T10 associations between PAC (mLO_2/min/kg) and physical activity (h/week) in asthmatics and controls.

oxygen consumption and HR [25]. The equation applied in this study was validated under the assumption of a linear relationship between VO_2 and HR and the submaximal method tended to underestimate PAC compared with laboratory monitored aerobic capacity [2]. Given such minor underestimation of the present PAC, there has not been an indication that this would have affected the groups in a differential way. Conversely, for the current full study population target heart rates were reached and hence the expected physiological stress levels.

The present results of the EIA-test indicated that lung function could have played a role in the asthmatic reduction of PAC. The decrease of the asthmatic lung function during the EIA-test potentially reflected the untreated nature of the asthmatic disease for half of the asthmatic children. Previous results of mild-to-moderate childhood asthma have shown that only sedentary children had impaired cardiopulmonary capacity [26]. The positive associations between physical activity and PAC that was seen for the asthmatics seemingly confirmed such results.

Earlier results published by my group found lower $HR_{steadystate}$ of the control group than of the asthma group to suggest that physical activity could have influenced HR differently in asthmatic and nonasthmatic children [2]. Even though regressions slopes for HR and VO_2 have been documented to alter with pulmonary disease [27], applying explanations like those to the present asthmatic PAC reductions would involve laboratory replication.

Although the present results have been generated from relatively small sample sizes, initial precautions were taken to power the study adequately. The longitudinal design served to demonstrate consistency of the results for PAC. While these data cannot ascertain causal associations between physical activity and PAC, they are nonetheless consistent with findings of others for both physical activity [19] and PAC [8, 9]. The reduced aerobic capacity of the asthmatic study group, consistent across observation times, may further add to the biological credibility of the current study hypothesis.

The extent to which the present asthmatic study population reported limitations from pulmonary symptoms disagreed with other asthmatic child populations studied [26]. Colleagues [26] investigated a large sample size and could report results of VO_{2max} from subgroups of sedentary and active (up to 2 hs/week) children that seemed comparable with the present results. The current sample, however, was not sufficiently sized to accommodate subgroup divisions. The frequent and largely untreated pulmonary symptoms reported to accompany physical activity by the asthmatic group could be a further explanation for the low asthmatic PAC that I found. Ultimately, the results may have been influenced by other known or unknown residual confounding factors that were not accounted for in this work.

BMI was higher than expected for the asthmatic group, which possibly indicated that the weight matching was not complete for the study population. VO_2 was derived from established data on VO_2 and running speed. Although baseline running speed showed no group differences, it cannot be excluded that the asthmatic children weighing slightly more than controls may have produced slower running speeds than controls at any one point during the ten months of observation time.

More recently, high BMI of asthmatic children and its relations with poor physical conditioning have been well acknowledged. Hence, the results suggested that rather than attempting to match participants on weight, future studies of asthmatic children might indeed generate important information from weight associations. In the light of the global weight burden with young people, the weight matching design may not be warranted when asthmatic children are under study.

In summary, the current results indicated that physical activity could be a risk factor for low PAC in the asthmatic children investigated. Although the results cannot necessarily be extrapolated to the global scene of asthmatic child populations, they underlined that joint monitoring of pulmonary symptoms and cardiopulmonary fitness of asthmatics may supply important information for prevention and treatment of those young suffering pulmonary symptoms by physical activity.

At a time when objective and individualised criteria to standardise exercise tests of asthmatic children are requested [3, 28], and where those that do exist have not been routinely implemented in paediatric asthma clinics, the public health implication of the current study is to target standardised monitoring of *pulmonary function* as well as *cardiopulmonary fitness* of asthmatic young; hence, to capture the variations of this burdening pulmonary childhood disease; the recommendations apply equally to Scandinavian and comparable populations of asthmatic children.

5. Conclusions

This study showed that the asthmatic children had consistently low PAC when observed across time. Physical activity was positively associated with PAC in the asthmatics.

Conflicts of Interest

The author has stated explicitly that there are no conflicts of interest in connection with this paper.

Acknowledgments

The study was financially supported by Danish Lung Association, Danish Health Insurance Foundation, Danish Physical Therapy Organisation, and Danish Asthma and Allergy Association. The author wishes to thank Dr. Aage Voelund, Principal Statistician Emeritus, Novo Nordisk A/S Copenhagen, Bagsvaerd, and Statistical Advisory Service, Department of Biostatistics, University of Copenhagen, Copenhagen, Denmark, for statistical guidance and data analysis. Dr. Vagn Braendholt, Associate Professor, Consultant, Zealand Region of Denmark, South Naestved Hospital, Naestved, Denmark, is thanked for the screening and enrolment of the asthmatic children and for his clinical assistance with the assessments by orchidometer. The current results contributed to the MPH thesis of the author: thesis no. 70, University of Copenhagen, Copenhagen, Denmark, 2001. In turn, this baseline study has been followed up by laboratory validation of the PAC-test. The follow-up study was published in the Clinical Respiratory Journal and made available at: http://dx.doi.org/10.1111/j.1752-699X.2008.00107.x.The baseline data for PAC have been included in detailed presentations of the follow-up study at International conventions as follows: World Congress of Asthma, Interasma, Guadalajara, Mexico, 15 October 2006; World Asthma Meeting, Istanbul, Turkey, 23 June 2007; European Respiratory Society, Annual Congress, Stockholm, Sweden, 19 September 2007; International Epidemiological Association, XVIII World Congress of Epidemiology, Porto Alegre, Brazil, 21 September 2008. On 10 December 2009, the comprehensive research project (1998–2009) was summarised at the International Meeting of Health and Environment, Rome, Italy.

References

[1] H. Milgrom and L. M. Taussig, "Keeping children with exercise-induced asthma active," *Pediatrics*, vol. 104, no. 3, p. e38, 1999.

[2] L. Lochte, M. Angermann, and B. Larsson, "Cardiorespiratory fitness of asthmatic children and validation of predicted aerobic capacity," *Clinical Respiratory Journal*, vol. 3, no. 1, pp. 42–50, 2009.

[3] C. J. Clark and L. M. Cochrane, "Physical activity and asthma," *Current Opinion in Pulmonary Medicine*, vol. 5, no. 1, pp. 68–75, 1999.

[4] J. M. Henriksen, *Exercise-induced asthma in children [DMSc Thesis]*, Allergy and Munksgaard International Publishers, Copenhagen, Denmark, 1990.

[5] K.-H. Carlsen, "Exercise induced asthma in children and adolescents and the relationship to sports," *Pediatric Allergy and Immunology*, vol. 9, no. 4, pp. 173–180, 1998.

[6] R. C. Strunk, D. A. Mrazek, J. T. Fukuhara, J. Masterson, S. K. Ludwick, and J. F. LaBrecque, "Cardiovascular fitness in children with asthma correlates with psychologic functioning of the child," *Pediatrics*, vol. 84, no. 3, pp. 460–464, 1989.

[7] L. Lochte, "Exercise capacity of asthmatic children validation in clinical Context," Thesis 70, University of Copenhagen, Copenhagen, Denmark, 2001.

[8] G. Hedlin, V. Graff-Lonnevig, and U. Freyschuss, "Working capacity and pulmonary gas exchange in children with exercise-induced asthma," *Acta Paediatrica Scandinavica*, vol. 75, no. 6, pp. 947–954, 1986.

[9] R. C. Strunk, D. Rubin, L. Kelly, B. Sherman, and J. Fukuhara, "Determination of fitness in children with asthma: use of standardized tests for functional endurance, body fat composition, flexibility, and abdominal strength," *American Journal of Diseases of Children*, vol. 142, no. 9, pp. 940–944, 1988.

[10] "The British guidelines on asthma management, 1995: review and position statement, British Thoracic Society," *Thorax*, vol. 52, supplement 1, pp. 1S–21S, 1997.

[11] M. I. Asher, U. Keil, H. R. Anderson et al., "International study of asthma and allergies in childhood (ISAAC): rationale and methods," *European Respiratory Journal*, vol. 8, no. 3, pp. 483–491, 1995.

[12] M. L. Booth, A. D. Okely, T. Chey, and A. Bauman, "The reliability and validity of the physical activity questions in the WHO health behaviour in schoolchildren (HBSC) survey: a population study," *British Journal of Sports Medicine*, vol. 35, no. 4, pp. 263–267, 2001.

[13] C. Currie, "Appendix 1: International standard version of the core questions of the 1997-98 survey," in *Health Behaviour in School-aged Children. Research Protocol for the 1997-98 Survey, A World Health Organization Cross-National Study*, vol. 20, University of Edinburgh, Edinburgh, UK, 1998.

[14] G. Polgar and V. Promadhat, *Pulmonary Function Testing in Children: Techniques and Standards*, W. B. Saunders, Philadelphia, Pa, USA, 1974.

[15] D. M. Styne, "The physiology of puberty," in *Clinical Paediatric Endocrinology*, C. G. D. Brook, Ed., pp. 234–252, Blackwell Science, Oxford, UK, 1995.

[16] M. M. Haby, J. K. Peat, C. M. Mellis, S. D. Anderson, and A. J. Woolcock, "An exercise challenge for epidemiological studies of childhood asthma: validity and repeatability," *European Respiratory Journal*, vol. 8, no. 5, pp. 729–736, 1995.

[17] D. C. Nieman, M. D. Austin, S. M. Chilcote, and L. Benezra, "Validation of a new handheld device for measuring resting metabolic rate and oxygen consumption in children," *International Journal of Sport Nutrition and Exercise Metabolism*, vol. 15, no. 2, pp. 186–194, 2005.

[18] K. Klausen, I. Hemmingsen, and B. Rasmussen, "Kondition og fysiologiske virkninger af konditionstraening," in *Almen Idraetsteori*, K. Klausen, I. Hemmingsen, and B. Rasmussen, Eds., pp. 81–96, Forum, Copenhagen, Denmark, 1985.

[19] W. Nystad, "The physical activity level in children with asthma based on a survey among 7-16-year-old school children," *Scandinavian Journal of Medicine and Science in Sports*, vol. 7, no. 6, pp. 331–335, 1997.

[20] T. W. Rowland, "Maturation of aerobic fitness," in *Developmental Exercise Physiology*, T. W. Rowland, Ed., p. 78, Human Kinetics, Champaign, Ill, USA, 1996.

[21] M. R. Sears, "Epidemiological trends in bronchial asthma," in *Asthma Its Pathology and Treatment*, M. A. Kalinger, P. J. Barnes, and C. G. A. Persson, Eds., pp. 1–49, Marcel Dekker, New York, NY, USA, 1991.

[22] G. Fink, C. Kaye, H. Blau, and S. A. Spitzer, "Assessment of exercise capacity in asthmatic children with various degrees of activity," *Pediatric Pulmonology*, vol. 15, no. 1, pp. 41–43, 1993.

[23] J. F. Sallis, J. J. Prochaska, and W. C. Taylor, "A review of correlates of physical activity of children and adolescents," *Medicine and Science in Sports and Exercise*, vol. 32, no. 5, pp. 963–975, 2000.

[24] L. Welsh, R. G. D. Roberts, and J. G. Kemp, "Fitness and physical activity in children with asthma," *Sports Medicine*, vol. 34, no. 13, pp. 861–870, 2004.

[25] M. A. Minor and J. C. Johnson, "Reliability and validity of a submaximal treadmill test to estimate aerobic capacity in women with rheumatic disease," *Journal of Rheumatology*, vol. 23, no. 9, pp. 1517–1523, 1996.

[26] P. Santuz, E. Baraldi, M. Filippone, and F. Zacchello, "Exercise performance in children with asthma: is it different from that of healthy controls?" *European Respiratory Journal*, vol. 10, no. 6, pp. 1254–1260, 1997.

[27] K. Wasserman, J. E. Hansen, D. Y. Sue, and B. J. Whipp, "Pathophysiology of disorders limiting exercise," in *Principles of Exercise Testing and Interpretation*, K. Wasserman, K. J. E. Hansen, D. Y. Sue, and B. J. Whipp, Eds., p. 53, Lea & Febiger, Philadelphia, Pa, USA, 1987.

[28] A. L. Varray, J. G. Mercier, C. M. Terral, and C. G. Prefaut, "Individualized aerobic and high intensity training for asthmatic children in an exercise readaptation program: is training always helpful for better adaptation to exercise?" *Chest*, vol. 99, no. 3, pp. 579–586, 1991.

31

Validity of Reporting Oxygen Uptake Efficiency Slope from Submaximal Exercise Using Respiratory Exchange Ratio as Secondary Criterion

Wilby Williamson,[1] Jonathan Fuld,[2] Kate Westgate,[1] Karl Sylvester,[2] Ulf Ekelund,[1] and Soren Brage[1]

[1] Medical Research Council Epidemiology Unit, Institute of Metabolic Science, Box 285, Addenbrooke's Hospital, Cambridge CB2 0QQ, UK

[2] Department of Respiratory Medicine, Cambridge University Hospitals, NHS Foundation Trust, Cambridge CB2 0QQ, UK

Correspondence should be addressed to Wilby Williamson, wilbywilliamson@hotmail.com

Academic Editor: Luke Howard

Background. Oxygen uptake efficiency slope (OUES) is a reproducible, objective marker of cardiopulmonary function. OUES is reported as being relatively independent of exercise intensity. Practical guidance and criteria for reporting OUES from submaximal tests has not been established. *Objective.* Evaluate the use of respiratory exchange ratio (RER) as a secondary criterion for reporting OUES. *Design.* 100 healthy volunteers (53 women) completed a ramped treadmill protocol to exhaustive exercise. OUES was calculated from data truncated to RER levels from 0.85 to 1.2 and compared to values generated from full test data. Results. Mean (sd) OUES from full test data and data truncated to RER 1.0 and RER 0.9 was 2814 (718), 2895 (730), and 2810 (789) mL/min per 10-fold increase in VE, respectively. Full test OUES was highly correlated with OUES from RER 1.0 ($r = 0.9$) and moderately correlated with OUES from RER 0.9 ($r = 0.79$). *Conclusion.* OUES values peaked in association with an RER level of 1.0. Submaximal OUES values are not independent of exercise intensity. There is a significant increase in OUES value as exercise moves from low to moderate intensity. RER can be used as a secondary criterion to define this transition.

1. Introduction

Exercise testing allows quantification of cardiopulmonary function providing valuable diagnostic and prognostic data. Peak and maximal cardiopulmonary exercise testing are gold standard modalities [1]. However, in clinical practice and field research reporting peak exercise parameters can be compromised by compliance and feasibility. There are a number of extrinsic factors, including financial restraints and risk mitigation protocols that can restrict exercise testing to submaximal intensities. Exercise testing in large-scale population studies has to ensure high participant turnover and maintain safety in often nonclinical, potentially resource-depleted environments. To maintain safety and efficiency, termination criteria are within the moderate, nonmaximal exercise intensity range. Tests stopped within 80–90% of maximal heart rate or when respiratory exchange ratio (RER)

reaches 0.9–1.0 [2, 3]. Terminating exercise within RER ranges of 0.9–1.0 places significant restrictions on the reporting of gas exchange data.

In clinical practice, the most frequently reported submaximal parameter is the ventilatory anaerobic threshold (VAT). However, reporting VAT is not without limitations, with potential for observer error or technical difficulties when defining values [4, 5]. These challenges are even more pronounced when using exercise tests with termination criteria of RER 0.9-1.0. Shorter test durations restrict the number of data points and intensity may not progress far enough beyond VAT to confidently report results using the recognised V-slope methods [6]. Under these conditions, it may also be more difficult to accommodate irregularities in breathing patterns. For example, hyperventilation that might be expected to settle as exercise progresses may compromise the reporting of graphical submaximal data points. These practical limitations provide an incentive to establish objective, reproducible submaximal gas exchange parameters with functional and prognostic value.

There are a number of potential parameters that can be reported from submaximal gas exchange data ranging from regressions of ventilation versus carbon dioxide exhalation to measures derived from oxygen uptake [7, 8]. The oxygen uptake efficiency slope (OUES) is a regression-derived parameter from the relationship between log-transformed minute ventilation (VE) and oxygen uptake (VO$_2$), with the coefficient "a" from the regression VO$_2 = a$ logVE $+ b$ being defined as the OUES. The coefficient "a" represents the rate of change in VO$_2$ in response to VE [9]. If an individual achieves a higher VO$_2$ with only a small increase in VE, this will produce a higher OUES and this is taken to represent more efficient oxygen uptake. OUES is regarded as an objective, reproducible marker of cardiopulmonary function calculated from sequential data points. Using sequential data points as opposed to time or intensity defined values has led to the suggestion that OUES represents a composite value for cardiopulmonary function inclusive of the physiological transition from low to vigorous intensity [9, 10].

In the context of maximal testing, OUES provides a similar marker of function and prognosis as Peak VO$_2$ [11–13]. However, the evidence that OUES remains relatively stable across moderate-to-high intensity exercise has promoted acceptance of OUES as a valid submaximal measure of function and disease prognosis [10]. Baba and coworkers were first to report the use of OUES in cardiovascular populations and identify the relative stability of OUES in the final quartile of a maximal test [9]. Hollenberg et al. then confirmed these results; OUES reported from 75% of the completed test differed by less than 2% of the OUES calculated from the full test [12]. These seminal papers provided the template to establish reporting criterion for submaximal OUES values and facilitate expansion into clinical practice. However, translation into the clinical domain has been slow despite the literature continuing to grow in support of OUES as a functional and prognostic parameter during peak and maximal tests [13, 14]. The majority of studies continue to report OUES defined by percentage data acknowledging that there is a strong correlation between submaximal and full test results [15]. Lending support to the statement that OUES is relatively independent of exercise intensity but not defining reporting criterion. Pogliaghi et al. explored defining submaximal OUES with regards to percentages of predicted heart rate reserve [16]. Heart rate is commonly used in noninvasive exercise testing to define intensity but the variance and potential error, especially in the clinical sitting, is well established [17]. Overall, there has been minimal progression in the literature on defining how to practically use OUES with reference to submaximal testing. This is potentially limiting the expansion of OUES in both the clinical and research domains.

Clinically, there is rarely the luxury of collecting peak exercise data, and in the context of submaximal tests, it is difficult to define percentage efforts. The same limitation holds for researchers working with large populations where field testing is limited by feasibility to submaximal tests. In both of these contexts OUES could be an ideal parameter to report. The objective of the current study is to report the reliability of using RER as a reporting criterion for OUES, exploring the question of whether there is a submaximal threshold below which OUES is not valid or incurs significant error when compared to true maximal data.

2. Methods

2.1. Participants. A total of 100 participants were recruited from the Cambridge area (UK). Participants were free from cardiopulmonary and metabolic diseases. Ethical approval for the study was obtained from the local research ethics committee. All participants provided written, informed consent.

2.2. Study Procedure. Participants were asked to refrain from eating, drinking (except water), smoking, and vigorous exercise for at least 2 hours before they arrived at the laboratory. Height and weight of participants in light clothing were recorded using a rigid stadiometer and calibrated scales, respectively.

2.3. Treadmill Test. A Jaeger Oxycon Pro system was configured to control a motorized treadmill (HP Cosmo Pulsar 4.0). The treadmill protocol was a nonindividualised ramp protocol adapted from an original epidemiological study protocol [18]. The original protocol was extended to include a 4th phase to ensure participants exercised to an exhaustive intensity. *Phase 1* (level walking) involved level walking with increasing speed (3 min at 3.2 km/h and then accelerating at 0.33 km·h^{-1} per min for the next 6 min), *phase 2* (graded walking) consisted of brisk walking (5.2–5.8 km/h) with increasing gradient (at a rate of 1.7% increased gradient/min for 6 min), *phase 3* (level running) involved level running with speed increasing from 9 to 12.5 km/h for 4.5 min (average acceleration of 0.78 km·h^{-1} per min), and phase 4 (uphill running) in which the gradient increased by 0.5% and the speed increased by 0.25 km·hr^{-1} every 15 seconds until exhaustion. Transition between *phases 2 and 3* was first a change in gradient by -10.2% over 30 seconds (now level), followed by a change in speed by 3.2 km/h over 30 seconds.

Continuous recording of respiratory gas exchange parameters was taken during the treadmill test and for 2 minutes during recovery after exercise test termination. Participants were asked to exercise until maximal exertion. Clinical indicators for terminating the treadmill test were onset of angina or angina-like symptoms or signs of poor perfusion including light-headedness, confusion, ataxia, pallor, cyanosis, nausea, or cold and clammy skin. In addition, tests were stopped following physical or verbal manifestations of severe fatigue, the volunteer requesting to stop despite verbal encouragement.

2.4. Respiratory Gas Analysis. Gas exchange data were acquired breath by breath and averaged over 20-second intervals for generation of graphic data and regression analysis for OUES and VE/VCO$_2$ [7]. Peak VO$_2$ and peak respiratory exchange ratio was expressed as the highest averaged values over sequential 30-second periods obtained from complete exercise data [11, 19]. Breath by breath averaging was expanded to 30 seconds in an attempt to reduce the effect of transient fluctuations in RER when calculating RER truncated OUES. RER data for each individual test was plotted against time to review trend. The VAT was determined by the V-slope method [6].

2.5. Determination of Oxygen Uptake Efficiency across Exercise Duration. OUES was calculated from complete and truncated gas exchange data according to a series of criteria.

(1) Defined as percentile of the complete test. OUES calculated from data taken from the first 25%, 50%, and 75% of time defined test data.

(2) Defined according to Ventilatory Anaerobic Threshold (VAT). Calculating OUES using data from start of test until time of VAT.

(3) Defined according to increasing Respiratory Exchange Ratio (RER). OUES values were calculated from test data limited to RER $\leq$ 0.85, RER $\leq$ 0.90, RER $\leq$ 0.95, RER $\leq$ 1.00, RER $\leq$ 1.10, and RER $\leq$ 1.20.

2.6. Gas Exchange Reference Values. Mean Peak VO$_2$, OUES, and VEVCO$_2$ results were compared with predicted reference ranges accounting for age, weight, height, and sex [7, 11, 19]. Peak VO$_2$ prediction equation:

Men: VO$_2$max = [50.2 − (0.394 (age (yrs)))],

Women: VO$_2$max = [42.83 − (0.371 (age (yrs)))].

OUES prediction equations:

Men: OUES [L/min/log(L/min)] = [−0.61 − 0.032 (age (yrs)) + 0.023(height (cm)) + 0.008 (weight (kg))],

Women: OUES [L/min/log(L/min)] = [−1.178 − 0.032 (age (yrs)) + 0.023 (height (cm)) + 0.008 (weight (kg))].

VE/VCO$_2$ prediction equations:

Men: VE/VCO$_2$ slope = 34.5 + 0.1 (age (yrs)) − 0.05 (height) (cm),

Women: VE/VCO$_2$ slope = 35.5 + 0.1(age (yrs)) − 0.05(height) (cm).

2.7. Statistics. Statistical analysis was performed using StataIC 11 (Stata Corp LP, TX).

Summary statistics for continuous variables are expressed as means with standard deviation ($\pm$SD). Relative and absolute agreement between the different measures of OUES were reported via correlation and Bland-Altman agreement analysis (including root mean square error). When displayed graphically, mean values are presented with

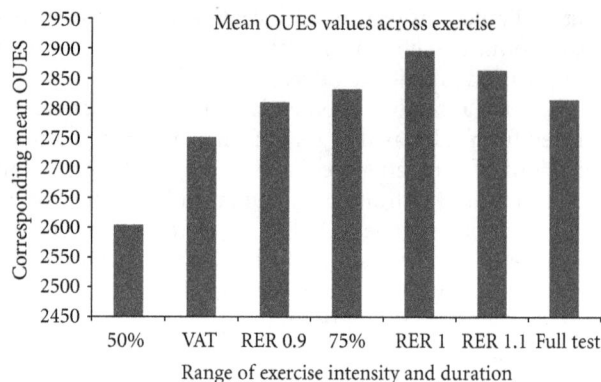

FIGURE 1: Mean OUES values between 50th percentile and full test defined by submaximal criteria. VAT Ventilatory Anaerobic Threshold, RER respiratory exchange ratio. Percentage of test defined by time to complete full test.

standard error bars. Subgroup analysis was performed using Student *t*-test and regression analysis.

3. Results

One hundred participants (53 women) underwent cardiopulmonary exercise testing (CPET) recording Peak VO$_2$, VAT, OUES, and VE/VCO$_2$ slope values. The group were healthy volunteers. The mean age was 41.4 yrs (range 22 to 65 yrs). Mean weight was 70.3 kg (range 44 to 109 kg) and mean height was 170.5 cm (range 144 to 195 cm).

Mean test duration was 1228 seconds (sd 152 s). Mean time to VAT was 821 seconds associated with an RER of 0.92 (sd 0.07). Only one individual passed the anaerobic threshold prior to 600 seconds. No participants were limited by clinical symptoms. Mean Peak VO$_2$ was 39.8 (sd 8.8) mL/kg/min; mean Peak RER was 1.19 (sd 0.11). Mean OUES using all available test data was 2814 (sd 718) (mL/min/logVE); mean VE/VCO$_2$ slope using all test data was 30.2 (sd 4.15). Exercise characteristics from the complete test are shown in Table 1. The results are consistent with high cardiovascular fitness within this sample; measured Peak VO$_2$ was 131.5% of the expected value.

3.1. OUES Values during Cardiopulmonary Exercise Testing. OUES values from complete test data were strongly correlated with Peak VO$_2$ ($r = 0.86$, $P < 0.0001$). OUES values were not independent of exercise intensity. The exercise test had to progress beyond 50% of the max duration and the ventilatory anaerobic threshold before OUES values approached that generated from full test data. Compared to full test data, the correlation increased and the error reduced for OUES values in association with increasing RER [Figures 2(a)–2(c)]. Using root mean squared error as a relative indicator of accuracy when reporting submaximal OUES, there is over 40% improvement reporting values from intensity corresponding with RER 1.0, compared with RER 0.85 (Figure 1). In the current study, OUES values peak in association with an RER of 1.0 (Table 2, Figure 1).

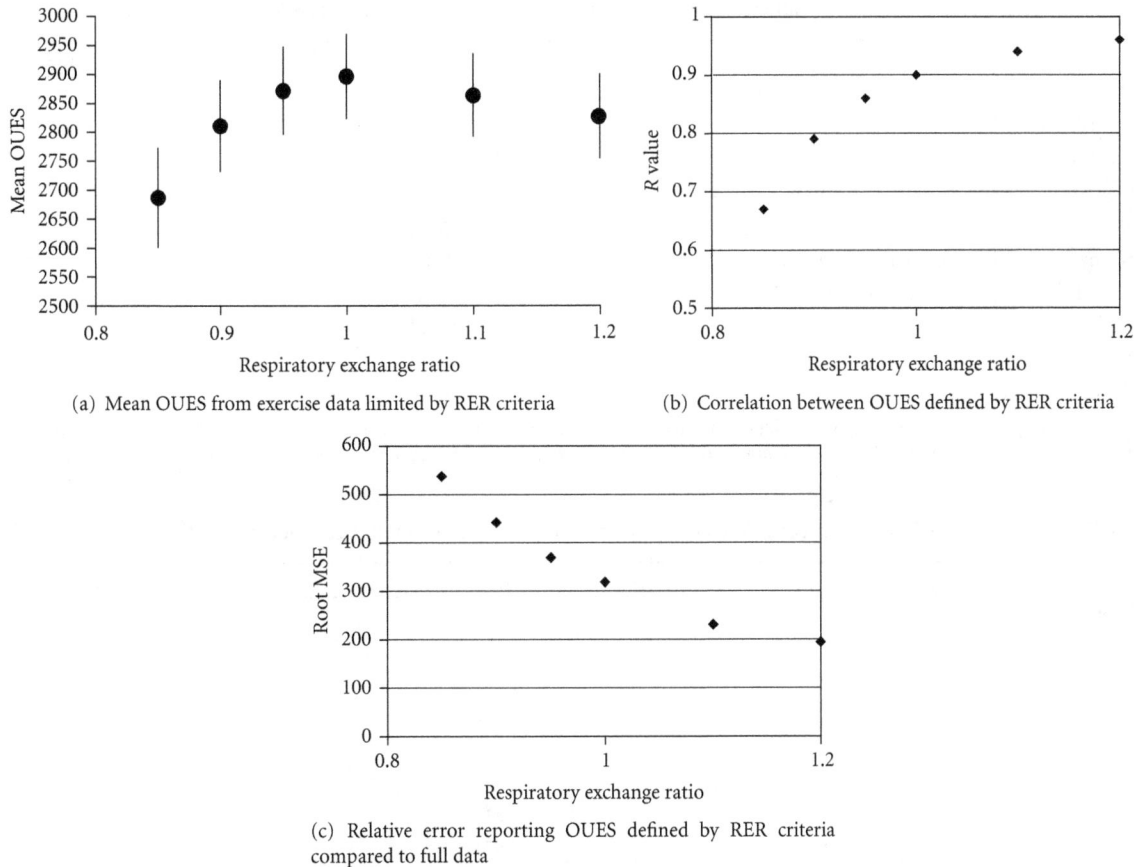

(a) Mean OUES from exercise data limited by RER criteria

(b) Correlation between OUES defined by RER criteria

(c) Relative error reporting OUES defined by RER criteria compared to full data

FIGURE 2: OUES values reported from exercise intensity defined by RER with associated correlation and relative error compared to full test data. Mean values are reported with standard error bars. (a) presents mean values of OUES generated from data associated with increasing RER. (b) presents the R value from Pearson Correlation comparing submaximal RER-defined exercise data with complete data. (c) shows the root mean squared error (RMSE) from the regression of the submaximal RER data versus complete exercise data. RMSE is presented as a value of the relative error reporting submaximal values as opposed to values from full test data.

4. Discussion

Using peak and maximal exercise tests, OUES has been shown to be a valid, reproducible parameter of cardiopulmonary function and prognosis [10]. It is believed that OUES parameterises the relationship between peripheral oxygen demand and the associated increases in cardiac output and alveolar ventilation. In a noninvasive setting, it provides a composite value for the efficiency of the cardiopulmonary system to oxygenate and perfuse peripheral tissues and subsequent oxygen utilisation [10].

Recent OUES literature explores the test-retest validity and functional outcomes in new clinical cohorts reporting favourable results [20, 21]. This is supporting a potential transition in preoperative and respiratory clinical practice to use OUES in preference to the ventilatory anaerobic threshold. However, the use of OUES largely remains confined to the research field. This may change if the value and reliability of OUES as a submaximal measure is reported in the context of secondary reporting criterion. In noninvasive exercise testing, clinicians and physiologists commonly use predetermined criteria including heart rate percentages, RER, and visual analogy scores to validate the test. However, there are

no established criteria for reporting OUES from submaximal tests.

The stability of OUES in submaximal ranges has been noted since it was first introduced in the literature [9]. This understanding has expanded to recognise that OUES from 50% of a completed test is comparable to the full test OUES in both healthy and noncyanotic disease groups [22]. Davies et al. were the first to report that OUES from the first 50% of a modified Bruce protocol exercise test could be used as a prognostic indicator in heart failure [13]. This was subsequently confirmed by Arena et al. [14]. In these studies the difference between OUES from the first 50% of a maximal test and full test OUES was 1% and 2.6%, respectively. In the current study, the difference was 7.5% between full test OUES and OUES from 50% of a complete test. Not surprisingly, the difference between OUES and submaximal measures increased with increasing truncation of data. OUES values reported using data from the first quarter of the test could be as much as 35% lower than the highest values and correlation with full test values was low ($r = 0.35$) (Figure 3).

The current study has presented the characteristics of OUES in relation to RER values. Using RER criteria, the

TABLE 1: Gas exchange parameters using the complete test to exhaustion data (peak exercise test data).

Variable	Mean	Standard deviation
Peak RER	1.19	0.11
Peak VO_2 mL/min	2796	783
Peak VO_2 mL/kg/min	39.8	8.8
Peak VO_2 as percentage of predicted VO_2max	131.5	20.4
VAT mL/kg/min	23.6	4.5
OUES mL/min per 10-fold ventilation increase	2814	718
OUES mL/min/kg per 10-fold ventilation increase	40.1	8.2
% Predicted OUES	130.7	34.2
VE/VCO_2 slope	30.2	4.15
Predicted VE/VCO_2 slope	30.6	1.56

Predicted values for VO_2max, OUES, and VE/VCO_2 slope generated from prediction equations. Abbreviations: RER, respiratory exchange ratio; VO_2, oxygen consumption; VE, minute ventilation; VCO_2, carbon dioxide production; VAT, ventilatory anaerobic threshold; OUES oxygen uptake efficiency slope.

TABLE 2: OUES values generated from restricting data points by percentile, respiratory exchange ratio, and ventilatory anaerobic threshold.

Submax criterion	Mean OUES	Standard deviation
Percentile of test data		
0–25%	1875	545
0–50%	2604	750
0–75%	2832	667
Respiratory exchange ratio		
<0.85	2687	860
<0.90	2810	789
<0.95	2871	759
<1.0	2895	730
<1.10	2863	719
<1.20	2824	734
Up to ventilatory anaerobic threshold	2672	687
Complete test data	2814	718

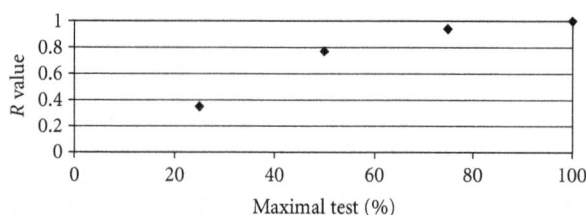

FIGURE 3: Correlation between submaximal and full test OUES values reported from percentiles of test data.

OUES has been identified to peak at submaximal intensities. The highest mean OUES value occurs in association with an RER of 1.0.

This is consistent with the reported patterns of oxygen uptake efficiency using other parameters. Sun et al. identified that the highest values for the ratio of minute ventilation to oxygen uptake (VE/VO_2) occurred in submaximal ranges [11].

Using RER criteria, there is less than a 3% difference between OUES values reported from full test data and data from start of test to RER 1.0 (Table 2). Bland-Altman plots help

to visualise the relationship between complete data OUES and results from RER 0.9, 0.95, and 1.1 (Figure 4). Mean difference between OUES from complete data and data up till RER 0.9 was less than 0.2% (3.86) with a correlation r value of 0.79. However, it should be noted that the limits of agreements contracted by over 50% when reporting OUES from RER 1.1 (limits −505 to 407) compared to using RER 0.9 (limits −961 to 969). Similar findings were reported by Van Laethem et al. when considering submaximal percentile data. Van Laethem also identified that test-retest reliability increased when OUES was calculated from peak exercise compared to submaximal [15]. Therefore, there are thresholds of reliability and reproducibility for reporting submaximal OUES values. In the current study, reporting OUES as RER increases above 0.9 provides values more reflective of the full test value.

4.1. The Validity of RER as Secondary Criterion for Reporting OUES. At rest and low intensity exercise, there are multiple extrinsic determinants of the RER ranging from dietary intake to previous exercise load. However, the determinants

(a)

(b)

(c)

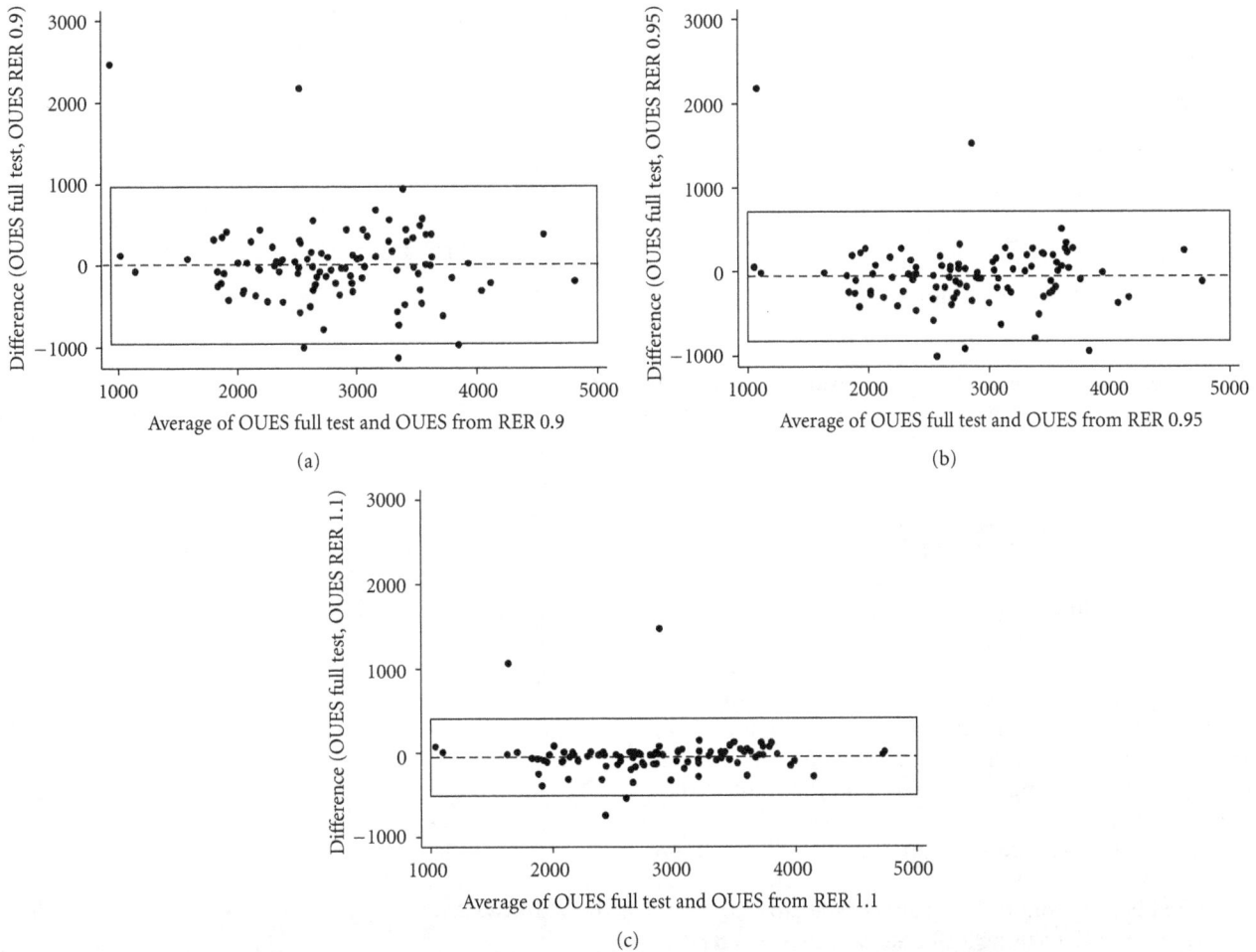

FIGURE 4: Bland Altman plots comparing full test data and data truncated using RER 0.9, 0.95, and 1.1 as cutoff criteria.

of RER become intrinsic to exercise-induced metabolism as intensity increases between 25% and 70% of peak work rate [23].

In the current study, phase 1 exercise (level walking) generated a mean RER of 0.85 at a relative intensity of 40% of peak exercise (mean VO_2 16.0 mL/kg/min sd 2.4), while phase 3 (level jogging/running) generated a mean RER of 0.94 reaching a relative intensity of 71% peak VO_2 (mean VO_2 28.4 mL/kg/min sd 3.5). These results are comparable to those of Goedecke who reported RER values of 0.86 (sd 0.037) and 0.976 (sd 0.043) during steady state 25% and 70% peak work rate (41% and 80% VO_2 Peak) [23]. This would suggest that provided exercise intensity progresses beyond 40% of the predicted peak value of VO_2 that RER can be used as valid criterion for identifying moderate intensity exercise.

RER is commonly used as a secondary criterion for satisfying the attainment of Peak VO_2. This has recently been challenged with reports that there could be as much as a 27% difference in the Peak VO_2 values recorded between an RER of 1.1 and maximal data [24]. The current study would suggest that the same concerns do not exist for reporting OUES. There is less than a 3% difference in comparison of the mean values across the RER range from 0.9 to 1.2 (Figure 2(a)).

In the current study, four individuals (4%) had peak RER less than 1.0 and there were a total of 16 individuals with peak RER values less than 1.1. It could be argued that these 16 individuals did not achieve true peak exercise. This prompted a review of the exercise characteristics of this group. Mean test duration completed by the group was 1087 seconds (sd 149). Although this test duration is lower than the full study group, all these low peak RER individuals continued to exercise beyond the start of phase 3 and 5 individuals entered the final stage of the protocol. The mean VAT of the group was 1516 mL/min (sd 509); this was not significantly different from the group with peak RER > 1.1. From the graphical data, 7 of the 16 individuals in this lower peak RER group attained a plateau in the VO_2 curve including the individual with the lowest peak RER. The exercise characteristics of this subgroup do not raise immediate concern about the validity of these test results. They represent the normal distribution of peak RER identified by Goedecke et al. [23] and highlight the difficulties of defining maximal tests under noninvasive conditions.

As a sub-analysis the study group was divided into three groups dependent on the peak RER: group 1 peak RER less than 1.1 ($n = 16$), group 2 peak RER 1.1 to 1.2 ($n = 42$), and group 3 peak RER > 1.2 ($n = 42$). Statistical analysis of

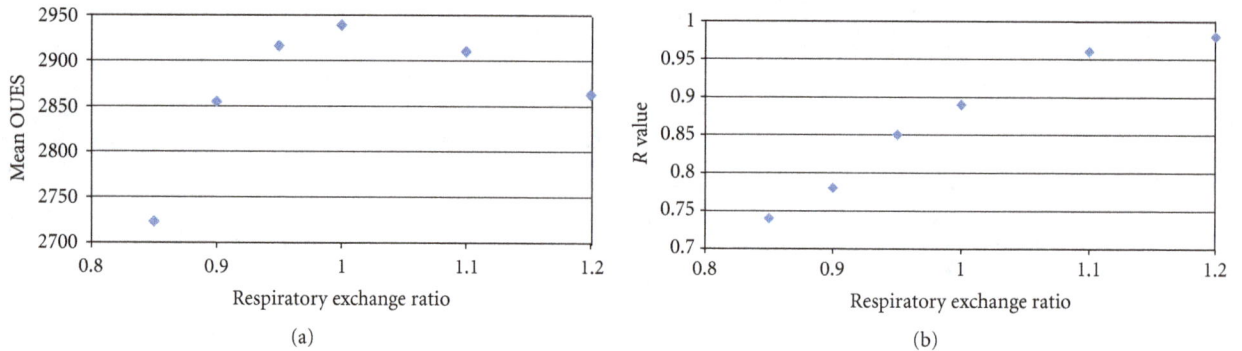

FIGURE 5: Subgroup analysis of 84 individuals with Peak RER > 1.1. (a) Mean OUES from exercise data limited by RER criteria. Group data for 84 individuals with peak RER > 1.1. (b) Correlation between OUES defined by RER criteria. Group data for 84 individuals with peak RER > 1.1.

the group OUES values identified no significant differences between the group means. Group 1 mean OUES 2711 (sd 970), Group 2 mean OUES 2742 (sd 688), and Group 3 mean OUES 2926 (sd 636). Combining groups 2 and 3 to represent a maximal group (peak RER > 1.1), a further sensitivity analysis was performed identifying the same patterns as Figures 2(a) and 2(b) with regards to change in mean OUES with RER. OUES peaks in association with RER 1.0 (mean 2939 sd 682) with an associated r value of 0.89 compared to full test results, reflecting the pattern from the whole group (Figures 5(a) and 5(b)).

These subanalyses show that maximal OUES values do not vary significantly with the normal distribution of peak RER in a fit healthy cohort. There are not the same concerns about reporting OUES using RER criteria as there is a reporting peak VO_2. The normal distribution of RER may raise concern that low peak RER individuals would be excluded if applying threshold exclusion criteria. However, in the present study only one individual had a peak RER less than 0.97. Further research is required to explore the characteristics and determinants of peak OUES at submaximal intensities; the highest value in this study occurred at RER 1.0 not with maximal data. The clinical relevance of using the highest value of OUES has not been explored. One of the rationales for using OUES is that it provides a composite value of cardiopulmonary fitness from across the spectrum of exercise intensity. Therefore, the assumption is that OUES reported from full test data would remain superior as a prognostic marker. These considerations require further formal investigation using invasive physiological measures.

4.2. Limitations. This study explored the validity of reporting submaximal values for OUES in healthy adults. It provides an indication of the variability in submaximal reporting, but it is limited by not being inclusive of a disease population. The relatively high peak VO_2 suggests that the sample is biased towards inclusion of fitter individuals. It could be argued that using RER as reporting criterion with submaximal data would need a prospective validation within a disease population.

The RER levels defining the submaximal criteria were arbitrarily selected. Mean RER in the first 25% of the test

was not below 0.85. To accurately define the cascade of physiological events in association with OUES, invasive monitoring and sampling would be required.

When combined with a rest test, the treadmill test protocol was designed to be representative of the intensity spectrum of physical activity encountered in daily living. The rise in intensity (ramp slope) is slower in comparison to other established protocols. This may affect the validity of the results; however, gas exchange patterns on the Wasserman plots were consistent with protocols of shorter test duration [8].

5. Conclusion

Cardiopulmonary exercise testing is a valuable research and clinical tool. Sub-maximal exercise testing produces a discrete set of limitations on the parameters that can be reliably reported. The ventilatory anaerobic threshold is often the preferred submaximal parameter. However, using VAT introduces potential observational error and can be time consuming to validate. The oxygen uptake efficiency slopes are validated as a prognostic indicator of cardiopulmonary disease that has the advantage of being objectively derived.

Previous studies reported that OUES can be regarded as independent of exercise intensity. This study identifies that there are certain caveats to that statement. OUES values change significantly during the transition from low to moderate intensity. There are definable reliability thresholds above 40% of peak exercise intensity, above 50% of time defined test, and in proximity of the VAT. During a ramp exercise protocol using RER as a reporting criterion, the current results predict higher confidence and reliability in an OUES value reported above an RER threshold of 1.0

Acknowledgments

The authors thank all participants for giving up their time and the field team of the MRC Epidemiology Unit for collecting the data, also special thanks to Stephanie Mayle for all her help and support. This paper was funded by the Medical Research Council.

References

[1] G. J. Balady, R. Arena, K. Sietsema et al., "Clinician's guide to cardiopulmonary exercise testing in adults: a scientific statement from the American heart association," *Circulation*, vol. 122, no. 2, pp. 191–225, 2010.

[2] D. C. Lee, E. G. Artero, X. Sui, and S. N. Blair, "Mortality trends in the general population: the importance of cardiorespiratory fitness," *Journal of Psychopharmacology*, vol. 24, no. 4, pp. 27–35, 2010.

[3] T. Tammelin, S. Näyhä, and H. Rintamäki, "Cardiorespiratory fitness of males and females of Northern Finland birth cohort of 1966 at age 31," *International Journal of Sports Medicine*, vol. 25, no. 7, pp. 547–552, 2004.

[4] M. P. Yeh, R. M. Gardner, and T. D. Adams, "Anaerobic threshold: problems of determination and validation," *Journal of Applied Physiology*, vol. 55, no. 4, pp. 1178–1186, 1983.

[5] J. G. Hopker, S. A. Jobson, and J. J. Pandit, "Controversies in the physiological basis of the 'anaerobic threshold' and their implications for clinical cardiopulmonary exercise testing," *Anaesthesia*, vol. 66, no. 2, pp. 111–123, 2011.

[6] W. L. Beaver, K. Wasserman, and B. J. Whipp, "A new method for detecting anaerobic threshold by gas exchange," *Journal of Applied Physiology*, vol. 60, no. 6, pp. 2020–2027, 1986.

[7] C. B. Cooper and T. W. Storer, *Exercise Testing and Interpretation a Practical Approach*, Cambridge University Press, Cambridge, UK, 2001.

[8] K. Wasserman, J. E. Hansen, D. Y. Sue, W. Stringer, and B. J. Whipp, *Principles of Exercise Testing and Interpretation*, Lippincott Williams & Wilkins, Philadelphia, Pa, USA, 4th edition, 2005.

[9] R. Baba, M. Nagashima, M. Goto et al., "Oxygen intake efficiency slope: a new index of cardiorespiratory functional reserve derived from the relationship between oxygen consumption and minute ventilation during incremental exercise.," *Nagoya Journal of Medical Science*, vol. 59, no. 1-2, pp. 55–62, 1996.

[10] M. Akkerman, M. Van Brussel, E. Hulzebos, L. Vanhees, P. J. M. Helders, and T. TakkenT, "The oxygen uptake efficiency slope: what do we know?" *Journal of Cardiopulmonary Rehabilitation and Prevention*, vol. 30, no. 6, pp. 357–373, 2010.

[11] X. G. Sun, J. E. Hansen, W. W. Stringer et al., "Oxygen uptake efficiency plateau: physiology and reference values," *European Journal of Applied Physiology*, vol. 112, no. 3, pp. 919–928, 2012.

[12] M. Hollenberg and I. B. Tager, "Oxygen uptake efficiency slope: an index of exercise performance and cardiopulmonary reserve requiring only submaximal exercise," *Journal of the American College of Cardiology*, vol. 36, no. 1, pp. 194–201, 2000.

[13] L. C. Davies, R. Wensel, P. Georgiadou et al., "Enhanced prognostic value from cardiopulmonary exercise testing in chronic heart failure by non-linear analysis: oxygen uptake efficiency slope," *European Heart Journal*, vol. 27, no. 6, pp. 684–690, 2006.

[14] R. Arena, J. Myers, L. Hsu et al., "The Minute Ventilation/Carbon Dioxide Production Slope is Prognostically Superior to the Oxygen Uptake Efficiency Slope," *Journal of Cardiac Failure*, vol. 13, no. 6, pp. 462–469, 2007.

[15] C. Van Laethem, J. De Sutter, W. Peersman, and P. Calders, "Intratest reliability and test-retest reproducibility of the oxygen uptake efficiency slope in healthy participants," *European Journal of Cardiovascular Prevention and Rehabilitation*, vol. 16, no. 4, pp. 493–498, 2009.

[16] S. Pogliaghi, E. Dussin, C. Tarperi, A. Cevese, and F. Schena, "Calculation of oxygen uptake efficiency slope based on heart rate reserve end-points in healthy elderly subjects," *European Journal of Applied Physiology*, vol. 101, no. 6, pp. 691–696, 2007.

[17] H. Tanaka, K. D. Monahan, and D. R. Seals, "Age-predicted maximal heart rate revisited," *Journal of the American College of Cardiology*, vol. 37, no. 1, pp. 153–156, 2001.

[18] S. Brage, U. Ekelund, N. Brage et al., "Hierarchy of individual calibration levels for heart rate and accelerometry to measure physical activity," *Journal of Applied Physiology*, vol. 103, no. 2, pp. 682–692, 2007.

[19] X. G. Sun, J. E. Hansen, N. Garatachea, T. W. Storer, and K. Wasserman, "Ventilatory efficiency during exercise in healthy subjects," *American Journal of Respiratory and Critical Care Medicine*, vol. 166, no. 11, pp. 1443–1448, 2002.

[20] M. Gruet, J. Brisswalter, L. Mely, and J. M. Vallier, "Clinical utility of the oxygen uptake efficiency slope in cystic fibrosis patients," *Journal of Cystic Fibrosis*, vol. 9, no. 5, pp. 307–313, 2010.

[21] B. J. Phypers, D. Robiony-Rogers, R. M. Pickering, and A. L. Garden, "Test-retest reliability of the oxygen uptake efficiency slope in surgical patients," *Anaesthesia*, vol. 66, no. 8, pp. 659–666, 2011.

[22] A. Giardini, S. Specchia, G. Gargiulo, D. Sangiorgi, and F. M. Picchio, "Accuracy of oxygen uptake efficiency slope in adults with congenital heart disease," *International Journal of Cardiology*, vol. 133, no. 1, pp. 74–79, 2009.

[23] J. H. Goedecke, A. St Clair Gibson, L. Grobler, M. Collins, T. D. Noakes, and E. V. Lambert, "Determinants of the variability in respiratory exchange ratio at rest and during exercise in trained athletes," *American Journal of Physiology—Endocrinology and Metabolism*, vol. 279, no. 6, pp. E1325–E1334, 2000.

[24] D. C. Poole, D. P. Wilkerson, and A. M. Jones, "Validity of criteria for establishing maximal O_2 uptake during ramp exercise tests," *European Journal of Applied Physiology*, vol. 102, no. 4, pp. 403–410, 2008.

32

Abdominal Adiposity Correlates with Adenotonsillectomy Outcome in Obese Adolescents with Severe Obstructive Sleep Apnea

Gustavo Nino,[1, 2, 3] **Maria J. Gutierrez,**[2, 4] **Anjani Ravindra,**[2] **Cesar L. Nino,**[5]
and Carlos E. Rodriguez-Martinez[6, 7, 8]

[1] *Penn State Sleep Research and Treatment Center, Pennsylvania State University College of Medicine, Hershey, PA, USA*
[2] *Department of Pediatrics, Pennsylvania State University College of Medicine, Hershey, PA, USA*
[3] *Division of Pediatric Pulmonary and Sleep Medicine, Penn State Hershey Children's Hospital,*
  Pennsylvania State University College of Medicine, 500 University Drive, Hershey, PA 17033-0850, USA
[4] *Division of Allergy and Immunology, Pennsylvania State University College of Medicine, Hershey, PA, USA*
[5] *Department of Electronics Engineering, Javeriana University, Bogota, Colombia*
[6] *Department of Pediatrics, School of Medicine, Universidad Nacional de Colombia, Bogota, Colombia*
[7] *Department of Pediatric Pulmonology and Pediatric Critical Care Medicine, School of Medicine,*
  Universidad El Bosque, Bogota, Colombia
[8] *Research Unit, Military Hospital of Colombia, Bogota, Colombia*

Correspondence should be addressed to Gustavo Nino, nino.gustavo@gmail.com

Academic Editor: Graham Roberts

Background. Obese adolescents with Obstructive Sleep Apnea (OSA) have a unique pathophysiology that combines adenotonsillar hypertrophy and increased visceral fat distribution. We hypothesized that in this population waist circumference (WC), as a clinical marker of abdominal fat distribution, correlates with the likelihood of response to AT. *Methods*. We conducted a retrospective cohort study of obese adolescents (BMI $\geq$ 97th percentile) that underwent AT for therapy of severe OSA ($n = 21$). We contrasted WC and covariates in a group of subjects that had complete resolution of severe OSA after AT ($n = 7$) with those obtained in subjects with residual OSA after AT ($n = 14$). Multivariate linear and logistic models were built to control possible confounders. *Results*. WC correlated negatively with a positive AT response in young adolescents and the percentage of improvement in obstructive apnea-hypopnea index (OAHI) after AT ($P \leq 0.01$). Extended multivariate analysis demonstrated that the link between WC and AT response was independent of demographic variables, OSA severity, clinical upper airway assessment, obesity severity (BMI), and neck circumference (NC). *Conclusion*. The results suggest that in obese adolescents, abdominal fat distribution determined by WC may be a useful clinical predictor for residual OSA after AT.

1. Introduction

Obstructive Sleep Apnea (OSA) is characterized by recurrent episodes of partial or complete upper airway obstruction, resulting in oxygen desaturation and sleep disruption [1]. A number of risk factors likely influence airway patency during sleep, and thus the susceptibility for OSA. Adenotonsillar enlargement is the most commonly recognized anatomic cause for pediatric OSA [1], and obesity is the major risk factor during adulthood [2, 3]. As a result, adenotonsillectomy

(AT) is considered the first line of therapy in most cases of pediatric OSA [4] but it is seldom effective in the adult population [5, 6], particularly in those who are obese [6, 7]. Obesity also increases the risk of residual OSA after AT in the pediatric population [8], however, the obesity features associated with decreased response to AT in children and adolescents are largely unknown.

The anatomic and functional risk factors relating obesity to OSA are complex. Obesity leads to upper airway narrowing due to enlargement of soft palate, lateral pharyngeal walls, tongue, and parapharyngeal fat pads [9–13]. Along with these upper airway changes, obesity causes restrictive respiratory physiology primarily attributed to abdominal visceral fat accumulation [14]. The combination of narrow upper airway and lung restriction promotes a smaller and more collapse-prone upper airway that significantly increases OSA risk in all ages [15]. Indeed, in extremely obese adolescents (BMI ≥ 40 kg/m^2), the reported prevalence of OSA is 55% [16]; in extremely obese adults the prevalence increases to 98% [17]. Interestingly, in the pediatric population visceral fat distribution is predictive of OSA severity independently of body mass index (BMI), which may explain why some obese children develop OSA and some do not [18].

In this context, there is emerging evidence suggesting that obese adolescents have a unique OSA pathophysiology. For instance, a recent study in young obese adolescents (mean age 12.5 ± 2.8 yr.) identified generalized overgrowth of adenoids and tonsils leading to upper airway restriction in subjects with OSA [19]. In the same study, there were no differences in soft palate, tongue, and mandible sizes in obese individuals with OSA compared to those without OSA. In contrast, obese adolescents with OSA had increased size of parapharyngeal fat pads and abdominal visceral fat, although the size of these tissues did not correlate with severity of OSA [19]. Collectively, these data suggested an important pathogenic role for adenotonsillar enlargement and body fat distribution in young obese adolescents with OSA. Our current work focused on how the clinical assessment of these factors may predict AT response in this population.

The primary goal of this study was to identify the clinical features that may predict response to AT in obese adolescents. Specifically, we hypothesized that in this population waist circumference (WC), as a clinical marker of abdominal fat distribution, correlates with the likelihood of response to AT independently of BMI. Secondary analysis evaluated the role of the clinical assessment of neck size, tonsillar size, and oropharyngeal narrowing (Mallampati score) predicting AT response in obese adolescents. Our hypotheses were tested using multivariate analysis contrasting WC and covariates in a group of subjects that had complete resolution of severe OSA after AT with those obtained in obese adolescents with severe OSA that did not resolve after AT. The resolution of OSA was clearly documented with clinical and polysomnographic objective evaluations before and after AT. The impact of the presented data is that it provides new information that may aid in the clinical assessment of obese adolescents with severe OSA, particularly in regard to likelihood of cure after AT.

2. Methods

2.1. Subjects. We conducted a retrospective cohort study. Our study population included young adolescents (10–16 years old) selected from our database of all children that underwent routine overnight polysomnography (PSG) at the Penn State Sleep Research and Treatment Center between September 2009 and October 2011. Patients of both genders and all ethnicities were eligible for the study if: (1) they were obese (BMI ≥ 97th percentile for age and sex according

to 2000 CDC growth charts for the United States), (2) had diagnosis of severe OSA defined as apnea–hypopnea index (OAHI) ≥ 10 events per hour on their initial PSG, (3) underwent AT for therapy of OSA, (4) had undergone a PSG within 6 months after AT, and (5) had documented clinical assessment of upper airway and fat distribution (neck, waist, and hip size) prior to AT. Patients were excluded if they had respiratory failure, central hypoventilation syndromes, congenital heart disease, severe developmental delay, cerebral palsy, craniofacial abnormalities, and neuromuscular disorders. Subjects were subdivided in those with "OSA resolution after AT" ($n = 7$) and those that did not have complete resolution of OSA after AT ($n = 14$). "OSA resolution after AT" was defined as the presence of all the following: (1) ≥90% reduction in obstructive apnea-hypopnea index (OAHI) after AT, (2) post-AT OAHI ≤5 events/hour, and (3) subjective improvement of OSA symptoms (i.e., snoring and excessive daytime sleepiness) in post-AT clinical visit. This study was approved by the Institutional Review Board of Penn State College of Medicine.

2.2. Sleep and Respiratory Recordings

2.2.1. PSG Protocol. Standard pediatric overnight PSG was performed on all patients. For 9-10 hours, the patient's sleep was continuously recorded to a computerized system (Twin PSG software; Grass Technologies. Inc., West Warwick, RI, USA) and scored manually in 30-second epochs according to standardized criteria [20]. Polysomnography measurements included electroencephalograms (EEG) (C4-A1, O2-A1), right and left electrooculograms (EOG), electrocardiogram (ECG), mental-submental electromyogram (EMG), leg EMG, thoracic and abdominal wall motion (respiratory inductance plethysmography), pulse oximetry (with 2-s averaging time), end-tidal carbon dioxide monitoring (RespSense Capnograph, Grass Technologies. Inc., West Warwick, RI, USA), combined nasal/oral thermistor and nasal pressure (model TCT R, Grass-Telefactor, Inc.). Objective estimate of snoring during the PSG was obtained with a microphone attached to the neck (model 1250G Grass Technologies Inc., West Warwick, RI, USA). Body position and movements were determined by a sensor and confirmed by direct observation throughout the night along with routine infrared video monitoring.

2.2.2. PSG Scoring and Analysis. Sleep stages, arousal index, sleep efficiency, and respiratory events were scored according to standardized criteria [20]. Five sleep stages were identified (wake stage = W, stage 1 = N1, stage 2 = N2, stage 3 = N3, and stage REM = R). The OAHI included obstructive apneas, hypopneas, and mixed apneas. The minimum respiratory event duration was ≥2 respiratory cycles. Obstructive apneas were scored if there was an absence of airflow with continued respiratory effort. Obstructive hypopneas were scored if there was a discernible decrease in airflow of approximately 50% associated with either a ≥3% SaO2 desaturation and/or an arousal. Mixed apneas were scored if there was a discernible decrease in airflow with a period of no respiratory effort and a period of continued respiratory effort associated with either a $\geq 3\%$ SaO2 desaturation and/or an arousal.

2.3. Clinical Fat Distribution and Upper Airway Variables

2.3.1. Obesity Anthropometric Measurements. Anthropometric data were obtained from electronic medical records (EMR) as they are performed routinely during PSG visit in our Sleep Research and Treatment Center (SRTC). Standing height and weight were obtained while patients were wearing lightweight clothing without shoes. Body mass index (BMI) was calculated using the formula weight (kg) divided by the square of height (m^2). A nonelastic flexible tape measure was used to measure neck, waist, and hip circumference. Waist circumference (WC) was measured at the level of the umbilicus with the participants standing at the end of normal expiration. The hip circumference (HC) was measured at the greater trochanter. Neck circumference (NC) was measured horizontally at the level of the thyroid cartilage with head erect and eyes facing forward. Waist-to-hip ratio was calculated as WC divided by HC.

2.3.2. Oropharynx and Tonsillar Size Clinical Assessment. Upper airway variables were obtained from EMR data recorded during the clinical visit prior to PSG in Penn State Children's Hospital and Penn State SRTC. In our institution oropharynx and tonsillar size are routinely assessed using a standardized grading system. Oropharynx is evaluated using Mallampati's classification [1–4] with the tongue kept in place without the use of a tongue depressor, as previously described [21]. In grade 1, the tonsils, pillars, pharynx, and soft palate are clearly visible. In grade 2, the uvula and only the upper part of the pillars and tonsils are visible between the palate and the tongue. In grade 3, only the soft and hard palate are visible, while the tonsils, pillars, pharynx, and base of the uvula were hidden behind the tongue. In grade 4, only the hard palate is visible. Tonsillar size is also routinely evaluated using a grading system [1–4] as previously described [22]. In grade 1, the tonsils are hidden in the tonsillar fossa behind the anterior pillars. In grade 2, the tonsils are visible beyond the anterior pillars and occupy $\leq 50\%$ of the pharyngeal space (the distance between the medial borders of the anterior pillars). In grade 3, the tonsils occupy between 50 and 75% of the pharyngeal space. In grade 4, the tonsils occupied $\geq 75\%$ of the pharyngeal space (kissing tonsils).

2.4. Statistical Analysis.
Data were analyzed using the software SAS version 9.2 or later (SAS Institute Inc., Cary, NC, USA). Means and proportions of main demographic and PSG variables (i.e., OAHI pre- and post-AT) were calculated for the entire study population, as well as stratified according to AT response status. The effect of the upper airway variables (Mallampati score and tonsillar size) and obesity parameters (BMI, WC, HC, NC and W/H ratio) were first described by summary statistics (mean/standard deviation) for individuals that responded to AT and those that did not respond to AT. For pair-wise relationships, two-sample t-test was used to compare the mean value of the continuous

outcome measures; and chi-square test or Fisher's exact test were used to compare the proportion of positive signals for binary outcomes. Multivariate general linear models were built to study the joint effect of obesity parameters (predictors) in the percentage of OAHI improvement (linear regression models) or probability of resolution of OSA (logistic regression models) subsequent to AT surgery, with control of some possible confounders such as gender, age, BMI, and upper airway variables. Significance was taken at the $P < 0.05$ level.

3. Results

3.1. Study Population. Our study population ($n = 21$) was subdivided into one group that responded to AT ($n = 7$) and another group without OSA resolution after AT ($n = 14$). Response to AT was defined as obstructive apnea-hypopnea index (OAHI) reduction after AT of $\geq 90\%$, post-AT OAHI of ≤ 5 events/hour, and subjective improvement of OSA symptoms post-AT. Accordingly, one group included subjects with a dramatic OAHI mean reduction of 94% (pre-AT OAHI = 34.4/hour and post-AT OAHI = 1.32/hour) and the other group included subjects with a moderate OAHI mean improvement of 35% (pre-AT OAHI = 31.1/hour and post-AT OAHI = 19.7/hour). Comparison of demographic variables in these two groups revealed no significant differences (Table 1(a)). Baseline polysomnographic parameters such as obstructive apnea-hypopnea index (OAHI), arousal index, and oxygen desaturation nadir were comparable in both groups (Table 1(b)).

3.2. Abdominal Adiposity Correlates Negatively with AT Response in Young Adolescents. To investigate the role of clinical fat distribution in predicting AT response in young adolescents, we first compared neck, waist and hip circumferences in the group of obese adolescents with OSA resolution after AT with that seen in individuals without complete resolution of OSA after AT. As illustrated in Table 2(b), waist, and hip circumferences were significantly larger in the obese group that did not respond to AT ($P \leq 0.01$) but neck size and waist-to-hip ratio were not significantly different. Univariate regression analysis revealed that waist circumference (WC) correlated negatively with the percentage of improvement in OAHI after AT (Adj $R^2 = 39.7\%$, $\beta = -1.64 \pm$ SE 0.4, $P \leq 0.01$) (Figure 1(a)) but neck circumference (NC) did not correlate significantly with AT response (Figure 1(b)). Extended analysis included multivariate predictive models built to assess the confounder effect of body mass index (BMI), gender, age, race, and neck size in the relationship between WC and the percentage of OAHI improvement (linear model) and the probability of OSA resolution (logistic model) following AT (Table 3). After adjusting for these covariables we found that the effect of WC in OSA resolution after AT is independent of BMI, gender, age, race, and neck size in young obese adolescents with severe OSA. The relationship between WC and AT response was not independent from waist-to-hip ratio as hip circumference (HC) also correlated negatively

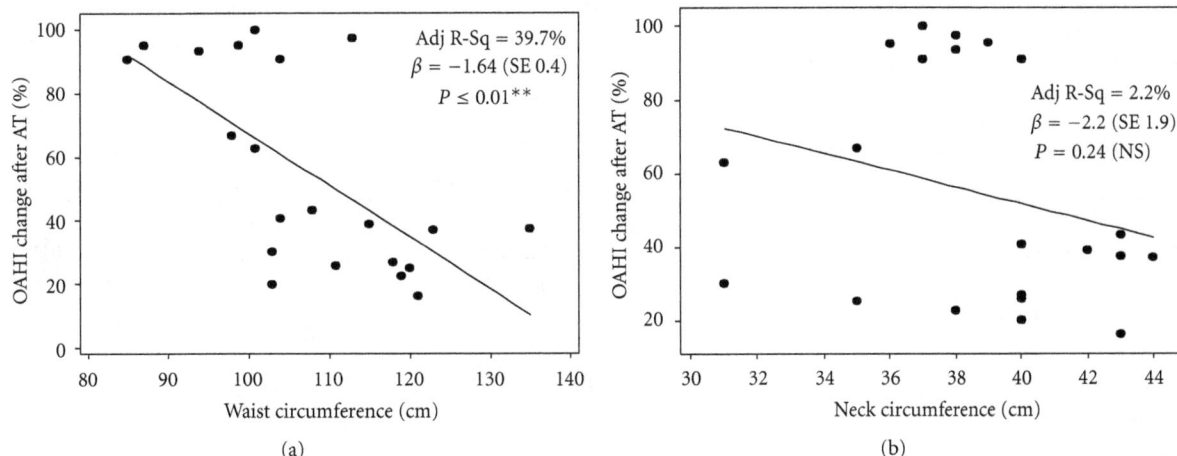

FIGURE 1: Univariate linear regression model (Fat distribution). Graphs demonstrate the correlation between either waist circumference (a) or neck circumference (b) and the percentage of apnea-hypopnea index (OAHI) change after adenotonsillectomy (AT) in obese adolescents. Adj R-Sq: adjusted coefficient of determination. β: parameter estimate. ± standard error (SE).

TABLE 1: Demographic and polysomnographic profile of subjects. For quantitative variables, data are presented as mean ± standard error (SE). AT: adenotonsillectomy; OAHI: obstructive apnea-hypopnea index. For categorical variables, data are presented as count number (column percentage). P values are obtained by either two-sample t-test or chi-square test, depending on the type of variables.

Factors/variables	Response to AT ($n = 7$)	No response to AT ($n = 14$)	P value
(A) Demographic variables			
Gender			
Female	2 (28.6%)	3 (21.5%)	0.725
Male	5 (71.4%)	11 (78.5%)	0.725
Age (years): mean (SE)	12.1 (0.4)	12.7 (0.6)	0.478
Ethnicity			
White	4 (57.1%)	8 (57.1%)	1.0
Others	3 (42.9%)	6 (42.9%)	1.0
(B) Sleep study parameters			
OSA severity			
Pre-AT OAHI: mean (SE)	34.4 (11.6)	31.1 (2)	0.789
Post-AT OAHI: mean (SE)	**1.32 (0.3)**	**19.7 (1.8)**	**< 0.01****
% OAHI improvement after AT	**94.6 (1.3)**	**35.2 (4.0)**	**< 0.01****
Sleep efficiency (%): mean (SE)	80.3 (4.6)	83.3 (2.5)	0.580
Arousal index (events per hr): mean(SE)	15.7 (3.5)	13.6 (2.4)	0.627
SaO2 nadir (%): mean (SE)	84 (3.0)	83.9 (1.4)	0.983

(**$P \leq 0.01$).

TABLE 2: Upper airway and obesity variables. For quantitative variables, data are presented as mean ± standard error (SE). BMI: body mass index. P values are obtained by two-sample t-test.

Factors/variables	Response to AT ($n = 7$)	No response to AT ($n = 14$)	P value
(A) Upper airway variables			
Tonsilar size 1–4: mean (SE)	2.43 (0.2)	2.36 (0.1)	0.773
Mallampati score 1–4: mean (SE)	2.71 (0.1)	2.86 (0.2)	0.551
(B) Obesity parameters			
BMI (kg/m^2): mean(SE)	33.5 (2.1)	37.6 (1.5)	0.131
Neck size (cm): mean (SE)	37.8 (0.51)	38.2 (1.2)	0.411
Waist size (cm): mean (SE)	**97.6 (3.7)**	**112.8 (2.8)**	**<0.01****
Hip size (cm): mean (SE)	**100.1 (2.7)**	**116.2 (3.3)**	**<0.01****
Waist-hip ratio: mean (SE)	0.97 (0.03)	0.97 (0.01)	0.972

(**$P \leq 0.01$).

TABLE 3: Multivariate regression analysis. Either regular linear regression or binary logistic regression was performed, depending on the type of outcome variable in the statistical model. For logistic regression, the odds ratios (OR) and their P values are reported; while for regular linear regression, the parameter estimates and their P values are reported.

Waist size predictive model variables adjusted	Response to AT (Y/N) OR, P value (by multivariate logistic regression)	% of AHI change after AT Parameter estimate, P value (by multiple linear regression)
(A) Demographic		
Waist circumference	**1.23, $P \leq 0.05$***	**−1.92, $P \leq 0.01$****
Age	0.78, $P = 0.54$	2.18, $P = 0.49$
Gender		
Female#		
Male	1.34, $P = 0.42$	−3.3, $P = 0.82$
Ethnicity		
White#		
Other	1.33, $P = 0.33$	−17, $P = 0.23$
(B) Obesity parameters		
Waist circumference	**1.25, $P \leq 0.05$***	**−1.35, $P \leq 0.05$***
BMI	0.94, $P = 0.68$	−1.32, $P = 0.34$
Neck size	0.89, $P = 0.60$	0.63, $P = 0.86$
(C) Upper airway variables		
Waist circumference	**1.18, $P \leq 0.05$***	**−1.65, $P \leq 0.01$****
Mallampati score	1.43, $P = 0.8$	−16.8, $P = 0.12$
Tonsilar size	0.55, $P = 0.64$	4.1, $P = 0.7$
(D) OSA variables		
Waist circumference	**1.33, $P \leq 0.05$***	**−1.96, $P \leq 0.01$****
Obstructive AHI	0.96, $P = 0.29$	0.30, $P = 0.34$
SaO2 nocturnal nadir	1.04, $P = 0.78$	9.2, $P = 0.18$
Snoring severity	0.29, $P = 0.34$	−0.53, $P = 0.61$

Note: #reference level.
(**$P \leq 0.01$,*$P \leq 0.05$).

with OSA resolution after AT (data not shown). Collectively, these results suggest that clinical abdominal adiposity correlates negatively with AT response in young adolescents independently of demographic variables, obesity severity (BMI), and clinical neck fat distribution, as evaluated by NC.

3.3. The Link between Abdominal Adiposity and AT Response Is Independent of Clinical Upper Airway Assessment. We next considered the role of clinical tonsillar size [1–4] and Mallampati scores [1–4] in predicting AT response in obese adolescents with severe OSA. Table 2(a) illustrates that there were no significant differences in the clinical grading of tonsillar hypertrophy and oropharyngeal narrowing (Mallampati score) in the group with OSA resolution after AT relative to that seen in individuals without complete resolution of OSA after AT (Table 2(a)). Univariate analysis demonstrated that neither clinical tonsillar size nor Mallampati grading correlated with OSA outcome following AT (data not shown). Moreover, multivariate predictive models demonstrated that these upper airway variables did not modify the relationship between abdominal adiposity (WC) and AT response in obese adolescents with severe OSA (Table 3).

3.4. OSA Severity (OAHI) Does Not Correlate with AT Outcome in Young Adolescents. To evaluate if OSA severity is a predictor of AT response in young adolescents, we compared OAHI in the group of obese adolescents with OSA resolution after AT with that seen in individuals without complete resolution of OSA after AT. Table 1(b) indicates that the PSG parameters indicative of OSA severity (i.e., OAHI) were comparable in both groups. Univariate regression analysis revealed that OAHI does not correlate with the percentage of improvement in OAHI after AT (Figure 2). Moreover, multivariate analysis demonstrated that OAHI and other PSG variables (i.e., oxygen desaturation nadir) did not modify the relationship between abdominal adiposity (WC) and AT outcome in obese adolescents with severe OSA (Table 3).

4. Discussion

Prior investigations have focused on determining the effectiveness of adenotonsillectomy (AT) in the entire population of obese children and adolescents with Obstructive Sleep Apnea (OSA). These studies have demonstrated that AT improves OSA to some extent, but it does not resolve OSA in the majority of obese, pediatric patients [23]. Our study

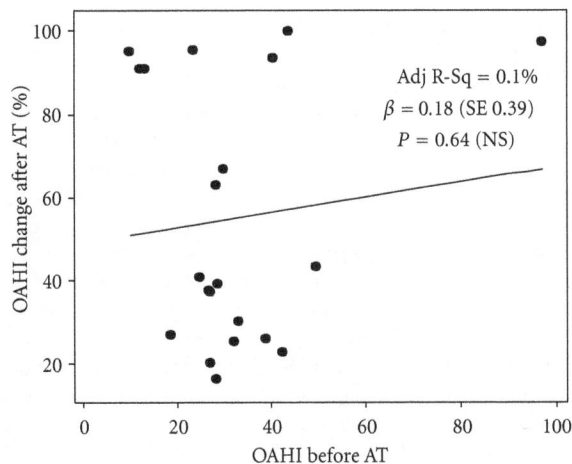

FIGURE 2: Univariate linear regression model (OSA severity). Graph demonstrates the correlation between obstructive apnea-hypopnea index (OAHI) before AT and the percentage of OAHI change after adenotonsillectomy (AT) in obese adolescents. Adj R-Sq: adjusted coefficient of determination. β: parameter estimate. $\pm$ standard error (SE).

was designed to extend the knowledge of this relationship by focusing on the group of obese adolescents with OSA for whom AT seems to be a viable cure. Specifically, we aimed to identify the clinical features that may predict which obese adolescents with severe OSA may have a beneficial response to AT. For this purpose, we compared a subpopulation of obese adolescents who had complete resolution of severe OSA after AT with another group of obese adolescents who had residual OSA after undergoing AT. The main finding of this study was that the circumference of the subject's waist (WC) had a negative correlation with a positive response to AT in obese adolescents. Extended, multivariate analysis also identified that the effect of WC was independent of the severity of OSA, the severity of obesity (as measured by body mass index (BMI), clinical tonsillar size, oropharyngeal narrowing (Mallampati score), and the circumference of the neck (NC). Accordingly, these results suggested that markers of abdominal adiposity, that is, WC, may be useful clinical predictors for residual OSA after AT in this population. In addition, the lack of correlation of other clinical parameters with AT outcome highlights the need for novel, diagnostic tools to better identify obese adolescents who have the potential for being cured by AT.

During this investigation, we evaluated three parameters in obese adolescents with severe OSA, that is, (1) *Clinical upper airway assessment:* consistent on pre-AT Mallampati score for oropharyngeal patency (grades 1–4) and standardized palatine tonsillar size (grades 1–4); (2) *Obesity parameters:* including BMI, neck circumference (NC), waist circumference (WC), hip circumference (HC), and waist-to-hip ratio; and (3) *OSA parameters in polysomnography (PSG):* including obstructive apnea-hypopnea index (OAHI), the severity of snoring, oxygen nadir desaturation, and the degree of sleep fragmentation, expressed as arousal index (AI). We compared these parameters in obese adolescents

who's AT treatment was successful with the same parameters in obese adolescents who had residual OSA after AT. As illustrated in Tables 1 and 2, no significant differences were observed in the clinical assessment of the airway, the severity of obesity (BMI), or PSG parameters between the two groups. Conversely, we found that abdominal adiposity, determined by WC, had a significant correlation with the patients' reduced response to AT. These findings are in general agreement with the prevailing notion that clinical adenotonsillar size does not correlate with the severity of OSA in obese children [24] and that BMI values alone do not seem to predict the severity of OSA in the pediatric population [25, 26]. In contrast, studies using magnetic resonance imaging (MRI) spectroscopy to quantify fat distribution in obese children with OSA [18] have identified a strong relationship between visceral adiposity and OSA, which is independent of BMI [18]. Interestingly, BMI does correlate with the severity of OSA in adults [27], which suggests that the pathogenic effects of obesity on OSA are different in children than in adults.

In this context, it is noteworthy that NC, a parameter of neck fat distribution associated with the severity of OSA in adults [27, 28], was not correlated with AT outcome in our population of obese adolescents. The latter results may reflect maturational changes that modulate the upper airway tone and patency in children, adolescents, and adults [1, 29]. In this regard, prior investigations of the upper airway of young adolescents identified that the slope of the pressure-flow curve (SPF), which relates to the collapsibility of the upper airway [29], is significantly more flat in adolescents than it is in adults [29]. In other words, it is expected that the upper airway of young adolescents can tolerate the load of neck adiposity better than that of adults because the adolescents' upper airway is less likely to collapse. Conversely, our data supported the concept that abdominal adiposity is a critical obesity factor for OSA in adolescents and adults [30–32], and, thus, it may be a useful clinical parameter to predict residual OSA following AT, independently of age.

Another important finding of this study was that obese adolescents had a heterogeneous response to AT. We identified that some obese teenagers with OSA can be cured completely by AT, regardless of their BMI, NC, oropharyngeal patency, or severity of OSA. For instance, an obese individual (BMI = 35 kg/m^2) with very severe OSA (OAHI = 97/hour) had complete resolution of OSA after AT (97% decrease in OAHI) (outlier in Figure 2). This heterogeneity in the response of obese adolescents to AT suggests a unique OSA pathophysiology in this age group. Indeed, Arens et al. recently identified overgrowth of the upper airway lymphoid tissues in obese pediatric subjects with OSA [19]. In contrast to obese adults, this study revealed that the soft palate and tongue are not different in obese children with OSA relative to pediatric obese individuals without OSA [19]. The latter evidence, together with our current data describing the role of abdominal adiposity in obese adolescents with OSA, suggests that OSA in this population is a multifactorial condition that involves pediatric elements (overgrowth of upper airway lymphoid tissues) and adult OSA features (enhanced visceral adiposity distribution), resulting in a very heterogeneous phenotype that requires individualized assessment.

In summary, in this study, we investigated the clinical features that may predict response to AT in young obese adolescents with severe OSA. Although the sample size was small, our strength is that we limited this investigation to individuals with PSG-documented resolution of OSA. Our results demonstrated that: (1) abdominal adiposity, as measured by WC, is correlated negatively with AT response in young adolescents and (2) the effect of abdominal adiposity is independent of the severity of OSA, the severity of obesity (BMI), clinically-determined tonsillar size, oropharyngeal narrowing (Mallampati score), and the distribution of neck fat (NC). The latter information suggests that abdominal fat distribution plays a pivotal role in the pathogenesis of OSA in obese adolescents, and, thus, it may be a useful clinical parameter for predicting residual OSA after AT. Our data also illustrated the unique phenotypical variability of OSA in obese adolescents and highlighted the need for novel, diagnostic approaches for this population. Emergent techniques, such as three-dimensional MRI spectroscopy, can delineate upper airway structures and body-fat composition [9–13, 18, 19], and, thus, they could be used to investigate the specific phenotypical features of OSA in obese adolescents, including their responsiveness to AT.

References

[1] R. Arens and C. L. Marcus, "Pathophysiology of upper airway obstruction: a developmental perspective," *Sleep*, vol. 27, no. 5, pp. 997–1019, 2004.

[2] L. J. Palmer, S. G. Buxbaum, E. Larkin et al., "A whole-genome scan for obstructive sleep apnea and obesity," *American Journal of Human Genetics*, vol. 72, no. 2, pp. 340–350, 2003.

[3] A. R. Schwartz, S. P. Patil, S. Squier, H. Schneider, J. P. Kirkness, and P. L. Smith, "Obesity and upper airway control during sleep," *Journal of Applied Physiology*, vol. 108, no. 2, pp. 430–435, 2010.

[4] American Academy of Pediatrics, "Clinical practice guideline: diagnosis and management of childhood obstructive sleep apnea syndrome," *Pediatrics*, vol. 109, no. 4, pp. 704–712, 2002.

[5] S. M. Caples, J. A. Rowley, J. R. Prinsell et al., "Surgical modifications of the upper airway for obstructive sleep apnea in adults: a systematic review and meta-analysis," *Sleep*, vol. 33, no. 10, pp. 1396–1407, 2010.

[6] A. Dündar, M. Gerek, A. Özünlü, and S. Yetişer, "Patient selection and surgical results in obstructive sleep apnea," *European Archives of Oto-Rhino-Laryngology*, vol. 254, supplement 1, pp. S157–S161, 1997.

[7] L. H. Larsson, B. Carlsson-Nordlander, and E. Svanborg, "Four-year follow-up after uvulopalatopharyngoplasty in 50 unselected patients with obstructive sleep apnea syndrome," *Laryngoscope*, vol. 104, no. 11, part 1, pp. 1362–1368, 1994.

[8] R. Bhattacharjee, L. Kheirandish-Gozal, K. Spruyt et al., "Adenotonsillectomy outcomes in treatment of obstructive sleep apnea in children: a multicenter retrospective study," *American Journal of Respiratory and Critical Care Medicine*, vol. 182, no. 5, pp. 676–683, 2010.

[9] L. Chi, F. L. Comyn, N. Mitra et al., "Identification of craniofacial risk factors for obstructive sleep apnoea using three-dimensional MRI," *European Respiratory Journal*, vol. 38, no. 2, pp. 348–358, 2011.

[10] R. L. Horner, R. H. Mohiaddin, D. G. Lowell et al., "Sites and sizes of fat deposits around the pharynx in obese patients with obstructive sleep apnoea and weight matched controls," *European Respiratory Journal*, vol. 2, no. 7, pp. 613–622, 1989.

[11] R. J. Schwab, K. B. Gupta, W. B. Gefter, L. J. Metzger, E. A. Hoffman, and A. I. Pack, "Upper airway and soft tissue anatomy in normal subjects and patients with sleep-disordered breathing: significance of the lateral pharyngeal walls," *American Journal of Respiratory and Critical Care Medicine*, vol. 152, no. 5 I, pp. 1673–1689, 1995.

[12] R. J. Schwab, M. Pasirstein, R. Pierson et al., "Identification of upper airway anatomic risk factors for obstructive sleep apnea with volumetric magnetic resonance imaging," *American Journal of Respiratory and Critical Care Medicine*, vol. 168, no. 5, pp. 522–530, 2003.

[13] K. E. Shelton, H. Woodson, S. Gay, and P. M. Suratt, "Pharyngeal fat in obstructive sleep apnea," *American Review of Respiratory Disease*, vol. 148, no. 2, pp. 462–466, 1993.

[14] J. C. H. Yap, R. A. Watson, S. Gilbey, and N. B. Pride, "Effects of posture on respiratory mechanics in obesity," *Journal of Applied Physiology*, vol. 79, no. 4, pp. 1199–1205, 1995.

[15] V. Hoffstein, N. Zamel, and E. A. Phillipson, "Lung volume dependence of pharyngeal cross-sectional area in patients with obstructive sleep apnea," *American Review of Respiratory Disease*, vol. 130, no. 2, pp. 175–178, 1984.

[16] M. Kalra, T. Inge, V. Garcia et al., "Obstructive sleep apnea in extremely overweight adolescents undergoing bariatric surgery," *Obesity Research*, vol. 13, no. 7, pp. 1175–1179, 2005.

[17] M. Valencia-Flores, A. Orea, V. A. Castaño et al., "Prevalence of sleep apnea and electrocardiographic disturbances in morbidly obese patients," *Obesity Research*, vol. 8, no. 3, pp. 262–269, 2000.

[18] C. A. Canapari, A. G. Hoppin, T. B. Kinane, B. J. Thomas, M. Torriani, and E. S. Katz, "Relationship between sleep apnea, fat distribution, and insulin resistance in obese children," *Journal of Clinical Sleep Medicine*, vol. 7, no. 3, pp. 268–273, 2011.

[19] R. Arens, S. Sin, K. Nandalike et al., "Upper airway structure and body fat composition in obese children with obstructive sleep apnea syndrome," *American Journal of Respiratory and Critical Care Medicine*, vol. 183, no. 6, pp. 782–787, 2011.

[20] C. Iber, S. Ancoli-Israel, A. L. Chesson Jr., and S. F. Quan, The AASM Manual for the Scoring of Sleep and Associated Events: Rules, Terminology and Technical Specifications, Westchester, Ill, USA, American Academy of Sleep Medicine, 2007.

[21] G. Liistro, P. Rombaux, C. Belge, M. Dury, G. Aubert, and D. O. Rodenstein, "High Mallampati score and nasal obstruction are associated risk factors for obstructive sleep apnoea," *European Respiratory Journal*, vol. 21, no. 2, pp. 248–252, 2003.

[22] Z. Xu, D. K. L. Cheuk, and S. L. Lee, "Clinical evaluation in predicting childhood obstructive sleep apnea," *Chest*, vol. 130, no. 6, pp. 1765–1771, 2006.

[23] D. J. Costa and R. Mitchell, "Adenotonsillectomy for obstructive sleep apnea in obese children: a meta-analysis," *Otolaryngology—Head and Neck Surgery*, vol. 140, no. 4, pp. 455–460, 2009.

[24] E. Dayyat, L. Kheirandish-Gozal, O. Sans Capdevila, M. M. A. Maarafeya, and D. Gozal, "Obstructive sleep apnea in children: relative contributions of body mass index and adenotonsillar hypertrophy," *Chest*, vol. 136, no. 1, pp. 137–144, 2009.

[25] A. G. Kaditis, E. I. Alexopoulos, F. Hatzi et al., "Adiposity in relation to age as predictor of severity of sleep apnea in

children with snoring," *Sleep and Breathing*, vol. 12, no. 1, pp. 25–31, 2008.

[26] M. T. Apostolidou, E. I. Alexopoulos, K. Chaidas et al., "Obesity and persisting sleep apnea after adenotonsillectomy in Greek children," *Chest*, vol. 134, no. 6, pp. 1149–1155, 2008.

[27] J. B. Dixon, L. M. Schachter, and P. E. O'Brien, "Predicting sleep apnea and excessive day sleepiness in the severely obese: indicators for polysomnography," *Chest*, vol. 123, no. 4, pp. 1134–1141, 2003.

[28] K. A. Ferguson, T. Ono, A. A. Lowe, C. F. Ryan, and J. A. Fleetham, "The relationship between obesity and craniofacial structure in obstructive sleep apnea," *Chest*, vol. 108, no. 2, pp. 375–381, 1995.

[29] P. Bandla, J. Huang, L. Karamessinis et al., "Puberty and upper airway dynamics during sleep," *Sleep*, vol. 31, no. 4, pp. 534–541, 2008.

[30] P. D. Levinson, S. T. McGarvey, C. C. Carlisle, S. E. Eveloff, P. N. Herbert, and R. P. Millman, "Adiposity and cardiovascular risk factors in men with obstructive sleep apnea," *Chest*, vol. 103, no. 5, pp. 1336–1342, 1993.

[31] E. Shinohara, S. Kihara, S. Yamashita et al., "Visceral fat accumulation as an important risk factor for obstructive sleep apnoea syndrome in obese subjects," *Journal of Internal Medicine*, vol. 241, no. 1, pp. 11–18, 1997.

[32] O. Oğretmenoğlu, A. E. Süslü, O. T. Yücel, T. M. Onerci, and A. Sahin, "Body fat composition: a predictive factor for obstructive sleep apnea," *Laryngoscope*, vol. 115, no. 8, pp. 1493–1498, 2005.

33

Utilization of CT Pulmonary Angiography in Suspected Pulmonary Embolism in a Major Urban Emergency Department

Adil Shujaat,[1,2] Janet M. Shapiro,[3] and Edward Eden[3]

[1] Division of Pulmonary and Critical Care Medicine, College of Medicine at Jacksonville, University of Florida, Jacksonville, FL, USA
[2] University of Florida, Shands Clinical Center, 655 West 8th Street, Suite 7-088, Jacksonville, FL 32209, USA
[3] Division of Pulmonary and Critical Care Medicine, St. Luke's and Roosevelt Hospitals of Columbia University, New York, NY, USA

Correspondence should be addressed to Adil Shujaat; adil.shujaat@jax.ufl.edu

Academic Editor: Nicole S. L. Goh

Objectives. We conducted a study to answer 3 questions: (1) is CT pulmonary angiography (CTPA) overutilized in suspected pulmonary embolism (PE)? (2) What alternative diagnoses are provided by CTPA? (3) Can CTPA be used to evaluate right ventricular dilatation (RVD)? *Methods.* We retrospectively reviewed the clinical information of 231 consecutive emergency department patients who underwent CTPA for suspected PE over a one-year period. *Results.* The mean age of our patients was 53 years, and 58.4% were women. The prevalence of PE was 20.7%. Among the 136 patients with low clinical probability of PE, a d-dimer test was done in 54.4%, and it was normal in 24.3%; none of these patients had PE. The most common alternative findings on CTPA were emphysema (7.6%), pneumonia (7%), atelectasis (5.5%), bronchiectasis (3.8%), and congestive heart failure (3.3%). The sensitivity and negative predictive value of CTPA for (RVD) was 92% and 80%, respectively. *Conclusions.* PE could have been excluded without CTPA in ~1 out of 4 patients with low clinical probability of PE, if a formal assessment of probability and d-dimer test had been done. In patients without PE, CTPA did not provide an alternative diagnosis in 65%. In patients with PE, CTPA showed the potential to evaluate RVD.

1. Introduction

The paradox in the diagnosis of pulmonary embolism (PE) is that it tends to be both underdiagnosed and overinvestigated. The prevalence of PE-varies from 10% to 25% in different studies [1–5]. The vast majority (94%) of PE related deaths are because of a failure of diagnosis [6]. The consequences of missing the diagnosis and the ease of recalling prior serious cases may lead to an overestimation of the probability of PE and lower the threshold for initiating a cascade of diagnostic testing, a phenomenon described as the availability heuristics in cognitive psychology [7, 8]. The widespread round-the-clock availability, excellent accuracy [9, 10] of CT pulmonary angiography (CTPA), and ability to provide an alternative diagnosis [11, 12] may further lower the threshold for performing this imaging study and result in its overuse. On the other hand, outcome studies using clinical prediction rules to refine diagnostic certainty have shown that PE can be safely excluded in patients with low clinical probability and normal

d-dimer levels without an imaging study [1, 2, 5]. However, the impact of such evidence-based strategies on actual clinical practice is not known. In this era of evidence-based decision making and cost-effective utilization of resources, it is imperative to diagnose and risk-stratify emergency department (ED) patients with pulmonary embolism in a more objective manner. We conducted a study to determine if the utilization of CTPA in suspected PE could be refined. We sought to answer these three questions: (1) is CTPA overutilized? (2) What alternative or incidental diagnoses are provided by CTPA? (3) Can CTPA be used to evaluate right ventricular dilatation (RVD)?

2. Methods

We retrospectively reviewed the clinical information of 231 consecutive ED patients who were suspected of PE and underwent a CTPA during the one-year period, January 2005 to December 2005 at St. Luke's Hospital which is a university affiliated hospital in New York City. The study was approved by the Institutional Review Board of St. Luke's and Roosevelt Hospitals.

We collected information on age, gender, presenting complaints, PE risk factors, physical examination, chest radiographs, electrocardiogram, arterial blood gas, d-dimer levels, CTPA, and echocardiography. The immunoturbidimetric STA-Lia test was used for plasma d-dimer. The VITRO ECi immunoassay was used for plasma troponin I. All CTPA studies were done on Toshiba's Aquilion MULTI (a 34-row detector CT scanner). The diagnosis of PE was excluded if CTPA did not show any evidence of PE.

One investigator retrospectively applied Wells' simplified clinical prediction model [13] without knowledge of results of the d-dimer levels and the CTPA (Table 1). One investigator reviewed the CTPA of patients without PE for alternative or incidental findings. One investigator reviewed the CTPA of those with PE for evidence of right ventricular dilatation (RVD) without knowledge of the echocardiography results. RVD was defined as the short axis of the right ventricle is larger than that of the left ventricle when measured between the inner surface of the free wall and the surface of the interventricular septum on a single axial image where both appeared maximally distended [14].

3. Results

3.1. Clinical Characteristics of the Patients. The mean age of the patients was 53 years, and 58.4% were women. The most common presenting complaints were dyspnea, chest pain, or both. Only 2 patients had hemoptysis. The most common risk factors for PE were malignancy, a previous history of deep vein thrombosis or PE, and immobilization or surgery (Table 2).

3.2. Probability Groups and Prevalence of PE. Of the 231 patients suspected of PE in which a CTPA was performed, 48 (20.7%) had evidence of PE. The prevalence of PE was 7.3%, 42.2%, and 100% in the low, moderate, and high probability groups, respectively (Tables 3 and 4).

3.3. Accuracy of d-Dimer. The sensitivity, specificity, negative predictive value and positive predictive value, of d-dimer were 90.4%, 34.5%, 94.8%, and 21.3%, respectively.

3.4. Alternative Findings on CTPA. The CTPA did not reveal an alternative finding in the majority (65%) of the patients. The most common alternative findings on CTPA were emphysema (7.6%), pneumonia (7.1%), and atelectasis (5.5%) (Table 5).

3.5. Prevalence of RVD. Of the 23 patients with PE who had echocardiography, 12 (52%) had evidence of RVD. The prevalence of RVD on CTPA was 55% (26/47 patients).

3.6. Accuracy of CTPA for RVD. The sensitivity, specificity, negative predictive value, and positive predictive value of

TABLE 1: Wells' simplified clinical prediction model.

Parameter	Points
Clinical symptoms or signs of deep vein thrombosis (DVT)	3
Heart rate > 100 beats per minute	1.5
Immobilization (for 3 or more days) or surgery in the last 4 weeks	1.5
Previous history of DVT or PE	1.5
Hemoptysis	1
Malignancy (diagnosed in the last 6 months, under active or palliative treatment)	1
Alternative diagnosis less likely than PE (based on presenting history, physical examination, CXR, EKG, and ABG)	3
Clinical probability of PE	Score
Low	<2
Moderate	2–6
High	>6

TABLE 2: Clinical characteristics of 231 patients suspected of having a PE in whom CTPA was ordered.

Age in years (mean)	53	
	N	%
Female gender	135	58.4
Pregnant	3	1.3
Dyspnea	73	31.6
Chest pain	58	25
Dyspnea and chest pain	22	9.5
Syncope	9	3.8
Near-syncope/dizziness	7	3
Leg pain/swelling	14	6
Heart rate > 100 beats/minute	78	33.7
Immobilization or surgery	12	5.2
Previous DVT or PE	19	8.2
Hemoptysis	2	0.86
Malignancy	24	10.3

TABLE 3: Clinical probability groups based on Wells' simplified prediction model.

Probability group	n/N	%
Low clinical probability	136/231	58.8
Moderate clinical probability	71/231	30.7
High clinical probability	8/231	3.5
Unknown	16/231	6.9

CTPA for RVD were 90.9%, 44.4%, 80%, and 66.6%, respectively.

3.7. Utilization of Diagnostic Studies. Of the 231 patients who were suspected of PE and underwent CTPA, 136 (58.8%) had a low clinical probability of PE. Of these patients, only 74

TABLE 4: Probability groups and prevalence of PE.

Prevalence of PE	n/N	%
Overall	48/231	20.7
Low clinical probability group	10/136	7.3
Moderate clinical probability group	30/71	42.2
High clinical probability group	8/8	100
Unknown	0/16	0

TABLE 5: Most common alternative or incidental findings on CTPA of patients without PE ($N = 183$).

	N	%
Emphysema	14	7.6
Pneumonia	13	7.1
Atelectasis	10	5.5
Bronchiectasis	7	3.8
Air trapping	6	3.3
Congestive heart failure	6	3.3
Pleural effusion	5	2.7
New pulmonary nodule/mass	3	1.6
No alternative finding	119	65

(54.4%) had a d-dimer sample sent as part of the diagnostic evaluation for PE. Of these 74 patients, 18 (24.3%) had normal d-dimer levels (<0.58 μg/mL). None of these patients had evidence of PE on CTPA.

If a clinical probability of PE had been assigned to all the ED patients suspected of PE and all the patients with a low clinical probability of PE had had a d-dimer sample sent, approximately one out of four CTPAs could have been avoided.

4. Discussion

The prevalence of PE in our study (20%) is comparable to that reported in the medical literature (10–25%) [1–5]. Similarly, the proportion of patients determined to have a low clinical probability (52%) is comparable to that cited in the literature (53–58%) [3]. However, a d-dimer sample was sent in only 54% of the patients with a low clinical probability, and it was normal in only 24% of these patients. Outcome studies have shown that PE can be excluded in patients with a low clinical probability and a low d-dimer result without the need for a CTPA [1, 2, 5]. Our study supports the hypothesis that CTPA is being overused and d-dimer underutilized in the diagnostic evaluation of ED patients suspected of PE. It shows that in a major urban ED like ours, where no clinical practice guideline for evaluation of PE was in place, if a clinical prediction model is used to assign a probability to ED patients suspected of PE and a d-dimer sample is sent in all the patients with a low clinical probability of PE, a CTPA can be avoided in approximately one-quarter of such patients.

An accurate determination of clinical probability of PE is important because the interpretation of diagnostic studies depends upon this probability. The presenting symptoms and signs of PE are nonspecific, and only 10–25% of the patients suspected of PE actually turn out to have it [1–5]. The accuracy and interobserver reliability of an empiric clinical probability assessment of PE by overall impression are poor [15] and inversely proportional to clinical experience [15, 16]. Recently two derived clinical prediction models have been externally validated and evaluated in outcome studies [1–5]. The Canadian Wells' simplified clinical prediction model [13] has the advantage over the Geneva model [17] of having been studied in both inpatients and outpatients and of having a moderate to substantial inter-observer agreement.

The sensitivity and negative predictive value of STA-Lia test d-dimer in our study were 90.4% and 94.8%, which are comparable to the sensitivity and negative predictive value of 98% and 97% cited in studies evaluating this assay [18, 19].

CTPA has replaced ventilation-perfusion scan as the imaging test of choice in patients suspected of PE. Outcome studies have shown it to be comparable to the "gold standard" conventional pulmonary angiography, which is seldom performed [10, 11]. It is available round the clock and also carries the potential advantage of providing an alternative diagnosis in those who turn out to not have PE. Few studies have examined the frequency and validity of alternative diagnoses in those who turn out to not have PE [12, 13]. Our study shows that CTPA revealed alternative findings in only 35% of such patients. The most common alternative findings were emphysema (7.6%), pneumonia (7.1%), atelectasis (5.5%), bronchiectasis (3.8%), air-trapping (3.3%), and pulmonary edema (3.3%).

CTPA is not without its drawbacks. There is a finite risk of general adverse reactions to iodinated contrast dye. The incidence of acute general adverse reactions varies and is 15% for mild reactions (nausea, vomiting, limited urticaria, and pallor), 1-2% for moderate ones (severe vomiting, extensive urticaria, laryngeal edema, and dyspnea), 0.2% for severe ones (pulmonary edema, arrhythmia, cardiac arrest, and circulatory collapse) [20]. There is also a risk of contrast-induced nephropathy that varies from 1% in patients with normal renal function to 50% in those with diabetic nephropathy [20], especially in patients congestive heart failure and with cor pulmonale who are on diuretics and are at high risk for PE. In contrast, when d-dimer is normal the probability of PE is low, and CTPA is not performed, the risk of PE during 3-month followup is only 0.2% [1]. Similarly, when d-dimer is normal PE is unlikely, and CTPA is not performed, the risk of nonfatal venous thromboembolism is only 0.5% [5].

More importantly, there is an underappreciated risk of radiation exposure from CTPA, which cannot be ignored in young women smokers on oral contraceptive pills and pregnant women who comprise a high-risk group for PE. Moreover, 60% of CTPA studies performed over a 2-year period at one institution were on women [21]. Interestingly, a similar proportion of CTPA studies done in our study were on women. CTPA delivers a minimum radiation dose of 2.0 rad (20 mGy) to each breast in an average-sized woman. By contrast, ventilation-perfusion scan delivers a dose of 0.28 mGy [21]. A 20-year-old woman receiving a dose of

40 mGy from a single CTPA study has been estimated to be at 68% greater risk for breast cancer by age 35 years than a 20-year-old woman without such exposure [22]. Because the thyroid, breast, and lungs are among the most cancer-susceptible organs in the body and are included in chest CT scan, the large scale of use may have epidemiologic significance. Estimates suggest that 6,800 future cancers may be attributable to chest CT scans performed in 2007 alone [23] and that 0.7% to 2% of all future cancers in the United States may be caused by radiation from CT scan [24, 25]. Nevertheless, CTPA is preferred over ventilation-perfusion scan for suspected PE in pregnant patients when venous ultrasonography of the legs is unrevealing. Although CTPA delivers a higher dose of radiation to the mother, it delivers a lower dose to the fetus than a ventilation-perfusion scan [26]. Lastly, use of CTPA for suspected PE without a formal assessment of probability of PE and d-dimer levels is not a cost-effective approach. Lee et al. performed a cost-effectiveness analysis of diagnostic strategies in suspected PE and showed that the strategy combining clinical probability assessment, highly sensitive rapid d-dimer assay (97% sensitivity), and multidetector CTPA had the lowest cost per life saved [27]. Moreover, the cost per life saved was $1258 when the clinical probability of PE was low compared to $3122 and $5496 when it was intermediate and high, respectively [27].

PE is a heterogeneous disorder that carries a highly variable mortality depending on its presentation and the patient's underlying cardiopulmonary status. Mortality varies from 1.5% in the case of a hemodynamically stable patient treated with anticoagulation alone [6] to almost certain death in the case of a cardiopulmonary arrest. There is a select group of hemodynamically stable PE patients with evidence of right ventricular dysfunction that need to be identified. Ten percent of such patients can decompensate and half of these can die [28]. Recognition of this group of patients at risk of hemodynamic deterioration is important in order to transfer them to the medical intensive care unit for closer monitoring and consideration of thrombolysis if necessary. Reliance on the availability and expertise of echocardiography for identifying such patients especially in the after-hours can lead to delay in triage and result in crowding in the ED. A few studies have suggested that CTPA can be used to evaluate RVD in PE patients [14, 29, 30]. Although we did not evaluate the outcome of patients who turned out to have PE, our study suggests that CTPA has the potential to evaluate RVD in such patients. The prevalence of RVD in the patients who turned out to have PE was 52% (12/23 patients) on echocardiography and 55% (26/47 patients) on CTPA. This is not much different from the ~30 to 55% prevalence cited in the literature [21, 31–33]. The high sensitivity (91.6%) of CTPA for RVD in our study is similar to that reported in a retrospective study of 110 consecutive patients suspected of PE. However, our study shows a lower specificity (44.4%) compared to that study (100%) [14]. This could be for a number of reasons: firstly, Lim et al. studied only patients with acute massive pulmonary embolism, whereas we studied all the patients with PE. Secondly, there were a significant number (44%) of technically difficult echocardiographic studies in our patients. Thirdly, 36% of the echocardiographic

studies were done more than 24 hours after the CTPA by which time RVD may have resolved.

5. Limitations

Our study is not without limitations. The retrospective nature of our study made it difficult to calculate the Wells' simplified model score in 16 (~7%) of the 231 patients because of missing data. However, none of these patients was diagnosed with PE on the CTPA. We did not follow up on the patients in whom PE was excluded. However, outcome studies have shown that the clinical validity of using a CTPA to rule out PE is similar to that reported for conventional pulmonary angiography. Although our study shows that CTPA revealed alternative findings in only 35% of such patients, we did not correlate the findings with the actual alternative diagnoses given to these patients. Our study suggests that CTPA has the potential to evaluate right ventricular dilatation. However, right ventricular *dilatation* alone may not reflect right ventricular *dysfunction*, and studies have defined right ventricular *dysfunction* on echocardiography as right ventricular hypokinesia or using composite criteria that included right ventricular *dilatation* with a threshold for right ventricular end-diastolic diameter/left ventricular end-diastolic diameter ratio of 0.6–1 [34, 35]. More importantly, we did not follow up the outcome of patients with RVD to determine the direct role of CTPA in risk-stratification. Lastly, we did not evaluate those ED patients who were suspected of PE but did not undergo a CTPA.

6. Conclusions

The choice of clinical prediction model is not as important as the fundamental principle of using such a model to accurately determine the clinical probability in each patient with suspected PE because the interpretation of diagnostic tests depends upon an accurate assessment of clinical probability. Since PE can be safely excluded without a CTPA in patients with a low clinical probability and a normal d-dimer level, application of a prediction model and use of d-dimer can refine diagnostic certainty and reduce the disproportionate number of CTPAs being done in such patients. Moreover, contrary to popular belief, CTPA did not reveal an alternative finding in 65% of the patients without PE. The usefulness of CTPA to evaluate RVD can potentially risk-stratify ED patients with PE, especially in the after-hours when availability of echocardiography is limited.

Abbreviations

CT: Computed tomography
CTPA: CT pulmonary angiography
PE: Pulmonary embolism
RVD: Right ventricular dilatation
ED: Emergency department.

Conflict of Interests

None of the authors has any conflict of interests with the content of this paper.

References

[1] P. S. Wells, D. R. Anderson, M. Rodger et al., "Excluding pulmonary embolism at the bedside without diagnostic imaging: management of patients with suspected pulmonary embolism presenting to the emergency department by using a simple clinical model and D-dimer," *Annals of Internal Medicine*, vol. 135, no. 2, pp. 98–107, 2001.

[2] M. J. H. A. Kruip, M. J. Slob, J. H. E. M. Schijen, C. van der Heul, and H. R. Büller, "Use of a clinical decision rule in combination with D-dimer concentration in diagnostic workup of patients with suspected pulmonary embolism: a prospective management study," *Archives of Internal Medicine*, vol. 162, no. 14, pp. 1631–1635, 2002.

[3] I. Chagnon, H. Bounameaux, D. Aujesky et al., "Comparison of two clinical prediction rules and implicit assessment among patients with suspected pulmonary embolism," *The American Journal of Medicine*, vol. 113, no. 4, pp. 269–275, 2002.

[4] S. J. Wolf, T. R. McCubbin, K. M. Feldhaus, J. P. Faragher, and D. M. Adcock, "Prospective validation of wells criteria in the evaluation of patients with suspected pulmonary embolism," *Annals of Emergency Medicine*, vol. 44, no. 5, pp. 503–510, 2004.

[5] A. van Belle, H. R. Büller, M. V. Huisman, P. M. Huisman et al., "Effectiveness of managing suspected pulmonary embolism using an algorithm combining clinical probability, D-dimer testing, and computed tomography," *Journal of the American Medical Association*, vol. 295, no. 2, pp. 172–179, 2006.

[6] J. E. Dalen, "Pulmonary embolism: what have we learned since Virchow? Natural history, pathophysiology, and diagnosis," *Chest*, vol. 122, no. 4, pp. 1440–1456, 2002.

[7] S. Iles, L. Beckert, M. Than, and G. I. Town, "Making a diagnosis of pulmonary embolism: new methods and clinical issues," *New Zealand Medical Journal*, vol. 116, no. 1177, 2003.

[8] H. C. Sox, M. A. Blatt, M. C. Higgins et al., *Medical Decision Making*, Butterworth-Heineman, Woburn, Mass, USA, 1988.

[9] L. K. Moores, W. L. Jackson Jr., A. F. Shorr, and J. L. Jackson, "Meta-analysis: outcomes in patients with suspected pulmonary embolism managed with computed tomographic pulmonary angiography," *Annals of Internal Medicine*, vol. 141, no. 11, pp. 866–874, 2004.

[10] R. Quiroz, N. Kucher, K. H. Zou et al., "Clinical validity of a negative computed tomography scan in patients with suspected pulmonary embolism: a systematic review," *Journal of the American Medical Association*, vol. 293, no. 16, pp. 2012–2017, 2005.

[11] M. J. L. van Strijen, J. L. Bloem, W. de Monye et al., "Helical computed tomography and alternative diagnosis in patients with excluded pulmonary embolism," *Journal of Thrombosis and Haemostasis*, vol. 3, no. 11, pp. 2449–2456, 2005.

[12] K.-L. Tsai, E. Gupta, and L. B. Haramati, "Pulmonary atelectasis: a frequent alternative diagnosis in patients undergoing CT-PA for suspected pulmonary embolism," *Emergency Radiology*, vol. 10, no. 5, pp. 282–286, 2004.

[13] P. S. Wells, D. R. Anderson, M. Rodger et al., "Derivation of a simple clinical model to categorize patients probability of pulmonary embolism: increasing the models utility with the SimpliRED D-dimer," *Thrombosis and Haemostasis*, vol. 83, no. 3, pp. 416–420, 2000.

[14] K.-E. Lim, C.-Y. Chan, P.-H. Chu, Y.-Y. Hsu, and W.-C. Hsu, "Right ventricular dysfunction secondary to acute massive pulmonary embolism detected by helical computed tomography pulmonary angiography," *Clinical Imaging*, vol. 29, no. 1, pp. 16–21, 2005.

[15] M. A. Rodger, E. Maser, I. Stiell, H. E. A. Howley, and P. S. Wells, "The interobserver reliability of pretest probability assessment in patients with suspected pulmonary embolism," *Thrombosis Research*, vol. 116, no. 2, pp. 101–107, 2005.

[16] S. Iles, A. M. Hodges, J. R. Darley et al., "Clinical experience and pre-test probability scores in the diagnosis of pulmonary embolism," *Monthly Journal of the Association of Physicians*, vol. 96, no. 3, pp. 211–215, 2003.

[17] J. Wicki, T. V. Perneger, A. F. Junod, H. Bounameaux, and A. Perrier, "Assessing clinical probability of pulmonary embolism in the emergency ward: a simple score," *Archives of Internal Medicine*, vol. 161, no. 1, pp. 92–97, 2001.

[18] G. Waser, S. Kathriner, and W. A. Wuillemin, "Performance of the automated and rapid STA Liatest D-dimer on the STA-R analyzer," *Thrombosis Research*, vol. 116, no. 2, pp. 165–170, 2005.

[19] R. E. G. Schutgens, F. J. L. M. Haas, W. B. M. Gerritsen, F. van der Horst, H. K. Nieuwenhuis, and D. H. Biesma, "The usefulness of five D-dimer assays in the exclusion of deep venous thrombosis," *Journal of Thrombosis and Haemostasis*, vol. 1, no. 5, pp. 976–981, 2003.

[20] S. Namasivayam, M. K. Kalra, W. E. Torres, and W. C. Small, "Adverse reactions to intravenous iodinated contrast media: a primer for radiologists," *Emergency Radiology*, vol. 12, no. 5, pp. 210–215, 2006.

[21] M. S. Parker, F. K. Hui, M. A. Camacho, J. K. Chung, D. W. Broga, and N. N. Sethi, "Female breast radiation exposure during CT pulmonary angiography," *The American Journal of Roentgenology*, vol. 185, no. 5, pp. 1228–1233, 2005.

[22] L. M. Hurwitz, T. Yoshizumi, R. E. Reiman et al., "Radiation dose to the fetus from body MDCT during early gestation," *The American Journal of Roentgenology*, vol. 186, no. 3, pp. 871–876, 2006.

[23] A. Berrington de González, M. Mahesh, K.-P. Kim et al., "Projected cancer risks from computed tomographic scans performed in the United States in 2007," *Archives of Internal Medicine*, vol. 169, no. 22, pp. 2071–2077, 2009.

[24] D. J. Brenner and E. J. Hall, "Computed tomography: an increasing source of radiation exposure," *The New England Journal of Medicine*, vol. 357, no. 22, pp. 2277–2284, 2007.

[25] A. Sodickson, P. F. Baeyens, K. P. Andriole et al., "Recurrent CT, cumulative radiation exposure, and associated radiation-induced cancer risks from CT of adults," *Radiology*, vol. 251, no. 1, pp. 175–184, 2009.

[26] H. T. Winer-Muram, J. M. Boone, H. L. Brown, S. G. Jennings, W. C. Mabie, and G. T. Lombardo, "Pulmonary embolism in pregnant patients: fetal radiation dose with helical CT," *Radiology*, vol. 224, no. 2, pp. 487–492, 2002.

[27] J.-A. Lee, B. K. Zierler, C.-F. Liu, and M. K. Chapko, "Cost-effective diagnostic strategies in patients with a high, intermediate, or low clinical probability of pulmonary embolism," *Vascular and Endovascular Surgery*, vol. 45, no. 2, pp. 113–121, 2011.

[28] S. Grifoni, I. Olivotto, P. Cecchini et al., "Short-term clinical outcome of patients with acute pulmonary embolism, normal blood pressure, and echocardiographic right ventricular dysfunction," *Circulation*, vol. 101, no. 24, pp. 2817–2822, 2000.

[29] N. Mansencal, T. Joseph, A. Vieillard-Baron et al., "Diagnosis of right ventricular dysfunction in acute pulmonary embolism using helical computed tomography," *The American Journal of Cardiology*, vol. 95, no. 10, pp. 1260–1263, 2005.

[30] A. Ghuysen, B. Ghaye, V. Willems et al., "Computed tomographic pulmonary angiography and prognostic significance in patients with acute pulmonary embolism," *Thorax*, vol. 60, no. 11, pp. 956–961, 2005.

[31] W. Kasper, S. Konstantinides, A. Geibel, N. Tiede, T. Krause, and H. Just, "Prognostic significance of right ventricular afterload stress detected by echocardiography in patients with clinically suspected pulmonary embolism," *Heart*, vol. 77, no. 4, pp. 346–349, 1997.

[32] S. Z. Goldhaber, W. D. Haire, M. L. Feldstein et al., "Alteplase versus heparin in acute pulmonary embolism: randomised trial assessing right-ventricular function and pulmonary perfusion," *The Lancet*, vol. 341, no. 8844, pp. 507–511, 1993.

[33] A. Ribeiro, P. Lindmarker, A. Juhlin-Dannfelt, H. Johnsson, and L. Jorfeldt, "Echocardiography Doppler in pulmonary embolism: right ventricular dysfunction as a predictor of mortality rate," *The American Heart Journal*, vol. 134, no. 3, pp. 479–487, 1997.

[34] O. Sanchez, L. Trinquart, I. Colombet et al., "Prognostic value of right ventricular dysfunction in patients with haemodynamically stable pulmonary embolism: a systematic review," *European Heart Journal*, vol. 29, no. 12, pp. 1569–1577, 2008.

[35] G. Coutance, E. Cauderlier, J. Ehtisham, M. Hamon, and M. Hamon, "The prognostic value of markers of right ventricular dysfunction in pulmonary embolism: a meta-analysis," *Critical Care*, vol. 15, no. 2, article R103, 2011.

34

Determination of Best Criteria to Determine Final and Initial Speeds within Ramp Exercise Testing Protocols

Sidney C. da Silva,[1] Walace D. Monteiro,[2,3] Felipe A. Cunha,[2,4] Jonathan Myers,[5] and Paulo T. V. Farinatti[2,3]

[1] *Department of Sports Science, Brazilian Olympic Committee, Avenida das Américas 899, 22631-000 Rio de Janeiro, RJ, Brazil*

[2] *Laboratory of Physical Activity and Health Promotion, Rio de Janeiro State University, Rua São Francisco Xavier 524, Sala 8121F, 20550-900 Rio de Janeiro, RJ, Brazil*

[3] *Graduate Program in Sciences of Physical Activity, Salgado de Oliveira University, Rua Marechal Deodoro 217, No. 2 Andar, 24030-060 Niteroi, RJ, Brazil*

[4] *Graduate Program in Medical Sciences, Rio de Janeiro State University, Avenida Professor Manoel de Abreu, 444/No. 2 Andar, Vila Isabel, 20550-170 Rio de Janeiro, RJ, Brazil*

[5] *Cardiology Division, Palo Alto VA Health Care System, Cardiology 111C, 3801 Miranda Avenue, Palo Alto, CA 94304, USA*

Correspondence should be addressed to Paulo T. V. Farinatti, pfarinatti@gmail.com

Academic Editor: Darcy D. Marciniuk

This study compared strategies to define final and initial speeds for designing ramp protocols. $V_{O_2 \max}$ was directly assessed in 117 subjects (29 ± 8 yrs) and estimated by three nonexercise models: (1) Veterans Specific Activity Questionnaire (VSAQ); (2) Rating of Perceived Capacity (RPC); (3) Questionnaire of Cardiorespiratory Fitness (CRF). Thirty seven subjects (30 ± 9 yrs) performed three additional tests with initial speeds corresponding to 50% of estimated $V_{O_2 \max}$ and 50% and 60% of measured $V_{O_2 \max}$. Significant differences ($P < 0.001$) were found between $V_{O_2 \max}$ measured (41.5 ± 6.6 mL·kg^{-1}·min^{-1}) and estimated by VSAQ (36.6 ± 6.6 mL·kg^{-1}·min^{-1}) and CRF (45.0 ± 5.3 mL·kg^{-1}·min^{-1}), but not RPC (41.3 ± 6.2 mL·kg^{-1}·min^{-1}). The CRF had the highest ICC, the lowest SEE, and better limits of agreement with $V_{O_2 \max}$ compared to the other instruments. Initial speeds from 50%–60% $V_{O_2 \max}$ estimated by CRF or measured produced similar $V_{O_2 \max}$ (40.7 ± 5.9; 40.0 ± 5.6; 40.3 ± 5.5 mL·kg^{-1}·min^{-1} resp., $P = 0.14$). The closest relationship to identity line was found in tests beginning at 50% $V_{O_2 \max}$ estimated by CRF. In conclusion, CRF was the best option to estimate $V_{O_2 \max}$ and therefore to define the final speed for ramp protocols. The measured $V_{O_2 \max}$ was independent of initial speeds, but speeds higher than 50% $V_{O_2 \max}$ produced poorer submaximal relationships between workload and V_{O_2}.

1. Introduction

Exercise capacity is an independent predictor of risk for cardiovascular disease and mortality among asymptomatic and symptomatic individuals [1–3]. Hence the determination of maximal oxygen uptake ($V_{O_2 \max}$) is considered to be one of the most important health-related parameters and has been widely used to evaluate cardiorespiratory fitness in health and illness [4–7].

However, the determination of exercise capacity is closely related to the test protocol employed [8]. An extensive body of evidence has shown that ramp exercise protocols offer advantages over traditional protocols, because the increase in external work occurs in a constant and continuous fashion, and when designing the protocol the rate of increase in workload can be individualized by a previous estimate of maximal exercise capacity [7, 9–12]. This is associated with greater linearity between V_{O_2} and work rate compared to traditional protocols with large and disproportionate work rate increments [9, 11, 13]. Moreover, ramp protocols induce more uniform hemodynamic and respiratory responses, facilitating the acquisition of information at submaximal intensities, such as the ventilatory threshold [9, 13].

Despite the apparent advantages over traditional exercise testing, standardized criteria to guide the application of ramp protocols remain sparse. For instance, a limitation of ramp protocols is the requirement to estimate maximal exercise capacity from an activity scale and then adjust the ramp rate accordingly [14]. In practical terms, an underestimation of maximal exercise capacity will result in a prolonged total test duration, while an overestimation will result in premature test termination and, therefore, inappropriate test protocol for eliciting a true $V_{O_2 max}$ [15]. However, there is no consensus in the literature concerning this issue. Available recommendations are generally vague and largely limited to the premise that tests should last between 8 and 12 min [4, 7, 14–17]. The same occurs with regard to the initial work rate of the test—actually we could not find recommendations of standard procedures for its determination [18].

Thus, the first objective of the present study was to compare three nonexercise models to predict maximal exercise capacity as criteria to determine the final speed of maximal treadmill ramp protocols. A second purpose was to investigate how different initial speeds calculated from $\%V_{O_2 max}$ influenced the $V_{O_2 max}$ measured in the tests.

2. Material and Methods

2.1. Subjects. A group of 117 subjects (47 women) aged between 18 and 51 years (mean: 29.1 ± 7.6 yrs), with no previous experience in high performance physical training, volunteered for the study. Exclusion criteria included a clinical diagnosis of any clinical condition that could limit exercise performance and the use of any medication with potential cardiovascular influence. All participants were fully informed about the procedures and potential risks before giving written consent to take part in the study, which was approved by the local Institutional Research Ethics Committee.

2.2. Procedures. A flowchart of the 1st and 2nd studies is presented in Figure 1, detailing the procedures adopted to determine the workload increments using the nonexercise models (1st study—final speed) and different percent $V_{O_2 max}$ intensities (2nd study—initial speed).

All 117 subjects enrolled in the first study. After signing the informed consent, the subjects performed the following procedures in a single visit to the laboratory: (a) anthropometric measurements; (b) application of three nonexercise models to estimate $V_{O_2 max}$ (Veterans Specific Activity Questionnaire (VSAQ), [19, 20]; Rating of Perceived Capacity (RPC) [21]; Questionnaire of Cardio-respiratory Fitness (CRF) [22]); (c) cardiopulmonary exercise testing.

The VSAQ was originally developed by Myers et al. [19, 20] with the specific purpose of individualizing ramp protocols. The VSAQ includes a list of physical activities

with scores ranging from 1 to 13. The responder indicates which of the listed activities would cause fatigue or shortness of breath. Subjects evaluated in the initial studies with the VSAQ had low cardiorespiratory fitness and a high prevalence of overweight/obesity, hypertension, or coronary disease. Even though further studies have demonstrated that the instrument also provided adequate estimation of $V_{O_2 max}$ in healthy active populations [5, 8], there is a lack of research specifically designed to assess its validity within the application of ramp protocols in healthy subjects. The RPC may be considered a variation of the VSAQ [21], presenting different maximal MET levels (ranging from 1 to 20), which are linked to physical activities of several intensities. Subjects rate their perceived capacity by choosing the most strenuous activity they could sustain for 30 min. However, the RPC has been not validated through direct comparison with exercise capacity using cardiopulmonary exercise testing. The CRF was not specifically developed to design ramp protocols, but it has been extensively applied as a nonexercise model to estimate the maximal cardiorespiratory capacity [22]. It is a progressive scale with scores for the intensity of the activities ranging from 0 to 7. The subjects must select the most appropriate score according to the physical activities performed in the last 30 days. The CRF was selected because of the unusual methodological meticulousness applied to its development. A large sample ($N = 799$) of men and women aged 19 to 79 years was tested. The estimated $V_{O_2 max}$ was compared to directly measured data, and the questionnaire was cross-validated with another population, which is uncommon in studies assessing such instruments [23, 24].

In the first study, the increase in work rate within the cardiopulmonary exercise test (CPET1) was individualized to elicit each subject's limit of tolerance in 10 min, and treadmill grade was set at 0%. Final and initial speeds were determined using ACSM equations for treadmill running [7], considering the intensities corresponding to the highest $V_{O_2 max}$ estimated by the non-exercise models (final speed) and 50% of this value (initial speed). The choice of 50% of the estimated $V_{O_2 max}$ to determine the initial speed was based on a previous pilot study involving 35 subjects. In this pilot study, the initial speed was set at 1/3 of the estimated $V_{O_2 max}$, which corresponded to a mean speed of 4.3 km·h^{-1} and a work rate increase of 0.88 km·h^{-1} each minute. The protocols lasted approximately 12 min (11.3 ± 2.2 min) and subjects remained walking, for about 4 min. Thus, an intensity of 50% $V_{O_2 max}$ would probably shorten the test and increase the time in which the subjects would be actually running.

A subgroup of 37 subjects (17 women; age: 29.1 ± 7.6 yrs) was randomly selected to participate in the second study. These subjects performed three additional cardiopulmonary exercise tests, separated by 72 to 120 h intervals. The increase in work rate and treadmill grade were the same applied in CPET1. In the first test (CPET1bis), the final speed was determined using the best non-exercise model as defined in the first study, and the initial speed set at 50% of this value. The other tests (CPET2 and CPET3) were then performed using the results of CPET1bis as reference. In brief,

1st study ($N = 117$)	2nd study ($N = 37$)		
CPET1	CPET1bis	CPET2	CPET3
• Anthropometric measurements. • Final speed calculated from the highest $V_{O_2 \, max}$ estimated by the three questionnaires (VSAQ, RPC, and CRF). • Initial speed calculated from 50% of the estimated value.	• Final speed calculated from the $V_{O_2 \, max}$ estimated by CRF. • Initial speed calculated from 50% of the estimated value.	• Final speed calculated from the $V_{O_2 \, max}$ measured during CPET1bis. • Initial speed calculated from 50% of the measured value.	• Final speed calculated from the $V_{O_2 \, max}$ measured during CPET1bis. • Initial speed calculated from 60% of the measured value.

Stages for determining the final and initial test speeds

(i) $\text{Speed}_{final} = (V_{O_2 \, max} - 3.5) \times 100\%/(0.2 + 0.9 \times G)$

• V_{O_2} is reported as $mL \cdot kg^{-1} \cdot min^{-1}$

• Speed in $m \cdot min^{-1}$ (converted to $km \cdot h^{-1}$)

• G = grade expressed in decimal form

(ii) $\text{Speed}_{initial} = \text{speed}_{final} \times \text{percentage}$

(iii) Increment ratio = $(\text{speed}_{final} - \text{speed}_{initial})/10 \, minutes$

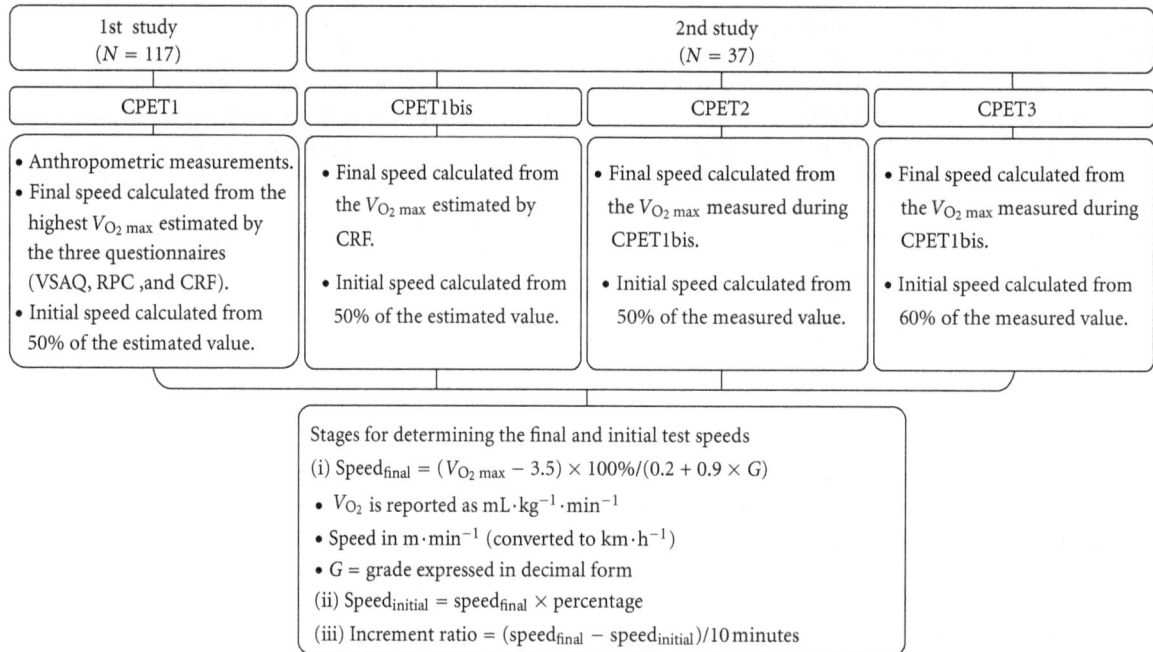

FIGURE 1: Flowchart of the 1st and 2nd studies including the procedures adopted to determine the workload increments, using nonexercise models to estimate $V_{O_2 \, max}$ and ACSM running equation to calculate the treadmill speeds. $V_{O_2 \, max}$: maximal oxygen uptake; CPET: cardiopulmonary exercise test; VSAQ: Veterans Specific Activity Questionnaire; RPC: Rating of Perceived Capacity; CRF: Questionnaire of Cardiorespiratory Fitness.

the final speed in CPET1bis was estimated from the maximal exercise capacity provided by CRF, whereas in both CPET2 and CPET3 it corresponded to the speed associated with the $V_{O_2 \, max}$ assessed in CPET1bis. The initial speeds corresponded to 50% $V_{O_2 \, max}$ estimated (CPET1bis), 50% $V_{O_2 \, max}$ measured (CPET2), and 60% $V_{O_2 \, max}$ measured (CPET3). This approach allowed to observe whether initial speeds ranging from 50 to 60% $V_{O_2 \, max}$ (estimated or measured) influenced the results of the tests.

In the first study the CPET1 was applied by a researcher blinded for the results of the non-exercise models. In the second study, the sequence of tests was defined by a counterbalanced crossover design. The participants were blinded for the %V_{O_2} used to establish the initial speeds, and the evaluator was blinded for the purposes of the study.

The cardiopulmonary exercise test protocols were performed using a super-ATL treadmill (Inbramed, Florianopolis, SC, Brazil), and V_{O_2} was averaged and recorded every 30 s. The 30 s time average provided a good compromise between removing noise from V_{O_2} data while maintaining the underlying trend [25]. Data was assessed using a mouthpiece and noseclip. Gas exchange was assessed using a VO2000 analyzer (Medical Graphics, Saint Louis, MO, USA), which was calibrated with a certified standard mixture of oxygen (17.01%) and carbon dioxide (5.00%), balanced with nitrogen. The flows and volumes for the pneumotachograph were calibrated with a 3 L syringe (Hans Rudolph, Kansas, MO, USA). Heart rate was monitored using a Polar S-810 device (Polar, Kempele, Finland). Mean

ambient temperature and relative humidity during testing were $22.4 \pm 1.8°C$ (range 18–23) and $62.5 \pm 4.1\%$ (range 50–75%), respectively.

The criteria for test interruption followed the recommendations of the American College of Sports Medicine [7]. The test was considered to achieve peak capacity when at least three of the following criteria were observed [26]: (a) maximum voluntary exhaustion as reflected by a score of 10 on the Borg CR-10 scale; (b) ≥95% predicted HR max (220—age) or presence of an HR plateau (ΔHR between two consecutive work rates ≤4 beats·min^{-1}); (c) presence of a V_{O_2} plateau (ΔV_{O_2} between two consecutive work rates <2.1 mL·$kg^{-1} \cdot min^{-1}$); (d) respiratory exchange ratio > 1.15. Participants were verbally encouraged to achieve maximal effort. Holding onto the side or front rails of the treadmill was not permitted.

2.3. Statistical Analyses. Data normality was confirmed by univariate analysis. Therefore the intraclass correlation coefficient (ICC) was used to verify the concordance between the $V_{O_2 \, max}$ assessed in CPET1 and the $V_{O_2 \, max}$ estimated by the non-exercise models. Limits of agreement and bias for measured and estimated $V_{O_2 \, max}$ were determined according to the Bland and Altman method [27]. Intraclass correlation (ICC), R-square coefficients (r^2), and standard errors of estimate (SEE) between actual and estimated $V_{O_2 \, max}$ were also calculated.

The $V_{O_2 \, max}$ values obtained in CPET1bis, CPET2, and CPET3 were compared by repeated measures ANOVA.

Additionally, linear regression was performed for each subject on each protocol in order to compare the relationships between workload and V_{O_2}, considering data in every 30 s of exercise. Mean ± SD values of intercepts and slopes were determined for each linear regression model. Student t-tests for paired samples were used to test whether the intercepts and slopes were significantly different from 0 and 1, respectively [12], and to test possible differences between the regression lines, as described in detail elsewhere [28]. The r^2 and SEE for the regression models obtained in all tests were calculated as supplementary criteria to define the best initial speed. Two-tailed statistical significance for all tests was accepted as $P \le 0.05$. All statistical analyses were performed using Statistica 7.0 (Statsoft, Tulsa, OK, USA) and SPSS 8.0 (IBM, Chicago, IL, USA) statistical analysis software.

3. Results

An achieved statistical power of 0.96 for an effect size of 0.25 was obtained by performing a post hoc power analysis (GPower version 3.0.10, Kiel, University of Kiel, Germany) based on the sample size, P value, number of repeated measures, and groups. Table 1 presents the characteristics of the samples comparing strategies to define final and initial speeds. Table 2 presents values for the assessed $V_{O_2 max}$ ($mL \cdot kg^{-1} \cdot min^{-1}$) by age and sex groups.

In the first study, mean duration of CPET1 was 13.3 ± 2.1 min for initial and final speeds of 5.9 ± 0.9 km·h^{-1} and 14.7 ± 2.1 km·h^{-1}, respectively. Significant differences were detected between $V_{O_2 max}$ assessed in CPET1 (41.5 ± 6.6 mL·kg^{-1}·min^{-1}) and $V_{O_2 max}$ estimated from VSAQ and CRF ($V_{O_2 max}$ VSAQ = 36.6±6.6 mL·kg^{-1}·min^{-1}, $P < 0.0001$; $V_{O_2 max}$ CRF = 45.0 ± 5.3 mL·kg^{-1}·min^{-1}; $P < 0.0001$), but not from RPC ($V_{O_2 max}$ RPC = 41.3 ± 6.2 mL·kg^{-1}·min^{-1}, $P = 0.99$).

Figure 2 shows the Bland-Altman analysis, including the limits of agreement for estimated and measured $V_{O_2 max}$. Table 3 presents values for R-square, SEE, and ICC between $V_{O_2 max}$ measured and estimated by the questionnaires. The RPC provided the lowest mean difference between $V_{O_2 max}$ directly assessed in CPET1 and estimated from the questionnaires (RPC = 0.24 mL·kg^{-1}·min^{-1}; CRF = −3.54 mL·kg^{-1}·min^{-1}; VSAQ = 4.94 mL·kg^{-1}·min^{-1}; $P = 0.05$). However, the CRF exhibited better limits of agreement compared to the other instruments. The higher values obtained for CRF with regard to R-square and ICC were consistent with the results of the Bland-Altman analysis. The SEE between assessed and estimated $V_{O_2 max}$ was also lower in CRF compared to VSAQ and RPC.

Table 4 shows the distribution of $V_{O_2 max}$ assessed in CPET1 according to tertiles, as well the percent agreement between estimated and measured $V_{O_2 max}$ in each tertile. The nonparametric Kendall's tau-b correlation between tertiles was similar across the three questionnaires and measured $V_{O_2 max}$. However the correlation using the CRF was higher over RPC and VSAQ—the proportion of subjects assigned

in the same tertile category was superior for CRF compared to the other questionnaires, and the distribution was more homogeneous.

With regard to the second study, mean durations of CPET1bis, CPET2, and CPET3 were 13.7 ± 1.8 min, 10.7 ± 1.9 min, and 10.6 ± 0.9 min, respectively. No differences were detected between $V_{O_2 max}$ assessed in CPET1bis (used as reference to define final and initial speeds in CPET2 and CPET3), CPET2, and CPET3 (CPET1bis = 40.7 ± 5.9 mL·kg^{-1}·min^{-1}; CPET2 = 39.8 ± 5.6 mL·kg^{-1}·min^{-1}; CPET3 = 40.3 ± 5.5 mL·kg^{-1}·min^{-1}; $P = 0.142$). Mean initial speeds applied in CPET1bis, CPET2, and CPET3 were 5.7 ± 0.8 km·h^{-1}, 8.1 ± 0.9 km·h^{-1}, and 9.1 ± 1.1 km·h^{-1}, respectively. Table 5 shows the relationships between workload and V_{O_2} in the ramp test protocols initiating with speeds corresponding to 50% and 60% $V_{O_2 max}$ either measured or estimated (slopes, intercepts, R-square, and SEE). CPET1bis showed the closest relationship with the theoretical identity line (slope = 1 and intercept = 0), with the highest R-square and lowest SEE in comparison with CPET2 and CPET3.

4. Discussion

The present study aimed to compare different strategies to define final and initial speeds when designing ramp exercise testing protocols for healthy young populations. Three nonexercise models were employed to estimate maximal cardiorespiratory capacity and therefore the final speed. The choice of VSAQ, RPC, and CRF to estimate the $V_{O_2 max}$ was due to the fact that these instruments have been frequently applied in previous studies and have been shown to have good potential to estimate the maximal cardiorespiratory capacity in different populations [23, 24]. Two relative intensities (%$V_{O_2 max}$) using different initial treadmill speeds were tested.

The values obtained for the $V_{O_2 max}$ assessed in CPET1 are consistent with reference values reported by previous research [4, 7, 14, 16]. Our findings on the ICC, R-square, SEE, and dispersion in the Bland-Altman plot (see Figure 2) suggest that there are advantages in using the CRF to determine the final speed, in comparison with the other instruments. In contrast, the VSAQ had the poorest precision and highest variability with respect to $V_{O_2 max}$ estimation. In their original study, Myers et al. [19] reported a stronger association between estimated and achieved cardiorespiratory capacity over the present data ($r = 0.79$; SEE = 4.97 mL·kg^{-1}·min^{-1}; $P = 0.001$ versus $r = 0.40$; SEE = 7.63 mL·kg^{-1}·min^{-1}; $P = 0.0001$, resp.). However, subjects in the two studies differed considerably in terms of clinical and fitness status, which may have contributed to such discrepancy, since poor conditioned individuals are more likely to interrupt earlier the test due to peripheral fatigue. Moreover, Myers et al. [19] did not directly assess the $V_{O_2 max}$ in their original research. In a later study, these investigators [20] validated the VSAQ measuring $V_{O_2 max}$ directly in a larger sample ($n = 337$). Subjects had similar characteristics as those in the original study, but the results were more

TABLE 1: Characteristics of the subjects participating in the comparisons regarding the final ($N = 117$) and initial ($N = 37$) speeds.

| | Age (years) | | | | Body mass (kg) | | | | Height (cm) | | | | Body fat (%) | | | | $V_{O_2\,max}$ (mL·kg^{-1}·min^{-1}) | | | |
	G	M	F	G2	G	M	F	G2	G	M	F	G2	G	M	F	G2	G	M	F	G2
Mean	29.1	29.8	28.2	29.7	71.7	79.7	59.7	72.4	171.2	176.7	163.1	170.4	15.2	11.7	20.4	16.8	41.5	43.9	37.8	40.7
SD	7.6	7.9	7.0	8.6	14.9	12.6	8.8	17.9	9.1	5.9	6.5	10.0	7.0	5.8	5.3	6.5	6.6	5.8	6.1	5.9
Minimum	18	18	19	18	46.7	57.4	46.7	46.5	150.0	163.3	150.0	150.5	2.9	2.9	11.2	6.0	25.6	32.8	25.6	28.5
Maximum	51	47	51	51	92.9	92.9	91.8	90.3	190.0	190.0	176.0	190.0	32.8	27.1	32.8	28.3	61.6	61.6	54.8	52.4

G: total sample ($n = 117$); M: males ($n = 70$); F: females ($n = 47$); G2: subgroup for initial speed comparison ($n = 37$).

TABLE 2: Descriptive values for $V_{O_2 max}$ ($mL \cdot kg^{-1} \cdot min^{-1}$) by age and sex groups.

| | Age (years) | | | | | |
| | Males ($N = 70$) | | | Females ($N = 47$) | | |
	18–29 ($N = 39$)	30–39 ($N = 20$)	>40 ($N = 11$)	18–29 ($N = 32$)	30–39 ($N = 10$)	>40 ($N = 5$)
Mean	46.2	41.1	39.4	39.0	34.3	37.0
SD	5.8	4.4	3.9	5.9	6.3	4.6
Minimum	36.5	32.8	34.0	26.2	25.6	29.5
Maximum	61.5	47.9	44.2	54.8	45.3	40.4

TABLE 3: Mean difference ($mL \cdot kg^{-1} \cdot min^{-1}$), R-square coefficient, standard error of estimate, and intraclass correlation between $V_{O_2 max}$ assessed and estimated by three non-exercise models ($N = 117$).

| | Total ($N = 117$) | | | | | Males ($N = 70$) | | | | | Females ($N = 47$) | | | | |
| | $V_{O_2 max}$ | | | | | $V_{O_2 max}$ | | | | | $V_{O_2 max}$ | | | | |
	Mean difference	r^2	SEE	ICC	P	Mean difference	r^2	SEE	ICC	P	Mean difference	r^2	SEE	ICC	P
VSAQ	4.94 (11.9%)	0.16	7.63	0.57	<0.0001	−1.81 (−4.1%)	0.05	7.92	0.36	<0.0317	−1.24 (−3.3%)	0.07	7.17	0.42	<0.040
RPC	0.24 (1.0%)	0.09	7.60	0.46	<0.001	3.22 (7.3%)	0.17	1.70	0.58	<0.0001	−3.49 (−9.2%)	0.07	8.35	0.42	<0.035
CRF	−3.54 (−8.5%)	0.53	5.75	0.83	<0.0001	−3.89 (−8.9%)	0.37	6.01	0.76	<0.0001	−2.90 (−7.7%)	0.47	5.36	0.81	<0.0001

VSAQ: Veteran Specific Activity Questionnaire using the following equation: V_{O_2} ($mL \cdot kg^{-1} \cdot min^{-1}$) = (4.7 + 0.97 (VSAQ) − 0.06 (age) × 3.5); for women this value was multiplied by 0.85 [8]; RPC: Rating of Perceived Capacity; CRF: Cardiorespiratory Fitness.

similar to our findings ($r = 0.42$; SEE = 9.1 $mL \cdot kg^{-1} \cdot min^{-1}$; $P = 0.001$).

Maeder et al. [5] compared the $V_{O_2 max}$ obtained in tests using cycle ergometer and treadmill with the exercise capacity estimated by the VSAQ in healthy subjects. The correlations were similar to our data (cycle ergometer: $r = 0.46$ and treadmill: $r = 0.50$; $P < 0.0001$). More recently, Maeder et al. [8] used the VSAQ to select the optimal treadmill ramp protocol in highly trained individuals and reported a similar correlation between estimated and measured $V_{O_2 max}$ ($r = 0.47$), even when using the VSAQ modified nomogram ($r = 0.56$).

Although the VSAQ was developed to facilitate the individualization of ramp protocols, previous research has not ratified this purpose in all populations. Actually, the available evidence does not support its use in determining the final speed within ramp protocols in healthy and well-conditioned populations. Actually the VSAQ has been shown to be more appropriate to estimate the $V_{O_2 max}$ in unfit individuals [20, 29]. The present results confirm this idea. Precision using the VSAQ was lower compared to the other instruments, and the same categorization was obtained in less than 40% of cases. Furthermore, the Bland-Altman plots suggested that in our sample the $V_{O_2 max}$ was systematically overestimated by the VSAQ.

The RPC closely paralleled $V_{O_2 max}$ assessed in CPET1 (mean difference of 0.24 $mL \cdot kg^{-1} \cdot min^{-1}$ or 1%), but exhibited high variability, as evidenced by the Bland-Altman method and SEE (7.60 $mL \cdot kg^{-1} \cdot min^{-1}$). This variation accounted for the relatively low ICC and R-square values. It is noteworthy that RPC was developed in a sample of 87 young, healthy women (age = 48.4 ± 17.4 years) [21]. However, our experience with this method suggests that strong agreement between estimated and actual $V_{O_2 max}$ can be also obtained in men. Interestingly, although our sample consisted of young

women (age = 28.2 ± 7.0 years), the comparison between $V_{O_2 max}$ directly measured and estimated by RPC showed greater concordance (ICC) and lower variation (SEE) among men versus women (ICC = 0.58 versus 0.42 and SEE = 1.70 $mL \cdot kg^{-1} \cdot min^{-1}$ versus 8.35 $mL \cdot kg^{-1} \cdot min^{-1}$, resp.). A possible explanation for this is that in the original RPC study the $V_{O_2 max}$ was estimated from the work performed on cycle ergometer, and not directly measured. The $V_{O_2 max}$ was estimated using maximal work and body mass, assuming as constants the amount of oxygen required for each Watt of power during ramp cycling (10.93 $mL \cdot min^{-1} \cdot W^{-1}$) and V_{O_2} at rest when sitting on the cycle (4.3 $mL \cdot min^{-1}$). However these unpublished data have been previously determined in a group of healthy men [21], and no information was provided with regard to their possible application in females.

The CRF has been widely used to estimate maximal cardiorespiratory capacity [12, 30–35]. Although it was not originally developed to help designing ramp protocols, our results indicate that it works well for this purpose. The original study by Matthews et al. [22] showed a higher correlation between $V_{O_2 max}$ measured and estimated from CRF than the present study, in a sample of 390 men ($r = 0.82$ versus $r = 0.61$, resp.) and 409 women ($r = 0.83$ versus $r = 0.69$, resp.). However, the SEEs in the total sample (5.7 $mL \cdot kg^{-1} \cdot min^{-1}$ versus 5.8 $mL \cdot kg^{-1} \cdot min^{-1}$) and in gender subgroups (men: 6.3 $mL \cdot kg^{-1} \cdot min^{-1}$ versus 6.0 $mL \cdot kg^{-1} \cdot min^{-1}$; women: 5.0 $mL \cdot kg^{-1} \cdot min^{-1}$ versus 5.4 $mL \cdot kg^{-1} \cdot min^{-1}$) were similar in the two studies. The Bland-Altman analysis showed limits of agreement higher over VSAQ and comparable to RPC, but the CRF had the greatest ICC. In addition, the tertile classifications obtained from CRF were more accurate compared to the other nonexercise models.

Overall, CRF showed higher concordance with measured $V_{O_2 max}$, lower dispersion, and better capacity to discriminate

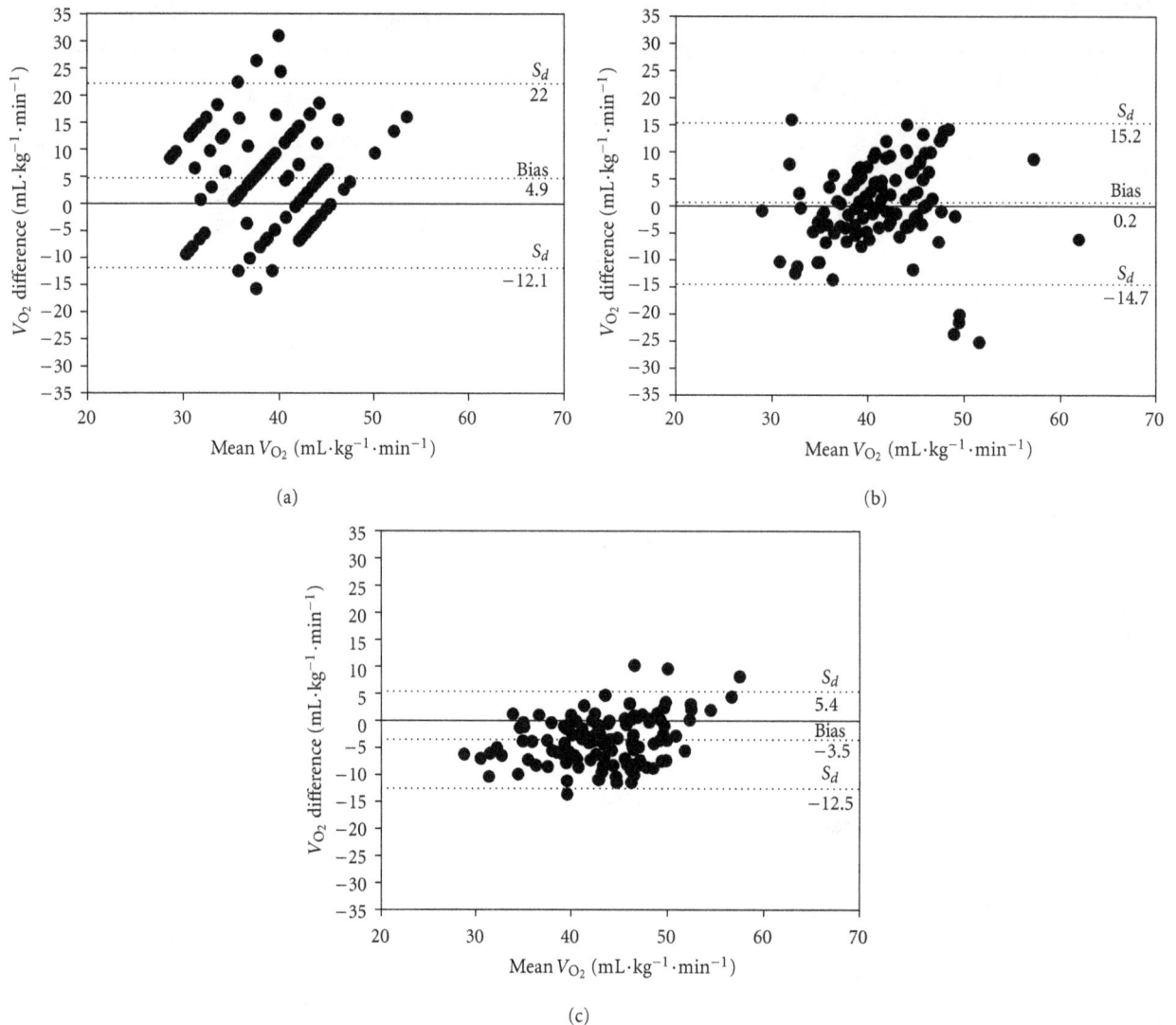

(a)

(b)

(c)

FIGURE 2: Bland-Altman plot for the individual differences between $V_{O_2 max}$ assessed in CPET1 and $V_{O_2 max}$ estimated by VSAQ (a), RPC (b), and CRF (c). The first and third horizontal dashed lines in each graph represent the 95% limits of agreement for VSAQ, RPC, CRF, and VSAQ, corresponding, respectively, to −12.1 to 22.0 (−29.1 to 53.0%); −14.7 to 15.2 (−35.5 to 36.6%); −12.5 to 5.4 (−30,0% to 13,0%). S_d: standard deviation of the differences.

TABLE 4: Percentage of participants ranked in the same tertile, percentage of total agreement, tau-b correlation coefficients between $V_{O_2 max}$ measured and estimated by three non-exercise models (VSAQ, RPC, and CRF) ($N = 117$).

	1st Tertile ($n = 39$)	2nd Tertile ($n = 39$)	3rd Tertile ($n = 39$)	Total ($N = 117$)	R (tau-b)
$V_{O_2 max}$ versus VSAQ	66.66% (26)	5.12% (2)	38.46% (15)	36.75% (43)	0.833
$V_{O_2 max}$ versus RPC	43.58% (17)	25.64% (10)	43.58% (17)	37.60% (44)	0.992
$V_{O_2 max}$ versus CRF	69.23% (27)	41.02% (16)	58.97% (23)	56.41% (66)	0.983

VSAQ: Veteran Specific Activity Questionnaire; RPC: Rating of Perceived Capacity; CRF: Questionnaire of Cardiorespiratory Fitness.

subjects with high and low cardio-respiratory capacity in comparison to VSAQ and RPC. Notably, the CRF may be limited when assessing cardiorespiratory capacity in subjects with $V_{O_2 max} > 55.0 \, mL \cdot kg^{-1} \cdot min^{-1}$ [29], which could be a problem when designing ramp protocols in highly fit individuals. However, fewer than 20% of ordinary healthy individuals achieve this level [7]. It therefore seems unlikely

that the final speed would be wrongly determined from inaccurate estimation of $V_{O_2 max}$ estimation, at least in most healthy nonathletic subjects.

In what concerns the second study, the literature is mixed regarding criteria to determine the initial speed for ramp testing [9, 11]. Recommendations from different expert panels are also ambiguous with regard to this issue

TABLE 5: Intercept, slope, R-square (r^2), and standard error of estimate (SEE) for the regression models obtained in ramp protocols initiating with speeds corresponding to 50% of the estimated $V_{O_2 \max}$ (CPET1bis), 50% of the measured $V_{O_2 \max}$ (CPET2), and 60% of the measure $V_{O_2 \max}$ (CPET3).

	Y intercept	Slope	r-Square	SEE ($mL \cdot kg^{-1} \cdot min^{-1}$)
V_{O_2} versus speed in CPET1bis	$-4.882 \pm 2.696^{*}$	$0.96 \pm 0.027^{\S}$	0.93 ± 0.050	2.14 ± 0.67
V_{O_2} versus speed in CPET2	$-8.270 \pm 6.312^{*}$	$0.94 \pm 0.029^{\S}$	0.89 ± 0.054	2.19 ± 0.55
V_{O_2} versus speed in CPET3	$-14.666 \pm 8.958^{*}$	$0.92 \pm 0.036^{\S}$	0.86 ± 0.065	2.48 ± 0.67

* Intercept significantly different from zero ($P < 0.0001$).
§ Slope significantly different from 1.0 ($P < 0.0001$).

[4, 7, 14, 15], and no formal criteria are available on this important aspect of ramp protocols. Our findings suggested that initial speeds within the range corresponding to 50% to 60% $V_{O_2 \max}$ influenced the duration of the test (CPET1bis = 13.7 ± 1.8 min > CPET2 = 10.7 ± 0.9 min ≅ CPET3 = 10.6 ± 0.9 min, P < 0.0001), but not the achieved $V_{O_2 \max}$ (CPET1bis = 40.7 ± 5.9 $mL \cdot kg^{-1} \cdot min^{-1}$ ≅ CPET2 = 40.0 ± 5.6 $mL \cdot kg^{-1} \cdot min^{-1}$ ≅ CPET3 = 40.3 ± 5.5 $mL \cdot kg^{-1} \cdot min^{-1}$, P = 0.14). From these results, any initial speed within this range would be appropriate for performing ramp tests. In contrast, the relationship between workload and V_{O_2} among the tests was affected by the initial speed. Considering the identity line as a reference for the ideal regression between workload and V_{O_2}, the current results suggest that higher initial speed produced the lowest R-squares (e.g., poorest adjustment to the identity line) (CPET3—60% $V_{O_2 \max}$ < CPET2—50% $V_{O_2 \max}$ < CPET1bis—50% $V_{O_2 \max}$).

Early research confirms the concept that the initial speed applied does not influence measured $V_{O_2 \max}$. Kang et al. compared three incremental treadmill protocols (Åstrand, Bruce, and Costill/Fox) in 25 sedentary subjects (10 women) [36]. The protocols began with speeds of 9.7 $km \cdot h^{-1}$, 2.5 $km \cdot h^{-1}$, and 14.4 $km \cdot h^{-1}$, respectively, and no differences in $V_{O_2 \max}$ were detected. The relationship between workload and V_{O_2} was not specifically addressed, but the authors considered that this could have been good, at least in the Costill/Fox protocol. The high initial speed significantly shortened the tests (to about 5 min) and precluded the identification of the ventilatory threshold.

In 1991, Myers et al. compared $V_{O_2 \max}$ obtained during ramp and conventional staged protocols (Bruce and Balke modified), which were very different with regard to the combination of initial speed, treadmill grade, and workload increment. The duration of tests was significantly different (Bruce: 6.6 ± 1.5 min versus Balke: 10.4 ± 3.4 min and Ramp: 9.1 ± 1.4 min, P < 0.05), with little impact on $V_{O_2 \max}$ (Bruce: 22.3 ± 8.0 $mL \cdot kg^{-1} \cdot min^{-1}$ versus Balke: 21.1 ± 8.0 $mL \cdot kg^{-1} \cdot min^{-1}$ and Ramp: 21.0 ± 8.0 $mL \cdot kg^{-1} \cdot min^{-1}$, P < 0.05). However, slopes and SEE for the regression curves between workload and V_{O_2} showed more linear relationships in the ramp protocol (Bruce: slope = 0.62 and SEE = 4.0 $mL \cdot kg^{-1} \cdot min^{-1}$; Balke: Slope = 0.79 and SEE = 3.4 $mL \cdot kg^{-1} \cdot min^{-1}$; Ramp: Slope = 0.80 and SEE = 2.5 $mL \cdot kg^{-1} \cdot min^{-1}$). In other words, differences

in the protocol design may reflect on physiological relationships in submaximal workloads, but not necessarily on the assessed $V_{O_2 \max}$. Our findings seem to ratify this idea.

In conclusion, CRF was superior in comparison with RPC and VSAQ to estimate maximal cardio-respiratory capacity and should be preferred when attempting to determine an appropriate speed for ramp testing. Initial speeds within the range corresponding to 50–60% $V_{O_2 \max}$ estimated or measured did not affect assessed $V_{O_2 \max}$. Nevertheless, speeds higher than 50% $V_{O_2 \max}$ may influence the quality of submaximal relationships between work rate and V_{O_2}. Moreover, higher speeds applied at the beginning of ramp protocols may hinder the performance of subjects with poor fitness levels and compromise test results. This information should be considered when data from exercise testing is used to establish relative exercise intensities for exercise prescription.

Acknowledgments

This paper was supported by grants from FAPERJ (Carlos Chagas Foundation for the Research Support in the State of Rio de Janeiro, Rio de Janeiro, Brazil) and CNPq (Brazilian Council for the Technological and Scientifical Development, Brasília, Brazil).

References

[1] S. Mora, R. F. Redberg, Y. Cui et al., "Ability of exercise testing to predict cardiovascular and all-cause death in asymptomatic women: a 20-year follow-up of the lipid research clinics prevalence study," *JAMA*, vol. 290, no. 12, pp. 1600–1607, 2003.

[2] M. Gulati, H. R. Black, L. J. Shaw et al., "The prognostic value of a nomogram for exercise capacity in women," *The New England Journal of Medicine*, vol. 353, no. 5, pp. 468–475, 2005.

[3] E. S. H. Kim, H. Ishwaran, E. Blackstone, and M. S. Lauer, "External prognostic validations and comparisons of age- and gender-adjusted exercise capacity predictions," *Journal of the American College of Cardiology*, vol. 50, no. 19, pp. 1867–1875, 2007.

[4] R. J. Gibbons, G. J. Balady, J. T. Bricker et al., "ACC/AHA 2002 guideline update for exercise testing: summary article. A report of the American College of Cardiology/American Heart Association Task Force on Practice Guidelines (Committee to update the 1997 exercise testing guidelines)," *Journal of the

American College of Cardiology, vol. 40, no. 8, pp. 1531–1540, 2002.

[5] M. Maeder, T. Wolber, R. Atefy et al., "Impact of the exercise mode on exercise capacity: bicycle testing revisited," *Chest*, vol. 128, no. 4, pp. 2804–2811, 2005.

[6] P. G. Snell, J. Stray-Gundersen, B. D. Levine, M. N. Hawkins, and P. B. Raven, "Maximal oxygen uptake as a parametric measure of cardiorespiratory capacity," *Medicine and Science in Sports and Exercise*, vol. 39, no. 1, pp. 103–107, 2007.

[7] American College of Sports Medicine (ACSM), *Guidelines of Exercise Testing and Exercise Prescription*, Lea & Febiger, Philadelphia, Pa, USA, 8nd edition, 2009.

[8] M. Maeder, T. Wolber, R. Atefy et al., "A nomogram to select the optimal treadmill ramp protocol in subjects with high exercise capacity: validation and comparison with the Bruce protocol," *Journal of Cardiopulmonary Rehabilitation*, vol. 26, no. 1, pp. 16–23, 2006.

[9] J. Myers, N. Buchanan, D. Walsh et al., "Comparison of the ramp versus standard exercise protocols," *Journal of the American College of Cardiology*, vol. 17, no. 6, pp. 1334–1342, 1991.

[10] B. J. Whipp, J. A. Davis, F. Torres, and K. Wasserman, "A test to determine parameters of aerobic function during exercise," *Journal of Applied Physiology Respiratory Environmental and Exercise Physiology*, vol. 50, no. 1, pp. 217–221, 1981.

[11] J. Myers, N. Buchanan, D. Smith et al., "Individualized ramp treadmill; Observations on a new protocol," *Chest*, vol. 101, no. 5, pp. 236–241, 1992.

[12] F. A. Cunha, A. W. Midgley, W. D. Monteiro, and P. T. V. Farinatti, "Influence of cardiopulmonary exercise testing protocol and resting VO_2 Assessment on $\%HR_{2max}$, $\%HRR$, $\%VO_{2max}$ and $\%VO_2R$ Relationships," *International Journal of Sports Medicine*, vol. 31, no. 5, pp. 319–326, 2010.

[13] J. Myers and D. Bellin, "Ramp exercise protocols for clinical and cardiopulmonary exercise testing," *Sports Medicine*, vol. 30, no. 1, pp. 23–29, 2000.

[14] G. F. Fletcher, G. J. Balady, E. A. Amsterdam et al., "Exercise standards for testing and training: a statement for healthcare professionals from the American Heart Association," *Circulation*, vol. 104, no. 14, pp. 1694–1740, 2001.

[15] A. W. Midgley, D. J. Bentley, H. Luttikholt, L. R. McNaughton, and G. P. Millet, "Challenging a dogma of exercise physiology: does an incremental exercise test for valid V·O2max determination really need to last between 8 and 12 minutes?" *Sports Medicine*, vol. 38, no. 6, pp. 441–447, 2008.

[16] American Thoracic Society/American College of Chest Physicians, "ATS/ACCP Statement on cardiopulmonary exercise testing," *American Journal of Respiratory and Critical Care Medicine*, vol. 167, no. 2, pp. 211–277, 2003.

[17] A. Mezzani, P. Agostoni, A. Cohen-Solal et al., "Standards for the use of cardiopulmonary exercise testing for the functional evaluation of cardiac patients: a report from the exercise physiology section of the European association for cardiovascular prevention and rehabilitation," *European Journal of Cardiovascular Prevention and Rehabilitation*, vol. 16, no. 3, pp. 249–267, 2009.

[18] S. C. da Silva, W. D. Monteiro, and P. T. V. Farinatti, "Exercise maximum capacity assessment: a review on the traditional protocols and the evolution to individualized models," *Revista Brasileira de Medicina do Esporte*, vol. 17, no. 5, pp. 363–369, 2011.

[19] J. Myers, W. Herbert, P. Ribisl, and V. F. Froelicher, "A nomogram to predict exercise capacity from a specific activity questionnaire and clinical data," *American Journal of Cardiology*, vol. 73, no. 8, pp. 591–596, 1994.

[20] J. Myers, D. Bader, R. Madhavan, and V. Froelicher, "Validation of a specific activity questionnaire to estimate exercise tolerance in patients referred for exercise testing," *American Heart Journal*, vol. 142, no. 6, pp. 1041–1046, 2001.

[21] A. G. M. Wisén, R. G. Farazdaghi, and B. Wohlfart, "A novel rating scale to predict maximal exercise capacity," *European Journal of Applied Physiology*, vol. 87, no. 4-5, pp. 350–357, 2002.

[22] C. E. Matthews, D. P. Heil, P. S. Freedson, and H. Pastides, "Classification of cardiorespiratory fitness without exercise testing," *Medicine and Science in Sports and Exercise*, vol. 31, no. 3, pp. 486–493, 1999.

[23] G. A. Maranhão Neto, P. M. Lourenço, and P. T. Farinatti, "Prediction of aerobic fitness without stress testing and applicability to epidemiological studies: a systematic review," *Cadernos de Saúde Pública*, vol. 20, no. 1, pp. 48–56, 2004.

[24] G. De Albuquerque Maranhão Neto, A. C. M. P. De Leon, and P. De Tarso Veras Farinatti, "Cross-cultural equivalence of three scales used to estimate cardiorespiratory fitness in the elderly," *Cadernos de Saúde Pública*, vol. 24, no. 11, pp. 2499–2510, 2008.

[25] A. W. Midgley, L. R. Mcnaughton, and S. Carroll, "Effect of the $\dot{V}o2$ time-averaging interval on the reproducibility of $\dot{V}o2max$ in healthy athletic subjects," *Clinical Physiology and Functional Imaging*, vol. 27, no. 2, pp. 122–125, 2007.

[26] E. T. Howley, D. R. Bassett, and H. G. Welch, "Criteria for maximal oxygen uptake: review and commentary," *Medicine and Science in Sports and Exercise*, vol. 27, no. 9, pp. 1292–1301, 1995.

[27] J. M. Bland and D. G. Altman, "Statistical methods for assessing agreement between two methods of clinical measurement," *The Lancet*, vol. 1, no. 8476, pp. 307–310, 1986.

[28] J. H. Zar, *Comparing Simple Linear Regression Equations. Biostatistical Analysis*, Prentice-Hall, Englewoods Cliff, NJ,USA, 1984.

[29] P. McAuley, J. Myers, J. Abella, and V. Froelicher, "Evaluation of a specific activity questionnaire to predict mortality in men referred for exercise testing," *American Heart Journal*, vol. 151, no. 4, pp. 890.e1–890.e7, 2006.

[30] A. S. Jackson, S. N. Blair, M. T. Mahar, L. T. Wier, R. M. Ross, and J. E. Stuteville, "Prediction of functional aerobic capacity without exercise testing," *Medicine and Science in Sports and Exercise*, vol. 22, no. 6, pp. 863–870, 1990.

[31] D. P. Heil, P. S. Freedson, L. E. Ahlquist, J. Price, and J. M. Rippe, "Nonexercise regression models to estimate peak oxygen consumption," *Medicine and Science in Sports and Exercise*, vol. 27, no. 4, pp. 599–606, 1995.

[32] J. D. George, W. J. Stone, and L. N. Burkett, "Non-exercise VO2max estimation for physically active college students," *Medicine and Science in Sports and Exercise*, vol. 29, no. 3, pp. 415–423, 1997.

[33] R. Jurca, A. S. Jackson, M. J. LaMonte et al., "Assessing cardiorespiratory fitness without performing exercise testing," *American Journal of Preventive Medicine*, vol. 29, no. 3, pp. 185–193, 2005.

[34] D. I. Bradshaw, J. D. George, A. Hyde et al., "An accurate VO_{2max} nonexercise regression model for 18-65-year-old adults," *Research Quarterly for Exercise and Sport*, vol. 76, no. 4, pp. 426–432, 2005.

[35] L. T. Wier, A. S. Jackson, G. W. Ayers, and B. Arenare, "Nonexercise models for estimating V·O2max with waist

girth, percent fat, or BMI," *Medicine and Science in Sports and Exercise*, vol. 38, no. 3, pp. 555–561, 2006.

[36] J. Kang, E. C. Chaloupka, M. A. Mastrangelo, G. B. Biren, and R. J. Robertson, "Physiological comparisons among three maximal treadmill exercise protocols in trained and untrained individuals," *European Journal of Applied Physiology*, vol. 84, no. 4, pp. 291–295, 2001.

35

Decreased Apoptotic Rate of Alveolar Macrophages of Patients with Idiopathic Pulmonary Fibrosis

Fotios Drakopanagiotakis,[1] **Areti Xifteri,**[1] **Evaggelos Tsiambas,**[2]
Andreas Karameris,[2] **Konstantina Tsakanika,**[3] **Napoleon Karagiannidis,**[1]
Demetrios Mermigkis,[1] **Vlasis Polychronopoulos,**[1] **and Demosthenes Bouros**[4]

[1] *3rd Respiratory Medicine Department, Sismanoglio General Hospital, 15126 Marousi, Greece*
[2] *Department of Pathology and Computerized Image Analysis, 417 NIMTS Hospital, 11521 Athens, Greece*
[3] *Bronchoalveolar Lavage Unit, Sismanoglio General Hospital, 15126 Marousi, Greece*
[4] *Department of Pneumonology, University Hospital of Alexandroupolis and Medical School of Democritus University of Thrace,*
    68100 Alexandroupolis, Greece

Correspondence should be addressed to Demosthenes Bouros, bouros@med.duth.gr

Academic Editor: Stefano Centanni

Introduction. Increased apoptosis of epithelial cells and decreased apoptosis of myofibroblasts are involved in the pathogenesis of IPF. The apoptotic profile of alveolar macrophages (AMs) in IPF is unclear. *Aim*. To investigate whether AMs of patients with IPF exhibit a different apoptotic profile compared to normal subjects. *Methods*. We analyzed, by immunohistochemistry, the expression of the apoptotic markers fas, fas ligand , bcl-2, and bax in AM obtained from bronchoalveolar lavage fluid (BALF) of 20 newly diagnosed, treatment-naive IPF patients and of 16 controls. Apoptosis of AM was evaluated by Apoptag immunohistochemistry. IPF patients received either interferon-g and corticosteroids or azathioprine and corticosteroids for six months. *Results*. BALF AMs undergoing apoptosis were significantly less in IPF patients. No difference was found in the expression of fas or fas ligand, bcl-2 and bax between IPF and control group. No difference was found between the respiratory function parameters of the two treatment groups after six months. A positive correlation was found between the number of bcl-2 positive stained macrophages and DLCO after treatment. *Conclusions*. The decreased apoptotic rate of AM of patients with IPF is not associated with decreased expression of apoptosis mediators involved in the external or internal apoptotic pathway.

1. Introduction

Idiopathic pulmonary fibrosis (IPF) is a chronic diffuse lung disease, characterised by progressive deterioration which ultimately leads to death [1].

Apoptosis is an important physiological process for the development and the maintenance of tissue homeostasis which ensures a balance between cellular proliferation and turnover in nearly all tissues [2]. Apoptosis can be activated by two pathways.

(a) The extrinsic or death-receptor pathway which involves the activation of death receptors present in the cell membrane, which are activated by death ligands. Fas and TNF-receptor 1 are the two most known death receptors. Connection of death Ligand, such as Fas Ligand to its death receptor leads to receptor polymerisation and activation of adaptor proteins called "activated death domains" which activate procaspase molecules to caspases.

(b) The intrinsic pathway which is associated to an increase of mitochondrial permeability and is activated by cellular "stress." Cellular stress leads to reduced expression of antiapoptotic mitochondrial proteins (bcl-2, bcl-x) and to increased expression of proapoptotic mitochondrial proteins (bak, bax, bim). The reduction of anti-apoptotic proteins causes an increase in mitochondrial membrane permeability and subsequent outflux of cytochrome c to the cytoplasm.

Increased apoptosis of epithelial cells resulting to inefficient reepithelialization [3] and resistance to apoptosis of fibroblasts and myofibroblasts associated with increased fibrosis has been described in lung biopsies of patients with IPF [2].

Macrophages play an important role for the removal of apoptotic cells, a process called "efferocytosis" [4]. Apoptotic macrophages have been reported to induce the apoptosis of normal macrophages and exaggerate lung fibrosis in experimental models and participate in the pathogenesis of fibrotic lung diseases such as the Hermansky-Pudlak syndrome [5]. However, the apoptotic profile of macrophages in IPF is not clear.

Bronchoalveolar lavage is a useful tool for research purposes in patients with idiopathic pulmonary fibrosis. Different cell populations can be obtained from bronchoalveolar lavage, in order to be evaluated in relation to the cytokines and growth factors, which they produce, as well as to their apoptotic behavior [6].

In the current study we investigated the expression of apoptotic markers in naive alveolar macrophages obtained from BAL of IPF patients and of normal subjects. Furthermore, we tried to correlate apoptotic markers' expression with clinical parameters.

2. Materials and Methods

2.1. Subjects. The study group consisted of twenty patients with newly diagnosed IPF who were admitted to "Sismanoglio" hospital from 2003 until 2007. The patients had not received any prior treatment for IPF. The diagnosis of IPF was established either by a surgical biopsy showing a usual interstitial pneumonia pattern or using the criteria of the American Thoracic Society [7–9].

Patients with acute exacerbation of IPF, infection, or uncontrolled heart disease were not included in the study. The control group consisted of otherwise healthy individuals who were submitted to bronchoscopy for various reasons, mainly chronic cough and hemoptysis. No subject in the control group suffered from malignant, inflammatory, or interstitial lung disease.

2.2. Study Design. The twenty patients were randomised to receive a combination of interferon-g (IFNγ-1b) 200 μg subcutaneously 3 times per week and 10 mg of oral prednisolone daily or 150 mg of oral azathioprine (AZA) and 10 mg of oral prednisolone daily. The study was approved by the Bioethics Committee of Sismanoglio Hospital and all participants gave informed consent.

Patients were evaluated at the beginning, three months and six months after treatment. Lung function testing, HRCT, bronchoscopy, and bronchoalveolar lavage were performed prior to treatment. Lung function testing was performed six months after treatment.

The two patient groups were compared regarding lung function parameters, and their correlation to bronchoalveolar lavage apoptosis markers in AM prior to treatment.

2.3. Methods. Fiberoptic bronchoscopy with bronchoalveolar lavage was performed in the newly diagnosed, treatment-naive IPF patients and in the control group according to recommended guidelines and previous reports [10, 11]. Cells were separated from BAL by low-speed centrifugation at 300 g for five minutes at 4°C and were washed three times with cold minimal essential medium (MEM) containing 25 Mm Hepes buffer. Total cell counts were determined using an improved Neubauer counting chamber. Slide preparations for differential percentage counting of the cells were made with a Shandon cytocentrifuge (Cytospin II, Shandon Ltd, Runcorn, Cheshire, UK). The differential count was determined on a stained preparation stained by May-Grunwald Giemsa staining and Papanicolaou staining after counting more than 1000 cells.

2.4. Antibodies and Immunohistochemistry (IHC). We selected and applied monoclonal antibodies including anti-bcl2 (Dako-Cytomation, Danemark), anti-bax (Dako-Cytomation, Denmark), anti-Fas (CD95) (Novo-Castra, UK) and also anti-fas ligand (Novo-Castra, UK) according to the manufacturer instructions. For detection of apoptosis, we used the Apopt-Ag plus peroxidase in situ apoptosis detection kit (Chemicon International) [12].

2.5. Evaluation of IHC Results by Computerized Image Analysis (CIA). We performed CIA by using a semiutomated system with the following hardware features: Intel Pentium IV, MATROX II CARD FRAME GRABBER, CAMERA MICROWAVE SYSTEMS (resolution of 800 $\times$ 600), microscope Olympus BX-50 and the following software: Windows XP/Image Pro Plus version 3.0-Media Cybernetics 1997. Measurements regarding protein expression of the markers described above were performed in 5 optical fields per case and at magnification of 400 (40 $\times$ 10). The brightness values represent levels within a 256-level scale (0–255). In all examined cases, areas of significant cellularity including isolated macrophages or small clusters of them were considered to be eligible for measurements. Semiautomated segmentation was performed by splitting those small clusters. Furthermore, for the evaluation of ApopTag method, the total amount of signals per case was measured (area covering brown staining pattern) at the same magnification (Figure 1).

2.6. Statistical Analysis. Analysis of variance was used to assess differences of the *apopt ag signals, apopt ag area and bcl2, bax, fas and fasl density* between patients and controls. Prior to the analysis, the density, signals, and area values were transposed into natural logarithms in order to reduce the within-patient variability. Summary statistics are expressed as in means and 95% confidence intervals. Tests were 2-sided and level of statistical significance was set at 5%. $P < 0.05$ values were considered as significant. For statistical analysis, SPSS version 17 was used.

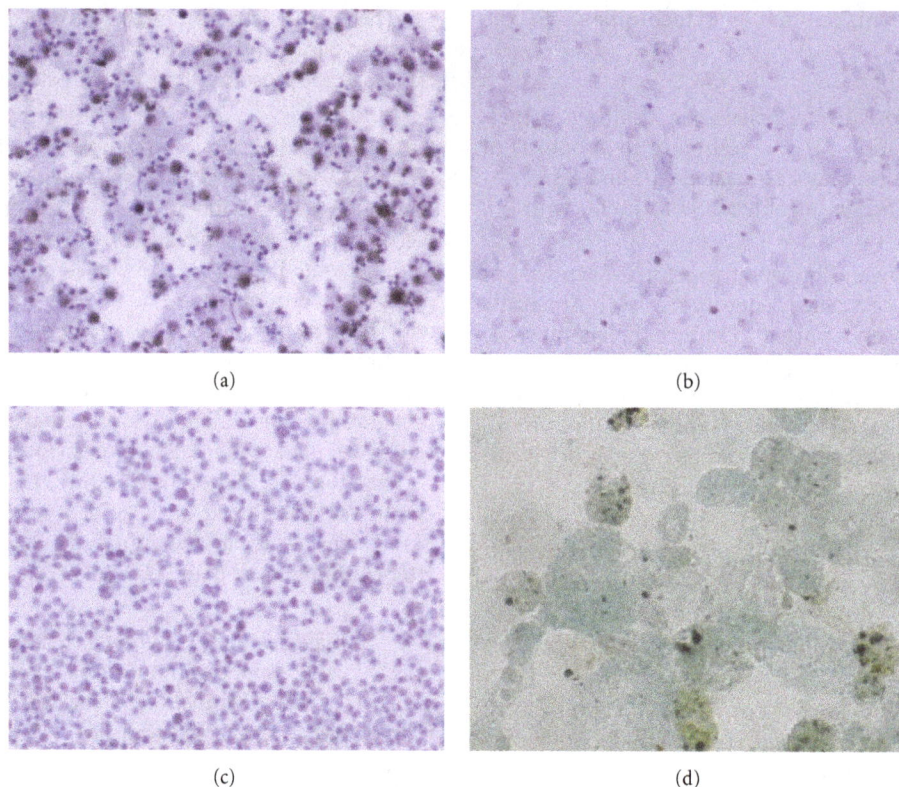

FIGURE 1: Computerized image analysis of stained BALF macrophages in patients with IPF. Brown colored dots represent the expression of apoptotic markers (objects) in BALF macrophages: (a) bax, (b) bcl-2, (c) fas, (d) ApoptAg.

TABLE 1: Patients' baseline characteristics.

	Minimum	Maximum	Mean	Std. deviation
Age	54,00	80,00	69,05	6,20
Symptoms' duration (months)	2,00	48,00	14,15	11,65
FVC%	37,00	99,00	71,1	19,1
DLCO%	6,00	122,00	55,2	27,9
PaO₂	58,00	95,00	72,09	11,54

3. Results

Baseline characteristics of the patients are shown in Table 1. Mean age was 69,05 years with a mean duration of symptoms of 14,15 months. Respiratory function was moderately impaired with a mean FVC 71,1% of predicted, diffusion capacity for carbon monoxide 55,2% of predicted and mean PaO_2 of 72,09 mm Hg.

Neutrophils, eosinophils, and mast cells were significantly increased in the BALF of patients with IPF compared to the control group. BALF of patients with IPF was also characterized by reduced percentage of macrophages (Table 2). There was no difference in bronchoalveolar lavage cell count between the two patient groups at baseline.

We examined the expression of specific apoptotic markers in BALF macrophages of treatment-naive patients and control group, representing activation of the extrinsic (fas, fas ligand) and the intrinsic pathway (bcl-2, bax) and total expression of apoptosis, based on expression of Apoptag; a statistically significant difference was found between the IPF group and control group at presentation regarding expression of Apoptag. Macrophages of patients with IPF showed reduced expression of Apoptag and reduced Apoptag stained area compared to macrophages of the control group (Table 3, Figures 2, 3, and 4).

Immunohistochemical staining showed no difference regarding the staining intensity of specific apoptotic markers of either the intrinsic (bcl-2, bax) or extrinsic apoptosis pathway (fas, fasl). However, the number of macrophages of IPF patients expressing the anti-apoptotic protein bcl-2 was significantly less compared to controls (Table 3, Figures 2, 3, and 5).

There were no differences between the interferon-g plus prednisone and azathioprine plus prednisone groups of patients regarding baseline demographic characteristics, smoking habit, clinical presentation, and respiratory function parameters.

Comparison of respiratory function parameters six months after treatment showed no difference between the two patient groups (Table 4).

We tried to correlate the expression of apoptotic markers in macrophages prior to treatment with respiratory function parameters (FVC, FEV1, DLCO) in patients with IPF before

TABLE 2: Bronchoalveolar lavage fluid parameters of IPF patients and control group at entry.

Cell type	IPF group (%) $n = 20$	Control group (%) $n = 10$	P value
Neutrophils	$24,6 \pm 4,6$	$6,1 \pm 3,8$	**0.001**
Macrophages	$55,9 \pm 6,9$	$81,4 \pm 5,4$	**0.001**
Lymphocytes	$5,7 \pm 3,7$	$12,6 \pm 2,8$	**0.001**
Eosinophils	$10,8 \pm 3,7$	$0,4 \pm 1,0$	**0.001**
Mast cells	$2,6 \pm 2,1$	0 ± 0	**0.001**
Total cell count ($\times 10^6$)	$20,06 \pm 3,03$	$26,3 \pm 4,9$	**0.001**

$P < 0.05$: statistically significant.

TABLE 3: Apoptotic markers' expression (CIA mean values) in patients before treatment and in control subjects.

	Control group [CI]	IPF group [CI]	P
ApoptAg density	100,1 [84,8–118,2]	124,8 [109,6–142,0]	**0.030**
ApoptAg area	580,03 [281,5–1193,7]	84,88 [40,8–175,2]	**<0.001**
ApoptAg (+) cells	78,8 [49,9–124,2]	11,1 [5,19–22,7]	**<0.001**
Bcl-2 density	149,8 [131,3–170,8]	151,7 [138,0–166,9]	0.883
Bcl-2 (+) cells	48,2 [26,1–88,5]	21,3 [12,9–34,5]	**0.030**
Bax density	134,6 [121,7–148,9]	131,0 [117,9–145,6]	0.771
Bax (+) cells	65,4 [37,2–114,5]	72,3 [53,9–96,7]	0.711
Fas ligand density	139,2 [129,2–150,1]	133,3 [126,1–140,9]	0.312
Fas ligand (+) cells	49,3 [30,1–80,5]	71,0 [51,7–97,3]	0.172
Fas density	163,5 [149,1–179,2]	151,3 [135,5–169,0]	0.291
Fas (+) cells	23,1 [13,5–39,1]	29,8 [18,9–46,7]	0.461

$P < 0.05$: statistically significant.

and after treatment. Expression of apoptotic markers in BALF did not correlate to pulmonary function parameters neither before nor after treatment with the exception of a positive relation between the number of bcl-2 positive stained macrophages and DLCO after treatment (r : 0.646, P : 0.032) (Table 5).

4. Discussion

In our study we demonstrated decreased apoptosis of bronchoalveolar lavage macrophages in patients with IPF compared to controls. This difference could not be attributed to the increased activation of the external apoptosis pathway, as measured by Fas, Fas ligand cellular expression, neither to increased expression of anti-apoptotic molecules of the intrinsic pathway such as bcl-2.

Alveolar macrophages are an important source of cytokines which participate in fibrogenesis. Little is known about the apoptotic profile of alveolar macrophages in IPF [4]. Intratracheal administration of apoptotic macrophages causes increased macrophage infiltration and apoptosis [13, 14] and in experimental models bleomycin induces alveolar macrophage apoptosis [15–17].

In lung biopsies of patients with IPF, fas was significantly expressed in macrophages compared to control [18]. In bleomycin-induced fibrosis increased macrophage expression of bcl-2 and bax proteins as well as caspases-1 and 3 has been described [19, 20]. In the present study, we did not find increased expression of bcl-2 or bax. This difference probably represents the discordance between bleomycin-induced fibrosis in animal models and pulmonary fibrosis in humans. Our present results are in accordance with previous observations of our group [21]. Moreover, immunochemistry depicts only a snapshot of a continuous, self-destructing process, without being able to describe the whole "pathogenesis story."

Cytokines can influence macrophage apoptotic death: macrophage apoptosis can be increased by interferon-gamma and reduced by IL-4, IL-10 and TGF-b [22]. Mice deficient for macrophage-colony stimulating factor (M-CSF) develop less pulmonary fibrosis and have a decreased number of macrophages in their lungs after bleomycin installation. M-CSF was significantly of higher levels in the bronchoalveolar lavage of patients with IPF [23].

Since macrophages participate so actively in cytokine production and the development of inflammation and fibrosis, increased removal of macrophages from the fibrosis sites might be beneficial, especially if this procedure could be realized by a noninflammatory process such as apoptosis. Recent studies support such a hypothesis, showing that alveolar macrophage depletion is associated with reduction of fibrosis in animal models [24]. We assume that the decreased apoptotic rate of macrophages shown in the present study could be involved in the preservation of pulmonary fibrosis.

TABLE 4: Pulmonary function parameters before and after treatment with IFNγ-1b or AZA.

	IFNγ-1b group			AZA group		
	Before treatment	After treatment	P	Before treatment	After treatment	P
FVC (%pred)	73.8 ± 18.6	64.0 ± 23.8	0.096	68.4 ± 21.6	68.5 ± 19.6	0.977
FEV$_1$ (%pred)	80.8 ± 19.4	70.7 ± 24.2	0.169	73.1 ± 19.5	72.1 ± 14.0	0.807
DLCO (%pred)	50.9 ± 39.4	37.5 ± 18.6	0.110	59.5 ± 15.7	61.8 ± 26.0	0.608
PO$_2$ at rest	76.09 ± 9,60	72.66 ± 12.97	0.490	68,10 ± 12,48	64.90 ± 8.68	0.360

$P < 0.05$: statistically significant.

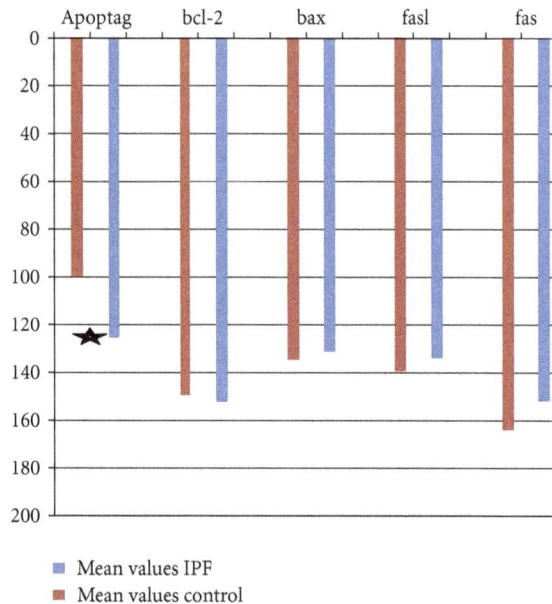

FIGURE 2: Mean staining densities for apoptotic markers between IPF patients (blue) and control (red). Values range between 0–255 A statistically significant increase in Apoptag density (reduced apoptosis expression) is observed in IPF patients.

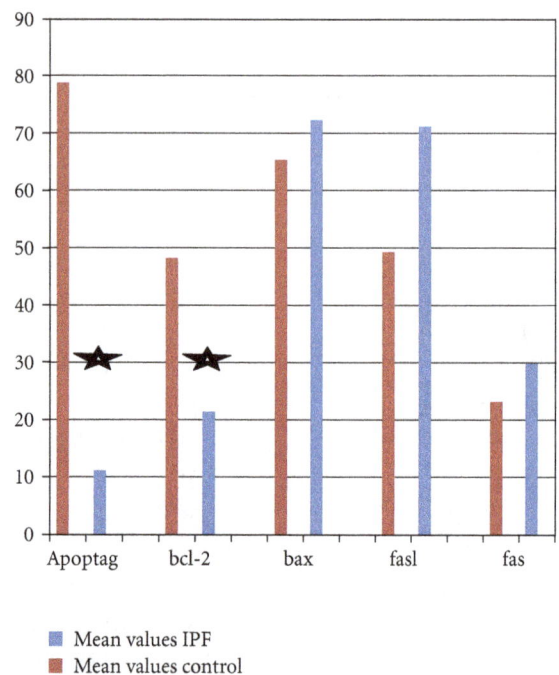

FIGURE 3: Mean number of positive objects (positive-stained cells) for apoptotic markers between IPF patients (blue) and control (red). A statistically significant increased number of Apoptag objects and of the antiapoptosis marker bcl-2 are observed in the control group compared to IPF patients.

Macrophages are the professional phagocytes of apoptotic cells which can engulf apoptotic remnants [25]. Macrophages ingesting apoptotic cells release the anti-inflammatory cytokines IL-10 and TGF-b1 [26, 27]. Furthermore, apoptotic cells can produce IL-10 and TGF-b1 as well, thus enhancing the phagocytic capacity of macrophages [28–30]. Macrophages which phagocytose apoptotic bodies can also release proapoptotic factors that induce apoptosis of adjacent cells [31].

Bronchoalveolar lavage is a useful research tool for the study of interstitial lung diseases [6]. An increase of neutrophils and eosinophils in the bronchoalveolar lavage of patients with IPF correlates to worse prognosis [32–34]. Such a difference was observed between IPF patients and the control group in our study.

Pharmacological therapies have not been shown to offer a survival benefit in patients with IPF [35–37]. We have also reported that interferon-g and azathioprine plus corticosteroids have proven equally nonefficacious in preventing deterioration in IPF in a six month period [38].

We tried to correlate apoptotic markers' expression with parameters of respiratory function, as an attempt to identify a potential biomarker of the disease. Such a correlation could not be established except for the relation of the antiapoptotic factor bcl-2 signals with diffusing capacity for carbon monoxide after treatment. This is the first report to our knowledge of such a correlation. However, this correlation should be regarded in caution and reassessed in larger studies as its physiological rationale is unclear. At present, better biomarkers for IPF do exist and they include KL-6, surfactant proteins A and D. Soluble Fas in bronchoalveolar lavage and in serum has also been related to IPF severity [39].

Important limitations apply to our study: first, the number of patients included is relatively small. However, IPF is a rare disease and bronchoscopy is not performed in all cases [7].

TABLE 5: Correlation of apoptotic markers' expression with respiratory function parameters before and after treatment in patients with IPF.

Before treatment		FVC	FVC%	FEV1	FEV1%	FEV1/FVC	DLCO	DLCO%	aFVC	aFVC%	aFEV1	aFEV1%	aFEV1/FVC	aDLCO	aDLCO%
ApoptAg (+) cells	Pearson	,010	-,215	,021	-,190	-,104	,046	,066	-,060	-,212	-,027	-,192	,139	-,219	-,234
	P	,966	,377	,931	,436	,672	,875	,821	,812	,398	,916	,446	,583	,473	,441
Apopt Ag area	Pearson	,021	-,206	,046	-,247	,134	-,377	-,340	-,069	-,236	-,002	-,242	,259	-,300	-,439
	P	,942	,460	,871	,374	,634	,283	,337	,806	,397	,994	,384	,351	,343	,153
ApoptAg density	Pearson	-,052	,177	,019	,240	,427	,042	,188	-,243	-,187	-,238	-,330	,348	-,517	-,538
	P	,854	,529	,947	,390	,113	,908	,602	,383	,504	,393	,230	,204	,086	,071
Bcl-2 (+) cells	Pearson	,388	,168	,365	,082	-,279	,204	,089	,449	,334	,462	,281	-,387	,557	,451
	P	,091	,479	,113	,730	,233	,466	,751	,054	,162	,046	,245	,102	,039	,106
Bcl-2 density	Pearson	-,196	-,082	-,215	-,071	,144	-,086	-,015	-,058	,075	-,048	,105	,188	-,439	-,421
	P	,467	,762	,425	,794	,594	,780	,961	,838	,792	,866	,709	,502	,204	,226
Bax (+) cells	Pearson	,039	-,199	-,086	-,314	-,643	,314	,265	,105	-,021	-,015	-,125	-,330	-,066	-,024
	P	,872	,401	,718	,178	,002	,255	,340	,667	,932	,951	,611	,168	,823	,936
Bax density	Pearson	-,072	-,257	-,125	-,379	,269	-,329	-,247	,183	,109	,198	,060	-,078	-,435	-,368
	P	,790	,337	,646	,148	,314	,250	,395	,513	,699	,479	,832	,781	,182	,266
Fas (+) cells	Pearson	,040	-,180	,070	-,217	-,268	,234	,241	,037	,000	,103	,044	-,011	,119	,157
	P	,866	,448	,769	,359	,254	,402	,386	,879	,999	,674	,857	,965	,686	,591
Fas density	Pearson	-,303	-,109	-,324	-,018	-,025	,258	,317	-,243	-,047	-,327	,009	,001	,124	,229
	P	,254	,688	,221	,947	,926	,395	,291	,383	,867	,234	,974	,997	,732	,524
Fasl (+) cells	Pearson	-,153	-,369	-,176	-,310	-,385	,073	,050	-,230	-,357	-,283	-,309	,089	-,081	-,028
	P	,520	,110	,459	,184	,094	,796	,861	,343	,133	,240	,198	,718	,782	,924
Fasl density	Pearson	,195	,172	,223	,195	-,077	,215	,152	,102	,053	,072	-,021	-,171	,548	,431
	P	,486	,541	,424	,487	,784	,501	,637	,729	,858	,807	,942	,558	,127	,247

$P < 0.05$: statistically significant.
FVC: forced vital capacity, FEV1: forced expiratory volume in one second, DLCO: diffusing capacity for carbon monoxide, a: after six months of treatment.

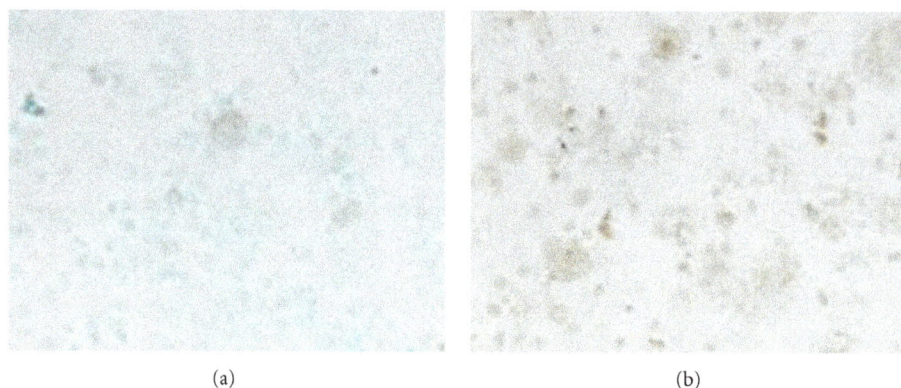

(a)   (b)

FIGURE 4: Decreased expression of apoptosis (Apoptag) in BALF macrophages of patients with IPF (a) compared to the control group (b).

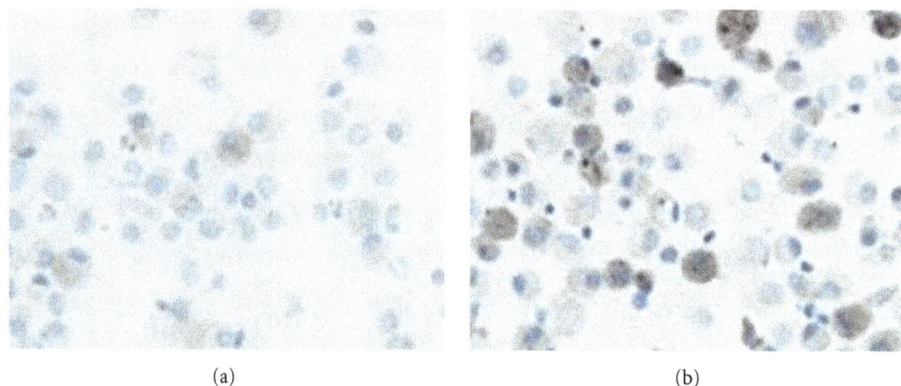

(a)   (b)

FIGURE 5: Decreased expression of the antiapoptotic bcl-2 protein in BALF macrophages of patients with IPF (a) compared to the control group (b).

Second, computerized image analysis is mainly applied in biopsies and there is limited data regarding its application in bronchoalveolar lavage. However, we preferred its use as it represents a more objective evaluation method compared to a semiquantitative measurement applied by the pathologist [40, 41]. In order to accumulate more data, not only did we measure staining intensity (which is more commonly measured in computerized image analysis) but also the total number of signals (objects) per optical field which represent positively stained cells.

Third, we did not examine the expression of other apoptotic factors such as TNF-a and TNF-a receptor or bak or bim of the extrinsic and intrinsic apoptotic pathway which might influence macrophage apoptosis [2]. We examined the expression of proteins that we thought would be more likely according to the literature, to be upregulated or downregulated in apoptosis of macrophages.

In conclusion, the present study showed that alveolar macrophages of patients with IPF exhibit a decreased apoptotic rate compared to normal subjects. We assume that macrophage resistance to apoptosis could be correlated to a continuous pathologic healing process observed in IPF.

References

[1] D. Bouros and K. M. Antoniou, "Current and future therapeutic approaches in idiopathic pulmonary fibrosis," *European Respiratory Journal*, vol. 26, no. 4, pp. 693–702, 2005.

[2] F. Drakopanagiotakis, A. Xifteri, V. Polychronopoulos, and D. Bouros, "Apoptosis in lung injury and fibrosis," *European Respiratory Journal*, vol. 32, no. 6, pp. 1631–1638, 2008.

[3] A. Tzouvelekis, A. Karameris, E. Tsiambas et al., "Telomerase in pulmonary fibrosis: a link to alveolar cell apoptosis and differentiation," *Pneumon*, vol. 23, no. 3, pp. 224–239, 2010.

[4] R. W. Vandivier, P. M. Henson, and I. S. Douglas, "Burying the dead: the impact of failed apoptotic cell removal (efferocytosis) on chronic inflammatory lung disease," *Chest*, vol. 129, no. 6, pp. 1673–1682, 2006.

[5] M. Brantly, N. A. Avila, V. Shotelersuk, C. Lucero, M. Huizing, and W. A. Gahl, "Pulmonary function and high-resolution CT findings in patients with an inherited form of pulmonary fibrosis, Hermansky-Pudlak syndrome, due to mutations in HPS-1," *Chest*, vol. 117, no. 1, pp. 129–136, 2000.

[6] S. Nagai, T. Handa, Y. Ito, M. Takeuchi, and T. Izumi, "Bronchoalveolar lavage in idiopathic interstitial lung diseases," *Seminars in Respiratory and Critical Care Medicine*, vol. 28, no. 5, pp. 496–503, 2007.

[7] "American Thoracic Society. Idiopathic pulmonary fibrosis: diagnosis and treatment. International consensus statement. American Thoracic Society (ATS), and the European Respiratory Society (ERS)," *American Journal of Respiratory and Critical Care Medicine*, vol. 161, no. 2, pp. 646–664, 2000.

[8] D. Bouros, "Idiopathic interstitial pneumonias: classification revision," *Pneumon*, vol. 23, no. 4, pp. 359–362, 2010.

[9] D. Bouros, "The new ATS/ERS/JRS IPF Guidelines," *Pneumon*, vol. 21, no. 2, pp. 117–120, 2008.

[10] H. Klech and W. Pohl, "Technical recommendations and guidelines for bronchoalveolar lavage (BAL)," *European Respiratory Journal*, vol. 2, no. 6, pp. 561–585, 1989.

[11] H. Klech and C. Hutter, "Clinical guidelines and indications for bronchoalveolar lavage (BAL): Report of the European Society of Pneumology Task Group on BAL," *European Respiratory Journal*, vol. 3, no. 8, pp. 937–969, 1990.

[12] Y. Gavrieli, Y. Sherman, and S. A. Ben-Sasson, "Identification of programmed cell death in situ via specific labeling of nuclear DNA fragmentation," *Journal of Cell Biology*, vol. 119, no. 3, pp. 493–501, 1992.

[13] L. Wang, J. M. Antonini, Y. Rojanasakul, V. Castranova, J. F. Scabilloni, and R. R. Mercer, "Potential role of apoptotic macrophages in pulmonary inflammation and fibrosis," *Journal of Cellular Physiology*, vol. 194, no. 2, pp. 215–224, 2003.

[14] L. Wang, J. F. Scabilloni, J. M. Antonini, Y. Rojanasakul, V. Castranova, and R. R. Mercer, "Induction of secondary apoptosis, inflammation, and lung fibrosis after intratracheal instillation of apoptotic cells in rats," *American Journal of Physiology*, vol. 290, no. 4, pp. L695–L702, 2006.

[15] R. F. Hamilton, L. Li, T. B. Felder, and A. Holian, "Bleomycin induces apoptosis in human alveolar macrophages," *American Journal of Physiology*, vol. 269, no. 3, pp. L318–L325, 1995.

[16] L. A. Ortiz, K. Moroz, J. Y. Liu et al., "Alveolar macrophage apoptosis and TNFf-α, but not p53, expression correlate with murine response to bleomycin," *American Journal of Physiology*, vol. 275, no. 6, pp. L1208–L1218, 1998.

[17] H. W. Zhao, S. Y. Hu, M. W. Barger, J. K. H. Ma, V. Castranova, and J. Y. C. Ma, "Time-dependent apoptosis of alveolar macrophages from rats exposed to bleomycin: involvement of TNF receptor 2," *Journal of Toxicology and Environmental Health A*, vol. 67, no. 17, pp. 1391–1406, 2004.

[18] K. Kuwano, H. Miyazaki, N. Hagimoto et al., "The involvement of Fas-Fas ligand pathway in fibrosing lung diseases," *American Journal of Respiratory Cell and Molecular Biology*, vol. 20, no. 1, pp. 53–60, 1999.

[19] K. Kuwano, N. Hagimoto, T. Tanaka et al., "Expression of apoptosis-regulatory genes in epithelial cells in pulmonary fibrosis in mice," *Journal of Pathology*, vol. 190, no. 2, pp. 221–229, 2000.

[20] K. Kuwano, R. Kunitake, T. Maeyama et al., "Attenuation of bleomycin-induced pneumopathy in mice by a caspase inhibitor," *American Journal of Physiology*, vol. 280, no. 2, pp. L316–L325, 2001.

[21] C. M. Mermigkis, K. Tsakanika, V. Polychronopoulos, N. Karagianidis, D. Mermigkis, and D. Bouros, "Expression of bcl-2 protein in bronchoalveolar lavage cell populations from patients with idiopathic pulmonary fibrosis," *Acta Cytologica*, vol. 45, no. 6, pp. 914–918, 2001.

[22] R. Bingisser, C. Stey, M. Weller, P. Groscurth, E. Russi, and K. Frei, "Apoptosis in human alveolar macrophages is induced by endotoxin and is modulated by cytokines," *American Journal of Respiratory Cell and Molecular Biology*, vol. 15, no. 1, pp. 64–70, 1996.

[23] C. P. Baran, J. M. Opalek, S. McMaken et al., "Important roles for macrophage colony-stimulating factor, CC chemokine ligand 2, and mononuclear phagocytes in the pathogenesis of pulmonary fibrosis," *American Journal of Respiratory and Critical Care Medicine*, vol. 176, no. 1, pp. 78–89, 2007.

[24] L. A. Murray, Q. Chen, M. S. Kramer et al., "TGF-beta driven lung fibrosis is macrophage dependent and blocked by Serum amyloid P," *International Journal of Biochemistry and Cell Biology*, vol. 43, no. 1, pp. 154–162, 2011.

[25] C. D. Gregory and A. Devitt, "The macrophage and the apoptotic cell: an innate immune interaction viewed simplistically?" *Immunology*, vol. 113, no. 1, pp. 1–14, 2004.

[26] R. E. Voll, M. Herrmann, E. A. Roth, C. Stach, J. R. Kalden, and I. Girkontaite, "Immunosuppressive effects of apoptotic cells," *Nature*, vol. 390, no. 6658, pp. 350–351, 1997.

[27] V. A. Fadok, D. L. Bratton, A. Konowal, P. W. Freed, J. Y. Westcott, and P. M. Henson, "Macrophages that have ingested apoptotic cells in vitro inhibit proinflammatory cytokine production through autocrine/paracrine mechanisms involving TGF-β, PGE2, and PAF," *Journal of Clinical Investigation*, vol. 101, no. 4, pp. 890–898, 1998.

[28] Y. Gao, J. M. Herndon, H. Zhang, T. S. Griffith, and T. A. Ferguson, "Antiinflammatory effects of CD95 ligand (FasL)-induced apoptosis," *Journal of Experimental Medicine*, vol. 188, no. 5, pp. 887–896, 1998.

[29] W. Chen, M. E. Frank, W. Jin, and S. M. Wahl, "TGF-β released by apoptotic T cells contributes to an immunosuppressive milieu," *Immunity*, vol. 14, no. 6, pp. 715–725, 2001.

[30] A. Byrne and D. J. Reen, "Lipopolysaccharide induces rapid production of IL-10 by monocytes in the presence of apoptotic neutrophils," *Journal of Immunology*, vol. 168, no. 4, pp. 1968–1977, 2002.

[31] S. B. Brown and J. Savill, "Phagocytosis triggers macrophage release of Fas ligand and induces apoptosis of bystander leukocytes," *Journal of Immunology*, vol. 162, no. 1, pp. 480–485, 1999.

[32] M. W. Peterson, M. Monick, and G. W. Hunninghake, "Prognostic role of eosinophils in pulmonary fibrosis," *Chest*, vol. 92, no. 1, pp. 51–56, 1987.

[33] L. C. Watters, T. E. King, and R. M. Cherniack, "Bronchoalveolar lavage fluid neutrophils increase after corticosteroid therapy in smokers with idiopathic pulmonary fibrosis," *American Review of Respiratory Disease*, vol. 133, no. 1, pp. 104–109, 1986.

[34] S. Yasuoka, T. Nakayama, and T. Kawano, "Comparison of cell profiles in bronchial and bronchoalveolar lavage fluids between normal subjects and patients with idiopathic pulmonary fibrosis," *Tohoku Journal of Experimental Medicine*, vol. 146, no. 1, pp. 33–45, 1985.

[35] M. Demedts, J. Behr, R. Buhl et al., "High-dose acetylcysteine in idiopathic pulmonary fibrosis," *New England Journal of Medicine*, vol. 353, no. 21, pp. 2229–2242, 2005.

[36] G. Raghu, K. K. Brown, W. Z. Bradford et al., "A placebo-controlled trial of interferon gamma-1b in patients with idiopathic pulmonary fibrosis," *New England Journal of Medicine*, vol. 350, no. 2, pp. 125–133, 2004.

[37] D. Bouros and A. Tzouvelekis, "Interferon-gamma for the treatment of idiopathic pulmonary fibrosis," *Pneumon*, vol. 22, no. 1, pp. 13–17, 2009.

[38] F. Drakopanagiotakis, D. Mermigkis, A. Xifteri et al., "A comparative study of treatment with azathioprine or interferon-g for patients with idiopathic pulmonary fibrosis," *Pneumon*, vol. 22, no. 3, pp. 240–253, 2009.

[39] A. Tzouvelekis, G. Kouliatsis, S. Anevlavis, and D. Bouros, "Serum biomarkers in interstitial lung diseases," *Respiratory Research*, vol. 6, article 78, 2005.

[40] M. Grunkin, J. Raundahl, and N. T. Foged, "Practical considerations of image analysis and quantification of signal transduction IHC staining," *Methods in Molecular Biology*, vol. 717, pp. 143–154, 2011.

[41] G. Kokolakis, L. Panagis, E. Stathopoulos, E. Giannikaki, A. Tosca, and S. Krüger-Krasagakis, "From the protein to the graph: how to quantify immunohistochemistry staining of the skin using digital imaging," *Journal of Immunological Methods*, vol. 331, no. 1-2, pp. 140–146, 2008.

36

A Multivariable Index for Grading Exercise Gas Exchange Severity in Patients with Pulmonary Arterial Hypertension and Heart Failure

Chul-Ho Kim, Steve Anderson, Dean MacCarter, and Bruce Johnson

Division of Cardiovascular Diseases, Mayo Clinic, Rochester, MN 55905, USA

Correspondence should be addressed to Chul-Ho Kim, kim.chulho@mayo.edu

Academic Editor: Jose Alberto Neder

Patients with pulmonary arterial hypertension (PAH) and heart failure (HF) display many abnormalities in respiratory gas exchange. These abnormalities are accentuated with exercise and track with disease severity. However, use of gas exchange measures in day-to-day clinical practice is limited by several issues, including the large number of variables available and difficulty in data interpretation. Moreover, maximal exercise testing has limitations in clinical populations due to their complexity, patient anxiety and variability in protocols and cost. Therefore, a multivariable gas exchange index (MVI) that integrates key gas exchange variables obtained during submaximal exercise into a severity score that ranges from normal to severe-very-severe is proposed. To demonstrate the usefulness of this index, we applied this to 2 groups (PAH, $n = 42$ and HF, $n = 47$) as well as to age matched healthy controls ($n = 25$). We demonstrate that this score tracks WHO classification and right ventricular systolic pressure in PAH ($r = 0.53$ and 0.73, $P \leq 0.01$) and NYHA and cardiac index in HF ($r = 0.49$ and 0.74, $P \leq 0.01$). This index demonstrates a stronger relationship than any single gas exchange variable alone. In conclusion, MVI obtained from light, submaximal exercise gas exchange is a useful approach to simplify data interpretation in PAH and HF populations.

1. Introduction

The lungs are linked hemodynamically in series with the heart, share a common surface area, are exposed to similar intrathoracic pressure changes during breathing, compete for intrathoracic space, and receive nearly 100% of the cardiac output. Receptors in the heart influence breathing patterns, while neural pathways in the lungs in turn may influence cardiac function (e.g., heart rate). Small increases in metabolic demand (e.g., exercise) enhance these cardiopulmonary interactions. Thus it is no surprise that diseases that primarily influence the lungs or the heart significantly impact the other organ system [1, 2]. This can be especially observed in patients with pulmonary arterial hypertension (PAH) where right heart failure evolves and in patients with left heart failure (HF) where significant changes occur in lung mechanics, ventilatory control, and ultimately in respiratory gas exchange. In both these patient groups gas exchange abnormalities are often present at rest, but are accentuated with the challenges of exercise. Thus,

noninvasive measures of cardiopulmonary gas exchange obtained during exercise have become a relatively common means to assess disease severity, prognosis, and response to therapy. However, despite the large availability of data confirming the utility of exercise gas exchange measures during exercise in these patients groups and the quickly improving and simplified approaches to testing, noninvasive respiratory gas exchange remains relatively poorly understood and underutilized in day to day clinical practice [3].

There have been a number of impediments to more extensive utilization of exercise respiratory gas exchange. This includes issues such as the large number of variables that are produced from typical commercially based systems, the somewhat broad range of normal values (influenced by age, gender, fitness, obesity, anxiety, body size, etc.), comorbidities that may influence the data, the complexities and expense that have been associated with comprehensive clinically based cardiopulmonary exercise testing, and difficulties and anxieties associated with maximal testing of often brittle patient populations [4].

TABLE 1: Model showing individual variables (individual variable index, IVI) that make up the multivariable scoring system. Normal values from literature with delta representing a risk cutoff for each IVI. (MVI = CUM IVI/6).

	Rest $PetCO_2$	$\Delta PetCO_2$	SaO_2	OUES	V_E/VCO_2 slope	P_{CAP}	
Normal value	40	3.6	94	1.6	26	400	
Delta	5	1.8	4	0.24	7	40	
Severity: IVI scores	Measured	Measured	Measured	Measured	Measured	Measured	CUM IVI
Normal: 0	40	3.6	94	1.6	26	360	0.00
Normal-mild: 1	35	1.8	90	1.36	33	320	6.00
Mild-moderate: 2	30	0	86	1.12	40	280	12.00
Moderate-severe: 3	25	−1.8	82	0.88	47	240	18.00
Severe-very severe: 4	20	−3.6	78	0.64	54	200	24.00

However, noninvasive commercially available gas exchange systems have been developed that are simpler, self-calibrating, with a lighter, less complicated patient interface [5]. In addition, it is becoming clear that gas exchange data other than peak oxygen consumption ($VO_{2\,max}$ or VO_{2peak}) that can be obtained from light or submaximal exercise (e.g., V_E/VCO_2 slope, OUES, and $PetCO_2$) as a slope or change from rest may be as good or in some cases more prognostic, reproducible, and sensitive than those obtained from maximal exercise testing and provoke less patient anxiety at reduced cost [6]. We have previously demonstrated that blending simpler devices with minimized, and submaximal protocols is well liked by patients, with the gas exchange data adequately separating both PAH and HF patients from healthy populations and according to disease severity [7–9].

To further simplify cardiopulmonary gas exchange for clinical use in the PAH and HF populations, we are further proposing a multivariable index (MVI) that takes into account the key gas exchange variables obtained during exercise that have been shown to be associated with these disease entities. The value of a multivariable index, or score, has been previously suggested and should have the following characteristics [10]: (1) utilizes variables that have been well documented in the literature for their normative ranges and prognostic value, (2) utilizes variables that have been associated with other clinical identifiers (e.g., disease classifications or common clinical metrics such as right heart pressures or cardiac index), (3) utilizes a model that can easily be adjusted as literature evolves, and (4) provides a simple conceptual framework for scoring that is similar to clinically intuitive scoring methods (e.g., WHO or NYHA classification), but provides a continuous variable which is more sensitive to changes in disease pathophysiology or to therapy than typical, more subjective scoring systems. This approach to creating a novel noninvasive gas exchange severity score from submaximal data for both PAH and HF is described and tested in these patient groups. We previously reported a gas exchange scoring system specific for PAH; however, we suggest this current more comprehensive and systematic approach provides a clearer framework for tracking PAH patients, appears to track disease status in the HF population, and provides a modifier for exercise induced PH [11–13].

2. Methods

2.1. Development of the Multivariable Index (MVI) for Scoring Gas Exchange Data.
Based on previously reported data from our laboratory as well as others, we identified 6 variables that have been shown to track disease severity and/or prognosis in PAH and in the HF populations which can be obtained from rest and light, submaximal exercise [8–10, 13–18]. Many of these variables have published cut off values or ranges that are associated with higher risk [16, 19]. This includes (1) the ventilatory equivalents for carbon dioxide production (V_E/VCO_2) or breathing efficiency [19], (2) the oxygen uptake efficiency slope (OUES) [17], (3) oxygen saturation (SaO_2) [20], (4) the resting $PetCO_2$ [21], (5) the change in $PetCO_2$ with exercise, and (6) a calculated gas exchange variable as an index for pulmonary capacitance (P_{CAP}) which is the oxygen pulse multiplied by $PetCO_2$ ($O_{2pulse} \times PetCO_2$) that tracks invasive measures of pulmonary capacitance [13] and a modifying variable based on the slope of change in the inflection of $PetCO_2$ from rest to light exercise [12]. This final modifier has been suggested to reflect more severe exercise-induced changes in pulmonary vascular pressure and/or potential shunting through a PFO or intrapulmonary shunts due to high pressures [12]. There is some redundancy purposefully built into the MVI for variables most strongly associated with clinical measures, but yet retaining the ultimate goal of a single score that quantifies the severity of derangement in gas exchange rather than a formal surrogate to these other clinical markers. In fact, we would propose that in many cases that gas exchange data from light exercise may give a more important measure of integrated central hemodynamic function than the more commonly used "gold standards" for assessing and quantifying disease severity.

Table 1 describes the variable set used, the normal values [3, 4, 22, 23], and the delta value or the difference between the normal value and the risk cutoff point. In the lower table, the rows under "measured" are measured values of the variable in that column ranging in severity from normal to severe-very severe. The first column is individual variable index (IVI) score following severity, and the last column is cumulative IVI scores in a row. It is noted that some variables vary directly in severity from low to high (e.g., V_E/VCO_2 slope) and some variables vary in severity inversely from high to low (e.g., OUES). In this manner, if the measured = NV

TABLE 2: Baseline multivariable index (MVI) scoring system.

CUM IVI	MVI = CUM IVI/6	Range	Severity	NYHA
0.00	0.00	<1	Normal	n/a
6.00	1.00	1 and <2	Normal-mild	I
12.00	2.00	2 and <3	Mild-moderate	II
18.00	3.00	3 and <4	Moderate-severe	III
24.00	4.00	≥4	Severe-very severe	IV

TABLE 3: MVI scoring system weighted for P_{CAP}.

CUM IVI	MVI = CUM IVI/7	Range	Severity	NYHA
0.00	0.00	<1	Normal	n/a
7.00	1.00	1 and <2	Normal-mild	I
14.00	2.00	2 and <3	Mild-moderate	II
21.00	3.00	3 and <4	Moderate-severe	III
28.00	4.00	≥4	Severe-very severe	IV

TABLE 4: MVI scoring system weighted for the slope of change and magnitude of change in PetCO$_2$ (indicative of exercise induced PH).

MVI$_{PH}$	Modifier
≥0	0.00
<0 and >−5	0.50
≥ −5 and > −10	0.75
≤ −10	1.00

(normal value), the value of the IVI = 0. If the measured equals the risk cutoff point, the value of IVI = 1. IVIs that result in MVIs greater than 4.0 are scored as severe-very severe. Hence, MVI is cumulative IVI divided by 6. Normal subjects have MVI values less than 1.0, and it can be seen that the 6 variable MVI values closely resemble the NYHA classification system as shown in Table 2.

2.2. Seven Variable Model with Weighting.

Another feature of the MVI classification system is the ability to impart a greater weight to IVIs. It is proposed that this feature would allow for the evolution of disease specific MVIs. For this paper, the individual IVI for P_{CAP} was "double counted." This metric was double weighted due to the ability of it to track pulmonary vascular capacitance, an important metric in gas exchange severity in both HF and PH. Therefore, the MVI was then obtained by dividing the cumulative IVI by 7, rather than 6 for the unweighted MVI. The effect of doing so can be observed in Table 3.

2.3. Additional Modifiers.

The MVI classification system also has the ability to apply modifiers. It has been demonstrated in the literature that an abrupt fall PetCO$_2$ (steep slope) with exercise is itself a gauge of severity of PH [12]. We therefore increased the MVI score by values proportional to the magnitude and slope of change in PetCO$_2$ during exercise (see Table 4). Adding the modifier for the PetCO$_2$ patterns increased the severity score for individual subjects without altering the MVI scale range. In addition, adding the MVI$_{PH}$ modifier to the MVI score consistently improved the correlations between the index and other clinical variables in both PAH and in the HF populations.

3. Results

3.1. Testing the Model in Patient Groups.

We examined the use of the final MVI score (CUM IVI/7 + additional modifier) in three populations from previously published studies (Table 5) [9, 24, 25]. This included patients with primarily PAH and classic systolic HF along with healthy subjects of similar age ranges. The PAH patients were recruited with known pulmonary hypertension through our PH clinic and performed a light submaximal 3 min step test after collecting 2 min of resting data, while the HF patients performed submaximal cycling ergometry (similar levels of perceived exertion). Control subjects performed a combination of the light step testing and submaximal cycle ergometry. Both patient groups had a range of disease severity levels and were typically on standard therapy. Breath by breath gas exchange data were collected for all populations using the Shape Medical Systems, Inc., simplified gas exchange system, and slopes (e.g., V_E/VCO_2) were determined by linear regression. Thirty second averages were used to calculate MVI variables.

The ranges for MVI for each database are illustrated in Figure 1(a) (PAH) and Figure 1(b) (HF). When compared to the WHO or NYHA classification for the respective patient cohorts, (Figures 2(a) and 2(b)), it can be seen that the clinical classification results in "data aliasing" versus the MVI score which gives a continuous variable. Figures 3 and 4 give examples of individual PAH and HF patients over the range of scores obtained by the final MVI model. This also includes a healthy normal individual. Figure 5 shows the ranges of MVI scores for the control, PAH, and HF populations. It should be noted that the patient populations presented have benefited from medical therapy, and thus overlap exists across populations.

Figure 6 shows an example of a PH patient and an HF patient before and after intervention (medication titration in the PH patient and cardiac resynchronization therapy in the HF patient). Both patients demonstrated benefits in clinical measures (RVSP, CI, and 6 min walk in PH patient and NT Pro BNP, NYHA class, and LVEF in the HF patient), with improvements in the MVI score. We also examined the overall relationship between the MVI score to RVSP and WHO classification in PAH (Figures 7(c) and 7(d)) and CI and NYHA class in HF (Figures 7(a) and 7(b)). The MVI demonstrated a good relationship with clinical indices, (e.g., WHO class and RVSP in PAH r = 0.53 and 0.73, resp., and NYHA and CI in HF r = 0.49 and 0.74, resp.; $P \leq 0.01$). The score was more highly correlated with the physiological measures versus the more subjective functional classifications. Individual correlations for the components of the MVI score with CI and RVSP are provided in Table 6. PetCO$_2$, OUES, V_E/VCO_2 slope, and P_{CAP} all demonstrated significant relationships with CI in HF and RVSP in PAH

TABLE 5: Subject characteristics.

	Controls	PAH	Heart failure
Number (% female)	25 (80%)	40 (80%)	45/(13%)
Age (years)	51 ± 15	50 ± 13	54 ± 8
Height (cm)	167.8 ± 8.2	167.7 ± 7.0	174.9 ± 8
Weight (kg)	70.1 ± 12.7	75.8 ± 16.5	86.6 ± 16.3
HF etiology			
Ischemic/dilated (n)			23/22
NYHA Class (I/II/III/IV)			5/7/23/10
LVEF (%)	61 ± 7	64 ± 7.3	20 ± 6
NT Pro BNP/BNP		770 ± 1239	852 ± 2341
Cardiac index	3.0 ± 0.3	3.1 ± 0.7	1.9 ± 0.6
PAH etiology			
Idiopathic	—	25 (63%)	
Hereditary	—	4 (10%)	
Associated with diet drug use	—	2 (5%)	
Portopulmonary hypertension	—	1 (2%)	
Associated with connective tissue disease	—	8 (20%)	
Functional class (WHO) (I/II/III/IV)	—	7/20/11/2	
RV pressure (mmHg)	26 ± 4	76 ± 23	49 ± 18

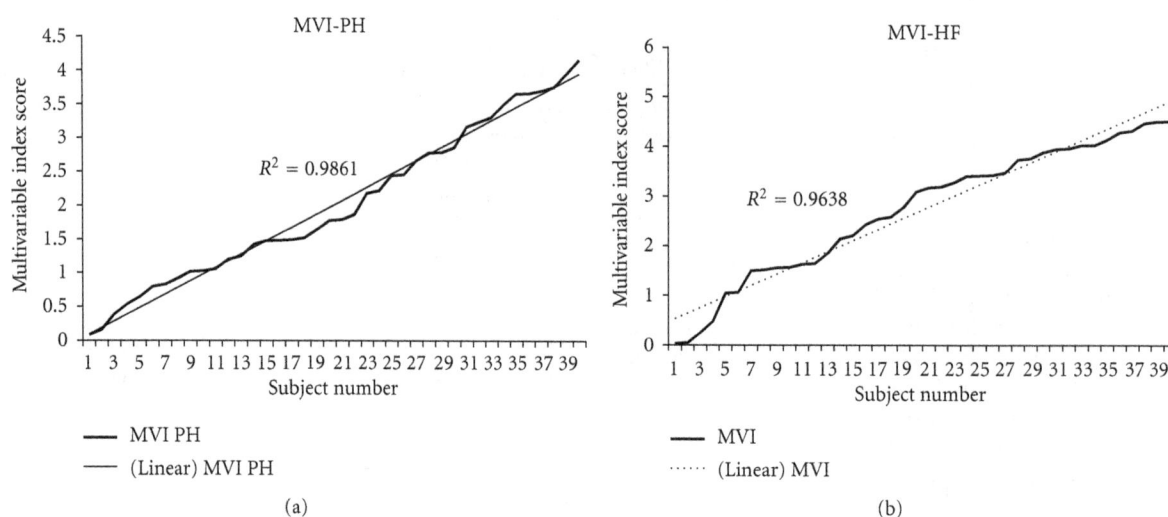

FIGURE 1: MVI score sorted and plotted for each subject for PAH and HF populations showing the score to be a continuous variable.

patients with less significant relationships between these gas exchange measures and NYHA or WHO classification. Modest improvements over the majority of variables were observed using the MVI score.

4. Discussion

4.1. Summary of Pertinent Findings. We propose a comprehensive multivariable index (MVI) scoring system to quantify gas exchange severity from light submaximal exercise data specific to populations with pulmonary vascular disease and demonstrate its utility in patients with PAH and systolic heart failure. The MVI allows a simple approach to integrating important gas exchange variables into a single conceptual score designed to track disease severity. The score

is further weighted towards variables that reflect more severe hemodynamic derangement during exercise and is based on exercise loads that are commonly experienced by patients in daily activities. This score while designed to reflect gas exchange abnormalities and not necessarily other clinical tracking variables shows a modest association with clinically used classification schemes as well as catheter or echo-based measures.

4.2. Rationale and Goals for Designing a MVI Scoring System for Exercise Gas Exchange in Chronic Disease. While methods for capturing noninvasive gas exchange during exercise have evolved to simple breath by breath systems, little advancement has been made in simplifying the approach to interpretation and applying this to clinical populations.

TABLE 6: Relationship of individual gas exchange measures with CI and RVSP in HF and PAH, respectively.

	HF cardiac index	NYHA	PAH RVSP	WHO
Rest $PetCO_2$	0.52	0.47	0.39	0.12
$\Delta PetCO_2$	0.42	0.23	0.62	0.55
SaO_2	0.05	0.23	0.47	0.15
OUES	0.66	0.40	0.46	0.47
V_E/VCO_2 slope	0.53	0.34	0.63	0.51
P_{CAP}	0.69	0.40	0.58	0.41
MVI score	0.74	0.49	0.73	0.53

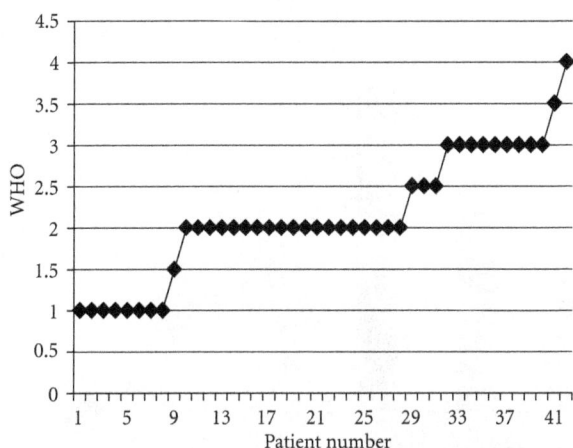

(a)

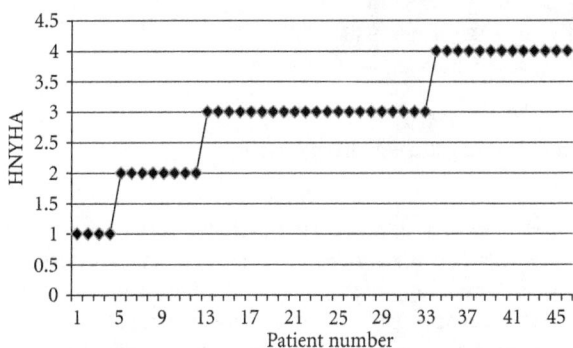

(b)

FIGURE 2: WHO classification for PH group and NYHA classification for HF group.

As a result, noninvasive measures of gas exchange during exercise remain underutilized in clinical practice [3, 4, 22]. A large number of variables are quantified during a typical test that include measures of breathing pattern, breath timing intervals, and gas exchange measures. Most established clinical exercise laboratories tend to focus on maximal testing and the classic assessment of peak oxygen consumption (VO_{2peak}). However, there are a number of limitations in this type of assessment. This includes issues regarding patient anxiety with maximal testing-balance problems

and uncertainties in their ability to push themselves to a true maximum. There is a need for more comprehensive monitoring equipment with the risks of maximal testing, often the need for multiple personnel for testing (increasing the cost), different use of protocols across centers as well as stopping criteria (making it hard to compare data), and the modest variability in the VO_{2peak} obtained. Over the last decade or more, it has become clear that a number of submaximal responses to exercise are as or more predictive for morbidity and mortality in the HF population, and many of these noninvasive submaximal measures are slopes or changes from rest and thus relatively insensitive to intensity of exercise, and in many cases being more reproducible [6]. Metrics that have been shown to be highly prognostic and sensitive to disease severity include the ventilatory efficiency, the oxygen uptake efficiency slope, the absolute or change in $PetCO_2$, the change in O_{2pulse}, (oxygen saturation, SaO_2) [8–10, 13–18].

Ventilatory efficiency has been linked to high dead space ventilation, due mostly to a more rapid shallow breathing pattern, combined with a greater relative hyperventilation. It increases progressively with disease severity in both PAH and HF [8, 9, 26]. $PetCO_2$ appears to track the rise in pulmonary vascular pressures with exercise, especially in PAH patients, likely not only due to both a pressure-induced increase in ventilation, but also due to increasing ventilation and perfusion inhomogeneities in the lungs and is typically inversely related with V_E/VCO_2 slope suggesting that in general they provide similar information [8, 9, 12]. Oxygen pulse (VO_2/HR) is essentially the stroke volume multiplied times oxygen extraction, but appears to track stroke volume relatively well [13]. Using invasive or technical echocardiography-based measures, various techniques have been used to quantify a value representing pulmonary vascular capacitance (change in stroke volume relative to change in pulmonary pressures), which has been shown to be predictive of mortality in the PAH population [27, 28]. We previously compared a noninvasive estimate of pulmonary capacitance based on the equation (O_{2pulse}, as an estimate of stroke volume) × ($PetCO_2$, as an estimate of pulmonary vascular pressure) to catheter based measures obtained during exercise and found a strong relationship in the HF population [13]. The gas exchange derived P_{CAP} also demonstrated a relatively strong relationship with our clinical metrics in this study with only modest improvements using the complete MVI score. However, many gas exchange variables tend to change in concert, and in particular measures of $PetCO_2$ and/or V_E/VCO_2 slope appear to be the variables that are most highly associated with clinical metrics and are counted or weighted heavily in the MVI scoring system, while at the same time allowing for other variables (e.g., SaO_2) to contribute in a positive or negative way to the final score. In addition, such an approach to amalgamating variables tends to reduce noise. Thus the MVI score is weighted heavily towards factors which elevate dead space ventilation, inhibit a rise in stroke volume, cause a more rapid, and shallow breathing pattern and to a lesser extent cause oxygen desaturation with exercise (e.g., shunt, low VA/Qc regions, and diffusion limitation). We also amplify the

	Normal	Normal-mild	Mild-moderate	Moderate-severe	Severe-very severe
Age (yr)	58	58	52	50	48
Weight (kg)	72	74	82	66	79
BNP		327	617	829	2100
Rest PetCO$_2$ (mmHg)	29.2	34.2	41.3	31.5	28.4
Delta PetCO$_2$ (mmHg)	5.1	−0.8	−4.1	−0.7	−5.5
SaO$_2$ (%)	95	91	95	97	94
OUES	2.1	1.5	1.1	0.7	0.8
V_E/VCO_2 slope	29.9	35.1	36	35.5	56.5
P_{CAP}	388	362	274	159	135
CUM IVI 7	0.17	7.44	13.69	20.42	28.2
CUM IVI/7	0.02	1.06	1.96	2.92	4.03
Modifier	0	0	0.25	0.25	0.5
MVI	0.02	1.06	2.21	3.17	4.53

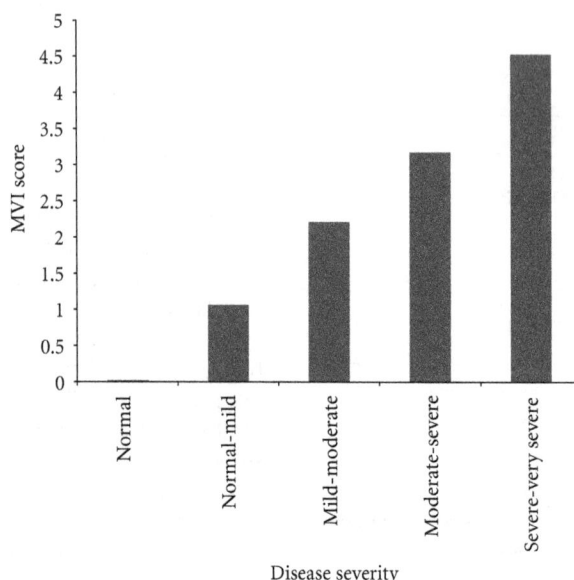

FIGURE 3: Final model with examples of *HF patients* according to gas exchange severity.

negative score if the rate of change in PetCO$_2$ with exercise is excessive.

4.3. Need for a Multivariable Gas Exchange Severity Score and Taking an Intuitive versus Statistical Approach.

The MVI score demonstrates a modest improvement in the association with clinical measures over any single variable. However, while the score was purposefully weighted to track disease severity in the PAH and HF populations, the original intent was to create a gas exchange severity score and thus to some extent to be independent of other clinical measures. Thus, while one would expect the MVI score to generally track other clinical or physiological measures associated with disease severity, one would not necessarily expect a strong relationship with these clinical measures for a variety of reasons. For example, in some PAH patients, creating artificial shunts may reduce symptoms, but at the same time cause greater gas exchange abnormalities with exercise, making the gas exchange severity score worse. Therefore we chose to take an intuitive approach rather than a statistical

approach to create the scoring system, as the score should be able to serve as an independent way to track disease and because there is no perfect gold standard for which to develop the statistical approach. In addition, other measures such as NYHA or WHO classification remain quite subjective.

Other problems exist with the current "gold standards," including a large variability in both echocardiogram and catheter-based measures, and both measures tend to have a number of limitations and often assumptions, particularly when cardiac hemodynamics are assessed during exercise. Thus our goal was to develop a comprehensive and adaptable gas exchange severity score based on the literature that is not dependent on maximal exercise values and provides an independent value for grading and tracking disease relative to other clinical measures.

4.4. Implications for the Future of Exercise Gas Exchange in Select Populations.

With simplified techniques for quantifying gas exchange and the growing awareness that values

	Normal	Normal-mild	Mild-moderate	Moderate-severe	Severe-very severe
Age (yr)	52	41	57	44	53
Weight (kg)	77	68	73	66	76
BNP		103	518	918	3056
Rest PetCO$_2$ (mmHg)	34.2	37.3	30.2	34.9	29.1
Delta PetCO$_2$ (mmHg)	3.7	−0.8	2.2	−1.8	−7.3
SaO$_2$ (%)	95	91	91	93	90
OUES	1.71	1.53	1.08	0.78	1.15
V_E/VCO$_2$ slope	29.4	35.1	33.7	36.2	61.0
P_{CAP}	396	362	226	242	166
CUM IVI 7	1.1	7.1	15.5	17	27.7
CUM IVI/7	0.16	1.02	2.21	2.43	3.96
Modifier	0	0	0	0.75	1
MVI	0.16	1.02	2.21	3.18	4.96

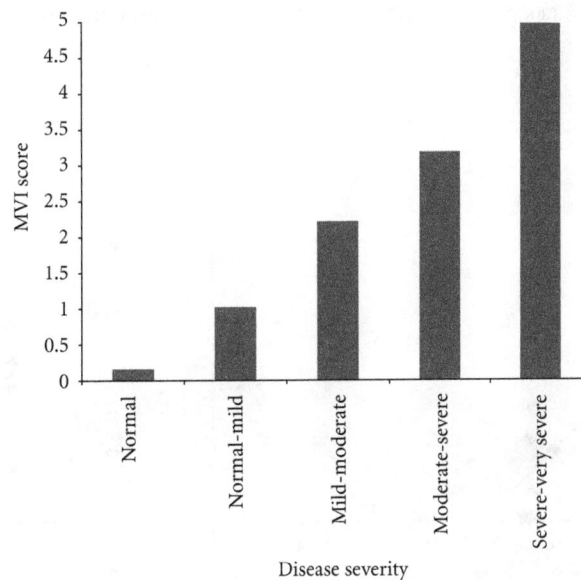

FIGURE 4: Final model with examples of *PAH patients* according to gas exchange severity.

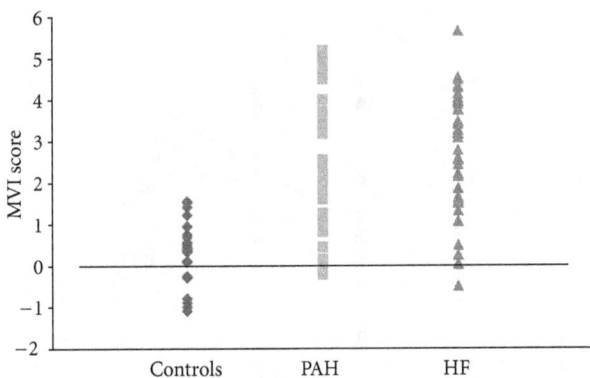

FIGURE 5: Range of MVI scores for patient groups and controls.

obtained with light submaximal exercise are as prognostic as maximally obtained values in several populations, cardiopulmonary gas exchange could be easily adapted to many clinical areas as more of a "vital sign" rather than the more comprehensive and elaborate approach to testing that has classically been used, particularly in the HF and PH populations where ischemia detection is not a primary end point. Adding a gas exchange severity score to this simplified approach for screening and tracking patients further simplifies testing and reduces the need for specific expertise in cardio respirator physiology. We would propose that having a scoring system such as the MVI would allow a more comprehensive metric than "VO$_{2peak}$" and a scaling system that is more similar to other scoring systems (e.g., NYHA or WHO classification) that are familiar to clinical experts.

4.5. Limitations. We have created a gas exchange severity score that is weighted towards abnormalities in gas exchange found in HF and PAH. We have not specifically tested this in large populations with multiple comorbidities (e.g., COPD), and thus its utility in these patient groups would need to be determined. However, the MVI system is easily adaptable to other patient groups and changed or weighted towards additional variables that are more specific to a given population.

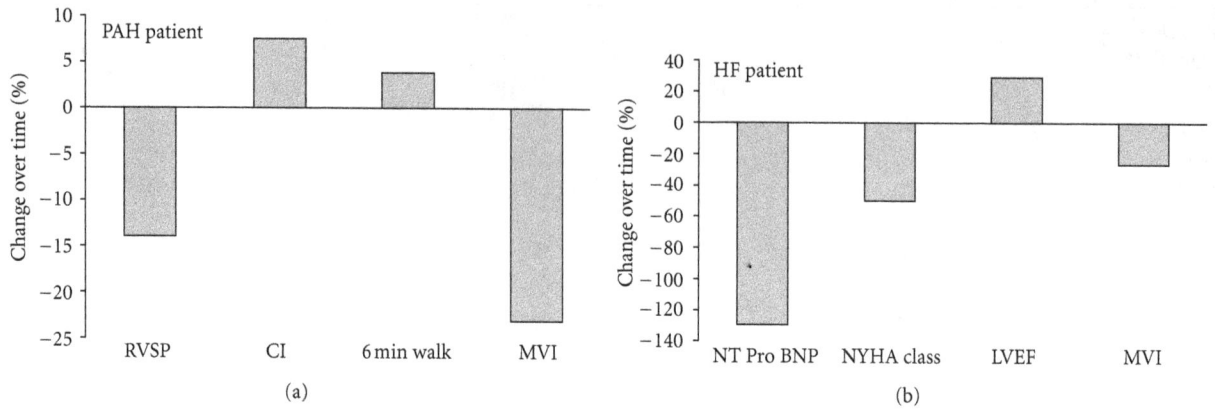

FIGURE 6: Tracking disease status over time, (a) PAH patient 3 mo. after treatment demonstrating modest improvements in clinical measures and the MVI score, (b) HF patients 3 mo. after CRT device implantation demonstrating similar directional changes in MVI score with clinical metrics.

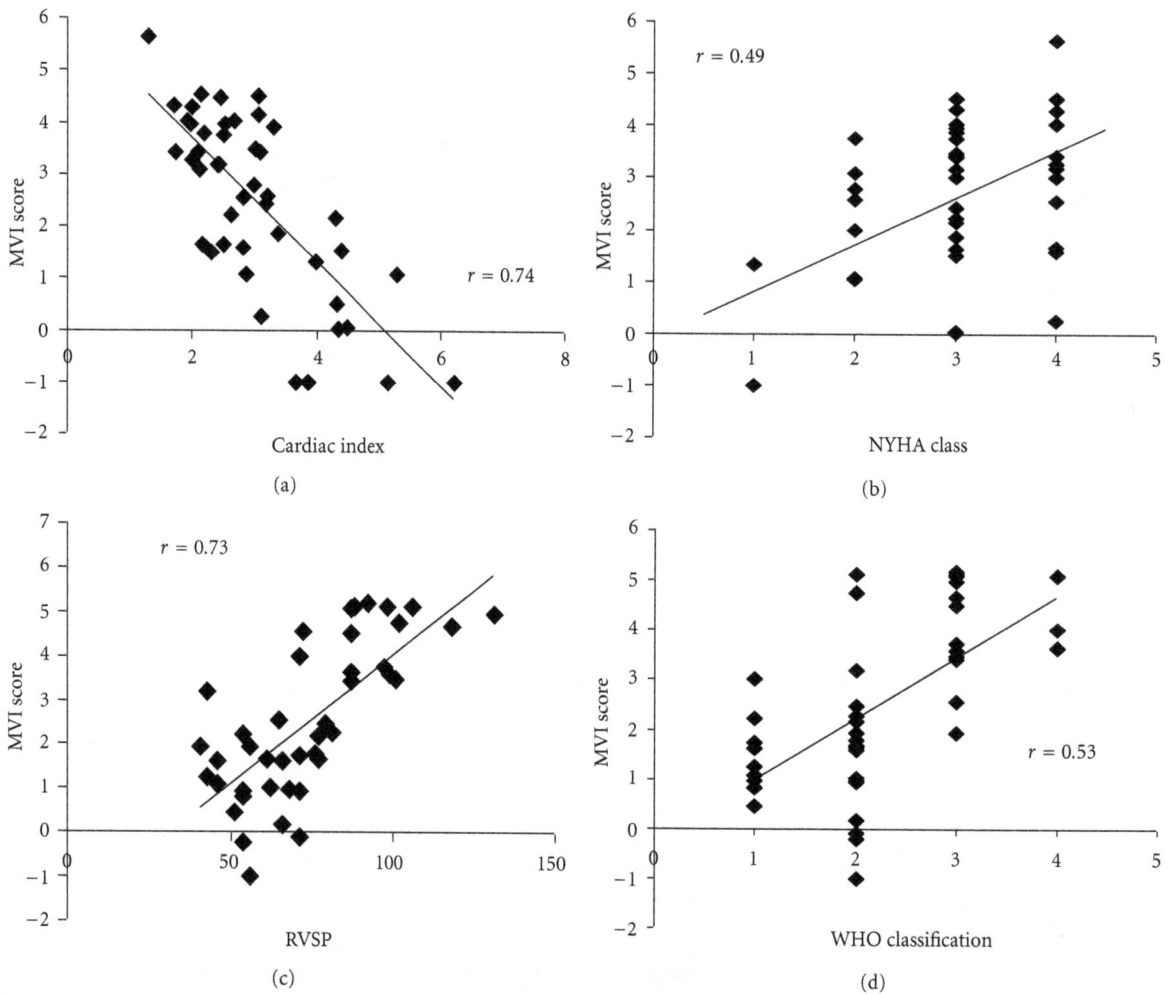

FIGURE 7: Relationships of MVI score with clinical parameters.

5. Conclusions

Measures of cardiopulmonary gas exchange with exercise have previously been underutilized due to their complexity and difficulty in interpretation. The MVI gas exchange severity score provides a simple means to rapidly assess disease risk and response to therapy in HF and PH patients and provides an overall assessment of integrative cardiac hemodynamics. The score reduces the complications of having to understand a large number of variables, eliminates the need for interpretation, accounts for variables with multiple directional changes, avoids noise that can be created by one value being abnormal versus the other values, and provides an easily identifiable numbering scheme for physicians to track.

References

[1] T. P. Olson, E. M. Snyder, and B. D. Johnson, "Exercise-disordered breathing in chronic heart failure," *Exercise and Sport Sciences Review*, vol. 34, no. 4, pp. 194–201, 2006.

[2] S. Lalande and B. D. Johnson, "Breathing strategy to preserve exercising cardiac function in patients with heart failure," *Medical Hypotheses*, vol. 74, no. 3, pp. 416–421, 2010.

[3] R. V. Milani, C. J. Lavie, M. R. Mehra, and H. O. Ventura, "Understanding the basics of cardiopulmonary exercise testing," *Mayo Clinic Proceedings*, vol. 81, no. 12, pp. 1603–1611, 2006.

[4] B. D. Johnson, P. D. Wagner, and J. A. Dempsey, "ATS/ACCP Statement on cardiopulmonary exercise testing," *American Journal of Respiratory and Critical Care Medicine*, vol. 167, no. 2, pp. 211–277, 2003.

[5] A. D. Miller, P. R. Woods, T. P. Olson et al., "Validation of a simplified, portable cardiopulmonary gas exchange system for submaximal exercise testing," *The Open Sports Medicine Journal*, vol. 4, pp. 34–40, 2010.

[6] J. E. Hansen, X. G. Sun, Y. Yasunobu et al., "Reproducibility of cardiopulmonary exercise measurements in patients with pulmonary arterial hypertension," *Chest*, vol. 126, no. 3, pp. 816–824, 2004.

[7] R. Arena, D. MacCarter, T. P. Olson et al., "Ventilatory expired gas at constant-rate low-intensity exercise predicts adverse events and is related to neurohormona markers in patients with heart failure," *Journal of Cardiac Failure*, vol. 15, no. 6, pp. 482–488, 2009.

[8] P. R. Woods, K. R. Bailey, C. M. Wood, and B. D. Johnson, "Submaximal exercise gas exchange is an important prognostic tool to predict adverse outcomes in heart failure," *European Journal of Heart Failure*, vol. 13, no. 3, pp. 303–310, 2011.

[9] P. R. Woods, R. P. Frantz, B. J. Taylor, and T. P. Olson, "The usefulness of submaximal exercise gas exchange to define pulmonary arterial hypertension," *The Journal of Heart and Lung Transplantation*, vol. 30, no. 10, pp. 1133–1142, 2011.

[10] J. Myers, R. Arena, F. Dewey et al., "A cardiopulmonary exercise testing score for predicting outcomes in patients with heart failure," *American Heart Journal*, vol. 156, no. 6, pp. 1177–1183, 2008.

[11] X. G. Sun, J. E. Hansen, R. J. Oudiz, and K. Wasserman, "Gas exchange detection of exercise-induced right-to-left shunt in patients with primary pulmonary hypertension," *Circulation*, vol. 105, no. 1, pp. 54–60, 2002.

[12] Y. Yasunobu, R. J. Oudiz, X. G. Sun, J. E. Hansen, and K. Wasserman, "End-tidal Pco_2 abnormality and exercise limitation in patients with primary pulmonary hypertension," *Chest*, vol. 127, no. 5, pp. 1637–1646, 2005.

[13] P. R. Woods, B. J. Taylor, R. P. Frantz, and B. D. Johnson, "A pulmonary hypertension gas exchange severity (PH-GXS) score to assist with the assessment and monitoring of pulmonary arterial hypertension," *American Journal of Cardiology*, vol. 109, no. 7, pp. 1066–1072, 2012.

[14] R. Arena, M. Guazzi, and J. Myers, "Prognostic value of end-tidal carbon dioxide during exercise testing in heart failure," *International Journal of Cardiology*, vol. 117, no. 1, pp. 103–108, 2007.

[15] R. Arena, J. Myers, L. Hsu et al., "The minute ventilation/carbon dioxide production slope is prognostically superior to the oxygen uptake efficiency slope," *Journal of Cardiac Failure*, vol. 13, no. 6, pp. 462–469, 2007.

[16] R. Arena, J. Myers, J. Abella et al., "The ventilatory classification system effectively predicts hospitalization in patients with heart failure," *Journal of Cardiopulmonary Rehabilitation and Prevention*, vol. 28, no. 3, pp. 195–198, 2008.

[17] R. Arena, J. Myers, J. Abella et al., "Prognostic significance of the oxygen uptake efficiency slope: percent-predicted versus actual value," *American Journal of Cardiology*, vol. 105, no. 5, pp. 757–758, 2010.

[18] M. Guazzi, "Alveolar gas diffusion abnormalities in heart failure," *Journal of Cardiac Failure*, vol. 14, no. 8, pp. 695–702, 2008.

[19] J. Myers, R. Arena, R. B. Oliveira et al., "The lowest VE/VCO_2 ratio during exercise as a predictor of outcomes in patients with heart failure," *Journal of Cardiac Failure*, vol. 15, no. 9, pp. 756–762, 2009.

[20] G. Paciocco, F. J. Martinez, E. Bossone, E. Pielsticker, B. Gillespie, and M. Rubenfire, "Oxygen desaturation on the six-minute walk test and mortality in untreated primary pulmonary hypertension," *European Respiratory Journal*, vol. 17, no. 4, pp. 647–652, 2001.

[21] R. Arena, M. A. Peberdy, J. Myers, M. Guazzi, and M. Tevald, "Prognostic value of resting end-tidal carbon dioxide in patients with heart failure," *International Journal of Cardiology*, vol. 109, no. 3, pp. 351–358, 2006.

[22] B. D. Johnson, B. Whipp, R. J. Zeballos et al., "Conceptual and physiological basis of cardiopulmonary exercise testing measurement. In the ATS/ACCP statement on cardiopulmonary exercise testing," *American Journal of Respiratory and Critical Care Medicine*, vol. 167, pp. 211–277, 2003.

[23] T. A. Goers, "Washington University School of Medicine Department of Surgery," *The Washington Manual of Surgery*, Wolters Kluwer Health/Lippincott Williams & Wilkins, Philadelphia, Pa, USA, 2008.

[24] P. R. Woods, R. P. Frantz, and B. D. Johnson, "The usefulness of submaximal exercise gas exchange in pulmonary arterial hypertension: a case series," *Clinical Medicine Insights*, vol. 4, no. 1, pp. 35–40, 2010.

[25] P. R. Woods, T. P. Olson, R. P. Frantz, and B. D. Johnson, "Causes of breathing inefficiency during exercise in heart failure," *Journal of Cardiac Failure*, vol. 16, no. 10, pp. 835–842, 2010.

[26] B. D. Johnson, K. C. Beck, L. J. Olson et al., "Ventilatory constraints during exercise in patients with chronic heart failure," *Chest*, vol. 117, no. 2, pp. 321–332, 2000.

[27] S. Mahapatra, R. A. Nishimura, P. Sorraja, S. Cha, and M. D. McGoon, "Pulmonary vascular capacitance predicts mortality

in pulmonary hypertension," *American College of Cardiology Foundation*, vol. 47, pp. 799–803, 2006.

[28] S. Mahapatra, R. A. Nishimura, J. K. Oh, and M. D. McGoon, "The prognostic value of pulmonary vascular capacitance determined by doppler echocardiography in patients with pulmonary arterial hypertension," *Journal of the American Society of Echocardiography*, vol. 19, no. 8, pp. 1045–1050, 2006.

Permissions

List of Contributors

Argyris Tzouvelekis, George Zacharis, Paschalis Ntolios, Andreas Koulelidis and Demosthenes Bouros
Department of Pneumonology, University Hospital of Alexandroupolis, Democritus University of Thrace, 68100 Alexandroupolis, Greece

Nikolaos Galanopoulos
Department of Rheumatology, University Hospital of Alexandroupolis, Democritus University of Thrace, 68100 Alexandroupolis, Greece

Evangelos Bouros and George Kolios
Laboratory of Pharmacology, Democritus University of Thrace, 68100 Alexandroupolis, Greece

Anastasia Oikonomou
Department of Radiology, University Hospital of Alexandroupolis, Democritus University of Thrace, 68100 Alexandroupolis, Greece

Kimberly B. Vera, Donald Moore, English Flack and Michael Liske
Division of Cardiology, Department of Pediatrics, Vanderbilt University School of Medicine, Nashville, TN 37232, USA

Marshall Summar
Center for Genetic Medicine Research, Children's National Medical Center, Washington, DC 20010, USA

Servet Kayhan, Halit Cinarka and Aziz Gumus
Department of Chest Disease, Faculty of Medicine, Recep Tayyip Erdogan University, 53100 Rize, Turkey

Umit Tutar
Department of Chest Disease, Hospital of Chest Disease and Thoracic Surgery, 55090 Samsun, Turkey

Nurhan Koksal
Department of Chest Disease, Faculty of Medicine, Ondokuz Mayis University, 55139 Samsun, Turkey

Wendy Thanassi
Department of Medicine, Veterans Affairs Palo Alto Health Care System, 3801 Miranda Avenue MC-, Palo Alto, CA 94304-1207, USA
Occupational Health Strategic Health Care Group, Office of Public Health, Veterans Health Administration, Washington, DC 20006, USA
Division of Emergency Medicine, Stanford University School of Medicine, Stanford, CA 94304, USA
War Related Illness and Injury Study Center (WRIISC) and Mental Illness Research Education and Clinical Center (MIRECC), Department of Veterans Affairs, Palo Alto, CA 94304, USA

Art Noda, Beatriz Hernandez, and Jerome A. Yesavage
War Related Illness and Injury Study Center (WRIISC) and Mental Illness Research Education and Clinical Center (MIRECC), Department of Veterans Affairs, Palo Alto, CA 94304, USA
Department of Psychiatry and Behavioral Sciences, Stanford University School of Medicine, Stanford, CA 94304, USA

Jeffery Newell
War Related Illness and Injury Study Center (WRIISC) and Mental Illness Research Education and Clinical Center (MIRECC), Department of Veterans Affairs, Palo Alto, CA 94304, USA

Paul Terpeluk
Department of Occupational Health, The Cleveland Clinic, Cleveland, OH 44195, USA

David Marder
University Health Services, University of Illinois Chicago, Chicago, IL 60612, USA

Robyn L. Chura and Scotty J. Butcher
School of Physical Therapy, University of Saskatchewan, 1121 College Dr, Saskatoon, SK, Canada S7N 0W3

Darcy D.Marciniuk and Ron Clemens
Respirology, Critical Care and Sleep Medicine, University of Saskatchewan, Canada

Lee Ingle Rebecca Sloan and Sean Carroll
Department of Sport, Health & Exercise Science, University of Hull, Cottingham Road, Kingston-upon-Hull HU6 7RX, UK

Kevin Goode, John G. Cleland and Andrew L. Clark
Department of Cardiology, Hull York Medical School, Daisy Building, University of Hull, Castle Hill Hospital, Cottingham, Kingston-upon-Hull HU16 5JQ, UK

Wataru Takahashi, Hideomi Yamashita, Kenshiro Shiraishi and Keiichi Nakagawa
Department of Radiology, University of Tokyo Hospital, 7-3-1, Hongo, Bunkyo-ku, Tokyo 113-8655, Japan

Yuzuru Niibe and Kazushige Hayakawa
Department of Radiology and Radiation Oncology, Kitasato Universtiy, Kanagawa 252-0374, Japan

Aaron Chidekel
Nemours Biomedical Research, Nemours Research Lung Center, Nemours/Alfred I. duPont Hospital for Children, 1600 Rockland Road, Wilmington, DE 19803, USA
Department of Pediatrics, Jefferson Medical College, Thomas Jefferson University, 1025 Walnut Street, Suite 700, Philadelphia, PA 19107, USA

Department of Pediatrics, Nemours/Alfred I. duPont Hospital for Children, 1600 Rockland Road, Wilmington, DE 19803, USA

Yan Zhu, JordanWang, John J. Mosko and Elena Rodriguez
Nemours Biomedical Research, Nemours Research Lung Center, Nemours/Alfred I. duPont Hospital for Children, 1600 Rockland Road, Wilmington, DE 19803, USA

Thomas H. Shaffer
Nemours Biomedical Research, Nemours Research Lung Center, Nemours/Alfred I. duPont Hospital for Children, 1600 Rockland Road, Wilmington, DE 19803, USA
Department of Pediatrics, Jefferson Medical College, Thomas Jefferson University, 1025 Walnut Street, Suite 700, Philadelphia, PA 19107, USA
Departments of Physiology and Pediatrics, Temple University School of Medicine, 3420 North Broad Street, Philadelphia, PA 19140, USA

BenoitWallaert, LidwineWemeau-Stervinou and Isabelle Tillie-Leblond
Clinique des Maladies Respiratoires, Centre de Compétence des Maladies Pulmonaires Rares, Hopital Calmette, Lille 2 University Boulevard Leclercq, CHRU, 59037 Lille, France

Julia Salleron
Unité de Biostatistiques, CHRU, 59037 Lille, France

Thierry Perez
Clinique des Maladies Respiratoires, Centre de Compétence des Maladies Pulmonaires Rares, Hopital Calmette, Lille 2 University Boulevard Leclercq, CHRU, 59037 Lille, France
Service d'Explorations Fonctionnelles Respiratoires, Hopital Calmette, CHRU, 59037 Lille, France

Christopher C. Griffith and Larry Nichols
Department of Pathology, University of Pittsburgh Medical Center, Pittsburgh, PA 15213, USA

Jay S. Raval
Department of Pathology, University of Pittsburgh Medical Center, Pittsburgh, PA 15213, USA
The Institute for Transfusion Medicine, Pittsburgh, PA 15220, USA

Tetsuya Inoue, Norio Katoh, Rikiya Onimaru and Hiroki Shirato
Department of Radiology, Hokkaido University Graduate School of Medicine, North 15 West 7, Kita-ku, Sapporo 060-8638, Japan

Sanghyuk S. Shin
San Diego State University, 5500 Campanile Drive, San Diego, CA 92182-4162, USA
Division of Global Public Health, Department of Medicine, School of Medicine, University of California San Diego, 9500 Gilman Drive, MC-0507, San Diego, CA 92093-0507, USA

Manuel Gallardo and Remedios Lozada
Patronato Pro-COMUSIDA, Ninos Heroes No. 697, Zona Centro, Tijuana, BC, Mexico

Daniela Abramovitz, Jose Luis Burgos, Timothy C. Rodwell, Steffanie A. Strathdee and Richard S. Garfein
Division of Global Public Health, Department of Medicine, School of Medicine, University of California

Rafael Laniado-Laborin
Parque Industrial Internacional, Universidad Autonoma de Baja California, Calzada Universidad 14418, Tijuana, BC, Mexico

Thomas E. Novotny
San Diego State University, 5500 Campanile Drive, San Diego, CA 92182-4162, USA San Diego, 9500 Gilman Drive, MC-0507, San Diego, CA 92093-0507, USA

Akihiko Ohwada
Ohwada Clinic, 4-7-13 Minamiyawata, Ichikawa, Chiba 272-0023, Japan
Department of Respiratory Medicine, Juntendo University School of Medicine, Tokyo 113-8421, Japan

Kazuhisa Takahashi
Department of Respiratory Medicine, Juntendo University School of Medicine, Tokyo 113-8421, Japan

Linnea Jarenbäck, Jaro Ankerst, Leif Bjermer and Ellen Tufvesson
Department of Clinical Sciences, RespiratoryMedicine and Allergology, Lund University, 221 84 Lund, Sweden

Gustavo Rocha and Hercília Guimarães
Division of Neonatology, Department of Pediatrics, Hospital de São João EPE, Faculty of Medicine of Porto University, 4202-451 Porto, Portugal

Maria João Baptista
Division of Pediatric Cardiology, Department of Pediatrics, Hospital de São João EPE, Faculty of Medicine of Porto University, 4202-451 Porto, Portugal

KaterinaManika, Vassilis Tsaoussis, Marina Antoniou and Ioannis Kioumis
Pulmonary Department, Aristotle University of Thessaloniki, "G. Papanikolaou" General Hospital, Exohi, 57010 Thessaloniki, Greece

Georgia G. Pitsiou, Afroditi K. Boutou, Nikolaos Chavouzis and Ioannis Stanopoulos
Respiratory Failure Unit, Aristotle University of Thessaloniki, "G. Papanikolaou" General Hospital, Exohi, 57010 Thessaloniki, Greece

Maria Fotoulaki
4th Department of Pediatrics, Aristotle University of Thessaloniki, "Papageorgiou" General Hospital, 56429 Thessaloniki, Greece

Kathleen L. Davenport
Department of Rehabilitation Medicine, University of Washington, 1959 Northeast Pacific Street, P.O. Box 356490, Seattle, WA 98195, USA

ChienHuiHuang
Department of Physical Therapy, Tzu Chi University, 701 Zhongyang Road, Section 3, Hualien 97004, Taiwan

Matthew P. Davenport
Department of Chemistry and Food Science, Framingham State University, 100 State Street, Framingham, MA 01701, USA

PaulW.Davenport
Department of Physiological Sciences, University of Florida, P.O. Box 100144 HSC, Gainesville, FL 32610, USA

Saria Tasnim and F. M. Anamul Hoque
Department of Obstetrics & Gynaecology, Institute of Child and Mother Health, Matuail, Dhaka 1362, Bangladesh

Aminur Rahman,
Centre for Injury Prevention Bangladesh, Bangladesh

Kei Nakajima
Division of Clinical Nutrition, Department of Medical Dietetics, Faculty of Pharmaceutical Sciences, Josai University, 1-1 Keyakidai, Sakado, Saitama 350-0295, Japan
Department of Internal Medicine, Social Insurance Omiya General Hospital, 453 Bonsai, Kita, Saitama 331-0805, Japan

Yulan Li
Division of Clinical Nutrition, Department of Medical Dietetics, Faculty of Pharmaceutical Sciences, Josai University, 1-1 Keyakidai, Sakado, Saitama 350-0295, Japan

Hiroshi Fuchigami
Department of Health Care Center, Social Insurance Omiya General Hospital, 453 Bonsai, Kita, Saitama 331-0805, Japan

HiromiMunakata
Department of Internal Medicine, Social Insurance Omiya General Hospital, 453 Bonsai, Kita, Saitama 331-0805, Japan

Ihsan Alloubi, Matthieu Thumerel, Jean-Marc Baste, Jean-François Velly and Jacques Jougon
Thoracic Surgery Department, Victor Segalen Bordeaux 2 University and Haut Lévêque Hospital, CHU de Bordeaux, 33604 Pessac Cedex, France

Hugues Bégueret
Pathology Department, Victor Segalen Bordeaux 2 University and Haut Lévêque Hospital, CHU de Bordeaux, 33604 Pessac Cedex, France

Hector A. Olvera
Center for Environmental Resource Management, University of Texas at El Paso, 500 W. University Avenue, El Paso, TX 79968, USA
Civil Engineering Department, University of Texas at El Paso, 500 W. University Avenue, El Paso, TX 79968, USA

Daniel Perez and Wen-Whai Li
Civil Engineering Department, University of Texas at El Paso, 500 W. University Avenue, El Paso, TX 79968, USA

JuanW. Clague
Geological Sciences Department, University of Texas at El Paso, 500 W. University Avenue, El Paso, TX 79968, USA

Yung-Sung Cheng
Aerosol and Dosimetry Program, Lovelace Respiratory Research Institute, 2425 Ridgecrest Dr. SE, Albuquerque, NM 87108-5127, USA

Maria A. Amaya
School of Nursing, University of Texas at El Paso, 500 W. University Avenue, El Paso, TX 79968, USA

ScottW. Burchiel and Marianne Berwick
Center for Environmental Health Sciences, University of New Mexico, Los Lunas, NM 87131, USA

Nicholas E. Pingitore
Geological Sciences Department, University of Texas at El Paso, 500 W. University Avenue, El Paso, TX 79968, USA
School of Nursing, University of Texas at El Paso, 500 W. University Avenue, El Paso, TX 79968, USA

Kathryn Giordano, Nicole Green, and MagdyW. Attia
Department of Emergency Medicine, Nemours/Alfred I. duPont Hospital for Children, Wilmington, DE 19803, USA

Elena Rodriguez and Milena Armani
Nemours Research Lung Center, Nemours/Alfred I. duPont Hospital for Children, Wilmington, DE 19803, SA

Joan Richards
Department of Respiratory Care, Nemours/Alfred I. duPont Hospital for Children, Wilmington, DE 19803, USA

Thomas H. Shaffer,2, 4, 5
Nemours Research Lung Center, Nemours/Alfred I. duPont Hospital for Children, Wilmington, DE 19803, USA
Department of Pediatrics, Jefferson Medical College, Philadelphia, PA 19107, USA
Departments of Physiology and Pediatrics, Temple University School of Medicine, Philadelphia, PA 19140, USA

Ken-ichi Tabata, Takefumi Satoh, Hideyasu Tsumura, Masaomi Ikeda, SatoruMinamida, Tetsuo Fujita, Daisuke Ishii, Masatsugu Iwamura and Shiro Baba
Department of Urology, Kitasato University School of Medicine, 1-15-1 Kitasato, Minami-ku, Sagamihara, Kanagawa 252-0375, Japan

Yuzuru Niibe and Kazushige Hayakawa
Department of Radiology and Radiation Oncology, Kitasato University School ofMedicine, 1-15-1 Kitasato,Minami-ku, Sagamihara, Kanagawa 252-0375, Japan

J.-Gonzalo Ocejo-Vinyals, Lucía Lavín-Alconero, Pablo Sańchez-Velasco, M.-Ańgeles Guerrero-Alonso, Fernando Ausıń and Francisco Leyva-Cobián
Servicio de Inmunología, Hospital Universitario Marqués de Valdecilla, Avenida de Valdecilla s/n, 39008 Santander, Spain

M.-Carmen Fariñas
Unidad de Enfermedades Infecciosas, Departamento de Medicina Interna, Hospital Universitario Marqu´es de Valdecilla, Universidad de Cantabria, 39011 Santander, Spain

Iukary Takenami
Advanced Laboratory of Public Health, Oswaldo Cruz Foundation, Gonçalo Moniz Research Center, Salvador, Bahia 40296 710, Brazil

Brook Finkmoore and Krisztina Emodi LeeW. Riley
Division of Infectious Diseases & Vaccinology, School of Public Health, University of California, Berkeley, CA 94720, USA

AlmérioMachado Jr.
Bahia School of Medicine and Public Health, Salvador, Bahia 40290 000, Brazil
Hospital Especializado Octávio Mangabeira, Secretary of Health of Bahia State, Salvador, Bahia 40320 350, Brazil

Sérgio Arruda
Advanced Laboratory of Public Health, Oswaldo Cruz Foundation, Gonçalo Moniz Research Center, Salvador, Bahia 40296 710, Brazil
Bahia School of Medicine and Public Health, Salvador, Bahia 40290 000, Brazil

H. Kupiainen and T. Laitinen
Department of Pulmonary Diseases and Clinical Allergology, Turku University Hospital and University of Turku, Kiinamyllynkatu 13, 20520 Turku, Finland
Clinical Research Unit for Pulmonary Diseases and Division of Pulmonology, Helsinki University Central Hospital, Tukholmankatu 8C, 00290 Helsinki, Finland

V. L. Kinnula and A. Lindqvist
Clinical Research Unit for Pulmonary Diseases and Division of Pulmonology, Helsinki University Central Hospital, Tukholmankatu 8C, 00290 Helsinki, Finland

D. S. Postma
Department of Pulmonology, University Medical Center Groningen, Hanzeplein 1, 9700 RB Groningen, The Netherlands

H. M. Boezen
Department of Epidemiology, University Medical Center Groningen, Hanzeplein 1, 9700 RB Groningen, The Netherlands

M. Kilpeläinen
Department of Pulmonary Diseases and Clinical Allergology, Turku University Hospital and University of Turku, Kiinamyllynkatu 13, 20520 Turku, Finland

Joshua Lawrenz, David Gasper, Jonathan Nitz and Richard C. Baybutt
Department of Applied Health Science, Wheaton College, 501 College Avenue, Wheaton, IL 60187, USA

Betty Herndon
Department of Basic Medical Sciences, School of Medicine, University of Missouri-Kansas City (UMKC), USA

Afrin Kamal, Daniel C. Dim, Cletus Baidoo and Agostino Molteni
Department of Pathology and Pharmacology, School of Medicine, University of Missouri-Kansas City (UMKC), 2411 Holmes Street, Kansas City, MO 64108, USA

AaronMehrer
Department of Anesthesiology, School of Medicine, University of Missouri-Kansas City (UMKC), Kansas City, MO 64108, USA

Adrian R. O'Hagan, RonaldMorton and Nemr Eid
Division of Pediatric Pulmonology, University of Louisville, Louisville, KY 40202, USA

Salamé Joseph
Faculty of Medical Sciences, Lebanese University, Beirut 961, Lebanon

Salameh Pascale
Faculties of Pharmacy and of Public Health, Lebanese University, Beirut 961, Lebanon

Khayat Georges
Hôtel-Dieu de France Hospital and Faculty of Medicine, Saint Joseph University, Beirut 961, Lebanon

WakedMirna
Saint George Hospital University Medical Center and Faculty of Medicine, Univerity of Balamand, Beirut 961, Lebanon

Lene Lochte
Centre for Child and Adolescent Health, Section of Aetiological Epidemiology, School of Social and Community Medicine, Faculty of Medicine and Dentistry, University of Bristol, Bristol BS8 2BN, UK

WilbyWilliamson, KateWestgate, Ulf Ekelund and Soren Brage
Medical Research Council Epidemiology Unit, Institute of Metabolic Science, Box 285, Addenbrooke's Hospital, Cambridge CB2 0QQ, UK

Karl Sylvester and Jonathan Fuld
Department of Respiratory Medicine, Cambridge University Hospitals, NHS Foundation Trust, Cambridge CB2 0QQ, UK

Gustavo Nino
Penn State Sleep Research and Treatment Center, Pennsylvania State University College of Medicine, Hershey, PA, USA
Department of Pediatrics, Pennsylvania State University College of Medicine, Hershey, PA, USA
Division of Pediatric Pulmonary and Sleep Medicine, Penn State Hershey Children's Hospital, Pennsylvania State University College of Medicine, 500 University Drive, Hershey, PA 17033-0850, USA

Maria J. Gutierrez
Department of Pediatrics, Pennsylvania State University College of Medicine, Hershey, PA, USA
Division of Allergy and Immunology, Pennsylvania State University College of Medicine, Hershey, PA, USA

Anjani Ravindra
Department of Pediatrics, Pennsylvania State University College of Medicine, Hershey, PA, USA

Cesar L. Nino
Department of Electronics Engineering, Javeriana University, Bogota, Colombia

Carlos E. Rodriguez-Martinez
Department of Pediatrics, School of Medicine, Universidad Nacional de Colombia, Bogota, Colombia
Department of Pediatric Pulmonology and Pediatric Critical Care Medicine, School of Medicine, Universidad El Bosque, Bogota, Colombia
Research Unit, Military Hospital of Colombia, Bogota, Colombia

Adil Shujaat
Division of Pulmonary and Critical Care Medicine, College of Medicine at Jacksonville, University of Florida, Jacksonville, FL, USA
University of Florida, Shands Clinical Center, 655West 8th Street, Suite 7-088, Jacksonville, FL 32209, USA

JanetM. Shapiro and Edward Eden
Division of Pulmonary and Critical Care Medicine, St. Luke's and Roosevelt Hospitals of Columbia University, New York, NY, USA

Sidney C. da Silva
Department of Sports Science, Brazilian Olympic Committee, Avenida das Américas 899, 22631-000 Rio de Janeiro, RJ, Brazil

Walace D. Monteiro and Paulo T. V. Farinatti
Laboratory of Physical Activity and Health Promotion, Rio de Janeiro State University, Rua São Francisco Xavier 524, Sala 8121F, 20550-900 Rio de Janeiro, RJ, Brazil
Graduate Program in Sciences of Physical Activity, Salgado de Oliveira University, Rua Marechal Deodoro 217, No. 2 Andar, 24030-060 Niteroi, RJ, Brazil

Felipe A. Cunha
Graduate Program in Sciences of Physical Activity, Salgado de Oliveira University, Rua Marechal Deodoro 217, No. 2 Andar, 24030-060 Niteroi, RJ, Brazil
Graduate Program in Medical Sciences, Rio de Janeiro State University, Avenida Professor Manoel de Abreu, 444/No. 2 Andar, Vila Isabel, 20550-170 Rio de Janeiro, RJ, Brazil

JonathanMyers
Cardiology Division, Palo Alto VA Health Care System, Cardiology 111C, 3801 Miranda Avenue, Palo Alto, CA 94304, USA

Fotios Drakopanagiotakis, Areti Xifteri, Napoleon Karagiannidis, DemetriosMermigkis and Vlasis Polychronopoulos
3rd Respiratory Medicine Department, Sismanoglio General Hospital, 15126 Marousi, Greece

Evaggelos Tsiambas and Andreas Karameris
Department of Pathology and Computerized Image Analysis, 417 NIMTS Hospital, 11521 Athens, Greece

Konstantina Tsakanika
Bronchoalveolar Lavage Unit, Sismanoglio General Hospital, 15126 Marousi, Greece

Demosthenes Bouros
Department of Pneumonology, University Hospital of Alexandroupolis and Medical School of Democritus University of Thrace, 68100 Alexandroupolis, Greece

Chul-Ho Kim, Steve Anderson, DeanMacCarter and Bruce Johnson
Division of Cardiovascular Diseases, Mayo Clinic, Rochester, MN 55905, USA